Computer-Aided Detection and Diagnosis in Medical Imaging

IMAGING IN MEDICAL DIAGNOSIS AND THERAPY

Series Editors: Andrew Karellas and Bruce R. Thomadsen

Published titles

Quality and Safety in Radiotherapy
Todd Pawlicki, Peter B. Dunscombe,
Arno J. Mundt, and Pierre Scalliet, Editors
ISBN: 978-1-4398-0436-0

Adaptive Radiation Therapy
X. Allen Li, Editor
ISBN: 978-1-4398-1634-9

Quantitative MRI in Cancer
Thomas E. Yankeelov, David R. Pickens,
and Ronald R. Price, Editors
ISBN: 978-1-4398-2057-5

Informatics in Medical Imaging
George C. Kagadis and Steve G. Langer, Editors
ISBN: 978-1-4398-3124-3

Adaptive Motion Compensation in Radiotherapy
Martin J. Murphy, Editor
ISBN: 978-1-4398-2193-0

Image-Guided Radiation Therapy
Daniel J. Bourland, Editor
ISBN: 978-1-4398-0273-1

Targeted Molecular Imaging
Michael J. Welch and William C. Eckelman,
Editors
ISBN: 978-1-4398-4195-0

Proton and Carbon Ion Therapy
C.-M. Charlie Ma and Tony Lomax, Editors
ISBN: 978-1-4398-1607-3

Comprehensive Brachytherapy: Physical and Clinical Aspects
Jack Venselaar, Dimos Baltas, Peter J. Hoskin,
and Ali Soleimani-Meigooni, Editors
ISBN: 978-1-4398-4498-4

Physics of Mammographic Imaging
Mia K. Markey, Editor
ISBN: 978-1-4398-7544-5

Physics of Thermal Therapy: Fundamentals and Clinical Applications
Eduardo Moros, Editor
ISBN: 978-1-4398-4890-6

Emerging Imaging Technologies in Medicine
Mark A. Anastasio and Patrick La Riviere, Editors
ISBN: 978-1-4398-8041-8

Cancer Nanotechnology: Principles and Applications in Radiation Oncology
Sang Hyun Cho and Sunil Krishnan, Editors
ISBN: 978-1-4398-7875-0

Monte Carlo Techniques in Radiation Therapy
Joao Seco and Frank Verhaegen, Editors
ISBN: 978-1-4665-0792-0

Image Processing in Radiation Therapy
Kristy Kay Brock, Editor
ISBN: 978-1-4398-3017-8

Informatics in Radiation Oncology
George Starkschall and R. Alfredo C. Siochi,
Editors
ISBN: 978-1-4398-2582-2

Cone Beam Computed Tomography
Chris C. Shaw, Editor
ISBN: 978-1-4398-4626-1

Tomosynthesis Imaging
Ingrid Reiser and Stephen Glick, Editors
ISBN: 978-1-4398-7870-5

Stereotactic Radiosurgery and Stereotactic Body Radiation Therapy
Stanley H. Benedict, David J. Schlesinger, Steven
J. Goetsch, and Brian D. Kavanagh, Editors
ISBN: 978-1-4398-4197-6

Computer-Aided Detection and Diagnosis in Medical Imaging
Qiang Li and Robert M. Nishikawa, Editors

IMAGING IN MEDICAL DIAGNOSIS AND THERAPY

Series Editors: Andrew Karellas and Bruce R. Thomadsen

Computer-Aided Detection and Diagnosis in Medical Imaging

Edited by

Qiang Li
Robert M. Nishikawa

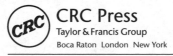

CRC Press
Taylor & Francis Group
Boca Raton London New York

CRC Press is an imprint of the
Taylor & Francis Group, an **informa** business

A TAYLOR & FRANCIS BOOK

CRC Press
Taylor & Francis Group
6000 Broken Sound Parkway NW, Suite 300
Boca Raton, FL 33487-2742

First issued in paperback 2021

© 2015 by Taylor & Francis Group, LLC
CRC Press is an imprint of Taylor & Francis Group, an Informa business

No claim to original U.S. Government works

Version Date: 20141103

ISBN 13: 978-0-367-78355-6 (pbk)
ISBN 13: 978-1-4398-7176-8 (hbk)

Library of Congress Cataloging-in-Publication Data

Computer-aided detection and diagnosis in medical imaging / [edited by] Qiang Li and Robert M. Nishikawa.
    p. ; cm. -- (Imaging in medical diagnosis and therapy)
    Includes bibliographical references and index.
    ISBN 978-1-4398-7176-8 (alk. paper)
    I. Li, Qiang, 1962- , editor. II. Nishikawa, Robert Mark, 1958- , editor. III. Series: Imaging in medical diagnosis and therapy.
    [DNLM: 1. Diagnostic Imaging. 2. Computer-Aided Design. 3. Image Processing, Computer-Assisted. WN 180]

RC78.7.D53
616.07'54--dc23   2014042751

Visit the Taylor & Francis Web site at
http://www.taylorandfrancis.com

and the CRC Press Web site at
http://www.crcpress.com

Contents

SECTION II   Computer-Aided Detection and Diagnosis in Chest and Abdominal Imaging

SECTION III   Emerging Computer-Aided Detection and Diagnosis

SECTION IV Assessment and Clinical Utility of Computer-Aided Detection and Diagnosis

Series Preface

Advances in the science and technology of medical imaging and radiation therapy are more profound and rapid than ever before, since their inception over a century ago. Further, the disciplines are increasingly cross-linked as imaging methods become more widely used for planning, guiding, monitoring, and assessing treatments in radiation therapy. Today, the technologies of medical imaging and radiation therapy are so complex and so computer driven that it is difficult for those (physicians and technologists) responsible for their clinical use to know exactly what is happening at the point of care when a patient is being examined or treated. Medical physicists are well equipped to understand the technologies and their applications, and they assume greater responsibilities in the clinical arena to ensure that what is intended for the patient is actually delivered in a safe and effective manner.

The growing responsibilities of medical physicists in the clinical arenas of medical imaging and radiation therapy are not without their challenges, however. Most medical physicists are knowledgeable in either radiation therapy or medical imaging and expert in one or a small number of areas within their discipline. They sustain their expertise in these areas by reading scientific articles and attending scientific talks at meetings. However, their responsibilities increasingly extend beyond their specific areas of expertise. To meet these responsibilities, medical physicists periodically must refresh their knowledge on the advances in medical imaging and radiation therapy, and they must be prepared to function at the intersection of these two fields. To accomplish these objectives is a challenge.

At the 2007 annual meeting of the American Association of Physicists in Medicine in Minneapolis, this challenge was the topic of conversation during a lunch hosted by Taylor & Francis Group and involving a group of senior medical physicists (Arthur L. Boyer, Joseph O. Deasy, C.-M. Charlie Ma, Todd A. Pawlicki, Ervin B. Podgorsak, Elke Reitzel, Anthony B. Wolbarst, and Ellen D. Yorke). The conclusion of the discussion was that a book series should be launched under the Taylor & Francis Group banner, with each book in the series addressing a rapidly advancing area of medical imaging or radiation therapy of importance to medical physicists. The aim would be for each book to provide medical physicists with the information needed to understand technologies driving rapid advances and their applications to safe and effective delivery of patient care.

Each book in the series is edited by one or more individuals with recognized expertise in the technological area encompassed by the book. The editors are responsible for selecting the authors of individual chapters and ensuring that the chapters are comprehensive and intelligible to someone without such expertise. The enthusiasm of the book editors and chapter authors has been gratifying and reinforces the conclusion of the Minneapolis luncheon that this series addresses a major need of medical physicists.

Imaging in Medical Diagnosis and Therapy would not have been possible without the encouragement and support of the series manager, Luna Han of Taylor & Francis Group. The editors and authors, and most of all I, are indebted to her steady guidance throughout the project.

William Hendee
Founding Series Editor
Rochester, Minnesota

Preface

Computer-aided detection (CADe) and computer-aided diagnosis (CADx) systems, collectively referred to as CAD systems, are playing increasingly important roles in aiding radiologists to improve their accuracy in the detection and diagnosis of various diseases, particularly cancers. The development of CAD systems requires multidisciplinary technologies from image processing, pattern recognition, artificial intelligence, to medical imaging. With the remarkable progress in these fields, CAD has advanced rapidly since the 1980s and has become one of the major research topics in medical imaging. CAD systems have been developed to detect and diagnose various diseases in various medical imaging modalities and in various body organs, from breast cancer in breast imaging, lung cancer in chest imaging, colon cancer in abdominal imaging, to brain tumor in brain imaging. This book presents the major technical advancements and methodologies in the development and clinical utility of CAD systems in breast imaging, chest imaging, abdominal imaging, and other emerging applications.

Recent years have seen a tremendous improvement in both the number and quality of CAD systems designed for the detection and diagnosis of various diseases in all major medical imaging modalities, including optical imaging, x-ray projection imaging, computed tomography (CT), magnetic resonance imaging (MRI), positron emission tomography (PET), and ultrasound. In 1998, the Food and Drug Administration (FDA) approved the first commercial CAD system to market in the United States—a CAD system developed by R2 Technology, Inc. to detect breast cancer. Since then, thousands of CAD systems for breast cancer have been installed worldwide. The utility of CAD systems is becoming a part of the routine clinical work for the detection of breast cancer in many hospitals. Other major medical systems companies, including General Electric (GE) Medical Systems, Siemens Medical Systems, and Philips Medical Systems, have developed and marketed their own versions of CAD systems. Major international conferences in medical imaging, such as the Radiological Society of North America Annual Meeting, SPIE Medical Imaging Conferences, and International Conferences on Computer-Assisted Radiology and Surgery, have held dedicated conferences/sessions on CAD in the past few years.

Despite the constant expansion of the CAD field over the past two to three decades, there is currently no single book dedicated to the development and utility of CAD systems. The lack of an authoritative book may thus deter the advancement and dissemination of CAD technologies. It is our belief that a book dedicated to the CAD field will provide readers with a comprehensive overview of CAD and bring together the available and emerging technologies in the field. This book aims to help promote a wide acceptance of the CAD concept and fast advancement in its technologies through the efforts of numerous researchers from several institutions.

This book is designed for individuals who are interested in CAD technologies, such as students, CAD system developers, basic scientists, and physician scientists in relevant research fields. Individuals who are relatively new to CAD research may use the book to systematically learn a variety of fundamental aspects in the process of CAD system development; individuals who are currently developing CAD systems may gain insights from others' work in the book to design a completely new or an improved CAD system; experienced researchers may also find the book useful in systematically providing up-to-date information and knowledge in available and emerging CAD technologies.

Chapter 1, by Kunio Doi, presents a historic overview of CAD, including early development of CAD schemes, a summary of recent CAD research, and application of CAD systems. The book is then divided into four major sections, each of which consists of a set of chapters. Section I presents the CAD technologies in breast imaging, which is the most advanced area of CAD application. This section includes chapters on detection and/or diagnosis of breast mass and microcalcifications in mammography and digital breast tomosynthesis, assessment of risk for breast cancer, case-based CAD systems in breast imaging, and a multimodality CAD system for breast cancer.

Section II discusses the CAD technologies in chest imaging and abdominal imaging. The six chapters in this section deal with detection and diagnosis of lung nodules in chest radiography and CT, detection and diagnosis of interstitial lung disease, measurement of changes in the size of lung nodules, establishment of a public lung image database, and detection of polyps in CT colonography.

Section III concerns emerging CAD technologies developed for a variety of diseases in a wide range of imaging modalities. The chapters in this section talk about detection and characterization of brain tumors and cerebrovascular diseases in brain imaging, detection of pulmonary embolisms, detection of eye diseases, detection and diagnosis of prostate cancer in MRI, detection and assessment of bone metastasis and other bone diseases, and the integration of CAD and picture archiving and communication systems (PACS).

Section IV describes the current utility of CAD systems in clinical practice. The chapters in this section discuss methodologies for the assessment of CAD systems and the clinical utility of CAD systems for breast cancer, lung cancer, and colon cancer. The final chapter, by Maryellen Giger, describes some lessons learned in CAD development and application as well as future perspectives on CAD development and research.

We thank the authors for their contributions to this book and Luna Han, editor at Taylor & Francis Group LLC, for her guidance in the preparation and writing of the book. Qiang Li is grateful for the support of the Department of Radiology, Duke University, and the Center of Advanced Medical Imaging Research, Shanghai Advanced Research Institute, Chinese Academy of Sciences. Robert Nishikawa acknowledges his many colleagues in the Department of Radiology at The University of Chicago, for their collegiality, insights, and support over a 24-year time span that has helped to form his thoughts and understanding of CAD.

Editors

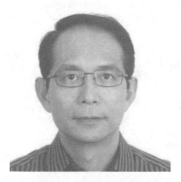 **Qiang Li** earned his BSc in computer science in 1983 from Xi'an Jiaotong University, Xi'an, Shaanxi, People's Republic of China; his MSc in computer science in 1986 from Huazhong University of Science and Technology, Wuhan, Hubei, People's Republic of China; and PhD in electrical engineering in 1998 from Kyoto Institute of Technology, Kyoto, Japan. He joined The University of Chicago in 1998 as a research associate and has developed computer-aided diagnosis (CAD) systems for detecting and diagnosing lung nodules in chest radiography and computed tomography. He moved to Duke University as an associate professor in 2008 and continued his research in the CAD field. He is now a professor at the Shanghai Advanced Research Institute, China, and an adjunct associate professor at Duke University. He holds six patents on CAD-related technologies and has published more than 60 peer-reviewed journal papers in CAD and medical imaging applications.

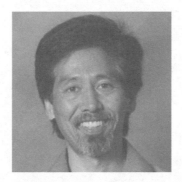 **Robert M. Nishikawa** earned his BSc in physics in 1981 and his MSc and PhD in medical biophysics in 1984 and 1990, respectively, all from the University of Toronto, Ontario, Canada. For his PhD thesis, he developed the initial digital mammography system in Martin Yaffe's laboratory and laid the theoretical groundwork upon which subsequent systems were developed. He then moved to The University of Chicago where, as a faculty member, he developed computer-aided diagnosis (CAD) systems for classifying and detecting clustered calcifications in mammograms and studied the clinical effectiveness of CAD systems for screening mammography. He holds seven patents on CAD-related technologies. He is currently a professor and director of the Clinical Translational Medical Physics Laboratory in the Department of Radiology at the University of Pittsburgh. He has won 24 awards, including two for *best* paper, two innovation awards, and one teaching award. He has more than 200 publications in breast imaging, many focusing on CAD. He is a fellow of the American Association of Physicists in Medicine (AAPM) and the Society of Breast Imaging.

Contributors

Robert Ambrosini
Department of Radiology
University of Rochester Medical Center
Rochester, New York

Samuel G. Armato III
Department of Radiology
The University of Chicago
Chicago, Illinois

Kazuto Ashizawa
Department of Clinical Oncology
Nagasaki University
Nagasaki, Japan

Sir Michael Brady
Department of Oncology
University of Oxford
Oxford, United Kingdom

Rachel F. Brem
Department of Radiology
The George Washington University
Washington, DC

Heang-Ping Chan
Department of Radiology
University of Michigan
Ann Arbor, Michigan

Abraham H. Dachman
Department of Radiology
The University of Chicago
Chicago, Illinois

Farid Dahi
Department of Radiology
University of Minnesota
Minneapolis, Minnesota

Delphine Davis
Department of Radiology
University of Rochester Medical Center
Rochester, New York

Kunio Doi
Kurt Rossmann Laboratories for Radiologic Image
    Research
Department of Radiology
The University of Chicago
Chicago, Illinois

and

Gunma Prefectural College of Health Sciences
Maebashi, Japan

Karen Drukker
Department of Radiology
The University of Chicago
Chicago, Illinois

Issam El Naqa
Department of Oncology
Montreal General Hospital
Montréal, Québéc, Canada

Matthew T. Freedman
Department of Oncology
Lombardi Comprehensive Cancer Center
Georgetown University
Washington, DC

Hiroshi Fujita
Department of Intelligent Image Information
Graduate School of Medicine
Gifu University
Gifu, Japan

Maryellen L. Giger
Department of Radiology
and
Committee on Medical Physics
The University of Chicago
Chicago, Illinois

Fiona J. Gilbert
School of Clinical Medicine
University of Cambridge
Cambridge, United Kingdom

Maureen G.C. Gillan
Aberdeen Biomedical Imaging Centre
University of Aberdeen
Aberdeen, United Kingdom

Ralph Highnam
Matakina Technology Limited
Wellington, New Zealand

H.K. Huang
Image Processing and Informatics Laboratory
Department of Biomedical Engineering
University of Southern California
Los Angeles, California

Henkjan Huisman
Department of Radiology and Nuclear Medicine
Radboud University Medical Center
Nijmegen, the Netherlands

Takayuki Ishida
Faculty of Health Sciences
Osaka University
Osaka, Japan

Mathews Jacob
Department of Electrical and Computer Engineering
University of Iowa
Iowa City, Iowa

Yulei Jiang
Department of Radiology
The University of Chicago
Chicago, Illinois

Hao Jing
Department of Biomedical Engineering
Illinois Institute of Technology
Chicago, Illinois

Nico Karssemeijer
Department of Radiology and Nuclear Medicine
Radboud University Medical Center
Nijmegen, the Netherlands

Shigehiko Katsuragawa
Faculty of Fukuoka Medical Technology
Teikyo University
Omuta, Japan

Anitha Priya Krishnan
Molecular Imaging Center
University of Southern California
Los Angeles, California

Anh Le
Image Processing and Informatics Laboratory
Department of Biomedical Engineering
University of Southern California
Los Angeles, California

Qiang Li
Department of Radiology
Duke University
Durham, North Carolina

and

Center for Medical Imaging Research
Shanghai Advanced Research Institute
Pudong, Shanghai, People's Republic of China

Jerome Zhengrong Liang
Department of Radiology
and
Department of Computer Science
and
Department of Biomedical Engineering
Stony Brook University
Stony Brook, New York

Geert Litjens
Department of Radiology and Nuclear Medicine
Radboud University Medical Center
Nijmegen, the Netherlands

Brent J. Liu
Image Processing and Informatics Laboratory
Department of Biomedical Engineering
University of Southern California
Los Angeles, California

Maciej A. Mazurowski
Department of Radiology
Duke University
Durham, North Carolina

Chisako Muramatsu
Department of Intelligent Image Information
Graduate School of Medicine
Gifu University
Gifu, Japan

Walter G. O'Dell
Department of Radiation Oncology
University of Florida
Gainesville, Florida

Jocelyn A. Rapelyea
Department of Radiology
The George Washington University
Washington, DC

Anthony Reeves
School of Electrical and Computer Engineering
Cornell University
Ithaca, New York

Charlene A. Sennett
Department of Radiology
The University of Chicago
Chicago, Illinois

Junji Shiraishi
Faculty of Life Sciences
Department of Medical Physics
Kumamoto University
Kumamoto, Japan

Georgia D. Tourassi
Biomedical Science and Engineering Center
Oak Ridge National Laboratory
Oak Ridge, Tennessee

Yoshikazu Uchiyama
Department of Radiological Technology
Kumamoto University
Kumamoto, Japan

Bram van Ginneken
Department of Radiology and Nuclear Medicine
Radboud University Medical Center
Nijmegen, the Netherlands

Pieter Vos
Department of Radiology and Nuclear Medicine
Radboud University Medical Center
Nijmegen, the Netherlands

Yongyi Yang
Department of Biomedical Engineering
Illinois Institute of Technology
Chicago, Illinois

Chuan Zhou
Department of Radiology
University of Michigan
Ann Arbor, Michigan

Chapter 1

Historical Overview

Kunio Doi

CONTENTS

1.1   INTRODUCTION

Computer-aided detection and/or diagnosis (CAD) has become a part of the routine clinical work for the detection of breast cancer on mammograms at many screening sites and medical centers (Giger et al., 2000; Warren-Burhenne et al., 2000; Freer and Ulissey, 2001; Butler et al., 2004; Destounis et al., 2004; Gur et al., 2004; Birdwell et al., 2005; Cupples et al., 2005; Dean and Ilvento, 2006; Gilbert et al., 2006, 2008; Morton et al., 2006; Gromet, 2008). With CAD, radiologists use the computer output as a *second opinion* and make the final decisions. It is likely that CAD is beginning to be applied widely in the detection and differential diagnosis of many different types of abnormalities in medical images obtained in various examinations by use of different imaging modalities. In fact, CAD has become one of the major research subjects in medical imaging and diagnostic radiology (Doi et al., 1992, 1999a,b; van Ginneken et al., 2001; Erickson and Bartholomai, 2002; Doi, 2003, 2004, 2005, 2006, 2007; Summers, 2003; Abe et al., 2004; Giger, 2004; Yoshida and Dachman, 2004; Li et al., 2005;

Hadjiiski et al., 2006; Bielen and Kiss, 2007; Nishikawa, 2007; Giger et al., 2008; de Boo et al., 2009; Elter and Horsch, 2009). Although early attempts at computerized analysis of medical images (Lodwick et al., 1963; Myers et al., 1964; Winsbarg et al., 1967) were made in the 1960s, serious and systematic investigation on CAD began in the 1980s with a fundamental change in the concept for the utilization of the computer output, from automated computer diagnosis to computer-aided diagnosis. In this chapter, the motivation and philosophy for the early development of CAD schemes are presented together with some of the important issues related to the future potential of CAD.

1.2   EARLY DEVELOPMENT OF CAD SCHEMES

Large-scale and systematic research and development of various CAD schemes were begun in the early 1980s at the Kurt Rossmann Laboratories for Radiologic Image Research in the Department of Radiology at the University of Chicago. Prior to and since that time, we have been engaged in some basic research on the effects of digital images on radiologic diagnosis (Ishida et al., 1982, 1983, 1984; Giger and Doi, 1984a,b, 1985; MacMahon et al., 1984, 1985, 1986; Fujita et al., 1985, 1986; Loo et al., 1985; Giger et al., 1986a,b; Kume et al., 1986; Ohara et al., 1986), and many investigators have become involved in research and development of some aspects of picture archiving and communication system (PACS) (Huang, 2010, 2011). Although PACS would be useful and advantageous in the management of radiologic images in radiology departments and might be beneficial economically to hospitals, it seemed unlikely at that time that PACS would bring a significant clinical benefit to radiologists. Therefore, we thought that a major benefit of digital images must be realized in radiologists' daily work. Of course, radiologists' daily work consists of image reading and radiologic diagnosis. Thus, we came to the question, "how can radiologists' diagnosis be helped by the benefits of digital images?" This led immediately to the concept of computer-aided diagnosis.

In the 1980s, the concept of automated diagnosis or automated computer diagnosis was already known from several studies (Lodwick et al., 1963; Myers et al., 1964; Winsbarg et al., 1967; Kruger et al., 1972, 1974; Toriwaki et al., 1973) in the 1960s and 1970s, but these early attempts were not successful. The difference between and the common aspects of automated diagnosis and computer-aided diagnosis are discussed in detail in Section 1.3. Thus, it appeared to be extremely difficult at that time to carry out a computer analysis on lesions studied in medical images. It was, therefore, uncertain whether the development of CAD schemes would be a success or a failure. Therefore, we thought that we should select research subjects that had the potential to have a major impact on medicine, if CAD could be developed successfully. Some of the most important subjects in medicine at that time were related to cardiovascular diseases, lung cancer, and breast cancer. Therefore, we decided to select three main research projects on these subjects, that is, for the detection and/or quantitative analysis of lesions involved in vascular imaging by Fujita et al. (1987) and Hoffmann et al. (1986), detection of lung nodules in chest radiographs by Giger et al. (1987, 1988), and detection of clustered microcalcifications in mammograms by Chan et al. (1987).

1.2.1 Strategies for Research and Development of CAD

In addition, our efforts on the research and development of CAD have been based on three fundamental strategies from the beginning to the present time, as described here. First, our basic strategy for the development of methods and

techniques for the detection and quantification of lesions in medical images has been based on the understanding of processes that would be involved in image readings by radiologists (Doi et al., 1992, 1999a; Doi, 2006). This strategy appeared quite logical and straightforward because radiologists are the ones who have been carrying out very complex and difficult tasks of image reading and radiologic diagnosis. Therefore, we assumed that computer algorithms should be developed based on the understanding of image readings, such as how radiologists can detect certain lesions, why they may miss some abnormalities, and how they can distinguish between benign and malignant lesions.

The second thought was related to the way in which the success of our efforts could be measured if we were successful in the development of CAD. It appeared that the best proof of our success would be the daily use of CAD in routine clinical work at many hospitals around the world. In order for us to realize this, it would be necessary for many industries to commercialize CAD products for the global medical market. Therefore, we decided to produce and protect intellectual properties related to basic technologies of CAD schemes in the form of patents and to promote these in communicating with many individuals in medical industries for potential efforts toward commercialization of CAD products. Subsequently, our first patent on CAD (Doi et al., 1990), filed in 1987, has become the most commonly cited patent in the field of CAD technology.

The third thought was to promote the wide acceptance of the CAD concept and to facilitate the global distribution of CAD research by many investigators at many different institutions. Because the success of CAD would require overwhelmingly large efforts on many aspects of CAD research such as the development of computerized schemes for many different types of lesions in many different modalities, observer performance studies, clinical trials, and commercialization, it appeared that we would not be successful if we were the only research group on CAD. Instead, we could be successful if many researchers from many institutions were involved in many aspects of CAD research. Therefore, all researchers on CAD should be considered as promoters and as our colleagues rather than as competitors. Therefore, for more than 20 years from the initial phase of CAD research, we have had large scientific exhibits at the Annual Meetings of the Radiological Society of North America (RSNA), which were held in Chicago, Illinois. In these exhibits, we have presented a comprehensive demonstration of CAD research in chest, breast, and vascular imaging.

In 1993, we set up a film digitizer and a computer for real-time demonstration of CAD for the detection of clustered microcalcifications on *unknown* new cases in mammograms. We invited in advance 118 breast radiologists to bring their films to the RSNA meeting for the testing of our CAD scheme. The results of this informal validation test were promising (Nishikawa et al., 1995a). From 1996 to 2001, we carried out observer performance studies with a large number of participants during the RSNA meetings for the detection of various lesions on chest images without and with the computer output, so that many radiologists would be able to have their own experience of using CAD. The usefulness of CAD discovered by many participants at the RSNA meetings was clearly demonstrated (MacMahon et al., 1999; Abe et al., 2003). These demonstrations appeared successful in promoting the CAD concept widely and quickly.

1.2.2   Initial CAD Schemes for the Detection of Lesions

Regarding CAD research on lung cancer, we attempted in the mid-1980s to develop a computerized scheme for the detection of lung nodules on chest radiographs. At that time and still now, it is well known that the visual detection of lung nodules is a difficult task for radiologists, who may miss up to 30% of the nodules. Radiologists have missed these lesions because of the overlap of normal anatomic structures with nodules, that is, the normal background in chest images tends to camouflage nodules (Kundel and Nodine, 1975; Kundel and Revesz, 1976; Kundel et al., 1978, 1979; Carmody et al., 1980). Therefore, it was predicted that the normal background structures in chest images would become a large obstacle in the detection of nodules, even by computer. Thus, the first step in the computerized scheme for the detection of lung nodules in chest images would be the removal or suppression of background structures in chest radiographs. A method for suppressing the background structures is the difference-image technique (Chan et al., 1987, 1990; Giger et al., 1987, 1988; Yin et al., 1993; Xu et al., 1997; Arimura et al., 2004; Shiraishi et al., 2006, 2007), in which the difference between a nodule-enhanced image and a nodule-suppressed image is obtained. This difference-image technique may be considered as the generalization of an edge enhancement technique and has been useful in enhancing lesions and suppressing the background not only for nodules in chest images (Xu et al., 1997; Shiraishi et al., 2006, 2007) but also for microcalcifications (Chan et al., 1987, 1990) and masses (Yin et al., 1993) in mammograms and for lung nodules in CT (Arimura et al., 2004).

Thus, at the Rossmann Laboratories in the mid-1980s, we had already developed basic schemes for the detection of lung nodules in chest images (Giger et al., 1987, 1988) and the detection of clustered microcalcifications in mammograms (Chan et al., 1987). Although the sensitivities of these schemes for the detection of lesions were relatively high even at that time, the number of false positives was very large. It was therefore quite uncertain and unpredictable whether the output of these computerized schemes could be used by radiologists in routine clinical work. For example,

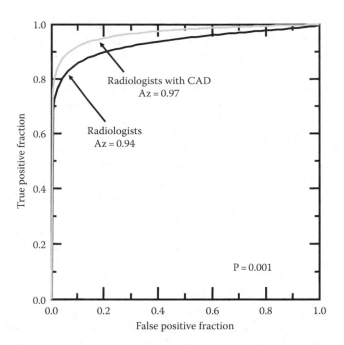

Figure 1.1   First scientific evidence of CAD in improving radiologists' ROC curve in the detection of clustered microcalcifications by the use of the computer output.

the average number of false positives was four per mammogram in the detection of clustered microcalcifications by computer, although the sensitivity was about 85%. However, in order to examine the possibility of practical uses of CAD in clinical situations, we carried out an observer performance study without and with computer output. To our surprise, radiologists' performance in detecting clustered microcalcifications was improved significantly when the computer output was available, even with such a large number of false positives. This result was published in 1990 by Chan et al. (1990) as the first scientific evidence that CAD could be useful in improving radiologists' performance in the detection of a lesion, as shown in Figure 1.1.

1.3   COMPUTER-AIDED DIAGNOSIS AND AUTOMATED COMPUTER DIAGNOSIS

1.3.1   Historical View on Computer Analysis of Medical Information and Images

Early studies on the quantitative analysis of medical images by computer (Lodwick et al., 1963; Myers et al., 1964; Winsbarg et al., 1967; Kruger et al., 1972, 1974; Toriwaki et al., 1973) were reported in the 1960s and 1970s. At that time, it was generally assumed that computers could replace radiologists in detecting abnormalities, because computers and machines are better at performing certain tasks than are human beings. Thus, the concept of computer diagnosis or automated diagnosis in radiology was established. Although interesting results were reported, these early attempts were not successful, because computers were not sufficiently powerful, advanced image-processing techniques were not available, and digital images were not easily accessible. However, a serious flaw was an excessively high expectation of computers. In fact, many different approaches to automated computer diagnosis have been attempted as aids in decision making in many fields of medicine since the 1950s. In the medical subspecialty of hematology, for example, Engle (1992), in 1992, in his review article on 30 years' experience, stated in his conclusion, "Thus, we do not see much promise in the development of computer programs to simulate the decision making of a physician. However, after many years we have concluded that we should stop trying to make computers act like diagnosticians."

In the 1980s, however, another approach emerged that assumed that the computer output could be utilized by radiologists, but not replace them. This concept is currently known as computer-aided diagnosis, which has spread widely and quickly. However, in the early phase of research on and development of CAD schemes, some computer scientists criticized CAD by saying that it simply would not work, which has been proved to be completely wrong. The reason for this strong criticism might have been related to an unsuccessful attempt in previous research efforts toward the development of automated computer diagnosis. This seems to indicate that a failure of a specific research project can lead to a strong *incorrect* bias toward another area of research that may look similar to the previous failed research.

However, these two concepts of automated computer diagnosis and computer-aided diagnosis clearly exist even at present. For example, some investigators have been working seriously on the development of automated computer diagnosis. In addition, there are many researchers who believe that the technology involved in the current CAD schemes could be applied as a means for primary diagnosis, which would be equivalent to automated computer diagnosis. During panel discussion sessions at two meetings, in 2002, of the Computer Assisted Radiology and Surgery in Paris, France, and the American Association of Physicists in Medicine in Montreal, Canada, about half of the participants voted for the possibility that CAD would be shifted to automated computer diagnosis within 50 years, whereas the other half voted against this prediction. Therefore, it may be useful to understand some of the common features and also the differences between CAD and automated computer diagnosis. The common approach to both CAD and automated computer diagnosis is that digital medical images are analyzed quantitatively by computers. Therefore, the development of computer algorithms is required for both CAD and computer diagnosis.

1.3.2 Clear Distinction between CAD and Computer Diagnosis

A major difference between CAD and computer diagnosis is the way in which the computer output is utilized for the diagnosis. With CAD, radiologists use the computer output as a *second opinion*, and radiologists make the final decisions. Therefore, for some clinical cases in which radiologists are confident about their judgments, radiologists may agree with the computer output, or disagree and then disregard the computer. However, for cases in which radiologists are less confident, it is expected that the final decision can be improved by use of the computer output. This improvement is possible, of course, only when the computer result is correct. The better the performance of the computer, the better the overall effect on the final diagnosis. However, the performance level of the computer does not have to be equal to or higher than that of radiologists. With CAD, the potential gain is due to the synergistic effect obtained by combining the radiologist's competence and the computer's capability. Because of these multiplicative benefits, the current CAD has become widely used in practical clinical situations.

With automated computer diagnosis, however, the performance level of the computer output is required to be very high. For example, if the sensitivity for the detection of lesions by computer would be lower than the average sensitivity of physicians, it would be difficult to justify the use of automated computer diagnosis. This is because the patients in most advanced countries would not be able to accept a level of diagnostic results by computer that is lower than the average level achievable by physicians. In addition, the reimbursement for the cost of an automated computer diagnosis may be refused by insurance companies. It would be difficult also to implement automated computer diagnosis if the number of false-positive detections by computer were large, such as one or more false positives per case. In such instances, because every case analyzed by computer would have a possibility of involving an abnormality, the physician would be required to verify all of the cases, and this would then not be considered an automated computer diagnosis. Therefore, high sensitivity and high specificity by computer are required for implementing automated computer diagnosis. This requirement is extremely difficult to meet for researchers who are developing computer algorithms for the detection of abnormalities on radiologic images. In fact, although CAD has been used widely for the detection of breast cancer on mammograms, it would not be possible for most advanced countries to employ the current computer results for automated computer diagnosis.

Another important and distinctive difference between CAD and automated computer diagnosis is the way that the performance and the usefulness would be evaluated quantitatively. The performance level of automated computer diagnosis is equal to the performance achieved by computer. However, the performance level of CAD is equal to the performance achieved by the physician who makes the final decision by using the computer output as a second opinion. Therefore, it is important and essential for CAD that the computer results be utilized effectively by physicians. It is thus necessary to evaluate quantitatively how much physicians can use the computer results to improve their overall performance. Even if the computer results are poor—for example, if both sensitivity and specificity are low—it is possible for physicians to incorporate the computer results efficiently. For example, if the computer could detect subtle lesions that might be difficult for physicians to detect, and also if physicians could disregard *obvious* computer false positives easily, it would be possible to realize CAD. However, if the computer results were poor, automated computer diagnosis could not be implemented.

1.3.3 Evaluation of Performances for CAD and Computer Diagnosis

Therefore, it is important for CAD to assess not only the computer performance, but also the performance of physicians. It is thus necessary to evaluate quantitatively and accurately by use of receiver operating characteristic (ROC) analysis (Metz, 1986, 1989, 2000; Shiraishi et al., 2009) whether the performance by physicians can be improved by use of computer results. In fact, even if the ROC curve for computer results in detecting clustered microcalcifications on mammograms is substantially lower than that by radiologists, the ROC curve obtained by radiologists using the computer results can be improved. The extent of this improvement due to CAD was confirmed to be statistically significant, as reported by Chan et al. (1990), thereby providing clear evidence for the benefits of CAD in the detection of clustered microcalcifications, as shown in Figure 1.1. Thereafter, a number of investigators have reported similar positive findings on the usefulness of CAD in detecting various lesions, including clustered microcalcifications (Chan et al., 1990) and masses (Chan et al., 1999; Moberg et al., 2001; Hadjiiski et al., 2004) in mammograms, breast lesions (Horsch et al., 2006; Sahiner et al., 2009) with multimodality imaging, lung nodules (Kobayashi et al., 1996; Kakeda et al., 2002, 2004, 2006; de Hoop et al., 2010) and interstitial opacities (Monnier-Cholley et al., 1998) in chest radiographs, lung nodules in CT (Li et al., 2005), intracranial aneurysms in magnetic resonance angiography (MRA)(Hirai et al., 2005), and polyps in CT colonography (Dachman et al., 2010). Thus, they have accelerated research and development on CAD schemes in many different types of examinations for the detection of various lesions.

In summary, although there are some common aspects of CAD and automated computer diagnosis, there are also distinct differences between them. Automated computer diagnosis is a concept based on computer algorithms, whereas CAD is a concept that has been established by taking into account the roles of physicians and computers equally. Because of this fundamental difference, the performance levels required for computer algorithms have resulted in a large difference between the two. With automated computer diagnosis, the performance by computers needs to be comparable to or better than that by physicians. With CAD, however, the performance by computers does not have to be comparable to or better than that by physicians, but needs to be complementary to that by physicians. In fact, a large number of CAD systems in the United States and Europe have been employed for assisting physicians in the early detection of breast cancers on mammograms. It should be noted that the overall performance level of these computers in CAD is far below the average performance level achievable by physicians, and yet it can be useful in practical clinical situations.

1.4 BRIEF SUMMARY OF RECENT CAD RESEARCH

The number of papers related to CAD research presented at the RSNA meetings from 2004 to 2010 is summarized in Table 1.1. This result may be helpful for grasping the overall research efforts in the field of CAD, although more details on specific subjects are discussed in subsequent chapters in this book. The majority of these presentations were concerned with three organs—chest, breast, and colon—but other organs such as brain, liver, and skeletal and vascular systems were also subjected to CAD research. It may be noted that the detection of cancer in the breast (Kobatake et al., 1999; Freer and Ulissey, 2001; Kita et al., 2002; Butler et al., 2004; Destounis et al., 2004; Gur et al., 2004; Hong et al., 2004; Birdwell et al., 2005; Brem et al., 2005; Cupples et al., 2005; Drukker et al., 2005; Dean and Ilvento, 2006; Gilbert et al., 2006, 2008; Morton et al., 2006; Rangayyan and Ayres, 2006; Jesneck et al., 2007; Gromet, 2008; Hupse and Karssemeijer, 2010; Yuan et al., 2010; Banik et al., 2011; Jing et al., 2011; Wei et al., 2011), lung (Kaneko et al., 1996; Sone et al., 1998; Henschke et al., 1999, 2002; Armato et al., 2002; Li et al., 2002; Kostis et al., 2003; Reeves et al., 2007; Hardie et al., 2008; Korfiatis et al., 2008; Chen et al., 2011; Freedman et al., 2011; Park et al., 2011), and colon (Yoshida et al., 2002a,b; Yao et al., 2005; Taylor et al., 2006; Sundaram et al., 2008; Suzuki et al., 2008; Dachman et al., 2010; Zhu et al., 2011) has been or is being subjected to screening examinations (Oken et al., 2005; Byers et al., 2006). A large

TABLE 1.1   NUMBER OF CAD PAPERS IN VARIOUS ORGANS PRESENTED AT THE RADIOLOGICAL SOCIETY OF NORTH AMERICA FROM 2004 TO 2010

	2004	2005	2006	2007	2008	2009	2010
Chest	70	48	62	72	73	45	42
Breast	48	49	47	39	51	42	37
Colon	15	30	25	32	24	14	21
Brain	9	17	12	13	20	3	11
Liver	9	9	8	8	22	8	15
Skeletal	8	5	7	11	6	4	3
Vascular, etc.[a]	2	7	6	17	31	16	27
Total	161	165	167	200	200	132	167

[a] Cardiac, prostate, pediatric, dental, and PACS.

fraction of these examinations give normal results, and the detection of only a small number of suspicious lesions by radiologists is considered both difficult and time consuming. Therefore, it appears reasonable that the initial phase of practical CAD in clinical situations has begun in these screening examinations. In fact, commercial CAD systems for the detection of these cancers are now available for clinical use. Figure 1.2 shows a comparison of the previous performance level (87% sensitivity at 1.0 false positive per image) in the detection of clustered microcalcifications by computer at the University of Chicago when the CAD technology was licensed to R2 Technology (now called Hologic Inc.) in 1993, with an estimated current performance level (98% sensitivity at 0.25 false positive per image) of the latest R2 CAD system. It is obvious from this result that a substantial improvement was possible due to efforts by people in industry, and thus a successful clinical CAD system has evolved. This may be a good example showing that a small positive seed that germinated at an academic institution can grow substantially by commercialization efforts in industry.

In mammography, investigators (Freer and Ulissey, 2001; Butler et al., 2004; Destounis et al., 2004; Gur et al., 2004; Birdwell et al., 2005; Cupples et al., 2005; Dean and Ilvento, 2006; Gilbert et al., 2006, 2008; Morton et al., 2006; Gromet, 2008) have reported results from retrospective and/or prospective studies on large numbers of screenees, ranging from 8,682 to 231,221, regarding the effect of CAD on the detection rate of breast cancer. Although there is a large variation in the results, it is important to note that all of these studies indicated an increase in the detection rates of breast cancer with the use of CAD. In addition, Cupples et al. (2005) reported a 164% increase in the detection of small (<1 cm) invasive cancers, and also a reduction of 5.3 years in the mean age of patients at the time of detection, when CAD was used in mammography. Among the total number of approximately 38 millions of mammographic examinations annually in the United States, it has been estimated that about 80% of these examinations have been studied with the use of CAD.

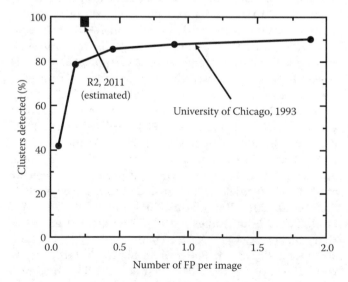

Figure 1.2 Comparison of free-response receiver operating characteristic (FROC) curves indicating a substantial improvement in the detection of clustered microcalcifications from the level of CAD scheme at the University of Chicago in 1993 to the estimated performance level of R2's ImageChecker in 2011.

1.5   EFFECT OF COMPUTER OUTPUT ON RADIOLOGISTS' PERFORMANCE

As described in Section 1.3, the unique aspect of CAD, compared with automated computer diagnosis, is the role of radiologists who can either use or disregard the computer output for final decisions. Therefore, it is critically important to understand why and how radiologists could utilize the computer output. Over the years, investigators have been developing two different types of CAD schemes, one for the detection of lesions and another for the differential diagnosis of detected lesions based on the classification between malignant and benign lesions, and also among different diseases such as different interstitial lung diseases. Although CAD schemes for the detection of lesions such as breast lesions on mammograms have been implemented successfully in clinical situations, no serious attempts have been made to apply CAD schemes for differential diagnosis to practical clinical situations, and no commercial systems for CAD for differential diagnosis are available at present. Therefore, it is important to note that there is a clear difference between the detection and the classification tasks regarding the effect of computer output on radiologists' performances, as discussed in the following text.

1.5.1   Effect of Computer Output on the Detection of Lesions

As Chan et al. (1990) demonstrated (Figure 1.1), for radiologists, the area under the ROC curve for the detection of clustered microcalcifications on mammograms was improved significantly when the computer output was available. The reason for this improvement was that, although a radiologist may miss some lesions at the first glance, he or /she may correct his or her their mistakes when they he or she sees the computer output pointing to the otherwise *missed* lesions. Some of computer false positives may not trouble radiologists, because most computer false positives are different from radiologists' false positives, and thus they can be disregarded by radiologists. However, an excessively large number of false positives are likely to discourage radiologists from paying serious attention to the computer output. Similar results on improved performance with the use of the computer output (Monnier-Cholley et al., 1998) were reported in the detection of interstitial opacities on chest radiographs. This improvement was possible because radiologists occasionally correct their *mistakes* when they recognize the *correct* computer output. In general, the extent of this type of improvement in the detection task with CAD was greater for nonexpert radiologists such as residents than for expert radiologists such as attendings (Kobayashi et al., 1996). Because the performance level of nonexperts without CAD is commonly lower than that of experts, one may consider that there is more room for improvement for nonexpert radiologists, and CAD may be able to help nonexperts more than they help experts. From all of these findings on the detection task in observer studies, it seems clear that radiologists can make proper judgments on most of the computer output by recognizing that it is a correct lesion or a false positive due to normal or benign patterns.

1.5.2   Effect of Computer Output on Differential Diagnosis

Although the performance levels of CAD schemes for differential diagnosis have been reported to be very high (Jiang et al., 1996, 1999; Ashizawa et al., 1999a,b; Chan et al., 1999; Aoyama et al., 2002, 2003; Huo et al., 2002; Hadjiiski et al., 2004; Li et al., 2004), no clinical CAD system for classification is available commercially at present. One of the reasons for this may be related to the assumption that the effect of the computer output on radiologists' classification task may be more complicated than the detection task. For example, Shiraishi et al. (2003) reported from an observer study on the distinction between benign and malignant nodules on chest radiographs that the Az value obtained from ROC curves, as shown in Figure 1.3, was improved from 0.743 to 0.817 with use of the computer output, which indicated the likelihood of malignancy (%). However, the performance (Az = 0.889) of the computer alone exceeded these results by a substantial margin. This indicates that radiologists were able to use the computer output to some extent, but were unable to take full advantage of all of the correct computer result. This probably reflects a lack of experience with the computer output and an underestimation of its reliability. Figure 1.4 shows the relationship between the likelihood measure of malignancy and the average change in the percentage confidence level by all of 16 radiologists for interpretation without and with the computer output. There was a large correlation coefficient

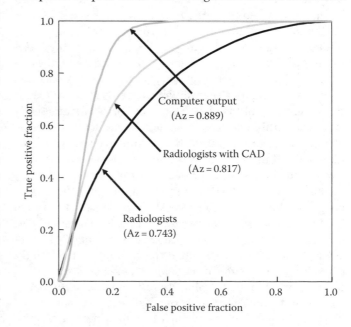

Figure 1.3   Comparison of ROC curves for the classification of benign and malignant nodules in chest radiographs by radiologists with and without the computer output and by computer alone.

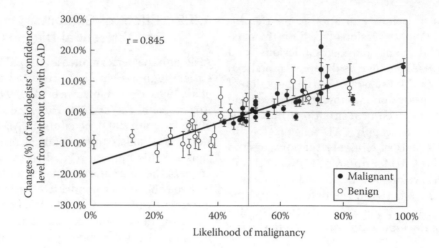

Figure 1.4   Effect of the likelihood of malignancy (%) on the change in radiologists' confidence level due to CAD on the classification of benign and malignant nodules in chest radiographs.

(r = 0.845) between them. The results in Figure 1.4 indicate that radiologists increased their confidence level when a large value of the likelihood measure of malignancy was provided by the computer, and they tended to decrease it with a small value of the likelihood measure of malignancy. Although decision making by radiologists was clearly influenced by the computer output, it is still unclear why and how radiologists use the computer output in their decision making for a differential diagnosis.

Another example is more promising for a CAD scheme (Aoyama et al., 2003; Li et al., 2004) for distinction between benign and malignant lung nodules on thoracic CT based on the determination of the likelihood of malignancy (%) of detected nodules. Li et al. (2004) demonstrated the usefulness of this scheme in observer performance studies, in which radiologists' performance with CAD (Az = 0.853) was greater than that of either radiologists alone (Az = 0.785) or the computer output alone (Az = 0.831), with statistically significant differences in Az values. The radiologists generally increased or decreased their confidence level when the likelihood of malignancy was above or below 50%, respectively, and the changes for most nodules tended toward a beneficial effect of the CAD output. Importantly, the correct computer output was able to assist radiologists in improving their decisions on many subtle cases. For some nodules, however, the radiologists' initial ratings without CAD were clearly correct, and even when the computer output indicated incorrect results, no serious detrimental effect due to CAD occurred in the radiologists' ratings. Thus, radiologists were able to maintain their own correct judgment when nodules appeared to be obviously benign or malignant even when the CAD output was incorrect. Therefore, this study indicated that a synergistic improvement in observers' interpretation by the use of a CAD scheme as a *second opinion* was possible, because the radiologists were able

to maintain their own correct opinions on some obvious cases, whereas the computer output assisted in improving their decisions in the majority of subtle cases.

1.6 POTENTIAL USEFULNESS OF SIMILAR IMAGES IN SUPPORT OF CAD

In order to assist radiologists further in their differential diagnosis in addition to providing the likelihood of malignancy (%), it would be useful to provide a set of benign and malignant images that are similar to an unknown new case under study. If the new case were considered very similar to one or more benign (or malignant) images by a radiologist, he/she would be more confident in deciding that the new case was benign (or malignant). Therefore, similar images (El-Naqa et al., 2004; Filev et al., 2005; Tourassi et al., 2007; Zheng et al., 2007; Mazurouski et al., 2008; Cho et al., 2011) may be employed as a supplement to the computed likelihood of malignancy for implementing CAD for a differential diagnosis. Figure 1.5 illustrates the comparison of an unknown case of a mass in a mammogram in the center with two benign masses on the left and two malignant masses on the right. In this simple example, most observers were able to identify the unknown case correctly as being more similar to malignant masses than to benign ones, because spiculations included in malignant cases are very similar to those in the unknown case.

The usefulness of similar images has been demonstrated in an observer performance study (Horsch et al., 2006; Muramatsu et al., 2006, 2007, 2010; Nakayama et al., 2009) in which the Az value for the ROC curves in the distinction between benign and malignant microcalcifications in mammograms was improved, as shown in Figure 1.6. Similar findings have been reported for the distinction between

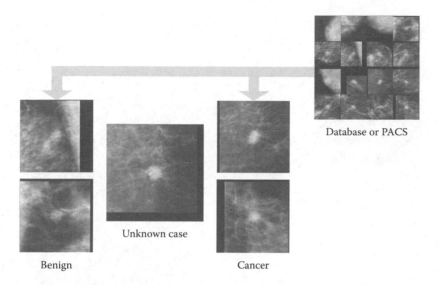

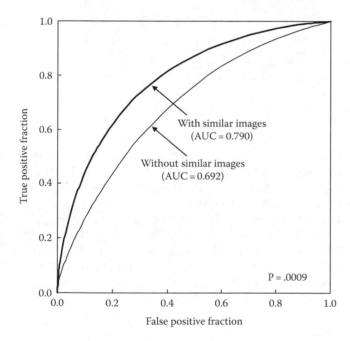

Database or PACS

Unknown case

Benign

Cancer

Figure 1.5 Illustration of potential usefulness of similar images for the classification of benign and malignant masses on mammograms.

Figure 1.6 Improvement in ROC curves for radiologists' classification of clustered microcalcifications with the use of similar images.

benign and malignant masses (Muramatsu et al., 2005), and also between benign and malignant nodules in thoracic CT (Li et al., 2003). There are at least two important issues related to the use of similar images in practical clinical situations. One is the need for a unique database that includes a large number of images that can be used as being similar to those of many unknown new cases, and another is a sensitive tool for finding images similar to an unknown case.

Although it may require considerable time and effort, a useful database for this purpose can be developed in the future by use of images stored in PACS.

At present, the majority of clinical images in PACS have not been used for clinical purposes, except for images of the same patients, such as in comparisons of a current image with previous images. Therefore, it would not be an overstatement to say that *the vast majority of images in PACS are currently sleeping* and need to be awakened in the future for daily use in many clinical situations. It would be possible to search for and retrieve very similar cases with similar images from PACS, if a reliable and useful method were developed for quantifying the similarity on a pair of images (or lesions) for visual comparison by radiologists. Recent studies indicated that the similarity of a pair of lung nodules in CT (Li et al., 2003) and of lesions in mammograms (Muramatsu et al., 2005, 2008, 2009, 2010) may be quantified by a psychophysical measure that can be obtained by the use of an artificial neural network trained with the corresponding image features and with subjective similarity ratings given by a group of radiologists. However, further investigations are required for examining the usefulness of this type of new tool for searching really similar images in PACS.

1.7 PROTOTYPE AND FIRST COMMERCIAL CAD SYSTEMS IN THE EARLY PHASE

For demonstration of the potential usefulness of CAD, the first prototype system of CAD for mammography (Nishikawa et al., 1995b) was developed in the

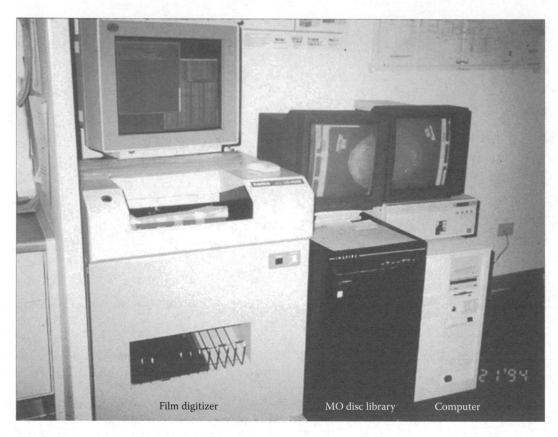

Film digitizer   MO disc library   Computer

Figure 1.7 First prototype CAD system for the detection of breast cancer on mammograms developed in 1994 at the University of Chicago.

Department of Radiology at the University of Chicago on November 8, 1994, 99 years since the discovery of X-rays by W.C. Roentgen, by the use of a laser scanner, a high-speed workstation, and a magnetic optical disk library with high-resolution monitors, as illustrated in Figure 1.7. The system included the software for the detection of both clustered microcalcifications and masses, and it was placed in the clinical section of breast imaging for prospective testing of consecutive clinical cases. In this study, 25,000 cases with more than 100,000 mammograms, including two views on both breasts, were digitized for the testing of CAD algorithms for the detection of microcalcifications and masses. One of the important findings from this study was that about onehalf of the *missed* breast cancers, which corresponded to previous mammograms made 1 or 2 years before the cancer was clinically confirmed, was detected by our prototype CAD system, thus indicating the potential for early detection of breast cancer with the use of CAD in mammography.

Although most major manufacturers of medical devices and equipment were well aware of considerable research efforts on CAD in academic institutions and their encouraging positive results, initial developments of commercial CAD systems were made by small venture companies. At present, all of the major companies have CAD products or activities related to CAD. The first commercial CAD system, ImageChecker, as shown in Figure 1.8, for the detection of breast cancer in mammography, was developed by R2 Technology based on the licensing of CAD technologies from the University of Chicago, and the first FDA approval of a CAD system for clinical use was obtained in 1998. For the detection of lung cancer on chest radiographs, the first CAD system, RapidScreen, as shown in Figure 1.9, was developed by Deus Technology (now called Riverain Medical), based on the licensing of CAD technologies from the University of Chicago, and in 2001, it received FDA approval for its clinical use. In addition, CAD technology developed at the University of Chicago was licensed to Median Technology, Mitsubishi Space Software Co., Toshiba Corporation, and General Electric Corporation. At present, many commercial CAD systems are available for the detection of various lesions obtained with various modalities. For example, there are more than 10 different commercial CAD systems for the detection of breast cancer in mammography, ultrasonography, and MRI of the breast.

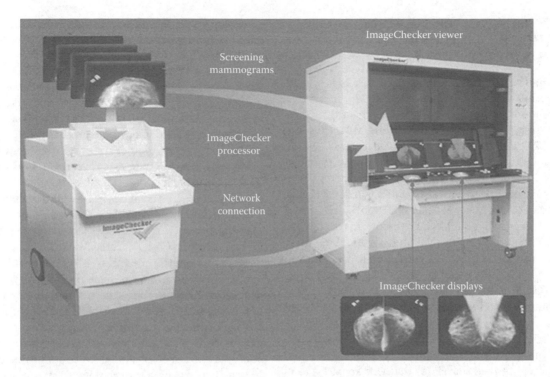

Figure 1.8   R2's ImageChecker system for the detection of breast cancer on mammograms in 1998.

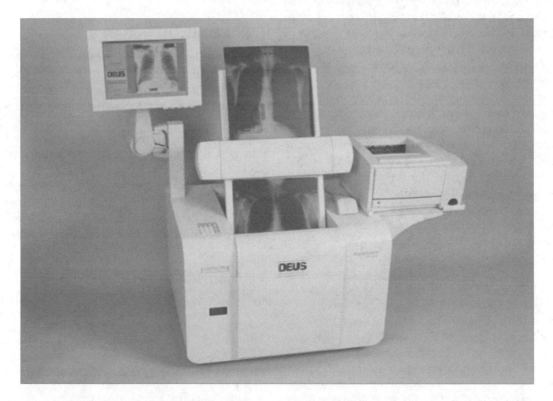

Figure 1.9   Deus's RapidScreen system for the detection of lung cancer on chest radiographs in 2001.

1.8 REEVALUATION OF READING METHODS FOR CAD IN THE PACS ENVIRONMENT

It is likely that, in the future, some CAD schemes will be included together with other software for image processing in workstations associated with some specific imaging modalities such as digital mammography, CT, and MRI. However, many other CAD schemes will be assembled as packages and will be implemented as a part of PACS. For example, the package for chest CAD may include the computerized detection of lung nodules (Xu et al., 1997; Shiraishi et al., 2006, 2007; Hardie et al., 2008; de Boo et al., 2009; Chen et al., 2011), interstitial opacities (Katsuragawa et al., 1988, 1989; Korfiatis et al., 2008; Park et al., 2011), cardiomegaly (Nakamori et al., 1990, 1991), vertebral fractures (Kasai et al., 2006, 2008), and interval changes (Kano et al., 1994; Ishida et al., 1999; Kakeda et al., 2002, 2006; Sasaki et al., 2011) in chest radiographs, as well as the computerized classification of benign and malignant nodules (Nakamura et al., 2000) and the differential diagnosis of interstitial lung diseases (Ashizawa et al., 1999a,b). All of the chest images taken for whatever purpose will be subjected to a computerized search for many different types of abnormalities included in the CAD package, and thus potential sites of lesions together with relevant information such as the likelihood of malignancy and the probability of a certain disease may be displayed on the workstation. For such a package to be used in clinical situations, it is important to reduce the number of false positives as much as possible so that radiologists will not be distracted by an excessive number of false positives, but will be prompted only or mainly by clinically significant abnormalities.

Radiologists may use this type of CAD package in the workstation in three different reading methods. One is first to read images without the computer output and then to request a display of the computer output before making the final decision; this *second-read* mode has been the condition that the FDA in the United States has required for the approval of a CAD system as a medical device. If radiologists keep their initial findings in some manner, this second-read mode may prevent a detrimental effect of the computer output on radiologists' initial diagnosis, such as incorrectly dismissing a subtle lesion because of the absence of computer output, although radiologists were very suspicious of this lesion initially. However, this second-read mode would increase the time required for radiologists' image reading, which is generally undesirable.

Another mode is to display the computer output first and then have the final decision made by a radiologist. With this *concurrent* mode, it is very likely that radiologists can reduce the reading time for image interpretations, but it is uncertain whether they may miss some lesions when no computer output was shown due to computer false negatives.

This negative effect can be reduced if the sensitivity in the detection of abnormalities is at a very high level, which may be possible with a package of a number of different, but complementary, CAD schemes. For example, although two CAD schemes may miss some lung nodules and other interstitial opacities on chest radiographs, it is possible that the temporal subtraction images obtained from the current and previous chest images demonstrate interval changes clearly, because the temporal subtraction technique is very sensitive to subtle changes between the two images. This would be one of the potential advantages in the packaging of a number of CAD schemes in the PACS environment.

The third method is called a *first-read* mode, with which radiologists would be required to examine only the locations marked by the computer. With this first-read mode, the sensitivity of the computer software must be extremely high, and if the number of false positives is not very high, the reading time may be reduced substantially. It is possible that, in the future, a certain type of radiologic examination that may commonly require a long reading time could be implemented by the concurrent-read mode or the first-read mode in a certain country due to economic and clinical reasons, such as a shortage of radiologist manpower. However, this would depend on the level of performance by the computer algorithm, and at present, it is difficult to predict what level of computer performance would make this possible.

1.9 CONCLUSION

Computer-aided diagnosis has become a part of clinical work in the detection of breast cancer by use of mammograms, but is still in its infancy of the development of its full potential for applications to many different types of lesions obtained with various modalities. CAD is a concept based on equal roles of physician and computer, and thus it is distinctly different from automated computer diagnosis. It is likely that, in the future, CAD schemes will be incorporated into PACS and that they will be assembled as a package for the detection of lesions and also for differential diagnosis. CAD will be employed as a useful tool for diagnostic examinations in daily clinical work.

REFERENCES

Abe H, MacMahon H, Engelmann R, Li Q, Shiraishi J, Katsuragawa S, Aoyama M, Ishida T, Ashizawa K, Metz C, Doi K. 2003. Computer-aided diagnosis in chest radiology: Results of large-scale observer tests performed at the 1996–2001 RSNA Scientific Assemblies. *RadioGraphics* 23: 255–265.

Abe H, MacMahon H, Shiraishi J, Li Q, Engelmann R, Doi K. 2004. Computer-aided diagnosis in chest radiography. *Semin Ultrasound CT MRI* 25: 432–437.

Aoyama M, Li Q, Katsuragawa S, Li F, Sone S, Doi K. 2003. Computerized scheme for determination of the likelihood measure of malignancy for pulmonary nodules on low-dose CT images. *Med Phys* 30: 387–394.

Aoyama M, Li Q, Katsuragawa S, MacMahon H, Doi K. 2002. Automated computerized scheme for distinction between benign and malignant solitary pulmonary nodules on chest images. *Med Phys* 29: 701–708.

Arimura H, Katsuragawa S, Suzuki K, Li F, Shiraishi J, Doi K. 2004. Computerized scheme for automated detection of lung nodules in low-dose CT images for lung cancer screening. *Acad Radiol* 11: 617–629.

Armato SG III, Li F, Giger ML, MacMahon H, Sone S, Doi K. 2002. Performance of automated lung nodule detection applied to cancers missed in a lung screening program. *Radiology* 225: 685–692.

Ashizawa K, Ishida T, MacMahon H, Vyborny CJ, Katsuragawa S, Doi K. 1999a. Artificial neural networks in chest radiographs: Application to differential diagnosis of interstitial lung disease. *Acad Radiol* 6: 2–9.

Ashizawa K, MacMahon H, Ishida T, Nakamura K, Vyborny CJ, Katsuragawa S, Doi K. 1999b. Effect of artificial neural network on radiologists' performance for differential diagnosis of interstitial lung disease on chest radiographs. *Am J Roentgenol* 172: 1311–1314.

Banik S, Rangayyan RM, Desautels JEL. 2011. Detection of architectural distortion in prior mammograms. *IEEE Trans Med Imaging* 30: 279–294.

Bielen D, Kiss G. 2007. CADe for CTC: Update. *Abdom Imaging* 32: 571–581.

Birdwell RL, Bandodkar P, Ikeda DM. 2005. Computer-aided detection with screening mammography in a university hospital setting. *Radiology* 236: 451–457.

Brem RF, Hoffmeister JW, Zisman G, DeSimio MP, Rogers SK. 2005. A computer-aided detection system for the evaluation of breast cancer by mammographic appearance and lesion size. *Am J Roentgenol* 184: 893–896.

Butler SA, Gabbay RJ, Kass DA, Siedler DE, O'Shaughnessy KF, Castellino RA. 2004. Computer-aided detection in diagnostic mammography: Detection of clinically unsuspected cancers. *Am J Roentgenol* 183: 1511–1515.

Byers T, Barrera E, Fontham ET et al. 2006. A midpoint assessment of the American Cancer Society challenge goal to halve the U.S. cancer mortality rates between the years 1990 and 2015. *Cancer* 107: 396–405.

Carmody DP, Nodine CF, Kundel HL. 1980. An analysis of perceptual and cognitive factors in radiographic interpretation. *Perception* 9: 339–344.

Chan HP, Doi K, Galhotra S, Vyborny CJ, MacMahon H, Jokich PM. 1987. Image feature analysis and computer-aided diagnosis in digital radiography. 1. Automated detection of microcalcifications in mammography. *Med Phys* 14: 538–548.

Chan HP, Doi K, Vyborny CJ, Schmidt RA, Metz CE, Lam KL, Ogura T, Wu Y, MacMahon H. 1990. Improvement in radiologists' detection of clustered microcalcifications on mammograms: The potential of computer-aided diagnosis. *Invest Radiol* 25: 1102–1110.

Chan HP, Sahiner B, Helvie MA, Petrick N, Roubidoux MA, Wilson TE, Adler DD, Paramagul C, Newman JS, Sanjay-Gopal S. 1999. Improvement of radiologists' characterization of mammographic masses by using computer-aided diagnosis: An ROC study. *Radiology* 212: 817–827.

Chen S, Suzuki K, MacMahon H. 2011. Development and evaluation of a computer aided diagnostic scheme for lung nodule detection in chest radiographs by means of two-stage nodule enhancement with support vector classification. *Med Phys* 38: 1844–1858.

Cho H-C, Hadjiiski LM, Sahiner B, Chan HP, Helvie M, Paramagul C, Nees AV. 2011. Similarity evaluation in a content-based image retrieval (CBIR) CADx system for characterization of breast masses on ultrasound images. *Med Phys* 38: 1820–1831.

Cupples TE, Cunningham JE, Reynolds JC. 2005. Impact of computer-aided detection in a regional screening mammography program. *Am J Roentgenol* 185: 944–950.

Dachman AH, Obchowski NA, Hoffmeister JW et al. 2010. Effect of computer-aided detection for CT colonography in multi-reader, muticase trial. *Radiology* 256: 827–835.

de Boo DW, Prokop M, Ulmann M, van Ginneken B, Schaefer-Prokop CM. 2009. Computer-aided detection (CAD) of lung nodules and small tumours on chest radiographs. *Eur J Radiol* 72: 218–225.

de Hoop B, de Boo DW, Gietema HA, van Hoorn F, Mearadji B, Schijf L, van Ginneken B, Prokop M, Schaefer-Prokop CM. 2010. Computer-aided detection of lung cancer on chest radiographs: Effect on observer performance. *Radiology* 257: 532–540.

Dean JC, Ilvento CC. 2006. Improved cancer detection using computer-aided detection with diagnostic and screening mammography: Prospective study of 104 cancers. *Am J Roentgenol* 187: 20–28.

Destounis SV, DiNitto P, Logan-Young W, Bonaccio E, Zuley ML, Willison KM. 2004. Can computer-aided detection with double reading of screening mammograms help decrease the false-negative rate? Initial experience. *Radiology* 232: 578–584.

Doi K. 2003. Computer-aided diagnosis in digital chest radiography. *Advances in Digital Radiography: RSNA Categorical Course in Diagnostic Radiology Physics 2003 Syllabus*, pp. 227–236.

Doi K. 2004. Overview on research and development of computer-aided diagnostic schemes. *Semin Ultrasound CT MRI* 25: 404–410.

Doi K. 2005. Current status and future potential of computer-aided diagnosis in medical imaging. *Brit J Radiol* 78: S3–S19 (Special Issue).

Doi K. 2006. Diagnostic imaging over the last 50 years: Research and development in medical imaging science and technology. *Phys Med Biol* 51: R5–R27.

Doi K. 2007. Computer-aided diagnosis in medical imaging: Historical review, current and future potential. *Comput Med Imaging Graph* 31: 198–211.

Doi K, Chan H-P, Giger ML. 1990. Method and system for enhancement and detection of abnormal anatomic regions in a digital image. United States Patent No. 4,907,156.

Doi K, Giger ML, MacMahon H et al. 1992. Computer-aided diagnosis: Development of automated schemes for quantitative analysis of radiographic images. *Semin Ultrasound CT MRI* 13: 140–152.

Doi K, MacMahon H, Giger ML, Hoffmann KR (eds.). 1999b. *Computer Aided Diagnosis in Medical Imaging*. Elsevier, Amsterdam, the Netherlands, pp. 3–560.

Doi K, MacMahon H, Katsuragawa S, Nishikawa RM, Jiang Y. 1999a. Computer-aided diagnosis in radiology: Potential and pitfalls. *Eur J Radiol* 31: 97–109.

Drukker K, Horsch K, Giger ML. 2005. Multimodality computerized diagnosis of breast lesions using mammography and sonography. *Acad Radiol* 8: 970–979.

El-Naqa I, Yang Y, Galasanos NP, Nishikawa RM, Wernick MN. 2004. A similarity learning approach to content based image retrieval: Application to digital mammography. *IEEE Trans Med Imaging* 23: 1233–1244.

Elter M, Horsch A. 2009. CADx of mammographic masses and clustered microcalcifications: A review. *Med Phys* 36: 2052–2068.

Engle RL. Winter 1992. Attempt to use computers as diagnostic aids in medical decision making: A thirty-year experience. *Perspect Biol Med* 35(2): 207–218 (The University of Chicago).

Erickson BJ, Bartholmai B. 2002. Computer-aided detection and diagnosis at the start of the third millennium. *J Dig Imaging* 15: 59–68.

Filev P, Hadjiiski LM, Sahiner B, Chan HP, Helvie M. 2005. Comparison of similarity measures for the task of template matching of masses on serial mammograms. *Med Phys* 32: 515–529.

Freedman MT, Lo BSC, Seibel JC, Bromley CM. 2011. Lung nodules: Improved detection with software that suppresses the rib and clavicle on chest radiographs. *Radiology* 260: 265–273.

Freer TW, Ulissey MJ. 2001. Screening mammography with computer-aided detection: Prospective study of 12,860 patients in a community breast center. *Radiology* 220: 781–786.

Fujita H, Doi K, Fencil LE, Chua KG. 1987. Image feature analysis and computer-aided diagnosis in digital radiography. 2. Computerized determination of vessel sizes in digital subtraction angiography. *Med Phys* 14: 549–556.

Fujita H, Doi K, Giger ML. 1985. Investigation of basic imaging properties in digital radiography. 6. MTFs of I.I.-TV digital imaging systems. *Med Phys* 12: 712–729.

Fujita H, Doi K, Giger ML, Chan HP. 1986. Investigation of basic imaging properties in digital radiography. 5. Characteristic curves of I.I.-TV digital systems. *Med Phys* 13: 13–18.

Giger ML. 2004. Computerized analysis of images in the detection and diagnosis of breast cancer. *Semin Ultrasound CT MRI* 25: 411–418.

Giger ML, Chan HP, Boone J. 2008. Anniversary paper: History and status of CAD and quantitative image analysis: The role of medical physics and AAPM. *Med Phys* 12: 5799–5820.

Giger ML, Doi K. 1984a. Investigation of basic imaging properties in digital radiography. Part 1: Modulation transfer function. *Med Phys* 11: 287–295.

Giger ML, Doi K. 1984b. Investigation of basic imaging properties in digital radiography. Part 2: Noise Wiener spectrum. *Med Phys* 11: 797–805.

Giger ML, Doi K. 1985. Investigation of basic imaging properties in digital radiography. Effect of pixel size on SNR and threshold contrast. *Med Phys* 12: 201–208.

Giger ML, Doi K, Fujita H. 1986a. Investigation of basic imaging properties in digital radiography. 7. Noise Wiener spectra of I.I.-TV digital imaging systems. *Med Phys* 13: 131–138.

Giger ML, Doi K, MacMahon H. 1987. Computerized detection of lung nodules in digital chest radiographs. *Proc SPIE* 767: 384–386.

Giger ML, Doi K, MacMahon H. 1988. Image feature analysis and computer-aided diagnosis in digital radiography. 3. Automated detection of nodules in peripheral lung fields. *Med Phys* 15: 158–166.

Giger ML, Huo Z, Kupinski MA, Vyborny CJ. 2000. Computer-aided diagnosis in mammography. In Fitzpatrick JM, Sonka M (eds.). *The Handbook of Medical Imaging. Medical Imaging Processing and Analysis*, Vol. 2. SPIE, pp. 915–1004.

Giger ML, Ohara K, Doi K. 1986b. Investigation of basic imaging properties in digital radiography. 9. Effect of displayed grey levels on signal detection. *Med Phys* 13: 312–318.

Gilbert FJ, Astley SM, Gillan MGC et al. 2008. Single reading with computer-aided detection for screening mammography. *New Engl J Med* 359: 1675–1684.

Gilbert FJ, Astley SM, McGee MA et al. 2006. Single reading with computer-aided detection and double reading of mammograms in the United Kingdom National Breast Screening Program. *Radiology* 241: 47–53.

Gromet M. 2008. Comparison of computer-aided detection to double reading of screening mammograms: Review of 231,221 mammograms. *Am J Roentgenol* 190: 854–859.

Gur D, Sumkin JH, Rockette HE, Ganott M, Hakim C, Hardesty L, Poller WR, Shah R, Wallace L. 2004. Changes in breast cancer detection and mammography recall rate after the introduction of a computer-aided detection system. *J Natl Cancer Inst* 96: 185–190.

Hadjiiski L, Chan HP, Sahiner B et al. 2004. Improvement in radiologists' characterization of malignant and benign breast masses on serial mammograms with computer-aided diagnosis: An ROC study. *Radiology* 233: 255–265.

Hadjiiski L, Sahiner B, Chan HP. 2006. Advances in computer-aided diagnosis for breast cancer. *Curr Opin Obstet Gynecol* 1: 64–70.

Hardie RC, Rogers SK, Wilson T, Rogers A. 2008. Performance analysis of a new computer aided detection system for identifying lung nodules on chest radiographs. *Med Image Anal* 12: 240–258.

Henschke CI, MacCauley DI, Yankelevitz DF, Naidich DP, McGuinness G, Miettinen OS, Libby DM, Pasmantier MW, Koizumi J, Altorki NK, Smith JP. 1999. Early lung cancer action project: Overall design and findings from baseline screening. *Lancet* 354: 99–105.

Henschke CI, Yankelevitz DF, Mirtcheva R, McGuinness G, McCauley D, Miettinen OS. 2002. CT screening for lung cancer: Frequency and significance of part-solid and nonsolid nodules. *Am J Roentgenol* 178: 1053–1057.

Hirai T, Korogi Y, Arimura H, Katsuragawa S, Kitajima M, Yamura M, Yamashita Y, Doi K. 2005. Intracranial aneurysms at MR angiography: Effect of computer-aided diagnosis on radiologists' detection performance. *Radiology* 237: 605–610.

Hoffmann KR, Doi K, Chan HP, Fencil L, Fujita H, Muraki A. 1986. Automated tracking of the vascular tree in DSA images using a double-square-box region-of-search algorithm. *Proc SPIE* 626: 326–333.

Hong AS, Baker JA, Lo JY, Nicholas JL, Soo MS. 2004. Computer-aided classification of breast masses using mammogram, ultrasound, and clinical inputs. *AJR* 4: 33.

Horsch K, Giger ML, Vyborny CJ, Lan L, Mendelson EB, Hendrick RE. 2006. Classification of breast lesions with multimodality computer-aided diagnosis: Observer study results on an independent clinical data set. *Radiology* 2: 357–368.

Huang HK. 2010. *PACS and Imaging Informatics: Principles and Applications*, 2nd edn. Wiley & Blackwell, Hoboken, NJ.

Huang HK. 2011. From PACS to web-based ePR system with image distribution for enterprise-level filmless healthcare delivery. *Radiol Phys Technol* 4: 91–108.

Huo Z, Giger ML, Vyborny CJ, Metz CE. 2002. Breast cancer: Effectiveness of computer-aided diagnosis-observer study with independent database of mammograms. *Radiology* 224: 560–568.

Hupse R, Karssemeijer N. 2010. The effect of feature selection methods on computer-aided detection of masses in mammograms. *Phys Med Biol* 55: 2893–2904.

Ishida M, Doi K, Loo LN, Metz CE, Lehr JL. 1984. Digital image processing: Effect on the detectability of simulated low-contrast radiographic patterns. *Radiology* 150: 569–575.

Ishida M, Frank PH, Doi K, Lehr JL. 1983. High-quality digital radiographic images: Improved detection of low-contrast objects and preliminary clinical studies. *RadioGraphics* 3: 325–338.

Ishida M, Kato H, Doi K, Frank PH. 1982. Development of a new digital radiographic image processing system. *Proc SPIE* 347: 42–48.

Ishida T, Katsuragawa S, Nakamura K, MacMahon H, Doi K. 1999. Iterative image warping technique for temporal subtraction of sequential chest radiographs to detect interval change. *Med Phys* 26: 1320–1329.

Jesneck JL, Lo JY, Baker JA. 2007. Breast mass lesions: Computer-aided diagnosis models with mammographic and sonographic descriptors. *Radiology* 2: 390–398.

Jiang Y, Nishikawa RM, Schmidt RA, Metz CE, Giger ML, Doi K. 1999. Improving breast cancer diagnosis with computer-aided diagnosis. *Acad Radiol* 6: 22–33.

Jiang Y, Nishikawa RM, Wolverton DE, Metz CE, Giger ML, Schmidt RA, Vyborny CJ, Doi K. 1996. Malignant and benign clustered microcalcifications: Automated feature analysis and classification. *Radiology* 198: 671–678.

Jing H, Yang Y, Nishikawa RM. 2011. Detection of clustered microcalcifications using spatial point process modeling. *Phys Med Biol* 56: 1–17.

Kakeda S, Kamada K, Hatakeyama Y, Aoki T, Ohguri T, Korogi Y, Katsuragawa S, Doi K. 2006. Effect of temporal subtraction of technique on reading time and diagnostic accuracy in the interpretation of chest radiographs. *AJR* 187: 1253–1259.

Kakeda S, Moriya J, Sato H, Aoki T, Watanabe H, Nakata H, Oda N, Katsuragawa S, Yamamoto K, Doi K. 2004. Improved detection of lung nodules with aid of computerized detection method: Evaluation of a commercial computer-aided diagnosis system. *AJR* 182: 505–510.

Kakeda S, Nakamura K, Kamada K, Watanabe H, Nakata H, Katsuragawa S, Doi K. 2002. Observer performance study on the usefulness of temporal subtraction in detection of lung nodules on digital chest images. *Radiology* 224: 145–151.

Kaneko M, Eguchi K, Ohmatsu H, Kakinuma R, Naruke T, Suemasu K, Moriyama N. 1996. Peripheral lung cancer: Screening and detection with low-dose spiral CT versus radiography. *Radiology* 201: 798–802.

Kano A, Doi K, MacMahon H, Hassell DD, Giger ML. 1994. Digital image subtraction of temporally sequential chest images for detection of interval change. *Med Phys* 21: 453–461.

Kasai S, Li F, Shiraishi J, Doi K. 2008. Usefulness of computer-aided detection schemes for vertebral fractures and lung nodules in chest radiographs: Observer performance study by use of ROC analysis without and with localization. *Am J Roentgenol* 191: 260–265.

Kasai S, Li F, Shiraishi J, Li Q, Doi K. 2006. Computerized detection of vertebral compression fractures on lateral chest radiographs: Preliminary results of a tool for early detection of osteoporosis. *Med Phys* 33: 4664–4676.

Katsuragawa S, Doi K, MacMahon H. 1988. Image feature analysis and computer-aided diagnosis in digital radiography: Detection and characterization of interstitial lung disease in digital chest radiographs. *Med Phys* 15: 311–319.

Katsuragawa S, Doi K, MacMahon H. 1989. Image feature analysis and computer-aided diagnosis in digital radiography: Classification of normal and abnormal lungs with interstitial disease in chest images. *Med Phys* 16: 38–44.

Kita Y, Tohno E, Highnam R, Brady M. 2002. A CAD system for the 3D location of lesions in mammograms. *Med Image Anal* 6: 267–273.

Kobatake H, Murakami M, Takeo H, Nawano S. 1999. Computerized detection of malignant tumors on digital mammograms. *IEEE Trans Med Imaging* 18: 369–378.

Kobayashi T, Xu X-W, MacMahon H, Metz CE, Doi K. 1996. Effect of a computer-aided diagnosis scheme on radiologists' performance in detection of lung nodules on radiographs. *Radiology* 199: 843–848.

Korfiatis P, Kalogeropoulou C, Karahaliou A, Kazantzi A, Skiadopoulos S, Costaridou L. 2008. Texture classification-based segmentation of lung affected by interstitial pneumonia in high-resolution CT. *Med Phys* 35: 5290–5302.

Kostis WJ, Reeves AP, Yankelevitz DF, Henschke CI. 2003. Three-dimensional segmentation and growth-rate estimation of small pulmonary nodules in helical CT images. *IEEE Trans Med Imaging* 22: 1259–1274.

Kruger RP, Thompson WB, Turner AF. January 1974. Computer diagnosis of pneumoconiosis. *IEEE Trans Syst Man Cybernet* SMC-4(1): 44–47.

Kruger RP, Towns JR, Hall DL et al. May 1972. Automated radiographic diagnosis via feature extraction and classification of cardiac size and shape descriptors. *IEEE Trans Biomed Eng* BME-19(3): 174–186.

Kume Y, Doi K, Ohara K, Giger ML. 1986. Investigation of basic imaging properties in digital radiography. 10. Structure mottle of I.I.-TV digital imaging systems. *Med Phys* 13: 843–849.

Kundel HL, Nodine CF. 1975. Interpreting chest radiographs without visual search. *Radiology* 116: 527–532.

Kundel HL, Nodine CF, Carmody D. 1978. Visual scanning, pattern recognition and decision-making in pulmonary nodule detection. *Invest Radiol* 13: 175–181.

Kundel HL, Revesz G. 1976. Lesion conspicuity, structured noise, and film reader error. *AJR* 126: 1233–1238.

Kundel HL, Revesz G, Toto L. 1979. Contrast gradient and the detection of lung nodules. *Invest Radiol* 14: 18–22.

Li F, Aoyama M, Shiraishi J, Abe H, Li Q, Suzuki K, Engelmann R, Sone S, MacMahon H, Doi K. 2004. Radiologists' performance for differentiating benign from malignant lung nodules on high-resolution CT by using computer-estimated likelihood of malignancy. *AJR* 183: 1209–1215.

Li F, Arimura H, Suzuki K, Shiraishi J, Li Q, Abe H, Engelmann R, Sone S, MacMahon H, Doi K. 2005. Computer-aided diagnosis for detection of missed peripheral lung cancers on CT: ROC and LROC analysis. *Radiology* 237: 684–690.

Li F, Sone S, Abe H, MacMahon H, Armato S, Doi K. 2002. Missed lung cancers in low-dose helical CT screening obtained from a general population. *Radiology* 225: 673–683.

Li Q, Li F, Armato SG III, Suzuki K, Shiraishi J, Abe H, Engelmann R, Nie Y, MacMahon H, Doi K. 2005. Computer-aided diagnosis in thoracic CT. *Semin Ultrasound CT MRI* 26: 357–363.

Li Q, Li F, Shiraishi J, Katsuragawa S, Sone S, Doi K. 2003. Investigation of new psychophysical measures for evaluation of similar images on thoracic CT for distinction between benign and malignant nodules. *Med Phys* 30: 2584–2593.

Lodwick GS, Haun CL, Smith WE et al. 1963. Computer diagnosis of primary bone tumor. *Radiology* 80: 273–275.

Loo LN, Doi K, Metz CE. 1985. Investigation of basic imaging properties in digital radiography. 4. Effect of unsharp masking on the detectability of simple patterns. *Med Phys* 12: 209–214.

MacMahon H, Engelmann R, Behlen F, Hoffmann KR, Ishida T, Roe C, Metz C, Doi K. 1999. Computer-aided diagnosis of pulmonary nodules: Results of a large-scale observer test. *Radiology* 213: 723–726.

MacMahon H, Vyborny CJ, Metz CE, Doi K, Sabeti V, Solomon SL. 1986. Digital radiography of subtle pulmonary abnormalities: An ROC study of the effect of pixel size on observer performance. *Radiology* 158: 21–26.

MacMahon H, Vyborny CJ, Powell G, Doi K, Metz CE. 1984. The effect of pixel size on the detection rate of early pulmonary sarcoidosis in digital chest radiographic systems. *Proc SPIE* 486: 14–20.

MacMahon H, Vyborny CJ, Sabeti V, Metz CE, Doi K. 1985. The effect of digital unsharp masking on the detectability of interstitial infiltrates and pneumothoraces. *Proc SPIE* 555: 246–252.

Mazurowski MA, Habas PA, Zurada JM, Tourassi GD. 2008. Decision optimization of case-based computer-aided decision systems using genetic algorithms with application to mammography. *Phys Med Biol* 53: 895–908.

Metz CE. 1986. ROC methodology in radiologic imaging. *Invest Radiol* 21: 720–733.

Metz CE. 1989. Some practical issues of experimental design and data analysis in radiological ROC studies. *Invest Radiol* 24: 234–245.

Metz CE. 2000. Fundamental ROC analysis. In Beutel J, Kundel HL, Van Metter RL (eds.). *Handbook of Medical Imaging*, Vol. 1. SPIE Press, The International Society for Optical Engineering, Bellingham, WA, pp. 751–770.

Moberg K, Bjurstam N, Wilczek B, Rostgard L, Egge E, Muren C. 2001. Computer assisted detection of interval breast cancers. *Eur J Radiol* 39: 104–110.

Monnier-Cholley L, MacMahon H, Katsuragawa S, Morishita J, Ishida T, Doi K. 1998. Computer aided diagnosis for detection of interstitial infiltrates in chest radiographs: Evaluation by means of ROC analysis. *Am J Roentgenol* 171: 1651–1656.

Morton MJ, Whaley DH, Brandt KR, Amrami KK. 2006. Screening mammograms: Interpretation with computer-aided detection-prospective evaluation. *Radiology* 239: 375–383.

Muramatsu C, Li Q, Schmidt RA et al. 2007. Determination of subjective similarity for pairs of masses and pairs of clustered microcalcifications on mammograms: Comparison of ranking scores and absolute similarity ratings. *Med Phys* 34: 2890–2895.

Muramatsu C, Li Q, Schmidt RA, Shiraishi J, Doi K. 2008. Investigation of psychophysical similarity measures for selection of similar images in the diagnosis of clustered microcalcifications on mammograms. *Med Phys* 35: 5695–5702.

Muramatsu C, Li Q, Schmidt RA, Shiraishi J, Doi K. 2009. Determination of similarity measures for pairs of mass lesions on mammograms by use of BI-RAD lesion descriptors and image features. *Acad Radiol* 16: 443–449.

Muramatsu C, Li Q, Schmidt RA, Suzuki K, Shiraishi J, Newstead GM, Doi K. 2006. Experimental determination of subjective similarity for pairs of clustered microcalcifications on mammograms: Observer study results. *Med Phys* 33: 3460–3468.

Muramatsu C, Li Q, Suzuki K, Schmidt RA, Shiraishi J, Newstead GM, Doi K. 2005. Investigation of psychophysical measure for evaluation of similar images for mammographic masses: Preliminary results. *Med Phys* 32: 2295–2304.

Muramatsu C, Schmidt RA, Shiraishi J, Li Q, Doi K. 2010. Presentation of similar images as a reference for distinction between benign and malignant masses on mammograms: Analysis of initial observer study. *J Dig Imaging* 23: 592–602.

Myers PH, Nice CM, Becker HC et al. 1964. Automated computer analysis of radiographic images. *Radiology* 83: 1029–1033.

Nakamori N, Doi K, MacMahon H, Sasaki Y, Montner S. 1991. Effect of heart size parameters computed from digital chest radiographs on detection of cardiomegaly: Potential usefulness for computer-aided diagnosis. *Invest Radiol* 26: 546–550.

Nakamori N, Doi K, Sabeti V, MacMahon H. 1990. Image feature analysis and computer-aided diagnosis in digital radiography: Automated analysis of sizes of heart and lung in digital chest images. *Med Phys* 17: 342–350.

Nakamura K, Yoshida H, Engelmann R, MacMahon H, Katsuragawa S, Ishida T, Ashizawa K, Doi K. 2000. Computerized analysis of the likelihood of malignancy in solitary pulmonary nodules with use of artificial neural networks. *Radiology* 214: 823–830.

Nakayama R, Abe H, Shiraishi J, Doi K. 2009. Potential usefulness of similar images in the differential diagnosis of clustered microcalcifications on mammograms. *Radiology* 253: 625–631.

Nishikawa RM. 2007. Current status and future directions of computer-aided diagnosis in mammography. *Comput Med Imaging Graph* 31: 224–235.

Nishikawa RM, Doi K, Giger ML et al. 1995a. Computerized detection of clustered microcalcifications: Evaluation of performance using mammograms from multiple centers. *RadioGraphics* 15: 443–452.

Nishikawa RM, Haldemann RC, Papaioannou J, Giger ML, Lu P, Schmidt RA, Wolverton DE, Bick U, Doi K. 1995b. Initial experience with a prototype clinical "intelligent" mammography workstation for computer-aided diagnosis. *Proc SPIE* 2434: 65–71.

Ohara K, Chan HP, Doi K, Fujita H, Giger ML. 1986. Investigation of basic imaging properties in digital radiography. 8. Detection of simulated low-contrast objects in DSA images. *Med Phys* 13: 304–311.

Oken MM, Marcus PM, Hu P et al. 2005. Baseline chest radiograph for lung cancer detection in the randomized prostate, lung, colorectal and ovarian cancer screening trial. *J Natl Cancer Inst* 97: 1832–1839.

Park SC, Tan J, Wang X et al. 2011. Computer-aided detection of early interstitial lung diseases using low-dose CT images. *Phys Med Biol* 56: 1139–1153.

Rangayyan RM, Ayres FJ. 2006. Gabor filters and phase portraits for the detection of architectural distortion in mammograms. *Med Biol Eng Comput* 44: 883–894.

Reeves AP, Biancardi AM, Apanasovich TV et al. 2007. The lung image database consortium (LIDC): A comparison of different size metrics for pulmonary nodule measurements. *Acad Radiol* 14: 1475–1485.

Sahiner B, Chan HP, Hadjiiski LM et al. 2009. Multi-modality CADx: ROC study of the effect on radiologists' accuracy in characterizing breast masses on mammograms and 3D ultrasound images. *Acad Radiol* 7: 810–818.

Sasaki Y, Abe K, Tabei M et al. 2011. Clinical usefulness of temporal subtraction method in screening digital chest radiography with a mobile computed radiography system. *Radiol Phys Technol* 4: 84–90.

Shiraishi J, Abe H, Engelmann R, Aoyama M, MacMahon H, Doi K. 2003. Computer-aided diagnosis to distinguish benign from malignant solitary pulmonary nodules on radiographs: ROC analysis of radiologists' performance-initial experience. *Radiology* 227: 469–474.

Shiraishi J, Li F, Doi, K. 2007. Computer-aided diagnosis for improved detection of lung nodules by use of PA and lateral chest radiographs. *Acad Radiol* 14: 28–37.

Shiraishi J, Li Q, Suzuki K, Engelmann R, Doi K. 2006. Computer-aided diagnostic scheme for the detection of lung nodules on chest radiographs: Localized search method based on anatomical classification. *Med Phys* 33: 2642–2653.

Shiraishi J, Pesce LL, Metz CE, Doi K. 2009. Experimental design and data analysis in receiver operating characteristic studies: Lessons learned from reports in radiology from 1997 to 2006. *Radiology* 253: 822–830.

Sone S, Takashima S, Li F, Yang Z, Honda T, Maruyama Y, Hasegawa M, Yamanda T, Kubo K, Hanamura K, Asakura K. 1998. Mass screening for lung cancer with mobile spiral computed tomography scanner. *Lancet* 351: 1242–1245.

Summers RM. 2003. Road maps for advancement of radiologic computer-aided detection in the 21st century. *Radiology* 229: 11–13.

Sundaram P, Zomorodian A, Beauleu C, Napel S. 2008. Colon polyp detection using smoothed shape operator: Preliminary results. *Med Image Anal* 12: 99–119.

Suzuki K, Yoshida H, Nappi J et al. 2008. Mixture of expert 3D massive-training ANNs for reduction of multiple types of false positives in CADe for detection of polyps in CTC. *Med Phys* 35: 694–703.

Taylor S, Halligan S, Burling D et al. 2006. Computer-assisted reader software versus expert reviewers for polyp detection on CTC. *AJR* 186: 696–702.

Toriwaki J, Suenaga Y, Negoro T et al. 1973. Pattern recognition of chest x-ray images. *Comput Graph Image Process* 2: 252–271.

Tourassi GD, Harrawood B, Singh S, Lo JY, Floyd CE. 2007. Evaluation of information-theoretic similarity measures for content-based retrieval and detection of masses in mammograms. *Med Phys* 34: 140–150.

van Ginneken B, ter Haar Romeny BM, Viergever MA. 2001. Computer-aided diagnosis in chest radiography: A survey. *IEEE Trans Med Imaging* 20: 1228–1241.

Warren-Burhenne LJ, Wood SA, D'Orsi CJ et al. 2000. Potential contribution of computer-aided detection to the sensitivity of screening mammography. *Radiology* 215: 554–562.

Wei J, Chan HP, Zhou C, Wu YT, Sahiner B, Hadjiiski LM, Roubidoux MA, Helvie MA. 2011. Computer-aided detection of breast masses: Four-view strategy for screening mammography. *Med Phys* 38: 1867–1876.

Winsbarg F, Elkin M, May J et al. 1967. Detection of radiographic abnormalities in mammograms by means of optical scanning and computer analysis. *Radiology* 89: 211–215.

Xu XW, Doi K, Kobayashi T, MacMahon H, Giger ML. 1997. Development of an improved CAD scheme for automated detection of lung nodules in digital chest images. *Med Phys* 24: 1395–1403.

Yao J, Summers R, Hara A. 2005. Optimizing the support vector machine committee configuration in a colonic polyp CADe system. *Proc SPIE Med Imaging* 5746: 384–392.

Yin FF, Giger ML, Vyborny CJ, Doi K, Schmidt RA. 1993. Comparison of bilateral-subtraction and single-image processing techniques in the computerized detection of mammographic masses. *Invest Radiol* 28: 473–481.

Yoshida H, Dachman AH. 2004. Computer-aided diagnosis for CT colonography. *Semin Ultrasound CT MRI* 25: 404–410.

Yoshida H, Masutani Y, MacEneaney P, Rubin D, Dachman AH. 2002a. Computerized detection of colonic polyps at CT colonography on the basis of volumetric features: Pilot study. *Radiology* 222: 327–336.

Yoshida H, Nappi J, MacEneaney P, Rubin D, Dachman AH. 2002b. Computer-aided diagnosis scheme for the detection of polyps at CT colonography. *RadioGraphics* 22: 963–979.

Yuan Y, Giger ML, Li H, Bhooshan N, Sennett CA. 2010. Multimodality computer-aided breast cancer diagnosis with FFDM and DCE-MRI. *Acad Radiol* 9: 1158–1167.

Zheng B, Mello-Thoms C, Wang X-H, Abrams GS, Sumkin JH, Chough DM, Ganott MA, Lu A, Gur D. 2007. Interactive computer-aided diagnosis of breast masses: Computerized selection of visually similar image sets from a reference library. *Acad Radiol* 14: 917–927.

Zhu H, Fan Y, Lu H, Liang Z. 2011. Improved curvature estimation for CADe of colonic polyps in CTC. *Acad Radiol* 18: 1024–1034.

Computer-Aided Detection and Diagnosis in Breast Imaging

Chapter 2

Detection and Diagnosis of Breast Masses in Mammography

Nico Karssemeijer

CONTENTS

2.1 INTRODUCTION

In many countries, regular breast cancer screening with mammography is offered to women over 40 or 50 years of age to detect early signs of breast cancer. Effectiveness of mammographic screening has been established by randomized controlled trials and by observation of a significant reduction in breast cancer mortality in the screened population in countries where large screening programs were established in the 1990s. In screening mammograms, clustered microcalcifications and breast masses are the most important signs of cancer in mammograms. While microcalcifications are most often associated with noninvasive in situ cancers, masses reflect the presence of invasive malignant processes. The majority of cancers in screening are detected by masses, and most palpable lesions in symptomatic women appear as masses.

In the widely adopted terminology of the American College of Radiology Breast Imaging Reporting and Data System (BI-RADS), a mass is a structure with convex outward borders visible in two different projections. A nonspecific dense region or potential mass seen in only one view is called an asymmetry. BI-RADS descriptors of masses are grouped into three categories: shape, margin, and density. If masses are circumscribed and have well-defined margins, they are more likely to be benign, while masses with ill-defined or spiculated margins are more likely to be malignant. Sometimes no

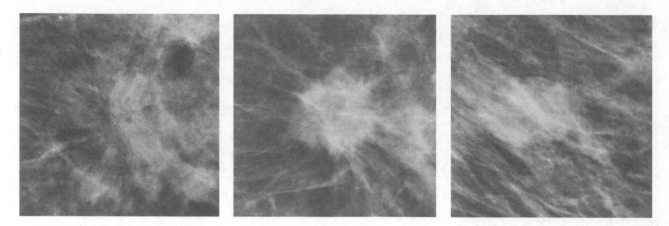

Figure 2.1   Examples of mammographic abnormalities. From left to right, an architectural distortion, a spiculated mass, and a partly obscured circumscribed mass are shown. While the mass on the right is benign, the other abnormalities are invasive ductal cancers.

definite mass is visible, but typical malignant mass margin features are present. In those cases, most often, the normal architecture of the breast is distorted by the presence of thin lines radiating from a point. These abnormalities are called architectural distortions (ADs). Some examples of masses and ADs are shown in Figure 2.1.

In practice, radiologists vary considerably in their classification of breast lesion features, because it is not always possible to clearly distinguish masses, AD, and asymmetry. In CAD research, it is common to develop algorithms that are aimed at the detection or classification of all mass-like abnormalities as a group. In short, these abnormalities are called *masses*, referring to all potentially malignant abnormalities other than microcalcification clusters. Also commercially available CAD systems present detection results in these two categories and include AD and asymmetries in the mass category.

Nearly all breast cancers originate in the ductal system, and as long as cancers remain inside the ducti or lobuli, mammography may reveal them only by the appearance of microcalcifications. As a general rule, only after cancers become invasive they may appear as masses. Obviously, in this phase, they should be detected as small as possible. Screening can be effective only when breast cancers are detected before they become palpable. Most masses detected in screening are within a range of 0.5–2 cm in diameter. In mammograms, masses smaller than 5 mm are rarely visible, while most masses larger than 2 cm are palpable. Invasive lobular cancers, accounting for about 10%–15% of invasive breast cancers, form an exception. Because they do not typically form a palpable lump and have more subtle characteristics in mammograms, they are often detected when they are larger.

Masses in mammograms can also be benign, and in mammograms, benign masses may be hard to distinguish from cancers. Benign masses usually appear more round or oval in shape and tend to have sharper boundaries, while malignant masses are more irregular in shape and

have more fuzzy or spiculated margins. Fibroadenomas and cysts are the most common types of benign masses. To determine if a mass is a cyst, additional ultrasound imaging is often used. Automated classification of breast masses is an active field of research. Extensive reviews of computerized analysis of masses in mammograms can be found in Oliver et al. (2010a, Tang et al., 2009).

2.2   MAMMOGRAPHIC IMAGING

In mammography, low-energy x-ray imaging is used to obtain images of the breast. To reduce thickness during the imaging procedure, the breast is compressed. This ensures better penetration, reduction of scatter, and reduction of motion artifacts. In most countries, it is standard practice to include two projections (views) of each breast in a mammogram, one in craniocaudal (CC) direction and one in a mediolateral oblique (MLO) projection, an angled side view in which the breast is compressed diagonally, and x-rays run from upper medial to lower lateral. The average angle between these two views is about 45°. Alternative views such as lateral projections are sometimes used. MLO views are preferred over lateral because of better coverage of the upper outer quadrant and the axilla (armpit). They can easily be recognized by the prominent presence of the pectoral muscle. In CC views, the glandular disk is generally projected better.

Masses in mammograms are compact structures appearing brighter than the tissue in which they are embedded. When the tissue surrounding a mass is fatty, detection is easy due to the much higher attenuation for x-rays of masses. Unfortunately, the attenuation of normal fibroglandular tissue, often referred to as dense tissue, and cancerous tissue is very similar. Because of this, masses may be hard to see or not detectable at all when they are projected in dense tissue.

Reducing the risk of missing breast cancer due to overlapping dense tissue is the most important reason for imaging the breast from two different angles in a mammogram.

Nowadays, in most screening facilities, digital mammography has replaced film-based mammography. Full-field digital mammography (FFDM), and to a lesser extent computed radiology, is widely used for capturing digital images. Most of the literature on computer-aided detection of breast cancer, however, is based on work with digitized film mammograms. There are some important differences. The most important is that, in digital imaging, manufacturers allow archival of raw images, in which the relation between pixel values and detector exposure is linear. Combined with information provided in the image headers, this allows a more quantitative approach to digital processing in CAD algorithms. Most digital CAD algorithms are designed to work on the raw data. Unfortunately, most clinics archive only processed mammograms, making it harder to acquire databases with raw data for CAD research. Large differences in image-processing techniques employed by manufacturers have resulted in a large variation of mammogram presentation styles. As processed images cannot be transformed back to the raw data format, development of CAD technology is hampered by this practice.

Although mammography is by far the most widely used breast imaging modality today, in particular, in screening, the sensitivity of mammography in dense breasts remains limited, despite advances of digital mammography and, more recently, the introduction of tomosynthesis. Additional imaging with ultrasound or MRI is recommended for screening in selected groups of women, for example, younger women in high-risk category.

2.3 SEGMENTATION AND IMAGE PROCESSING

2.3.1 Segmentation

Many CAD algorithms for the detection of masses require anatomical features in mammograms to be segmented and labeled. The location of normal structures appearing in mammograms can be used to restrict processing to relevant areas, to perform location-dependent processing, or to correlate findings in different views. Typical normal regions to be identified are background, breast tissue, pectoral muscle, skin-line projection, chest wall, and the nipple. Also a dense tissue region representing the projection of fibroglandular tissue may be segmented. In dense mammograms, this region may overlap with the pectoral muscle.

Segmentation of the background in a mammogram is relatively easy in digitally recorded mammograms. In the background, exposure to the detector is much higher than in the exposed tissue area. Therefore, by determining a suitable threshold, the background can be accurately segmented. In digitized film mammograms, segmentation is more difficult. The optical density of the background is high, and due to the poor response of the film at high optical densities, the contrast at the skin–air interface may be very low. On top of that, the response of film digitizers in dark areas of film can be very noisy. Because of this, accurate and robust segmentation of the background in digitized film mammograms requires application of more advanced techniques, such as dynamic multiple thresholding or atlas-based methods (Iglesias and Karssemeijer, 2009, Wu et al., 2010). Another problem is the presence of view identification markers in the background, which may overlap breast tissue in large breasts. When these are included in the breast tissue mask, subsequent processing may fail, and false-positive (FP) detections may result.

Several methods have been proposed for the segmentation of the pectoral muscle in MLO views. The pectoral muscle is commonly visible as a bright triangular area in the upper left or right quadrant of the image, depending on laterality, with a straight or gently curved boundary. In most cases, the pectoral muscle can be segmented easily using region growing or a combination of thresholding and connected component labeling, but in dense breasts, such methods tend to fail due to overlap of dense tissue with the pectoral. Making use of the fact that the pectoral line should be almost straight if the breast is positioned correctly, methods based on modifications of the Hough transform have been successfully applied (Karssemeijer, 1998, Ferrari et al., 2004b). A straight-line estimate can also be obtained by iterative thresholding and line fitting (Kwok et al., 2004) and can be used as an initial estimate for a more refined search, for instance, using dynamic programming (Yam et al., 2001). Methods that do not initialize segmentation by a straight line have also been proposed, using Gabor filtering or texture orientation (Ferrari et al., 2004b, Zhou et al., 2010).

Some mammogram analysis techniques require the location of the nipple to be known. To determine this location by approximation, one can choose the point on the skin–air interface that is furthest away from the pectoral boundary in MLO views or from the chest wall in CC views. In Chandrasekhar and Attikiouzel (1997), a method is described that uses analysis of average gradient strength perpendicular to the skin–air interface. Restricting the nipple location to the skin–air interface, classification methods have been used to accurately determine the nipple location using features representing intensity patterns near the nipple (van Engeland et al., 2003) and (Zhou et al., 2004).

For some mass detection methods, it is important to have a representation of dense tissue available. As dense tissue and masses have similar intensities, projections of dense tissue may mimic masses and as such are the major source of FPs in screening. Dense tissue may also partially obscure masses, making them hard to detect for both humans and computers. Knowing where the breast is projected, after background and pectoral muscle have been segmented, dense tissue segmentation can be restricted to the projected breast area. Currently, the most widely used method for the segmentation of dense tissue in mammograms is interactive thresholding. This method, which is implemented in the Cumulus software, has been used in major studies in which evidence for a strong association between the presence of dense tissue and breast cancer risk was obtained (Byng et al., 1994, Boyd et al., 2010). The method works well as long as the breast thickness is uniform in the compressed tissue area, as this results in a more or less uniform fatty tissue background against which densities that attenuate X-rays stronger clearly stand out. However, due to various sources of inhomogeneity, such as decreased thickness in the periphery of the breast, compression paddle tilt, and the anode heel effect, breast density measured by thresholding is often not accurate. Automated methods to segment breast density range from methods that automate threshold selection (Karssemeijer, 1998, Ferrari et al., 2004a) to methods acting more region based by incorporating texture measurements (Hein et al., 2008, Oliver et al., 2008, Lladó et al., 2009, Oliver et al., 2010c, Kallenberg et al., 2011). Efforts have also been made to estimate the volume fraction of dense tissue projected in each pixel, instead of making a binary classification by thresholding (Highnam and Brady, 1999, Pawluczyk et al., 2003, van Engeland et al., 2006a).

2.3.2 Image Enhancement and Normalization

Mammograms from various sources may differ strongly in appearance. This has to be taken into account when developing CAD algorithms, as ideally one wants to develop methods that work on any mammogram. Thus far, most algorithms for mammographic mass detection and characterization have been developed for digitized films. In these images, the exact relation between pixel values and the x-ray image formed by the attenuation pattern in the breast is nonlinear. While the imaging physics in mammography is well understood, quantitative analysis of digitized mammograms is hampered by the lack of calibration data, which makes it hard in practice to relate measurements to attenuation properties of the tissues. This has changed with the introduction of digital mammography. In the raw data produced by these systems, pixel values have a linear relation to x-ray exposure, which in principle allows a more quantitative approach. To this end, a model of the acquisition process has to be used, including effects of the energy spectrum and scatter (Highnam and Brady, 1999). Obviously, raw data have to be available to be able to use this approach.

The majority of CAD programs reported in the literature have been developed to work on digitized film. To deal with acquisition differences, images are often normalized before processing, interpolating them to a fixed resolution and intensity range. Computerized detection and characterization of masses are generally not performed at the highest resolution available in the source data. In most studies in the literature, processing is performed using 0.2 mm pixels or even larger. An intensity range less of 12 bit/pixel or higher is generally considered sufficient. In the development of CAD systems, raw data of digital systems should not be mixed directly with digitized film mammograms. However, raw images can be transformed to look similar to a conventional digitized mammogram, using a method mimicking the screen-film detector system and film digitizer (Kallenberg and Karssemeijer, 2008). This allows combining FFDM databases and digitized film databases in CAD development and evaluation. Unfortunately, such a transformation cannot be applied to mammograms processed by manufacturers, as processing algorithms of manufacturers are usually unknown and include nonlinear local contrast enhancement that cannot be reversed.

When acquiring a mammogram, the breast is compressed to approximately uniform thickness at locations where the compression paddle is in contact with the breast. In the periphery, however, breast thickness rapidly decreases, causing a strong gradient in image intensity perpendicular to the breast edge. This gradient may easily lead to inaccurate results of CAD algorithms. Therefore, correcting for breast thickness decrease in the peripheral zone of a mammogram is an important preprocessing step in CAD systems. Peripheral enhancement is also a common procedure when raw mammograms are processed for presentation to radiologists. An example is shown in Figure 2.2. In this case, the mammogram has been smoothed with a large Gaussian kernel, and at all sites i where the smoothed image had pixel values g_i lower that a threshold T, the original pixel values y_i were replaced by $y'_i = y_i - g_i + T$. The two parameters in this algorithm are the size of the Gaussian smoothing kernel and the value of the threshold T. The latter was chosen here as the mean pixel value in the mammogram. This procedure was first applied in Karssemeijer and te Brake (1996). A disadvantage of this rather simple approach is that ringing artifacts are introduced near the boundary of bright areas in the image. These can be reduced by using nonlinear smoothing methods. Another approach for thickness equalizing in the periphery of the breast is described by Byng et al. (1997), where the aim is the reduction of the dynamic range to improve image display. Model-based approaches for peripheral enhancement were also proposed (Snoeren and Karssemeijer, 2004, 2005). Contrast equalization can also be applied to the pectoral muscle, as shown in Figure 2.2.

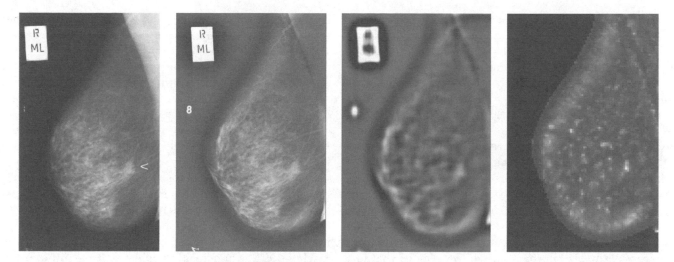

Figure 2.2   A digitized MLO view of the right breast shows an invasive cancer indicated by an arrow. Images from left to right show the result of a preprocessing step including peripheral and pectoral equalization, the output of a Laplacian filter matched to the size of the mass, and the result of a gradient field concentration filter.

Detection of masses is complicated by the rich structure of normal mammographic regions. A major component of this structure is comprised by linear structures representing fibroglandular tissue, ducts, and blood vessels. Although these structures are very different in appearance from mammographic masses, they may easily reduce the performance of mass detection methods. A simple way to remove linear structures is smoothing. However, smoothing also affects the edges of masses and may remove spiculation, which is an important feature of malignant masses. To preserve features related to a mass, it has been suggested to remove curvilinear structure in a preprocessing step (Cerneaz and Brady, 1994, Zwiggelaar et al., 1999). A map of pixels that are part of linear structures is formed first, and by subtraction or interpolation, the pixel values in this map are replaced by a local background estimates. To avoid that spiculation patterns are affected, classification of linear structures may be necessary (Zwiggelaar et al., 2004, Muralidhar et al., 2010).

2.4   DETECTING MASS CANDIDATES

Most mass detection methods consist of multiple stages, where in the initial stage, a set of candidate regions is selected for further analysis. In this initial stage, filters and segmentation methods are used that are sensitive for all types of mass-like abnormalities. Ideally, all potential masses are included in the result, as subsequent stages of the detection process are generally designed to reduce FPs and do not allow for new regions to be included.

Mass detection methods differ strongly in the approach they take in the initial stage. Some researchers approach initial detection as a segmentation problem, where the task is to distinguish pixels in masses from background pixels. In this way, detection of the location of a potential mass and segmentation of the mass are combined in one step. Using unsupervised region-based methods, contour-based techniques, or a combination of both, mammograms are partitioned in nonoverlapping mass candidate regions and background. The assumption is made that a mass is homogeneous with respect to some property, usually the pixel value or brightness itself. Brzakovic used a multiresolution segmentation scheme to identify regions (Brzakovic et al., 1990). A method based on adaptive thresholding, followed by a refinement stage using a Markov random field model, is described by Li et al. (1995). Using spatial interactions defined by the Markov model, this segmentation method can iteratively guide the segmentation process toward a solution that is composed of larger connected structures only. Constraints on the shape of these regions, however, cannot be imposed. The region growing was used by Chang et al. (1996), in a method where results of a number of different segmentation processes are combined by using the overlap of detected regions. Yin and Giger use local gray-level thresholding based on histograms in subimages (Yin et al., 1993). A segmentation method based on edge detection, after a contrast enhancement step, is used by Petrick et al. (1996). Hong and Sohn proposed to use a topographic representation, in which saliency of regions is measured topologically using hierarchical relations between contours and nesting depth (Hong and Sohn, 2010).

A disadvantage of methods using intensity-based segmentation techniques is that they are not very specific. Most mammograms contain many normal dense tissue regions, and if these are all included as candidate regions, this complicates subsequent stages of the detection process. Moreover, the segmentation methods mentioned earlier are not sensitive to characteristic abnormal patterns, such as spiculation, and cannot deal well with mass regions that are partially projected in dense tissue. Therefore, model-based supervised methods have been investigated as an alternative for candidate detection. Moving away from segmentation, the task is no longer to identify *mass* pixels correctly, but to generate a signal at the location of a mass. Accurate segmentation can be left to a subsequent stage when seed locations for potential abnormalities are selected. Supervised methods are well suited for this purpose. Using a set of training cases, machine learning can be used to develop detectors that are sensitive for specific features of mammographic masses. With this approach, it can be avoided that any bright area is detected regardless of its shape or that spiculated lesions are not detected well. Obviously, one has to make sure that relevant features are represented in the classification stage of the detector. One of the consequences of using more complex features in the initial pixel-level stage is that the computational load increases. To increase speed, images can be best processed in a sampling mode, where features are computed at a sequence of regularly spaced test sites. These should be distributed densely enough to avoid missing small masses.

Detection procedure is sufficient to generate potentially suspicious sites. Starting from these sites, regions can be segmented in the original image or in feature space, using techniques as region growing, active contours, or random field models.

Features that signal the presence of masses in mammograms can be computed by bandpass filters that selectively enhance areas that are brighter than their surroundings. One way to do this is by convolution of the image with filter functions that have a positive center and a negative surround, using either a single or multiresolution mode (Zheng et al., 1995, Karssemeijer and te Brake, 1996, Sahiner et al., 1996a). Examples of such a filter function are the Laplacian of the Gaussian (LoG) or a difference of two Gaussian (DoG) filters with a different scale. The latter approach of subtracting two images smoothed at a different spatial scale is often referred to as a difference image technique. In Figure 2.2, it is shown how a Laplacian filter responds well to a mass when the size of the mass fits the dimension of the central part of the kernel and when the contrast of the mass is high enough. However, application of this filter alone is not sufficient. The response to masses with low contrast of this type of detectors is poor, while the shape of the convolution filter function influences the detection of lesions. To tune the shape of filters to mammographic masses, it has been proposed to use a convolution neural network (Sahiner et al., 1996a) in which a set of filter kernels is learned from example

patterns during a training phase. Multiscale approaches using wavelets have also been investigated (Laine et al., 1994, Wei et al., 1995).

Methods based on convolution generally lead to detectors with an output proportional to the contrast of regions. This may not be desirable, as the contrast of mass lesions varies due to differences in lesion size, tissue properties, exposure conditions, and, in case of digitized film, the nonlinearity of the contrast transfer of a film/screen imaging system. Obviously, one wants to detect malignant lesions regardless of their size, while detection methods should be sensitive for both high- and low-contrast lesions. To avoid dependence on contrast, template matching can be used. This method was already applied in early papers on mass detection (Lai et al., 1989, Ng and Bischof, 1992), where mass templates with a uniform central region and a uniform surround were used at multiple scales. Potential locations of masses were determined by maxima of the normalized cross-correlation of the templates with the image. Detectors that are insensitive for contrast variation can also be constructed by using gradient orientation fields. In te Brake and Karssemeijer (1999), a statistical method is proposed in which a statistical measure of gradient convergence is used to detect masses. This approach appeared to be superior to multiscale Laplacian filtering and has advantages over methods based on template matching. An example is shown in Figure 2.2. Use of gradient orientation fields was also investigated by Kobatake, who proposed the adaptive iris filter (Kobatake et al., 1999).

Malignant masses are often spiculated. Sometimes, a radiating pattern of lines even is the most prominent sign of cancer. For instance, this may occur in dense breasts when the central invasive process of a cancer is obscured by fibroglandular tissue. Therefore, detection of spiculation should be part of the candidate detection process. In early papers on breast mass detection, it was already recognized that both aspects, detection of masses and spiculation, should be combined. Ng and Bischof (1992) describe three approaches for the detection of spiculation and combine these with a mass detection method using multiscale template matching. All three methods are based on use of the Hough transform. The idea is that by shooting straight lines through edge points in the direction normal to the local gradient, a peak of line density at centers of radiating structures can be obtained. Due to edges at the mass boundary, however, the response of this method appeared rather poor. To improve performance, the authors attempt to detect spicules first, based on their characteristic microstructure, though the low-resolution images used in their work hardly justified such an approach. Detection of spicules and subsequent accumulation of evidence for the presence of spiculated masses have been suggested by many authors since then (Zwiggelaar et al., 1999, Sampat et al., 2008). Because linear structures are found in normal mammographic patterns as well, explicit detection of spicules requires classification. In Zwiggelaar et al. (2004) and Muralidhar et al. (2010), methods for detecting linear structures in mammograms, and for classifying them into anatomical types (vessels, spicules, ducts, etc.), are described.

A statistical approach to detect stellate patterns was proposed in Karssemeijer and te Brake (1996). A feature representing the degree of convergence of an orientation field is defined, with local orientations derived from second-order Gaussian derivatives. The feature value is computed as the normalized number of pixels with directions pointing to a central location. A second feature measures uniformity of the orientation pattern surrounding the central location. Using both features, a classifier can be trained to detect radiating line patterns and to distinguish these from crossing line or vessel structures. Both features are statistically normalized using the variance and the expected value of the feature values in random noise patterns. These features can also be computed in a multiresolution mode, where window size changes adaptively, thus optimizing detection performance for lesions of varying diameters. Figure 2.3 gives an example of the response of the orientation convergence filter to a spiculated lesion. A method for the detection of spiculated masses without localization of individual spicules is also presented by Liu et al. (2001). In this method, converging line patterns are detected using wavelet-based texture filters in a multiresolution scheme.

Sometimes masses are located very close to the chest wall boundary of the image, and then it is not uncommon that they are partly outside the field of view of the image. This makes them hard to deal with in most algorithms. Therefore, it has been suggested to apply a separate method for such masses with partial loss of region (Hatanaka et al., 2001).

2.5 ARCHITECTURAL DISTORTIONS

AD is the third most common sign of breast cancer in screening mammograms. However, as no clear distinction can be made between masses and AD, the two groups are usually merged in the development of CAD algorithms. Most cases of AD can be described as radiating patterns of lines without central densities. Such patterns are also referred to as stellate lesions. Mass detection algorithms that are sensitive for spiculation generally do detect AD as well, even though they are not specifically designed for it. Baker performed a study in which the sensitivity of commercially available CAD systems for AD was determined (Bake et al., 2003). It was found that fewer than half of the cases of AD were detected by the two most widely available CAD systems at the time. Based on these results, it seems worthwhile to put more focus on the development of AD and to treat these abnormalities as a separate group. Relatively few papers in the literature are dedicated to this topic. In Karssemeijer and te Brake (1996), a detector for stellate mammographic distortions was developed based on the statistical analysis of line orientation fields computed using second-order Gaussian derivatives. Rangayyan and Ayres (2006) used Gabor filters and phase portraits for the detection of AD in mammograms, while in Tourassi et al. (2006), fractal analysis is used. More recently, various methods were combined using a Bayesian classifier, but high sensitivity could be obtained only at the cost of many FPs, indicating that further research is needed (Banik et al., 2011).

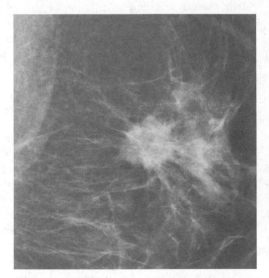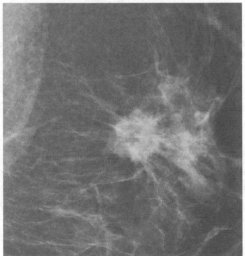

Figure 2.3 A spiculated mass is detected by the application of a filter designed to signal converging line patterns.

2.6 REGION CLASSIFICATION

Classification of mammographic regions based on local features has two important applications. The first is in systems intended to help radiologists with diagnosing lesions that have been detected, either with or without the aid of a computer. The input of these systems can take various forms, ranging from a single location to a manually drawn contour of the lesion. The classification stage can involve multiple classes, or it can be designed as a two-class benign versus malignant task. The second application of region classification is found in detection systems, where the task is to determine whether candidate lesions are real lesions or FPs. The true-positive (TP) class can include benign and malignant lesions, or it may be restricted to cancers only. Most region classification schemes require that a lesion is segmented, thus enabling feature computation methods to make use of a lesion boundary. In this section, mass lesion segmentation methods are described, followed by a description of feature extraction approaches. Next, region classification will be discussed.

2.6.1 Lesion Segmentation

When masses are circumscribed and projected in a homogeneous background of fatty tissue, their contours can be easily extracted, and most segmentation methods will work well. However, most mammograms contain patches of normal glandular tissue, and when these are overlapping or connected to the region to be segmented, the problem gets more difficult. Even for expert radiologists, it is often not possible to define an accurate boundary along the complete contour of a mass. Uncertainty in the true lesion extent may be not only due to obscuring dense tissue but also due to spiculation or an unsharp mass margin. Therefore, though sometimes researchers are taking manual delineations of masses as ground truth in studies evaluating mass segmentation methods, results of such comparisons should be interpreted with care. Task-based evaluations, in which the effect of various segmentation methods on the final result of a classification or detection task is determined, may be more appropriate. For example, the effect of the segmentation stage on the overall accuracy of a CAD system for the classification of benign and malignant masses was investigated in Sahiner et al. (2001b). It was found that though there was some difference between automated segmentation and the segmentations of two radiologists, there was no significant difference between the final ROC results of a classification experiment when human or automated segmentation was used.

Several variations of region-growing method have been proposed for the segmentation of masses in mammograms. Kupinski developed two techniques, respectively, based on a radial gradient index (RGI) feature and on a simple probabilistic model (Kupinski and Giger, 1998). In both methods, a series of image partitions is created using gray-level information as well as prior knowledge. Subsequently, the partition that maximizes a criterion function is selected as the final segmentation. The segmentation algorithms more closely matched radiologists' outlines of a set of lesions than a conventional region-growing algorithm, with best performance for the RGI-based method. te Brake compared a number of region-growing methods to a discrete dynamic contour method for finding mass boundaries (te Brake and Karssemeijer, 2001). In an evaluation in which both masses and ADs were included, the performance of the methods was compared using annotations made by a radiologist and using the segmentations in a CAD system. While comparable performance was obtained in the comparison to radiologists' annotations, the dynamic contour approach led to better performance in the discrimination task.

Mass segmentation methods differ in the way they deal with the problem of partly obscured lesions. In obscured sections of a mass, image information is insufficient to determine the exact location of a contour locally. To obtain a best-fitting solution, interpolation is required. For this purpose, Timp proposed to use a cost-optimization method using dynamic programming, where the cost function is defined after resampling the image in a polar coordinate system (Timp and Karssemeijer, 2004). The method performed better than two other automated segmentation methods, region-growing and a discrete contour model, on a dataset of 1210 masses using comparison with manual segmentations for evaluation. In addition, in a CAD system for classifying benign and malignant masses, the use of the dynamic programming method led to significantly better results than the other two methods. Dynamic programming was also used by Elter et al. (2010). In this work, segmentation is performed by automatically tracing the mass contour in between two manually provided landmark points on the contour, leading to better results than previous methods using a lesion center location as the starting point.

2.6.2 Feature Extraction

Once the boundaries of potential mass areas have been obtained, region-based features can be computed. By creating rich representations capturing the most relevant aspects of masses and normal tissue, classification schemes can be developed to discriminate regions. Features used in the literature can be grouped into different categories. Morphological features are used to represent the size and shape of regions; texture features represent gray-level statistics inside a mass, in absolute terms or in contrast with tissue surrounding the mass; and border features represent properties of the mass boundary, such as sharpness, smoothness, spiculatedness, or fuzziness. In general, one could say that two approaches are used. The first is to use general-purpose methods not specific to mammography. Usually, this leads to very large feature spaces, which can subsequently be reduced by feature selection or other dimensionality reduction techniques, such as principal component analysis. The second approach is to design features specifically for mammographic masses, guided by radiologists' descriptions such as provided by BI-RADS. This has the advantage that feature spaces remain smaller and that classification results obtained leave some room for interpretation in radiological terms.

The design of features can be guided by some general principles. Firstly, rotation invariance of features is usually desired, as masses in the breast have no preferred orientation. An exception to this rule may be formed by features making use of normal linear structures in the breast, which may better be analyzed with respect to the location of the nipple. Secondly, invariance of features to monotonic intensity transformations is a good property, in particular in systems designed to operate on digitized films, in which intensity and contrast of masses strongly depend on the nonlinear characteristics of the acquisition. In digital mammography, when raw data are available, features may be computed in the (log) exposure domain, and invariance to intensity transforms becomes less of an issue. Obviously, to obtain a robust system that may be applied to mammograms from a range of sources, the spatial resolution of mammograms has to be taken into account. In most published studies, images are down-sampled to a uniform resolution before processing.

Features developed specifically for detection and discrimination of mammographic masses include quantitative indicators of spiculation, which is a primary sign for malignancy. In Huo et al. (1995), Huo and colleagues presented a technique that quantifies the degree of spiculation using radial edge-gradient analysis. In a classification task, two measures computed from the surrounding periphery of a segmented mass led to similar results to that achieved when a radiologist's ratings of spiculation were used. Dedicated features for representing spiculation and morphology were also proposed by other authors (Rangayyan et al., 1997, Mudigonda et al., 2000, te Brake et al., 2000, Sahiner et al., 2001a). Border features representing the degree of sharpness, spiculation, and microlobulation of mass margins were investigated by Varela et al. (2006). The use of texture features has been explored by many authors. Multiresolution texture analysis was first investigated by Wei et al. (1995), who computed co-occurrence matrix features using the original image or wavelet coefficients as input. Sahiner et al. investigated texture feature computation after applying a rubber band straightening transform to the segmented mass region (Sahiner et al., 1998a), using spatial gray-level

dependence matrices and run-length statistics matrices. Evaluation was done for the entire region, a band of pixels surrounding the segmented mass, and the transformed image. Features extracted from the transformed band were found to be the most effective in a classification task. The use of local binary patterns for representing textural properties of masses was investigated in Lladó et al. (2009).

2.6.3 False-Positive Reduction

Region classification is applied to reduce FPs after candidate mass regions have been detected in an initial detection stage. The initial detection stage is usually designed in such a way that the risk of false negatives is minimized. Obviously, this goes at the cost of FPs, and a choice has to be made regarding the number of candidate regions one is willing to accept. In methods described in the literature, the number of candidate regions per image typically ranges from 5 to 25. To some extent, this number is arbitrary, and its choice may not have a strong impact on final detection results reported at low FP rates. Obviously, the larger the number of candidate regions is, the more computational power is needed to perform region classification. However, it is important to realize that by enlarging the number of candidate regions, the classification problem changes by making it more unbalanced with regard to the number of TP and FP training patterns. Some classification methods are not suitable for dealing with unbalanced datasets, while it is often needed to take the distribution of training samples over the classes into account when optimizing parameters in classification procedures.

To optimize mass detection and FP reduction methods, a relevant performance criterion has to be defined. If the goal is to apply a mass detection algorithm in a CAD system presenting prompts to the readers, performance can be related to the operating points at which these systems are used in clinical practice. As most radiologists do not tolerate a high FP rate, current systems operate in the range of 0.1–0.5 FP/image. Therefore, the sensitivity of a mass detection system in this range of operating points is a suitable measure. The task of FP reduction can then be defined, for example, as optimizing the sensitivity of CAD at a fixed operating point in the clinically relevant range, starting from an arbitrary number of candidate regions. The number of candidate regions one starts with, which can be adjusted in the initial stage, can be treated as a parameter in the optimization process.

Optimization of classifiers used in FP reduction may involve dimensionality reduction. Sahiner et al. (1996b) investigated feature selection using genetic algorithms in the problem of classification of mass and normal breast tissue, using a linear discriminant classifier (LDA) and a backpropagation neural network (BPN). The effect of feature selection methods on computer-aided detection of masses in mammograms using LDA or BPN classifiers was also studied by Hupse and Karssemeijer (2010). By optimizing the mean sensitivity of the system in a predefined range of the free-response receiver operating characteristics, it was found that feature selection leads to better performance when compared to a system in which all features were used. However, in a more recent study, it was found that by using support vector machines for classification, better results can be obtained without feature selection step (Lesniak et al., 2011), given that a large number of cases and features are available.

The composition of databases used to test and train computer-aided detection systems can have a profound effect on performance measures. Even when databases are very large and contain consecutive samples of mammograms from multiple sources, large differences may occur. In the first place, this is due to the fact that screening programs vary considerably. Recall rate, screening interval, type of reading (double or single), age range of the screened population, and breast density are examples of factors that influence the subtlety of screen-detected cancers. Secondly, databases may include prior screening mammograms of interval or screen-detected cancers and may be enriched with FPs of the readers. Nishikawa et al. (1994) investigated how the choice of cases used in the development of a breast mass detection system can affect the test results and concluded that because of the strong dependence of measured performance on the testing database, it is difficult to estimate the accuracy of a CAD scheme reliably and it is questionable to compare different CAD schemes when different cases are used for testing.

Apart from making it more difficult to compare CAD systems, the variation of databases also poses a challenge in the development of CAD systems, as it has to be investigated which composition of the training database is optimal for a given task. It has been attempted to address this problem by developing multiple classifiers trained with different subsets of the training data and to merge results in a final stage. Wei et al. (2006) described a dual system approach that combines a CAD system optimized with *average* masses with another CAD system optimized with *subtle* masses. A BPN classifier was trained to merge the scores from the two single CAD systems and differentiate true masses from normal tissue. With the dual system approach, better overall performance was obtained.

2.6.4 Classification and Diagnosis

Once a lesion is detected, it has to be characterized in order to make a correct decision regarding how to deal with it. These decisions take place at the screening stage, where the question is whether a woman should be recalled, and

in the diagnostic stage, where additional imaging or biopsies can be performed. In screening programs, where batch mode reading is common, the radiologists have to rely on the mammogram alone. In the diagnostic setting, the problem is quite different because assessment of lesions often includes ultrasound and/or MRI. The primary question is whether a lesion is malignant or not. In addition, both benign and malignant lesions can be categorized further. Important benign categories are cysts and fibroadenomas.

The problem of classifying benign and malignant masses has been well studied, and excellent results have been obtained. Observer studies have demonstrated that computer-aided diagnosis can potentially help radiologists improve their diagnostic accuracy in the task of differentiating between benign and malignant masses seen on mammogram (Chan et al., 1999, Huo et al., 2002). Also in a multimodal setting including mammography and ultrasound, it has been shown that the use of CAD can improve the performance of radiologists in mass classification (Horsch et al., 2006). However, despite these encouraging results, to date, these systems have not yet found an application in clinical practice.

Technically, the development of a CAD system for the characterization of mass lesions is quite similar to the development of a FP reduction stage as described earlier. Lesions indicated by the reader are segmented and using on a feature-based representation a supervised classifier can be trained to perform the task (Chan et al., 1998, Sahiner et al., 1998b, Hadjiiski et al., 1999, Mudigonda et al., 2000, Lim and Er, 2004, Varela et al., 2006). Feature selection was investigated in Sahiner et al. (1998c), where it was found that by using a genetic algorithm tailored to obtain good performance at a high sensitivity, a significantly better system could be obtained than by using a stepwise feature selection method. Optimization of classification performance at a predefined decision criterion is clinically relevant, as use of CAD to reduce biopsies could become an important application if the number of missed malignancies can be kept to an acceptable minimum. However, given current clinical practice, this should be done in a multimodal setting with ultrasound. Development of such a system was investigated by Drukker et al. (2005).

Using a computer-aided classification system, the probability of malignancy of a new lesion can be determined. However, this can be done accurately only if the dataset used for training the CAD system is representative for the environment in which CAD is used and if the prevalence of benign and malignant cases in this environment is the same as in the training data. Although prevalence differences can be taken into account when computing probabilities (Horsch et al., 2008), a problem is that clinical environments and potential applications of CAD in a clinical setting differ. Therefore, both the prevalence and subtlety of various categories of benign and malignant lesions are hard to determine beforehand. Due to these problems, presenting a probability of malignancy computed by CAD to the readers may be misleading and confusing. Alternatives are described in Horsch et al. (2006). For a given image of a lesion, CAD results can be presented by displaying similar images of known lesions automatically selected from reference libraries, based on a similarity index. Further exploration of this idea leads to content-based image retrieval (CBIR) systems, for which dedicated detection systems can be developed (El-Naqa et al., 2004, Tourassi et al., 2007). To present CAD results without the use of probabilities, one can also provide a numerical rating of the likelihood of malignancy on an arbitrary scale, where the reader has to learn to interpret the scale during a training phase. To facilitate interpretation, in Horsch et al. (2006), the rating for a given lesion is shown relative to the distributions of ratings of benign and malignant lesions in a training database.

In a recent study, seven similarity measures are considered for a CBIR system for the classification of breast masses (Cho et al., 2011). The similarity between query and retrieved masses was evaluated based on radiologists' visual similarity assessments. Classification performance of the similarity measures was also determined using ROC analysis. It was found that the CBIR system that was most effective in retrieving similar masses did not have the best classification performance, illustrating that these tasks are distinctly different. Methods to determine visual similarity of masses were also studied in Zheng et al. (2007), where the aim was to aid radiologists with a reference library in distinguishing TP from FP CAD marks in a detection system.

2.7 CONTEXT AND MULTIPLE VIEWS

2.7.1 Location and Context

The relative location of a mass and the mammographic context in which a suspect abnormality is embedded should be taken into account for its interpretation. Therefore, radiologists read mammographic views in combination, making correspondences between regions and judging to what extent a mass or AD can be explained by normal anatomy. Because of breast compression and deformation, this is a complex process. The importance of location follows from the existence of forbidden zones, a 3–4 cm wide strip running parallel to edge of pectoral muscle and the retro-glandular space. As these should normally not display dense tissue, unless breasts are very dense, small densities in these zones are highly suspect, in particular when they are asymmetric. To include such considerations in CAD systems, an internal frame of reference is needed in which locations of lesions can be represented. A common way is

to set up a Cartesian frame of reference, taking one axis as the line running along the chest wall (CC) or pectoral (MLO) boundary, and the other perpendicular to it toward the nipple (Paquerault et al., 2002, van Engeland et al., 2003, Zheng et al., 2006). However, these methods may become unreliable if the breast positioning is not adequate. In Pu et al. (2008), a method is presented in which the frame of reference is based on fitting an ellipse to the breast boundary. A non-Cartesian coordinate frame in which orientations of breast patterns may be represented in a more meaningful way is proposed in Brandt et al. (2011).

The mammographic image background, in particular the type of density pattern, has a large effect on the performance of both human readers and CAD algorithms for the detection of masses. When masses are partly obscured, segmentation becomes more difficult, leading to less reliable feature representations. In addition, dense breast patterns give rise to more candidate regions and thus increase the risk of FPs. This also holds for radiologists, as in screening programs, the FP rate increases in dense breasts. To optimize screening performance, the type of background has to be taken into account. This is done in Oliver et al. (2010b), where a method is proposed to use breast density in the training step of a CAD system for the detection of masses, using manual and automatic annotations. Experiments showed improved results when breast density information was used, while results obtained using automatic breast density estimation outperformed those based on the manual annotations provided by expert radiologists. Another approach to include density context was explored in Hupse and Karssemeijer (2009), where a set of context features was developed that represent suspiciousness of normal tissue in the same case. To this end, reference areas are defined in corresponding regions as the mass candidate in contra- and ipsilateral views. A significant improvement of detection performance was obtained, and context computed using multiple views yielded a better performance than context derived from only a single view.

2.7.2 Mammogram Registration

When reading mammograms, radiologists make multiple comparisons between mammographic views, in an exam and between exams. To learn a computer to perform such comparisons, mammograms have to be aligned or registered, such that regional correspondences can be defined. However, corresponding mammograms often differ considerably in appearance, due to variation in positioning, compression, and X-ray exposure, while natural changes in the breast over time and anatomic differences between the right and left breasts add to that. Therefore, correspondence between positions in two views can be determined only by approximation.

Various approaches to establish correspondence between mammographic views have been proposed. These are applicable when view types are corresponding, for example, both are MLO or CC. When views are different, no unique point-to-point correspondence can be established, except for locations where a lesion or another specific feature is present. Yin et al. (1991, 1993) applied a relatively simple rigid body transformation to align the skin line of two breast images with corresponding views. More elaborate methods generate a set of corresponding landmarks or control points in each breast, and apply some form of nonlinear interpolation. Lau and Bischof (1991) used a set of three control points defined on the skin line, including the estimated location of the nipple, while Vujovic used automatically generated control points targeted at cross sections of prominent ducts and vessels (Vujovic and Brzakovic, 1997). Warping based on corresponding features is also used in Sallam and Bowyer (1999). A registration method for aligning mammogram sequences based on landmarks and thinplate spline transformations was developed by Marias et al. (2005). The method first aligns the breast boundaries by calculating salient curvature points that conform to a breast model. Subsequently, registration is refined by adding a small number of robust internal landmarks defined using wavelet scale-space analysis. In a dataset of 36 mammogram pairs with 75 visually defined correspondences, an average registration error of 4 mm was obtained using breast boundary alignment, which was reduced to 3.5 mm using the internal landmarks. Registration can also be performed without explicit warping. In Brandt et al. (2011), a breast coordinate system is proposed to map locations in mammograms, based on the location of the pectoral muscle, the nipple, and the shape of the breast boundary.

In a study by van Engeland et al., four registration methods were compared using a dataset of 150 temporal mammograms with manually annotated correspondences, such as characteristic microcalcifications visible in both views (van Engeland et al., 2003). Best results were obtained when using a transformation involving translation, rotation, scaling, and vertical shearing, in combination with a mutual information criterion for optimization. After registration, the average distance between corresponding locations was 7.9 mm. A similar error was found by Hadjiiski et al. (2001), who reported on a two-stage temporal registration method for masses based on the breast boundary, using the nipple as a landmark. In the first global stage, the average error obtained in a series of 124 temporal mammograms was 8.4 mm, using manually identified nipple locations. In a subsequent refinement stage, the mismatch of temporal mass pairs was reduced by regional registration. This topic is discussed in the subsection on temporal analysis later. A quantitative evaluation of intensity-based image registration methods in mammography was also conducted

by Díez et al. (2011), using methods ranging from a global and rigid transformation to local deformable paradigms using various metrics and multiresolution approaches. In contrast to previous work, where local deformations often caused unrealistic distortions, the authors found that by using local multiresolution B-spline deformations, the most accurate registration results were obtained.

It should be noted that mammogram registration may be hampered by the fact that image intensity distributions can change considerably with changes of acquisition parameters, in particular kVp, while conditions get worse when temporal image pairs are obtained with equipment from different vendors. To alleviate problems, it has been proposed to combine geometric registration with an estimation of a gray-scale transform to match both mammograms, using a parametric model (Snoeren and Karssemeijer, 2007). This technique might be applied for the computation of features representing temporal change.

2.7.3 Asymmetry

Asymmetry between the left and right breasts is one of the signs used by radiologists to detect and diagnose breast cancer. The term asymmetry is generally used for nondistinct areas of density appearing in only one breast. An example is shown in Figure 2.4. Bilateral comparison was used in the earliest papers on computerized detection of abnormalities in mammograms (Lau and Bischof, 1991, Yin et al., 1991, 1993), where asymmetric regions were identified by bilateral subtraction and smoothing, after aligning the views. To make this method more effective, some form of normalization of the gray levels has to be applied, as exposure conditions may vary. For instance, mammograms can be normalized to the same levels of mean intensity and variance (Lau and Bischof, 1991), or can be calibrated by a more rigorous approach, taking all aspects of image acquisition into account (Highnam and Brady, 1999). The subtraction itself can also be performed in a nonlinear way, for instance, as described in Yin et al. (1991, 1993), where multiple thresholds were used prior to subtraction, setting pixels below the threshold to a constant value. In addition to subtraction of intensity levels, images representing texture differences in corresponding regions of an image pair can be computed as well (Lau and Bischof, 1991).

Another procedure for the analysis of left–right asymmetry in mammograms was proposed in Ferrari et al. (2001), using the detection of linear directional components in a wavelet representation. By selecting principal components of the filter responses, preserving only the most relevant directional elements appearing at all scales, a statistical analysis of bilateral differences of the oriented patterns was performed using phase images. Bilateral analysis was also used in a method to reduce FPs (Wu et al., 2007). For each

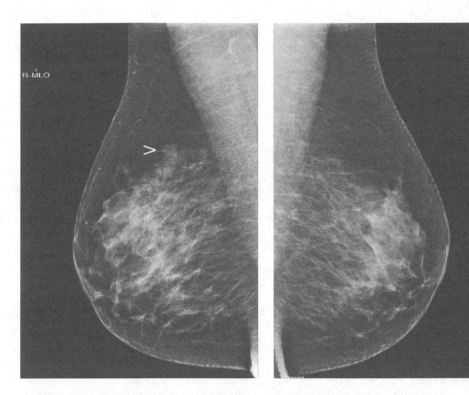

Figure 2.4   Example of an invasive ductal cancer detected in screening by the asymmetric density in the upper outer quadrant of the right breast.

detected candidate mass, a regional registration technique was used to define a region of interest that is symmetrical to the object location on the contralateral mammogram. Bilateral texture features were then derived from corresponding pairs of regions, leading to a significant improvement of detection performance.

2.7.4   Temporal Analysis

Density patterns in mammograms change over time, and monitoring these changes is an important aspect of reading screening mammograms. Small changes may reveal tumor formation or growth. Accurate serial comparison of mammograms is possible only if the positioning of the breast on the detector does not vary too much. Therefore, it is important that technicians are trained properly. While screening, radiologists compare current mammograms with one set of prior mammograms, usually those taken at the most recent prior screening. However, some readers prefer to use older priors for comparison because this makes it easier to observe gradual changes. This reading protocol was in fact dictated by the design of mammographic film alternators, which had place only for two rows of films. With digital technology, multiple priors can be accessed more easily, and serial mammogram reading may change. Strategies for using priors differ. Many radiologists use priors only when they see a potential abnormality in the current screening

mammogram, to find out if it is new or increasing in size. Some radiologists, though, are using priors also for primary detection by performing a regional comparison.

In CAD systems, temporal analysis for mass detection can be included in the initial detection stage, to improve the detection of candidate regions, or in the region analysis stage. The latter seems more appropriate as variation of positioning often makes accurate registration impossible, thus making pixel-based temporal comparison less feasible. One should realize that changes related to tumor growth are generally small compared to the volume of dense tissue in most breasts. On average, the volume of dense tissue in a breast is in the range of 50–100 cm^3, while a small mass detectable in screening mammograms may be less than 1 cm^3. Therefore, directly detecting small abnormalities by mammogram registration and subtraction is not a viable approach, as this leads to a large number of FPs, due to normal changes and misregistrations appearing in the difference image (Marias et al., 2005).

Once suspicious regions have been identified in mammograms by a CAD system, corresponding locations in prior mammograms can be examined to extract additional features for classification. Commonly, a two-stage approach is used, where a global mammogram registration method as described earlier is followed by a regional registration method focusing on the area of interest of a mass and its surroundings. In this way, the average registration error can be reduced to about 2.5 mm if the mass is visible in both views (Hadjiiski et al., 2001). To compare features of mass regions over time, it is important to establish correct correspondences. Therefore, it is relevant to evaluate registration methods by their ability to link temporal mass regions correctly. In Sanjay-Gopal et al. (1999), it was found that using a regional registration technique in 63 out of 74 temporal pairs, the region on the previous mammogram that corresponded to the mass on the current mammogram could be correctly identified, while the average distance of the target lesion to the registered mass centroid was 2.8 mm. Using a different approach, in Timp et al. (2005), it was reported that in a series of 389 temporal mass pairs, 82% of the lesions could be correctly linked. This method involved a similarity metric evaluated by moving the current mass region projected on the prior in the neighborhood of the registered location, where the similarity metric includes distance to the registered location, a template-based correlation, and the mass likelihood at the target location computed by a mass detection algorithm. Different similarity measures for matching regions in temporal mammogram pairs were compared in Filev et al. (2005).

When correspondence between regions in prior and current mammograms has been established, interval change analysis can be conducted to improve computer-aided detection or classification of masses. For instance, temporal features can be obtained by combining feature values from both regions. In Timp and Karssemeijer (2006), mass detection performance with and without the use of temporal features was studied using datasets from 938 patients. Temporal features were effective in reducing FPs, and a significant improvement in detection performance was obtained with the use of temporal features. Interestingly, detection improved both for cases in which the mass was already visible in the prior and for cases where no mass could be seen in the prior at the location of the tumor. In another study, interval change analysis was effectively used to improve characterization of mass lesions (Timp et al., 2007).

2.7.5 Matching Regions in CC and MLO Views

In mammography, it is standard practice to obtain MLO and CC projections of both breasts. As the breast is compressed from a different angle in MLO and CC views, and because each pixel represents a column of tissue, pixelwise registration of MLO and CC views is not possible. However, characteristic features visible in both views can be matched. Radiologists do this when they suspect abnormalities. They combine information from the two projections to make detection and diagnosis more reliable, and they derive the clock position from the projected locations of a lesion. This is an important aspect of reading mammograms that appears to be quite complicated to model in computer algorithms.

Most CAD systems for mass detection are currently based on independent analysis of single views.

Automated matching of corresponding regions in MLO and CC views has been studied by several researchers with the aim of improving mass detection results (Paquerault et al., 2002, van Engeland et al., 2006b, Qian et al., 2007, van Engeland and Karssemeijer, 2007, Samulski and Karssemeijer, 2011). Typically, the output of a single-view CAD system is used as a starting point, and a classifier is designed to compute a correspondence score indicating if regions in a pair correspond to the same mass. The classifier may be a two-class system, where incorrectly matched pairs are pairs containing an FP (Paquerault et al., 2002, van Engeland et al., 2006b), or a four-class system where TP, FP, TP–FP, and FP–TP pairs each form a separate class (Samulski and Karssemeijer, 2011). Region similarity features can be used to match mass regions, where the relative location of lesions provides one of the most important cues to decide if regions can be matched. To reduce computation, the number of region pairs to be evaluated can be restricted based on location alone. Distance to a projected set of plausible locations can be used together with region similarity features to determine a correspondence score.

Projective geometry may be used to predict plausible locations of a mass region in the ipsilateral view. In its simplest form, disregarding breast compression and assuming that the breast is rotated around an axis running from the nipple to the chest wall, this leads to a method where the projection of the rotation axis or centerline is determined in both views and where the distance of the nipple to the mass candidate regions projected onto this line is assumed to be the same. Thus, given a location in one view, the corresponding locations in the ipsilateral view form a straight line as depicted in Figure 2.5. An alternative method is also used, in which the distance of a mass to the nipple is assumed to be constant, leading to corresponding locations forming an arc in the ipsilateral view. Arguments for this approach are that the breast is strongly deformed and pulled away from the chest wall for optimal positioning, thus stretching the tissue between the nipple and the chest wall, and that it avoids the need to determine a centerline. The latter requires segmentation of the pectoral muscle in MLO views. Both methods and a combination of the two have been compared using large series of cases with annotated masses, and it was found that overall better results are obtained with the straight-line method (Zheng et al., 2009). It has also been attempted to take compression into account to find corresponding locations. In Kita et al. (2001, 2002), researchers used a breast deformation model in which curved epipolar lines are calculated using stereo camera geometry. Using such curved epipolar lines, the 3D location of a lesion can be estimated. Though promising, this method has not yet been evaluated thoroughly.

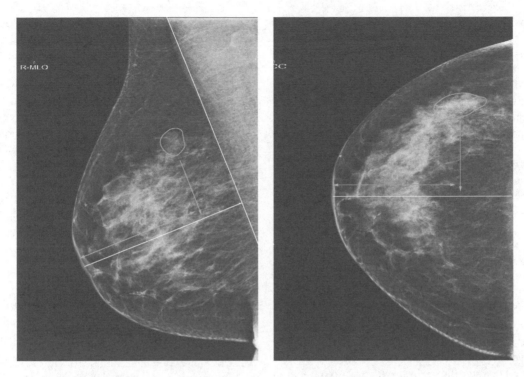

Figure 2.5 To match regions in MLO and CC views, a breast centerline is computed. When the regions are projected on this line, the distance to the nipple should be similar in both views.

2.8 CASE-BASED ANALYSIS

Case-based analysis may be the ultimate goal of CAD in screening applications. Automated interpretation of a mammogram as a whole, in combination with priors and additional information such as individual breast cancer risk, can lead to interesting applications of CAD that go well beyond current applications. In the end, the decision whether to recall a woman has to be optimized taking costs and benefits of breast screening into account. In the literature, first steps toward case-based analysis of mammograms can be found. These include temporal analysis and use of context, as described earlier, and combination of information from CC and MLO views. Most of this work is aimed at reducing FPs. A Bayesian network approach aimed at fusing information provided by a multiview CAD system at the patient level is described in Velikova et al. (2009).

To optimize mass detection results, combination of information from MLO and CC views is essential in screening. Radiologists compare the two ipsilateral mammographic views to decide whether a mass is present and actionable. If a suspicious region in one view correlates with features seen in the other view, the probability that the region is a true lesion gets higher. On the other hand, when a potential abnormality is visible in only one view, this generally reduces the chance that it is a true lesion. It should be noted,

however, that the reasoning taking place in multiview comparisons may be complex, because abnormalities can be (partly) obscured in one projection by overlapping glandular tissue. Thus, breast density and the location of lesions with respect to the main glandular components of the breast play an important role in the interpretation process. In addition, by superposition of normal breast structures, mass lesions may be simulated in one view, in which case the ipsilateral view may provide essential information to discard it, thus reducing FPs.

Methods to combine information from ipsilateral mammographic views to improve computer-aided detection of masses have been reported by several researchers. After correspondence between regions has been established, using one of the methods discussed earlier, information from the two views can be fused. Paquerault et al. (2002) proposed to rank the single view and correspondence scores within each image and to average them subsequently. A significant improvement of detection performance was obtained by using this scheme when abnormal cases with a mass visible in both views were used. Fusion schemes based on similarity features and classifiers were also proposed by other authors (van Engeland and Karssemeijer, 2007, Velikova et al., 2009, Wei et al., 2009). In these studies, a significant improvement of region-based detection performance was obtained. Unfortunately, however, case-based performance remained similar. In practice, case-based sensitivity, which considers a lesion to be detected if it is reported in at least one view, is more relevant, although there may be some benefit if CAD detects a region in both views, as studies suggest that readers are more likely to act on CAD prompts if a region is marked in both views. This motivated Zheng et al. (2006) to develop a multiview CAD system that aims to maintain the same case-based sensitivity while increasing the number of masses being detected on both ipsilateral views.

To improve case-based detection performance, Samulski investigated a new learning method for multiview CAD systems (Samulski and Karssemeijer, 2011). The method builds on a single-view lesion detection system and a correspondence classifier, which provides class probabilities for the various types of region pairs and correspondence features. In the learning scheme, the correspondence classifier output is used to bias the selection of training patterns for a multiview CAD system. This is done in such a way that learning focuses on improving classification of the most suspect candidate mass in a pair, thus avoiding that the additional information provided by similarity of the two views is predominantly used to improve the likelihood scores of the weaker regions. This approach led to a significant improvement of case-based detection performance, increasing the mean sensitivity in the range of 0.01–0.5 FPs per image by 4.7%.

By combining bilateral and ipsilateral analyses, a four-view CAD system for mass detection was developed by Wei et al. (2011). In the system, after the initial detection of breast masses on individual views, information of the ipsilateral views of the breast and information of the bilateral analysis are first fused separately. Subsequently, results are fused in the four-view stage with a decision tree, yielding a significant improvement in the initial single-view detection. The breast-based sensitivity at 0.5 FPs per image increased from 58% to 76%.

2.9   DISCUSSION

After two decades of development, CAD systems for the diagnosis of mammographic mass lesions are performing at a high level, which in some studies is shown to be comparable to that of radiologists. However, these systems have not yet been introduced in clinical practice. On the other hand, despite huge efforts to develop CAD systems for mass detection in screening mammograms, the performance of these systems is still well below that of trained human readers. But they are widely used in screening practice. Most mass detection systems have been developed to operate at a high sensitivity, which is achievable only if many FPs are accepted with current technology. Nevertheless, a gradual increase in the performance of CAD systems for mammographic mass detection can be observed in the literature, and if this trend

continues, it may be expected that CAD systems will match the performance of human readers in the future. Multiview methods and information fusion will become more important. This is a highly challenging topic for researchers. Contextual reasoning has to be modeled, which is known to be one of the most difficult aspects of image analysis, while human readers seem to do this almost effortlessly. On the other hand, with the introduction of digital mammography, computerized image analysis is gaining a new advantage: very large databases with digital screening mammograms are becoming available for the training of CAD systems, and analysis can become more quantitative by making use of the robust and stable characteristics of digital detectors.

REFERENCES

Baker, J. A., Rosen, E. L., Lo, J. Y., Gimenez, E. I., Walsh, R., and Soo, M. S. (2003). Computer-aided detection (CAD) in screening mammography: Sensitivity of commercial cad systems for detecting architectural distortion. *American Journal of Roentgenology*, 181(4):1083–1088.

Banik, S., Rangayyan, R. M., and Desautels, J. E. L. (2011). Detection of architectural distortion in prior mammograms. *IEEE Transactions on Medical Imaging*, 30(2):279–294.

Boyd, N. F., Martin, L. J., Bronskill, M., Yaffe, M. J., Duric, N., and Minkin, S. (2010). Breast tissue composition and susceptibility to breast cancer. *Journal of the National Cancer Institute*, 102(16):1224–1237.

Brandt, S., Karemore, G., Karssemeijer, N., and Nielsen, M. (2011). An anatomically oriented breast coordinate system for mammogram analysis. *IEEE Transactions on Medical Imaging*, 30(10):1841–1851.

Brzakovic, D., Luo, X. M., and Brzakovic, P. (1990). An approach to automated detection of tumors in mammograms. *IEEE Transactions on Medical Imaging*, 9(3):233–241.

Byng, J. W., Boyd, N. F., Fishell, E., Jong, R. A., and Yaffe, M. J. (1994). The quantitative analysis of mammographic densities. *Physics in Medicine and Biology*, 39(10):1629–1638.

Byng, J. W., Critten, J. P., and Yaffe, M. J. (1997). Thickness-equalization processing for mammographic images. *Radiology*, 203(2):564–568.

Cerneaz, N. and Brady, J. M. (1994). Enriching digital mammogram image analysis with a description of the curvi-linear structures. In Gale, A. G., Astley, S. M., Dance, D. R., and Cairns, A. Y., editors, *Digital Mammography*, pp. 297–306. Elsevier, Amsterdam, the Netherlands.

Chan, H. P., Sahiner, B., Helvie, M. A., Petrick, N., Roubidoux, M. A., Wilson, T. E., Adler, D. D., Paramagul, C., Newman, J. S., and Sanjay-Gopal, S. (1999). Improvement of radiologists' characterization of mammographic masses by using computer-aided diagnosis: An roc study. *Radiology*, 212(3):817–827.

Chan, H. P., Sahiner, B., Lam, K. L., Petrick, N., Helvie, M. A., Goodsitt, M. M., and Adler, D. D. (1998). Computerized analysis of mammographic microcalcifications in morphological and texture feature spaces. *Medical Physics*, 25(10):2007–2019.

Chandrasekhar, R. and Attikiouzel, Y. (1997). A simple method for automatically locating the nipple on mammograms. *IEEE Transactions on Medical Imaging*, 16(5):483–494.

Chang, Y. H., Zheng, B., and Gur, D. (1996). Computerized identification of suspicious regions for masses in digitized mammograms. *Investigative Radiology*, 31(3):146–153.

Cho, H.-C., Hadjiiski, L., Sahiner, B., Chan, H.-P., Helvie, M., Paramagul, C., and Nees, A. V. (2011). Similarity evaluation in a content-based image retrieval (cbir) cadx system for characterization of breast masses on ultrasound images. *Medical Physics*, 38(4):1820–1831.

Díez, Y., Oliver, A., Lladó, X., Freixenet, J., Martí, J., Vilanova, J. C., and Martí, R. (2011). Revisiting intensity-based image registration applied to mammography. *IEEE Transactions on Information Technology in Biomedicine*, 15(5):716–725.

Drukker, K., Horsch, K., and Giger, M. L. (2005). Multimodality computerized diagnosis of breast lesions using mammography and sonography. *Academic Radiology*, 12(8):970–979.

El-Naqa, I., Yang, Y., Galatsanos, N. P., Nishikawa, R. M., and Wernick, M. N. (2004). A similarity learning approach to content-based image retrieval: Application to digital mammography. *IEEE Transactions on Medical Imaging*, 23(10):1233–1244.

Elter, M., Held, C., and Wittenberg, T. (2010). Contour tracing for segmentation of mammographic masses. *Physics in Medicine and Biology*, 55(18):5299–5315.

Ferrari, R. J., Rangayyan, R. M., Borges, R. A., and Frre, A. F. (2004a). Segmentation of the fibro-glandular disc in mammograms using gaussian mixture modelling. *Medical and Biological Engineering and Computing*, 42(3):378–387.

Ferrari, R. J., Rangayyan, R. M., Desautels, J. E., and Frre, A. F. (2001). Analysis of asymmetry in mammograms via directional filtering with Gabor wavelets. *IEEE Transactions on Medical Imaging*, 20(9):953–964.

Ferrari, R. J., Rangayyan, R. M., Desautels, J. E. L., Borges, R. A., and Frere, A. F. (2004b). Automatic identification of the pectoral muscle in mammograms. *IEEE Transactions on Medical Imaging*, 23(2):232–245.

Filev, P., Hadjiiski, L., Sahiner, B., Chan, H.-P., and Helvie, M. A. (2005). Comparison of similarity measures for the task of template matching of masses on serial mammograms. *Medical Physics*, 32(2):515–529.

Hadjiiski, L., Chan, H. P., Sahiner, B., Petrick, N., and Helvie, M. A. (2001). Automated registration of breast lesions in temporal pairs of mammograms for interval change analysis–local affine transformation for improved localization. *Medical Physics*, 28(6):1070–1079.

Hadjiiski, L., Sahiner, B., Chan, H. P., Petrick, N., and Helvie, M. (1999). Classification of malignant and benign masses based on hybrid art2lda approach. *IEEE Transactions on Medical Imaging*, 18(12):1178–1187.

Hatanaka, Y., Hara, T., Fujita, H., Kasai, S., Endo, T., and Iwase, T. (2001). Development of an automated method for detecting mammographic masses with a partial loss of region. *IEEE Transactions on Medical Imaging*, 20(12):1209–1214.

Heine, J. J., Carston, M. J., Scott, C. G., Brandt, K. R., Wu, F.-F., Pankratz, V. S., Sellers, T. A., and Vachon, C. M. (2008). An automated approach for estimation of breast density. *Cancer Epidemiology Biomarkers and Prevention*, 17(11):3090–3097.

Highnam, R. and Brady, M. (1999). *Mammographic Image Analysis*. Kluwer Academic Publishers.

Hong, B.-W. and Sohn, B.-S. (2010). Segmentation of regions of interest in mammograms in a topographic approach. *IEEE Transactions on Information Technology in Biomedicine*, 14(1):129–139.

Horsch, K., Giger, M. L., and Metz, C. E. (2008). Prevalence scaling: Applications to an intelligent workstation for the diagnosis of breast cancer. *Academic Radiology*, 15(11):1446–1457.

Horsch, K., Giger, M. L., Vyborny, C. J., Lan, L., Mendelson, E. B., and Hendrick, R. E. (2006). Classification of breast lesions with multimodality computer-aided diagnosis: Observer study results on an independent clinical data set. *Radiology*, 240(2):357–368.

Huo, Z., Giger, M. L., Vyborny, C. J., Bick, U., Lu, P., Wolverton, D. E., and Schmidt, R. A. (1995). Analysis of spiculation in the computerized classification of mammographic masses. *Medical Physics*, 22(10):1569–1579.

Huo, Z., Giger, M. L., Vyborny, C. J., and Metz, C. E. (2002). Breast cancer: Effectiveness of computer-aided diagnosis observer study with independent database of mammograms. *Radiology*, 224(2):560–568.

Hupse, R. and Karssemeijer, N. (2009). Use of normal tissue context in computer-aided detection of masses in mammograms. *IEEE Transactions on Medical Imaging*, 28(12):2033–2041.

Hupse, R. and Karssemeijer, N. (2010). The effect of feature selection methods on computer-aided detection of masses in mammograms. *Physics in Medicine and Biology*, 55(10):2893–2904.

Iglesias, J. E. and Karssemeijer, N. (2009). Robust initial detection of landmarks in film-screen mammograms using multiple FFDM atlases. *IEEE Transactions on Medical Imaging*, 28(11):1815–1824.

Kallenberg, M. and Karssemeijer, N. (2008). Computer-aided detection of masses in full-field digital mammography using screen-film mammograms for training. *Physics in Medicine and Biology*, 53(23):6879–6891.

Kallenberg, M., Lokate, M., van Gils, C., and Karssemeijer, N. (2011). Automatic breast density segmentation based on pixel classification. In *Medical Imaging*, volume 7963 of *Proceedings of the SPIE*, p. 796307.

Karssemeijer, N. (1998). Automated classification of parenchymal patterns in mammograms. *Physics in Medicine and Biology*, 43(2):365–378.

Karssemeijer, N. and te Brake, G. M. (1996). Detection of stellate distortions in mammograms. *IEEE Transactions on Medical Imaging*, 15(5):611–619.

Kita, Y., Highnam, R., and Brady, M. (2001). Correspondence between different view breast x rays using curved epipolar lines. *Computer Vision and Image Understanding*, 83(1):38–56.

Kita, Y., Tohno, E., Highnam, R., and Brady, M. (2002). A cad system for the 3D location of lesions in mammograms. *Medical Image Analysis*, 6(3):267–273.

Kobatake, H., Murakami, M., Takeo, H., and Nawano, S. (1999). Computerized detection of malignant tumors on digital mammograms. *IEEE Transactions on Medical Imaging*, 18(5):369–378.

Kupinski, M. A. and Giger, M. L. (1998). Automated seeded lesion segmentation on digital mammograms. *IEEE Transactions on Medical Imaging*, 17(4):510–517.

Kwok, S. M., Chandrasekhar, R., Attikiouzel, Y., and Rickard, M. T. (2004). Automatic pectoral muscle segmentation on medio-lateral oblique view mammograms. *IEEE Transactions on Medical Imaging*, 23(9):1129–1140.

Lai, S. M., Li, X., and Bischof, W. F. (1989). On techniques for detecting circumscribed masses in mammograms. *IEEE Transactions on Medical Imaging*, 8(4):377–386.

Laine, A. F., Schuler, S., Fan, J., and Huda, W. (1994). Mammographic feature enhancement by multiscale analysis. *IEEE Transactions on Medical Imaging*, 13(4):725–740.

Lau, T. K. and Bischof, W. F. (1991). Automated detection of breast tumors using the asymmetry approach. *Computers and Biomedical Research*, 24(3):273–295.

Lesniak, J., Hupse, R., Kallenberg, M., Samulski, M., Blanc, R., Karssemeijer, N., and Székely, G. (2011). Computer aided detection of breast masses in mammography using support vector machine classification. In *Medical Imaging*, volume 7963 of *Proceedings of the SPIE*, p. 79631K.

Li, H. D., Kallergi, M., Clarke, L. P., Jain, V. K., and Clark, R. A. (1995). Markov random field for tumor detection in digital mammography. *IEEE Transactions on Medical Imaging*, 14(3):565–576.

Lim, W. K. and Er, M. J. (2004). Classification of mammographic masses using generalized dynamic fuzzy neural networks. *Medical Physics*, 31(5):1288–1295.

Liu, Y., Collins, R. T., and Rothfus, W. E. (2001). Robust midsagittal plane extraction from normal and pathological 3-D neuroradiology images. *IEEE Transactions on Medical Imaging*, 20(3):175–192.

Lladó, X., Oliver, A., Freixenet, J., Martí, R., and Martí, J. (2009). A textural approach for mass false positive reduction in mammography. *Computerized Medical Imaging and Graphics*, 33(6):415–422.

Marias, K., Behrenbruch, C., Parbhoo, S., Seifalian, A., and Brady, M. (2005). A registration framework for the comparison of mammogram sequences. *IEEE Transactions on Medical Imaging*, 24(6):782–790.

Mudigonda, N. R., Rangayyan, R. M., and Desautels, J. E. (2000). Gradient and texture analysis for the classification of mammographic masses. *IEEE Transactions on Medical Imaging*, 19(10):1032–1043.

Muralidhar, G. S., Bovik, A. C., Giese, J. D., Sampat, M. P., Whitman, G. J., Haygood, T. M., Stephens, T. W., and Markey, M. K. (2010). Snakules: A model-based active contour algorithm for the annotation of spicules on mammography. *IEEE Transactions on Medical Imaging*, 29(10):1768–1780.

Ng, S. L. and Bischof, W. F. (1992). Automated detection and classification of breast tumors. *Computers and Biomedical Research*, 25(3):218–237.

Nishikawa, R. M., Giger, M. L., Doi, K., Metz, C. E., Yin, F. F., Vyborny, C. J., and Schmidt, R. A. (1994). Effect of case selection on the performance of computer-aided detection schemes. *Medical Physics*, 21(2):265–269.

Oliver, A., Freixenet, J., Martí, J., Pérez, E., Pont, J., Denton, E. R. E., and Zwiggelaar, R. (2010a). A review of automatic mass detection and segmentation in mammographic images. *Medical Image Analysis*, 14(2):87–110.

Oliver, A., Freixenet, J., Martí, R., Pont, J., Pérez, E., Denton, E. R. E., and Zwiggelaar, R. (2008). A novel breast tissue density classification methodology. *IEEE Transactions on Information Technology in Biomedicine*, 12(1):55–65.

Oliver, A., Lladó, X., Freixenet, J., Martí, R., Pérez, E., Pont, J., and Zwiggelaar, R. (2010b). Influence of using manual or automatic breast density information in a mass detection cad system. *Academic Radiology*, 17(7):877–883.

Oliver, A., Lladó, X., Pérez, E., Pont, J., Denton, E. R. E., Freixenet, J., and Martí, J. (2010c). A statistical approach for breast density segmentation. *Journal of Digital Imaging*, 23(5):527–537.

Paquerault, S., Petrick, N., Chan, H.-P., Sahiner, B., and Helvie, M. A. (2002). Improvement of computerized mass detection on mammograms: Fusion of two-view information. *Medical Physics*, 29(2):238–247.

Pawluczyk, O., Augustine, B. J., Yaffe, M. J., Rico, D., Yang, J., Mawdsley, G. E., and Boyd, N. F. (2003). A volumetric method for estimation of breast density on digitized screen-film mammograms. *Medical Physics*, 30(3):352–364.

Petrick, N., Chan, H.-P., Sahiner, B., and Wei, D. (1996). An adaptive density-weighted contrast enhancement filter for mammographic breast mass detection. *IEEE Transactions on Medical Imaging*, 15(1):59–67.

Pu, J., Zheng, B., Leader, J. K., and Gur, D. (2008). An ellipse-fitting based method for efficient registration of breast masses on two mammographic views. *Medical Physics*, 35(2):487–494.

Qian, W., Song, D., Lei, M., Sankar, R., and Eikman, E. (2007). Computer-aided mass detection based on ipsilateral multiview mammograms. *Academic Radiology*, 14(5):530–538.

Rangayyan, R. M. and Ayres, F. J. (2006). Gabor filters and phase portraits for the detection of architectural distortion in mammograms. *Medical and Biological Engineering and Computing*, 44(10):883–894.

Rangayyan, R. M., El-Faramawy, N. M., Desautels, J. E. L., and Alim, O. A. (1997). Measures of acutance and shape for classification of breast tumors. *IEEE Transactions on Medical Imaging*, 16(6):799–810.

Sahiner, B., Chan, H. P., Petrick, N., Helvie, M. A., and Goodsitt, M. M. (1998a). Computerized characterization of masses on mammograms: The rubber band straightening transform and texture analysis. *Medical Physics*, 25(4):516–526.

Sahiner, B., Chan, H. P., Petrick, N., Helvie, M. A., and Goodsitt, M. M. (1998b). Computerized characterization of masses on mammograms: The rubber band straightening transform and texture analysis. *Medical Physics*, 25(4):516–526.

Sahiner, B., Chan, H. P., Petrick, N., Helvie, M. A., and Goodsitt, M. M. (1998c). Design of a high-sensitivity classifier based on a genetic algorithm: Application to computer-aided diagnosis. *Physics in Medicine and Biology*, 43(10):2853–2871.

Sahiner, B., Chan, H. P., Petrick, N., Helvie, M. A., and Hadjiiski, L. M. (2001a). Improvement of mammographic mass characterization using spiculation measures and morphological features. *Medical Physics*, 28(7):1455–1465.

Sahiner, B., Chan, H.-P., Petrick, N., Wei, D., Helvie, M. A., Adler, D. D., and Goodsitt, M. M. (1996a). Classification of mass and normal breast tissue: A convolution neural network classifier with spatial domain and texture images. *IEEE Transactions on Medical Imaging*, 15(5):598–610.

Sahiner, B., Chan, H. P., Wei, D., Petrick, N., Helvie, M. A., Adler, D. D., and Goodsitt, M. M. (1996b). Image feature selection by a genetic algorithm: Application to classification of mass and normal breast tissue. *Medical Physics*, 23(10):1671–1684.

Sahiner, B., Petrick, N., Chan, H. P., Hadjiiski, L. M., Paramagul, C., Helvie, M. A., and Gurcan, M. N. (2001b). Computer-aided characterization of mammographic masses: Accuracy of mass segmentation and its effects on characterization. *IEEE Transactions on Medical Imaging*, 20(12):1275–1284.

Sallam, M. Y. and Bowyer, K. W. (1999). Registration and difference analysis of corresponding mammogram images. *Medical Image Analysis*, 3(2):103–118.

Sampat, M. P., Bovik, A. C., Whitman, G. J., and Markey, M. K. (2008). A model-based framework for the detection of spiculated masses on mammography. *Medical Physics*, 35(5):2110–2123.

Samulski, M. and Karssemeijer, N. (2011). Optimizing Case-based Detection Performance in a Multiview CAD System for Mammography. *IEEE Transactions on Medical Imaging*, 30(4):1001–1009.

Sanjay-Gopal, S., Chan, H. P., Wilson, T., Helvie, M., Petrick, N., and Sahiner, B. (1999). A regional registration technique for automated interval change analysis of breast lesions on mammograms. *Medical Physics*, 26(12):2669–2679.

Snoeren, P. R. and Karssemeijer, N. (2004). Thickness correction of mammographic images by means of a global parameter model of the compressed breast. *IEEE Transactions on Medical Imaging*, 23(7):799–806.

Snoeren, P. R. and Karssemeijer, N. (2005). Thickness correction of mammographic images by anisotropic filtering and interpolation of dense tissue. In *Medical Imaging*, volume 5747 of *Proceedings of the SPIE*, pp. 1521–1527.

Snoeren, P. R. and Karssemeijer, N. (2007). Gray-scale and geometric registration of full-field digital and film-screen mammograms. *Medical Image Analysis*, 11(2):146–156.

Tang, J., Rangayyan, R. M., Xu, J., Naqa, I. E., and Yang, Y. (2009). Computer-aided detection and diagnosis of breast cancer with mammography: Recent advances. *IEEE Transactions on Information Technology in Biomedicine*, 13(2):236–251.

te Brake, G. M. and Karssemeijer, N. (1999). Single and multiscale detection of masses in digital mammograms. *IEEE Transactions on Medical Imaging*, 18(7):628–639.

te Brake, G. M. and Karssemeijer, N. (2001). Segmentation of suspicious densities in digital mammograms. *Medical Physics*, 28(2):259–266.

te Brake, G. M., Karssemeijer, N., and Hendriks, J. H. (2000). An automatic method to discriminate malignant masses from normal tissue in digital mammograms. *Physics in Medicine and Biology*, 45(10):2843–2857.

Timp, S. and Karssemeijer, N. (2004). A new 2D segmentation method based on dynamic programming applied to computer aided detection in mammography. *Medical Physics*, 31(5):958–971.

Timp, S. and Karssemeijer, N. (2006). Interval change analysis to improve computer aided detection in mammography. *Medical Image Analysis*, 10(1):82–95.

Timp, S., van Engeland, S., and Karssemeijer, N. (2005). A regional registration method to find corresponding mass lesions in temporal mammogram pairs. *Medical Physics*, 32(8):2629–2638.

Timp, S., Varela, C., and Karssemeijer, N. (2007). Temporal change analysis for characterization of mass lesions in mammography. *IEEE Transactions on Medical Imaging*, 26(7):945–953.

Tourassi, G. D., Delong, D. M., and Floyd, C. E. (2006). A study on the computerized fractal analysis of architectural distortion in screening mammograms. *Physics in Medicine and Biology*, 51(5):1299–1312.

Tourassi, G. D., Harrawood, B., Singh, S., Lo, J. Y., and Floyd, C. E. (2007). Evaluation of information-theoretic similarity measures for content-based retrieval and detection of masses in mammograms. *Medical Physics*, 34(1):140–150.

van Engeland, S. and Karssemeijer, N. (2007). Combining two mammographic projections in a computer aided mass detection method. *Medical Physics*, 34(3):898–905.

van Engeland, S., Snoeren, P., Hendriks, J., and Karssemeijer, N. (2003). A comparison of methods for mammogram registration. *IEEE Transactions on Medical Imaging*, 22(11):1436–1444.

van Engeland, S., Snoeren, P. R., Huisman, H., Boetes, C., and Karssemeijer, N. (2006a). Volumetric breast density estimation from full-field digital mammograms. *IEEE Transactions on Medical Imaging*, 25(3):273–282.

van Engeland, S., Timp, S., and Karssemeijer, N. (2006b). Finding corresponding regions of interest in mediolateral oblique and craniocaudal mammographic views. *Medical Physics*, 33(9):3203–3212.

Varela, C., Timp, S., and Karssemeijer, N. (2006). Use of border information in the classification of mammographic masses. *Physics in Medicine and Biology*, 51(2):425–441.

Velikova, M., Samulski, M., Lucas, P. J. F., and Karssemeijer, N. (2009). Improved mammographic CAD performance using multiview information: A Bayesian network framework. *Physics in Medicine and Biology*, 54(5):1131–1147.

Vujovic, N. and Brzakovic, D. (1997). Establishing the correspondence between control points in pairs of mammographic images. *IEEE Transactions on Image Processing*, 6(10):1388–1399.

Wei, D., Chan, H., Helvie, M. A., Sahiner, B., Petrick, N., Adler, D. D., and Goodsitt, M. M. (1995). Classification of mass and normal breast tissue on digital mammograms: Multiresolution texture analysis. *Medical Physics*, 22(9):1501–1513.

Wei, J., Chan, H.-P., Sahiner, B., Hadjiiski, L. M., Helvie, M. A., Roubidoux, M. A., Zhou, C., and Ge, J. (2006). Dual system approach to computer-aided detection of breast masses on mammograms. *Medical Physics*, 33(11):4157–4168.

Wei, J., Chan, H.-P., Sahiner, B., Zhou, C., Hadjiiski, L. M., Roubidoux, M. A., and Helvie, M. A. (2009). Computer-aided detection of breast masses on mammograms: Dual system approach with two-view analysis. *Medical Physics*, 36(10):4451–4460.

Wei, J., Chan, H.-P., Zhou, C., Wu, Y.-T., Sahiner, B., Hadjiiski, L. M., Roubidoux, M. A., and Helvie, M. A. (2011). Computer-aided detection of breast masses: Four-view strategy for screening mammography. *Medical Physics*, 38(4):1867–1876.

Wu, Y., Wei, J., Hadjiiski, L., Sahiner, B., Zhou, C., Ge, J., Shi, J., Zhang, Y., and Chan, H. (2007). Bilateral analysis based false positive reduction for computer-aided mass detection. *Medical Physics*, 34(8):3334–3344.

Wu, Y.-T., Zhou, C., Chan, H.-P., Paramagul, C., Hadjiiski, L. M., Daly, C. P., Douglas, J. A., Zhang, Y., Sahiner, B., Shi, J., and Wei, J. (2010). Dynamic multiple thresholding breast boundary detection algorithm for mammograms. *Medical Physics*, 37(1):391–401.

Yam, M., Brady, M., Highnam, R., Behrenbruch, C., English, R., and Kita, Y. (2001). Three-dimensional reconstruction of microcalcification clusters from two mammographic views. *IEEE Transactions on Medical Imaging*, 20(6):479–489.

Yin, F. F., Giger, M. L., Doi, K., Metz, C. E., Vyborny, C. J., and Schmidt, R. A. (1991). Computerized detection of masses in digital mammograms: Analysis of bilateral subtraction images. *Medical Physics*, 18(5):955–963.

Yin, F. F., Giger, M. L., Vyborny, C. J., Doi, K., and Schmidt, R. A. (1993). Comparison of bilateral-subtraction and single-image processing techniques in the computerized detection of mammographic masses. *Investigative Radiology*, 28(6):473–481.

Zheng, B., Chang, Y. H., Staiger, M., Good, W., and Gur, D. (1995). Computer-aided detection of clustered microcalcifications in digitized mammograms. *Academic Radiology*, 2(8):655–662.

Zheng, B., Leader, J. K., Abrams, G. S., Lu, A. H., Wallace, L. P., Maitz, G. S., and Gur, D. (2006). Multiview-based computer-aided detection scheme for breast masses. *Medical Physics*, 33(9):3135–3143.

Zheng, B., Mello-Thoms, C., Wang, X.-H., Abrams, G. S., Sumkin, J. H., Chough, D. M., Ganott, M. A., Lu, A., and Gur, D. (2007). Interactive computer-aided diagnosis of breast masses: Computerized selection of visually similar image sets from a reference library. *Academic Radiology*, 14(8):917–927.

Zheng, B., Tan, J., Ganott, M. A., Chough, D. M., and Gur, D. (2009). Matching breast masses depicted on different views a comparison of three methods. *Academic Radiology*, 16(11):1338–1347.

Zhou, C., Chan, H.-P., Paramagul, C., Roubidoux, M. A., Sahiner, B., Hadjiiski, L. M., and Petrick, N. (2004). Computerized nipple identification for multiple image analysis in computer-aided diagnosis. *Medical Physics*, 31(10):2871–2882.

Zhou, C., Wei, J., Chan, H.-P., Paramagul, C., Hadjiiski, L. M., Sahiner, B., and Douglas, J. A. (2010). Computerized image analysis: Texture-field orientation method for pectoral muscle identification on mlo-view mammograms. *Medical Physics*, 37(5):2289–2299.

Zwiggelaar, R., Astley, S. M., Boggis, C. R. M., and Taylor, C. J. (2004). Linear structures in mammographic images: Detection and classification. *IEEE Transactions on Medical Imaging*, 23(9):1077–1086.

Zwiggelaar, R., Parr, T. C., Schumm, J. E., Hutt, I. W., Taylor, C. J., Astley, S. M., and Boggis, C. R. (1999). Model-based detection of spiculated lesions in mammograms. *Medical Image Analysis*, 3(1):39–62.

Chapter 3

Detection and Diagnosis of Microcalcifications in Mammography

Hao Jing, Issam El Naqa, and Yongyi Yang

CONTENTS

3.1 INTRODUCTION

3.1.1 Breast Cancer and Mammography

Breast cancer remains the most frequently diagnosed non–skin cancer in women in the United States. According to the American Cancer Society (ACS), an estimated 232,670 new cases of breast cancers are expected to occur among women in the United States during 2014. Approximately 40,000 women are anticipated to die from the disease in the same year (ACS 2014). Early detection is known to be the key to successful treatment of breast cancer. The combination of early detection and improvements in available treatment options has led to 2%–3.2% decline per year in mortality rates among women in recent years.

Mammography is an imaging procedure in which low-energy X-ray images of the breast are taken. Typically, they are in the order of 0.7 mSv. A mammogram can detect a cancerous or precancerous tumor in the breast even before the tumor is large enough to feel. Despite advances in imaging technology, mammography remains the most cost-effective strategy for early detection of breast cancer in clinical practice. The sensitivity of mammography could be up to approximately 90% for patients without symptoms (Mushlin et al. 1998). However, this sensitivity is highly dependent on the patient's age, the size and conspicuity of the lesion, the hormone status of the tumor, the density of a woman's breasts, and the overall image quality and the interpretative skills of the radiologist (Urbain 2005). Therefore, the overall sensitivity of mammography could vary from 90% to 70% only (Kolb et al. 2002). Moreover, it is very difficult to distinguish mammographically benign lesions from malignant ones. It has been estimated that one-third of regularly screened women experience at least one false-positive (benign lesions being biopsied) screening mammogram over a period of 10 years (Elmore et al. 1998). A population-based study included about 27,394 screening mammograms that were interpreted by 1067 radiologists showed that the radiologists had substantial variations in the false-positive rates ranging from 1.5% to 24.1% (Tan et al. 2006). Unnecessary biopsy is often cited as one of the *risks* of screening mammography. Surgical, needle-core, and fine-needle aspiration biopsies are expensive, invasive, and traumatic for the patient.

3.1.2 Microcalcifications and Computer-Aided Diagnosis

Clustered microcalcifications (MCs) can be an important early sign of breast cancer in women. They are found in 30%–50% of mammographically diagnosed cases. MCs are calcium deposits of very small dimension and appear as a group of granular bright spots in a mammogram (e.g., Figure 3.1). Individual MCs are sometimes difficult to detect because of the surrounding breast tissue, their variation in shape, and

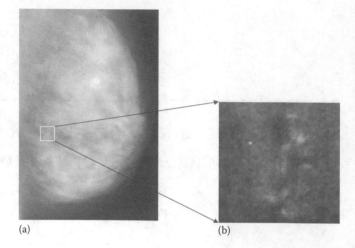

(a)   (b)

Figure 3.1 A mammogram image in MLO view (a) and a magnified view of a region containing clustered microcalcifications (b).

small dimension. It is also often difficult to distinguish benign from malignant MCs because of their subtlety in appearance.

Because of their importance in cancer diagnosis, there has been intensive research for the development of computerized methods for automatic detection and analysis of MCs in mammograms (Nishikawa 2007, Rangayyan et al. 2007, Sampat et al. 2005). Collectively, these methods are known as computer-aided diagnosis (CAD) schemes, which are developed as a potentially efficacious solution to improving radiologists' diagnostic accuracy in screening mammography and diagnostic workup. In these CAD schemes, the computer is intended to play the role of a virtual *second reader*, alerting the radiologist to potential lesions in an image for further review and evaluation or providing an estimate on diagnostic variables, such as probability of malignancy. The rest of this chapter will focus on the development of computerized methods for automatic detection and analysis of MCs in mammogram images.

3.1.3 Computer-Aided Detection versus Diagnosis

CAD schemes encompass computer-aided detection (CADe) and computer-aided diagnosis (CADx). Detection and diagnosis are two interrelated concepts in CAD. Detection aims to distinguish an object of interest (lesion) from its surrounding tissues in an image using pattern recognition techniques, while diagnosis is a process of staging of disease involvement to choose proper treatment approach. In the case of MCs, CADe would aim to identify clustered MCs in mammogram images, while CADx would be related to the clustering patterns indicating the degree of malignancy. For convenience, we describe computerized methods for MCs in mammogram images separately in CADe and CADx schemes in the following text.

3.2 COMPUTER-AIDED DETECTION OF MICROCALCIFICATIONS

3.2.1 Overview of CADe Methods

There have been many methods reported for MC detection in mammogram images in the literature (El-Naqa and Yang 2005, Nishikawa 2007, Sampat et al. 2005). Broadly, these methods can be divided into the following four categories: (1) basic image enhancement methods, (2) multiscale filtering methods, (3) stochastic modeling methods, and (4) machine learning methods. Such a categorization is mainly based on the employed image-processing techniques in different methods. It is not uncommon for a modern system to employ one or more of these techniques to achieve better detection accuracy. Nevertheless, we find such a categorization to be pedagogically convenient for the presentation of different methods.

3.2.1.1 Image Enhancement Methods

Methods in this category are motivated by the fact that MCs tend to be brighter than their surrounding breast tissue in a mammogram. Hence, the underlying principle for detection is to improve the contrast of MCs relative to their surrounding background and then apply thresholding to separate them. An example of this approach is the difference of Gaussians (DoG) detector (Dengler et al. 1993), which uses two Gaussian kernels of different widths. Another example is the image difference technique developed by Nishikawa et al. (1995). The method is based on a difference image technique followed by morphological erosion to reduce false positives. Similar to the DoG method, the difference image is produced by using two filters, one for enhancing the MCs and the other for suppressing them. More recently, a noise equalization scheme was proposed by Mcloughlin et al. (2004). In this method, it is assumed that the dominant source of noise in digital mammograms is due to limited quantum. This quantum noise is modeled by using a simple square-root law of gray levels. The local contrast is improved by removing this noise dependency on the gray level (McLoughlin et al. 2004). Qian et al. (2002) applied a region grouping approach for MC detection based on cluster analysis. A visual model in conjunction with anisotropic diffusion filtering was proposed by Linguraru et al. (2006).

The main advantage of these methods is in their simplicity, ease of implementation, and efficiency, which is a very desirable property for real-time application in a busy mammographic clinic. However, this also can come at the expense of reduced accuracy in many cases. For instance, the difference image approach is similar to a Laplacian edge detector, which is inherently sensitive to noise and may generate many false-positive signals. To overcome such problems, pre- or postprocessing techniques such as morphological operators are applied to reduce the number of false positives.

3.2.1.2 Multiscale Decomposition Methods

Methods in this category are based on the difference in frequency content of the bright MC spots from their surrounding background. Wavelet-based approaches fall into this category. They have been proposed in Yoshida et al. (1994, Strickland and Hahn 1996, 1997). In Yoshida et al. (1994), a decimated wavelet transform and supervised learning are combined for the detection of MCs, while in Strickland and Hahn (1996, 1997), an undecimated wavelet transform and optimal subband weighting are used. Besides the wavelet approaches, a detection scheme using multiscale analysis is proposed based on the Laplacian-of-Gaussian filter and a mathematical model describing an MC as a bright spot of a certain size and contrast (Netsch 1996). Bazzani et al. (2001) proposed a method for MC detection based on multiresolution filtering analysis and statistical testing, in which a support vector machine (SVM) classifier was used to reduce the false detection rate.

3.2.1.3 Stochastic Modeling Methods

Methods in this category aim to exploit the statistical difference (e.g., order statistics) between MCs and their surroundings. For instance, a pixel-wise Markov random field (MRF) framework was developed by Karssemeijer (1992) for the segmentation of MCs in a mammogram. The clustering property that MCs typically appear in tightly distributed clusters in small lesions in mammograms was demonstrated to be beneficial in this approach. In Gurcan et al. (1997), the difference in higher order statistics was used to discriminate between MCs and background tissues. An MRF approach was also used by Caputo et al. based on *spin glass* energy functions associated with generalized Gaussian kernels (Caputo et al. 2002). Gaussian mixture models were used for MC detection in Casaseca-de-Higuera et al. (2005). Recently, in Jing et al. (2011), a spatial point process (SPP) was used to model the distribution of clustered MCs. This approach will be described as an example later in Section 3.2.4.

3.2.1.4 Machine Learning Methods

Methods in this category use artificial intelligence techniques to learn dependencies from data. In the context of MC detection, the problem is typically posed as a binary classification problem, where the goal is to determine whether an MC is present at a pixel location (labeled: +1) or not (labeled: −1). Machine learning methods have received the largest share of research in recent developments. As an example, Yu and Guan proposed a two-stage neural network approach, where wavelet components, gray-level statistics, and shape features were used to train a two-stage network (Yu and Guan 2000). The first stage was used to identify potential MC pixels in the mammograms, and the second stage was used to detect individual MC objects. Neural networks were investigated for MC detection by multiple researchers (Bocchi et al. 2004, Gurcan et al. 2002, Sajda et al. 2002). However, the high nonlinearity associated with these methods may result in trapping in local minima and thus limiting their discrimination power. Methods based on evolutionary genetic algorithms (GAs) were proposed in Peng et al. (2006), where GAs were used to search for optimal bright spots in mammogram images that could be classified as MCs. A main challenge in evolutionary methods is their numerical instability and sensitivity to initialization procedures, which could be problematic in the case of MC detection. Another recent development in machine learning is a class of learning algorithms known as SVMs. Conceptually, an SVM utilizes an implicit nonlinear kernel mapping to a higher-dimensional space, where an optimal hyperplane classifier (which maximizes the separation margin between two classes) is applied. SVMs were recently demonstrated to achieve high accuracy for MC detection in the literature (El-Naqa et al. 2002b, Singh et al. 2006, Wei et al. 2005). El-Naqa et al. demonstrated that the prediction power could be further improved by applying a successive enhancement learning (SEL) procedure, where SVM training is adjusted iteratively by reincorporating misclassified samples. More recently, Wei et al. (2005) demonstrated that the computational efficiency could be improved significantly while maintaining the best prediction power by using a Bayesian learning approach known as relevance vector machine (RVM). This is an important issue for real-time processing of mammograms in a clinical setup. Machine learning methods have been demonstrated to generate powerful classifiers in many pattern recognition problems; however, in many instances, there is a risk of overfitting the data if these methods were not rigorously validated on independent datasets or tested using statistical resampling methods.

3.2.1.5 Pre- and Postprocessing Methods

Apart from the different approaches used for the detection of MCs, some pre- and postprocessing methods have also been investigated to improve the detection performance for MCs. For example, an adaptive approach based on region growing was proposed to enhance the mammographic features (Morrow et al. 1992). A noise equalization approach was studied by estimating the noise statistics at pixels with different gray levels (Mcloughlin et al. 2004, Veldkamp and Karssemeijer 2000). A fractal modeling approach was also applied for the enhancement of MCs, in which mammograms were modeled with deterministic fractal objects defined by 2D affine transformations. One factor that contributes to false-positive detections is the existence of linear or curve-like breast structures in mammograms. Removal of such breast structures can also lead to improvement in the detection performance of MCs.

3.2.2 Detection Performance Metrics

The performance of a CADe algorithm system for MC detection is typically evaluated using metrics based on the sensitivity (true-positive [TP] fraction) and specificity (true-negative fraction) at a particular operating threshold. Graphically, this could be presented in terms of a receiver-operating characteristic (ROC) curve over the continuum of the decision threshold. Due to the importance of the correct localization of the detected clusters in MC detection, a generalization of ROC known as free-response receiver-operating characteristic (FROC) (Bunch et al. 1978) plot is used to report the performance of the detection algorithm. An FROC curve provides a comprehensive summary of the trade-off between detection sensitivity and specificity. However, in the literature, there also exist several other strategies for the evaluation of detected clustered MCs, and caution should be taken when comparing the published results of different algorithms. The FROC curve for a detection algorithm can vary with the clustering criteria used, and there exist different criteria in the literature (Kallergi et al. 1999). Even for the same criterion, use of different parameters such as the distance allowance between MCs can also impact the resulting FROC curves. This effect was demonstrated in El-Naqa and Yang (2005), where a criterion recommended by Kallergi et al. was used for identifying MC clusters (Kallergi et al. 1999). Specifically, a group of objects classified as MCs is considered to be a TP cluster only if (1) the objects are connected with nearest-neighbor distances less than 0.2 cm and (2) at least three true MCs are detected by the algorithm within an area of 1 cm^2. Likewise, a group of objects classified as MCs is labeled as a false-positive cluster if the objects satisfy the cluster requirement but contain no true MCs. Such a criterion has been reported to yield more realistic performance than several other alternatives.

3.2.3 Example#1: Using Machine Learning Methods for MC Detection

In this section, we describe an example of using machine learning for MC detection in digital mammograms. We follow the approach first proposed in El-Naqa et al. (2002b), where an SVM classifier was trained through supervised learning to classify at each location in a mammogram image whether an MC object is either *present* (class 1) or *absent* (class 2).

Conceptually, an SVM classifier functions as follows: first, an implicit nonlinear mapping $\Phi(\mathbf{x})$ is applied to map an input vector $\mathbf{x}$ into a higher-dimensional space, then a linear classifier is designed in this mapped space according to the principle of maximum separation margin between the two classes. With the notion of a kernel function $K(\mathbf{x},\mathbf{y}) \triangleq \Phi(\mathbf{x})^T \Phi(\mathbf{x})$, the resulting SVM decision function can be written as

$$f_{SVM}(\mathbf{x}) = \sum_{i=1}^{N_s} \alpha_i K(\mathbf{x},\mathbf{s}_i) + b \qquad (3.1)$$

where $\mathbf{s}_i$, $i = 1,...,N_s$, denote the so-called support vectors, which are a small fraction of the training samples.

Both the support vectors and the parameters in the SVM function in Equation 3.1 are determined through minimization of the structural risk of the classifier, which is a trade-off between the separation margin between the two classes and the empirical error on the training samples. The purpose is to avoid overfitting, a situation in which the decision boundary too precisely corresponds to the training data and thereby fails to perform well on data outside the training set.

For the SVM kernel function, the radial basis function (RBF) is commonly used, which is defined as

$$K(\mathbf{x},\mathbf{y}) = \exp\left(-\frac{\|\mathbf{x}-\mathbf{y}\|^2}{2\sigma^2}\right) \qquad (3.2)$$

where $\sigma > 0$ is a constant that defines the kernel width.

As an input to the SVM classifier, a small $M \times M$ image window centered at the location of interest is used. Such a choice is motivated by the fact that individual MCs are well localized in a mammogram; therefore, to detect whether an MC is present at a given location, it is sufficient to examine the image content within a small neighborhood around that location. A small window size is also desirable for computational reasons. As examples, Figure 3.2 shows some image windows for the *MC present* class and the *MC absent* class. These *MC present* samples were selected from MCs indentified by experienced mammographers in a set of training images; similarly, the *MC absent* samples were selected from non-MC locations in the training images.

An interesting aspect in MC detection is that there are far more *MC absent* samples than *MC present* samples in the training images, because MCs occupy only a very small fraction of the image pixels in a mammogram. To take advantage of this, we developed an SEL procedure that could further improve the prediction power of the SVM classifier. With SEL, SVM training is adjusted iteratively by selecting the more difficult *MC absent* examples from all the available training images while keeping the total number of training examples small.

After training, the SVM classifier can then be applied to detect the presence of MCs in a mammogram image. In Figure 3.3, we show the output of the SVM classifier to a typical mammogram image, where the MCs are highlighted in the SVM classifier output. In Figure 3.4, we show the detection performance, summarized using FROC curves, achieved by the SVM classifier based on a set of 76 clinical mammogram images in an evaluation study (El-Naqa et al. 2002b). Results are also shown for several other MC detection methods, including the image difference technique filter (IDTF) (Nishikawa et al. 1995), the DoG (Dengler et al. 1993), multiscale decomposition by wavelets (Strickland and Hahn 1996), and machine learning methods using neural networks (Yu and Guan 2000). As can be seen, the machine learning–based methods achieve the best performance.

3.2.4 Example#2: Statistical Modeling Using Spatial Point Process for MC Detection

The conventional approach for MC detection has been to treat the individual MCs as an independent mammogram image. In this section, we describe a statistical modeling approach (Jing and Yang 2009, Jing et al. 2011) that can incorporate the spatial clustering property of MCs into the detection process and thereby improve the detection accuracy.

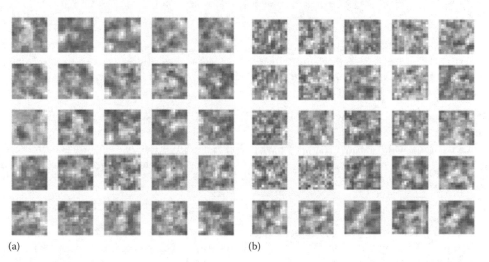

(a)   (b)

Figure 3.2 Examples of image windows of microcalcifications (a) and background regions (b).

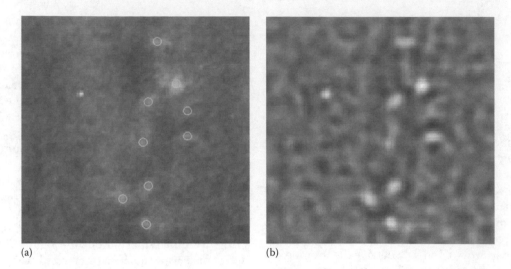

(a)   (b)

Figure 3.3   A mammogram region where microcalcifications are marked by circles (a) and the SVM classifier output (b).

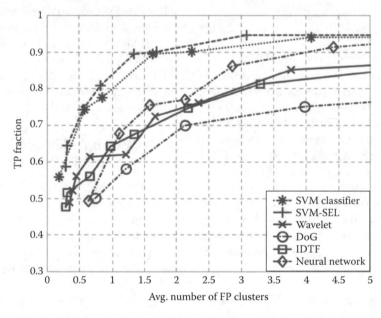

Figure 3.4   FROC results obtained by different methods, including (1) image enhancement methods, DoG and IDTF, (2) multiscale decomposition by wavelets (From Strickland, R.N. and Hahn, H.L. Wavelet transforms for detecting microcalcifications in mammograms, *IEEE Transactions on Medical Imaging*, 15, 218–229, 1996.), and (3) machine learning methods using neural networks. (From Yu, S. and Guan, L., *IEEE Trans. Med. Imag.*, 19, 115, 2000.)

In this method, the image $f(\mathbf{x})$ is modeled as a superposition of a number of MCs (signals) in a noisy background. Specifically, at pixel location $\mathbf{x} \in \Omega$, we have

$$f(\mathbf{x}) = \sum_{i=1}^{N} w_i K(\mathbf{x};\mathbf{x}_i) + n(\mathbf{x}) \qquad (3.3)$$

where

$K(\mathbf{x};\mathbf{x}_i)$ is the signal corresponding to the MC located at $\mathbf{x}_i$, which has strength (or amplitude) w_i
$n(\mathbf{x})$ denotes the background noise
N is the number of MCs

The MC signal $K(\mathbf{x};\mathbf{x}_i)$ is modeled by a truncated Gaussian kernel centered at $\mathbf{x}_i$.

The detection of MCs is then treated as an estimation problem of the following parameters of the image model in Equation 3.3:

$$\Theta = \left\{ N, \mathbf{x}_i, w_i, \; i = 1,...,N \right\} \qquad (3.4)$$

Assume a Gaussian noise model for the background noise $n(\mathbf{x})$ with mean μ_b and variance σ_b^2. Then, the likelihood function of the image data can be written as

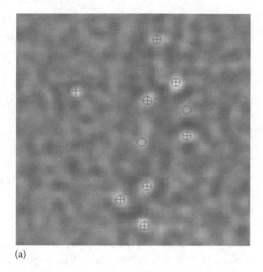

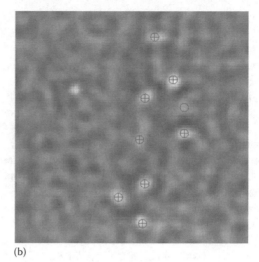

(a) (b)

Figure 3.5 Detection results by SVM (a) and SPP (b).

$$p(f(\mathbf{x})|\Theta) = \left(2\pi\sigma_b^2\right)^{-\frac{1}{2}} \exp\left\{-\frac{1}{2\sigma_b^2}\left[f(\mathbf{x}) - \sum_{i=1}^{N} w_i K(\mathbf{x}, \mathbf{x}_i) - \mu_b\right]^2\right\}$$

(3.5)

In reality, the background in a mammogram image is rarely stationary. In our experiments, a prefiltering step was first applied prior to detection as described in Mcloughlin et al. (2004) in order to remove the inhomogeneity in the background.

To characterize spatial clustering properties among a group of MC objects in a mammogram image, we model the spatial distribution of the MC objects by an SPP $\mathbf{s} = \{s_i, i = 1,...,N\}$, $s_i = (\mathbf{x}_i, w_i)$, where as in Equation 3.3, $\mathbf{x}_i$ denotes the spatial location of the ith MC and w_i denotes its amplitude. We model this process by using a Gibbs point process with a prior distribution of the following form:

$$p(\Theta) \propto \beta^N \prod_{s_i \in \mathbf{s}} g_1(s_i) g_2(s_i, \mathbf{s})$$

(3.6)

In Equation 3.6, the spatial distribution of MC objects is modeled by a Poisson process, and the density parameter β is associated with the average number of MCs in an image; the term $g_1(s_i)$ is used to characterize the property of individual MC objects (specifically, their amplitude); and the term $g_2(s_i, \mathbf{s})$ is used to model the spatial interactions between an MC s_i and its neighboring MCs. The interested reader is referred to Jing et al. (2011) for more details on the definition of these two terms.

The detection of MCs in this problem is solved by maximizing a posteriori estimation for Θ. That is,

$$\hat{\Theta} = \arg\max_{\Theta}\left\{p(\mathbf{f}|\Theta) p(\Theta)\right\}$$

(3.7)

This problem is noted to be not analytically tractable. The technique of reversible jump Markov chain Monte Carlo (RJMCMC) (Andrieu et al. 2003) is used for the solution, which can handle the difficulty that the number of MCs in a mammogram is not known a priori.

As an example, in Figure 3.5, we show the detection output by the SPP method for the image shown earlier in Figure 3.1. For comparison, the output is also shown for the SVM detector. In this figure, the detected MCs are indicated by + signs, and the ground truth is indicated by circles. As can be seen, there are one FP MC and two missed MCs in the SVM detection, and there are only one missed MC and no FP in the SPP detection. These results were shown for the two methods at the same FP level when tested on a set of images. In a test with 141 clinical mammograms, the improvement of the proposed method over the SVM classifier was demonstrated to be significant using a bootstrapping method for performance comparison (Jing et al. 2011).

3.3 COMPUTER-AIDED DIAGNOSIS (CADx) OF MICROCALCIFICATIONS

3.3.1 Overview of CADx Methods

Though commonly seen on mammograms, MC clusters are often difficult to diagnose. Because of their importance in cancer diagnosis, there has been significant research in CADx techniques for computerized diagnosis of clustered MCs. In CADx, the main purpose is the classification of MC clusters into two classes, benign or malignant, which is a two-class classification problem. A common approach to this problem is to apply supervised learning, in which a pattern classifier is first trained on a set of existing cases (called training samples), which is then applied to subsequent testing cases (unseen during trainings). In the literature, various machine learning methods such as artificial neural network (ANN) and linear discriminant analysis (LDA) have been used in the development of CADx classifiers for the diagnosis of clustered MCs.

In early work (Wu et al. 1993), Wu et al. designed a three-layer, feed-forward neural network trained with a back-propagation algorithm for mammographic lesion (including MCs and masses) interpretation, and the features used were extracted by experienced radiologists. Baker et al. constructed an ANN based on the standardized lexicon of the Breast Imaging Recording and Data System (BI-RADS) of the American College of Radiology and showed that the positive predictive value of biopsy can be improved by this approach (Baker et al. 1995). A computerized algorithm using ANN was developed by Jiang (1996) and was demonstrated to be more accurate than radiologists in the diagnosis of MC lesions. Markopoulos et al. (2001) showed that the use of an ANN-based approach could improve the diagnosis performance of radiologists for MCs. In Lo et al. (2002), an ANN using BI-RADS descriptors was tested on data from different institutions, and it was found that the performance decreased significantly for cross-institutional test. The ANN approach remains to be popular in CADx research in recent years. For example, in Kallergi (2004), a CAD system for MC lesions using ANN was shown to be superior to a similar visual analysis system and could be applied to images from different imaging systems and film digitizers. In Bocchi and Nori (2007), an ANN was used with shape features from Radon transom of MCs for classification.

Compared with ANN, LDA is a linear classifier and much more efficient to train. In early work (Chan et al. 1995), Chan et al. used LDA for the classification of benign and malignant MCs based on visibility and shape features. This approach was later extended to morphology and texture features (Chan et al. 1998). In Dhawan et al. (1996), LDA was compared with ANN using gray-level image structure features for the classification of benign and malignant MCs. In Lo et al. (2003), LDA was used to demonstrate the value of radiologist-extracted features as a source of information CAD of MC clusters. In Gupta et al. (2006), Gupta et al. compared the performance of an LDA classifier based on BI-RADS descriptors from one or two views and suggested that combining information from two mammographic views may improve the performance.

Besides ANN and LDA, other classifiers have also been explored, such as the kernel Fisher discriminant, SVMs, and RVMs in a comparison study in Wei et al. (2005), where the SVM was shown to yield improved performance. More recently, the classifiers of logistic regression (LR) (Chhatwal et al. 2009) and Bayesian network (Burnside et al. 2009) were also investigated.

3.3.2 MC Features in CADx

An important issue in CADx is the selection of features for characterizing the clustered MCs. Various types of features have been investigated in the literature for MC lesions (Cheng et al. 2003, Elter and Horsch 2009, Nishikawa 2007, Rangayyan et al. 2007, Sampat et al. 2005). These features are defined to reflect the gray-level or geometric properties of the MC lesions. They are extracted either from the individual MCs or from the entire lesion region. The features from individual MCs are then summarized using statistics to characterize an MC cluster.

3.3.2.1 Gray-Level Features

Among the gray-level features, the brightness, contrast, and gradient of individual MCs and the texture in the lesion region are commonly used. In Jiang et al. (1992), the effective thickness and effective volume were defined on the physical properties of the MCs and were shown to be useful in diagnosis classification. Texture features have also been widely investigated for the classification of MC lesions. In Thiele et al. (1996, Chan et al. 1998), the spatial gray-level dependence matrices (Haralick et al. 1973) were used to calculate texture features. It was shown that texture features could have significant discriminating power between benign and malignant lesions. These texture features are also called Haralick features. In Dhawan et al. (1996), texture features calculated from gray-level histogram and wavelet packets were studied. In Soltanian-Zadeh et al. (2004), wavelet features were compared with Haralick features and were shown to be more useful in classification.

3.3.2.2 Geometric Features

Different from the gray-level features, the geometric features are used to quantify the size and shape of individual MCs. There have been many such features investigated. For example, in Shen et al. (1994), compactness, moments, and Fourier descriptors were used to characterize the shape of MCs. In Jiang et al. (1996), the variation of the distance from the center of the MC to its boarder pixels along eight different orientations was used. More recently, the Radon transform was investigated and shown to be effective in discriminating between benign and malignant MCs by Bocchi and Nori (2007). The Radon transform was calculated along eight directions, similar to that in Jiang et al. (1996) intuitively. In Tay and Ma (2010), a shape feature using wavelet decomposition was shown to be effective. Other geometric features were also used to characterize the shape properties of individual MCs in the literature, including circularity, rectangularity, and eccentricity.

Besides individual MCs, geometric features are also used to characterize their cluster region. These include the number of MCs, area, shape, and spatial distributions of the cluster. The shape features of a cluster region can be computed similarly as for individual MCs, such as the circularity, rectangularity, and compactness. For characterizing the spatial distribution of MCs within a cluster, features include the density of MCs, the mean, and variance of the interdistance between MCs (Wei et al. 2005). The convex hull from the location of MCs was also used (Papadopoulos et al. 2005).

3.3.2.3 Other Features

The gray-level or geometric features described earlier are typically computed from the images. Apart from these features, some researchers have also investigated features extracted by human-readers. For example, 14 lesion descriptors provided by radiologists were used in Wu et al. (1993) with a neural network classifier. In Lo et al. (2002), Bilska-wolak and Floyd (2002), and Gupta et al. (2006), features based on the standardized BI-RADS lexicon were used.

3.3.2.4 Feature Selection

With many features extracted, another important issue is how to determine which features to use in a CADx classifier, which can have a significant impact on the classification performance. There can be several reasons for this. One is that some of the extracted features could be highly correlated with each other, and some of the extracted features may not even be relevant for the classification task. In such a case, using all the features together in the classifier may not necessarily be beneficial as far as the classification performance is concerned. Another reason is that the number of training samples is typically limited, and using too many features could potentially lead to overfitting during training (the curse of dimensionality).

To select the most salient features for the classifier, one approach is to use those features identified by experience radiologists who can provide important domain knowledge in their diagnosis. Another common approach is to apply a feature selection algorithm developed in the field

of machine learning by Guyon and Elisseeff (2003), which aims to optimize the classification performance. One such feature selection algorithm is the sequential forward/backward procedure that finds a subset of features by sequential searching. Such an approach is computationally efficient, but the solution can be suboptimal. Another approach is to use a statistical searching algorithm such as the GA (Chan et al. 1998, Zhang et al. 2004), which can avoid potential local optimum but is computationally more expensive.

3.3.3 Classification Performance Metrics

To evaluate the performance of CADx algorithms, the technique of ROC curve is now routinely used in medical applications (Metz 2008). An ROC curve depicts the classification performance by showing the trade-off between the true-positive rate (TPR or sensitivity) as the ordinate and the false-positive rate (FPR) as the abscissa. For a given classifier, it is obtained by continuously varying the threshold associated with its decision function. The area under the ROC curve (AUC) is used to summarize the diagnostic performance. Intuitively, a larger AUC means higher benefit (sensitivity) with lower cost (false classification) and hence indicates a better performance for a classifier.

While the AUC is often calculated as the AUC over the entire FPR range of [0,1], partial AUC is also used at times. In such a case, the AUC is calculated for FPR over a range that is more meaningful to clinical practice. For example, in Baker et al. (2001), the AUC was calculated for the FPR range corresponding to a biopsy recommendation.

There exist several software tools developed for the evaluation of AUC and statistical comparison between different ROC curves. Among them, the ROCKIT (Metz et al. 1998) is commonly used for CADx of MC lesions in the literature.

As in the case of FROC curves in MC detection, it should be noted that the diagnosis performance can vary with various factors. Even for the same CADx classifier, its performance can vary with the distribution of cases used for evaluation. Thus, caution should be taken when comparing different CADx algorithms using the published results when they were obtained from different datasets.

3.3.4 CBIR in CADx

In recent years content-based image retrieval (CBIR) has been studied as an alternative aid in diagnostic imaging (Muller et al. 2004, Rahman et al. 2004), of which the goal is to provide radiologists with examples of lesions with known pathology that are similar to the lesion being evaluated (to boost their diagnostic accuracy). In order for a CBIR system to be useful as a diagnostic aid, the retrieved images must be truly relevant to the query image as perceived by the radiologists, who otherwise may simply dismiss its use as a visual aid.

Since 2000 (El-Naqa et al. 2000, 2002b, 2004), we have proposed and investigated a supervised learning approach for modeling the notion of similarity used by radiologists when they interpret mammograms. The rationale behind this approach is that the similarity metric must conform closely to the perception of the radiologists and that simple mathematical distance metrics developed in the context of general-purpose image retrieval may not adequately characterize clinical notions of image relevance, which are complex assessments made by expert observers. Similarly, standard approaches used in the general CBIR field (e.g., using features based on intensity histograms) may also be inadequate for specialized clinical applications such as mammographic interpretation.

In Alto et al. (2005), Alto selected a set of features for retrieval according to their effectiveness in classifying the masses as benign or malignant. In Muramatsu et al. (2007), a psychophysical similarity measure learned from radiologists' similarity ratings using ANN was explored. In Oh et al. (2010), a relevance feedback approach based on incremental learning with SVM regression was proposed to improve the retrieval accuracy. In Cho et al. (2011), a set of similarity metrics were explored and compared based on the radiologists' assessment with masses in ultrasound images.

A CBIR system can be viewed as a CAD tool to provide evidence for case-based reasoning. With CBIR, the system first retrieves a set of cases similar to a query and subsequently derives a decision for the query based on the information from the retrieved cases (Holt et al. 2005). For example, in Floyd et al. (2000) and Bilska-Wolak and Floyd (2002), the prediction of the query was based on the ratio of malignant cases among all retrieved cases. In Zheng et al. (2006), the similarity levels between the query and retrieval cases were used as weighting factors for prediction. In Mazurowski et al. (2008), an information theory CAD approach was further extended by assigning importance weights learned using the GA.

In recent years, we have been investigating an approach of using retrieved images to boost the classification of a CADx classifier (Jing and Yang 2010, Wei et al. 2006, 2009). In conventional CADx, a pattern classifier was first trained on a set of training cases and then applied to subsequent testing cases. Deviating from approach, for a given case to be classified (i.e., query), we will first obtain a set of known cases with similar features to that of the query case from a reference database and use these retrieved cases to adapt the CADx classifier so as to improve its classification accuracy on the query case. We will illustrate this approach with an example later in Section 3.3.6.

3.3.5 Example#1: Machine Learning Methods for MC Classification

In this section, we demonstrate the use of two pattern classifiers for the classification of clustered MCs: one is a linear classifier based on LR and the other is a nonlinear SVM classifier (Wei et al. 2005). The SVM classifier has the same form as given earlier in Equation 3.1, in which the RBF kernel is used. We give a brief description of the linear classifier here.

3.3.5.1 Linear Classifier
Mathematically, a linear classifier is of the form

$$f(\mathbf{x}) = \mathbf{w}^T \mathbf{x} + b \qquad (3.8)$$

where

  $\mathbf{x}$ is a vector denoting the features of an input pattern (i.e., lesion)
  $f(\mathbf{x})$ is the output that is typically compared against an operating threshold for the classification of $\mathbf{x}$

In practice, the discriminant vector $\mathbf{w}$ and bias b are determined from a set of training samples: $\{(\mathbf{x}_i, y_i), i = 1, ..., N\}$, where the class label $y_i \in \{-1, +1\}$ is given for each sample. In LR, these parameters $\mathbf{w}$ and b are determined through maximization of the following log-likelihood function:

$$L(\mathbf{w}, b) = \sum_{i=1}^{N} \log p(y_i, \mathbf{x}_i; \mathbf{w}, b) \qquad (3.9)$$

where the probability term is given by

$$p(y_i = 1, \mathbf{x}_i; \mathbf{w}, b) = \left[1 + \exp(-\mathbf{w}^T \mathbf{x}_i - b) \right]^{-1} \qquad (3.10)$$

This optimization problem can be solved efficiently by the method of iteratively reweighted least square (IRLS) (Bishop 2006).

3.3.5.2 Dataset Description
For testing the classifiers, a dataset of 104 cases (46 malignant, 58 benign), all containing clustered MCs, is used. This dataset was collected at the University of Chicago. It consists of some cases that are difficult to classify; the average classification performance by a group of five attending radiologists on this dataset yielded a value of only 0.62 in the AUC (Jiang et al. 1996). The MCs in these mammograms have been marked by a group of expert readers.

For this dataset, a set of eight features were extracted to characterize MC clusters (Jiang et al. 1996): (1) the number of MCs in the cluster, (2) the mean effective volume (area times effective thickness) of individual MCs, (3) the area of the cluster, (4) the circularity of the cluster, (5) the relative standard deviation of the effective thickness, (6) the relative standard deviation of the effective volume, (7) the mean area of MCs, and (8) the second highest shape-irregularity measure.

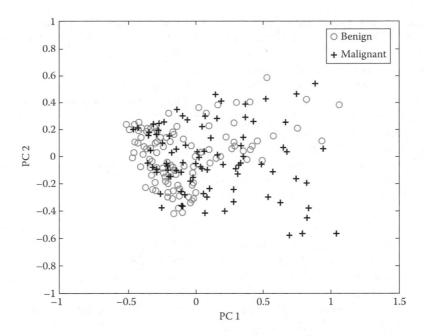

Figure 3.6   PCA plot of benign and malignant cases in the dataset.

These features were selected because they have meanings that are closely associated with features used by radiologists in the clinical diagnosis of MC lesions.

To illustrate the distribution of the cases in the dataset, we show in Figure 3.6 a scatter plot of the feature vectors of all the cases using PCA, where the first two PCA components are shown for the two classes, that is, benign and malignant. As can be seen, the samples from the two classes are mixed with each other, and there is no clear separation between the two classes. This indicates that the classification of this dataset can indeed be quite challenging.

3.3.5.3   Classification Performance
To evaluate the classifiers, a leave-one-out (LOO) procedure was applied to the 104 cases, during which each case was held out in turn for testing and the rest 103 cases were used for training the classifiers. In the end, the ROCKIT software was used to calculate the performance AUC. The linear classifier LR achieved AUC = 0.7174. In contrast, the SVM achieved AUC = 0.7373. From these results, it can be seen that the classification performance of the classifiers is far from being perfect. This highlights the difficulty in the diagnosis of MC lesions in mammograms.

3.3.6   Example#2: Using CBIR for Case-Adaptive CADx

In this section, we demonstrate the use of retrieved cases to achieve case-adaptive classification with a CADx classifier. Here we describe this approach using a linear classifier with LR (Jing and Yang 2010).

3.3.6.1   Case-Adaptive Classification Boosted with CBIR
Assume that a baseline classifier $f(\mathbf{x})$ has been already been trained with LR on a set of training samples: $\{(\mathbf{x}_i, y_i), i = 1, ..., N\}$. Now, consider a query lesion $\mathbf{x}$ to be classified. Let $\{(\mathbf{x}_i^{(r)}, y_i^{(r)}), i = 1, ..., N_r\}$ be a set of N_r retrieved cases that are similar to $\mathbf{x}$. In this approach, we use the retrieved samples $\{(\mathbf{x}_i^{(r)}, y_i^{(r)}), i = 1, ..., N_r\}$ to adapt the classifier $f(\mathbf{x})$. Specifically, the objective function in Equation 3.9 is modified as

$$L(\mathbf{w}) = \sum_{i=1}^{N} \log p(y_i, \mathbf{x}_i; \mathbf{w}) + \sum_{i=1}^{N_r} \beta_i \log p(y_i^{(r)}, \mathbf{x}_i^{(r)}; \mathbf{w}) \quad (3.11)$$

In Equation 3.11, the weighting factors β_i are adjusted according to the similarity of $\mathbf{x}_i^{(r)}$ to the query $\mathbf{x}$. The idea is to put more emphasis on those retrieved samples that are more similar to the query, with the goal of refining the decision boundary of the classifier in the neighborhood of the query. That is, the retrieved samples are now used to steer the classifier toward the neighborhood of the query $\mathbf{x}$

3.3.6.2   Dataset Description
To demonstrate this approach, a set of 589 cases, all containing MC lesions, were extracted from the benign and cancer volumes in the DDSM database maintained at the University of South Florida (Heath et al. 2001). Among these cases, 331 are benign and 258 are malignant. The extracted mammogram images were adjusted to correspond to the

same optical density and to have a uniform resolution of 0.05 mm/pixel. To quantify the MC lesions in these mammogram images, we first applied an MC detection algorithm using an SVM classifier (El-Naqa et al. 2004) to automatically locate the MCs in each lesion region provided by the dataset. To help suppress the false positives in the detection, the images were first processed with the isotropic normalization technique prior to the detection (Mcloughlin et al. 2004). The detected MCs were grouped into clusters.

Afterward, a set of descriptive features was computed for the clustered MCs, and the following nine features were selected by a sequential backward selection procedure (Guyon and Elisseeff 2003): (1) area of the cluster, (2) compactness of the cluster, (3) density of the cluster represented by the number of MCs in a unit area, (4) standard deviation of the interdistance between neighboring MCs, (5) number of MCs in the cluster, (6) sum of the size of all MC objects in the cluster, (7) mean of the average brightness in each MC object, (8) mean of the intensity standard deviation in each MC object, and (9) the compactness of the second most irregular MC object in the cluster. These features were used to form a vector **x** for each lesion in the dataset.

3.3.6.3   Classification Results

To evaluate the classifiers, an LOO procedure was applied to the cases in the dataset. In Figure 3.7, we show the performance results achieved by the case-adaptive classifier and the baseline classifier; for the adaptive classifier, the AUC value is shown with different numbers of retrieved cases N_r. From Figure 3.7, it can be seen that the best performance (AUC = 0.7755) was obtained by the adaptive classifier when $N_r = 20$, compared to AUC = 0.6848 for the baseline classifier

(p-value < 0.0001). The performance is also noted to deteriorate somewhat with increased N_r. This is because the number of similar cases for a given query is typically small due to the limited number of cases in the reference library. With large N_r, some of the retrieved cases will become less similar to the query and will not help the classification on the query.

3.4   CONCLUSION REMARKS

In recent years, many computerized methods have been developed for use in CAD schemes as a diagnostic aid to improving radiologists' diagnostic accuracy in mammography. Thanks to the intense research and development efforts, CADe systems have now been introduced clinically to screening mammography (Brem et al. 2005, Burhenne et al. 2000). There also exist clinical studies that show that CADe results in higher sensitivity with a small increase in recall rate (Birdwell et al. 2005, Cupples et al. 2005, Freer and Ulissey 2001). This is consistent with results from laboratory observer (i.e., simulated clinical reading) studies (Chan et al. 1990, Kegelmeyer et al. 1994), although one clinical study also found no apparent increase in cancer detection compared to historical control (Gur et al. 2004).

In CADx, the computer predicts the likelihood that a lesion is malignant, which is presented to the radiologist as a second opinion. Laboratory observer studies have shown that with CADx, radiologists can improve their biopsy recommendation by sending more cancer cases and fewer benign cases to biopsy (Chan et al. 1999, Hadjiiski et al. 2004, Horsch et al. 2006, Huo et al. 2002, Jiang et al. 1999).

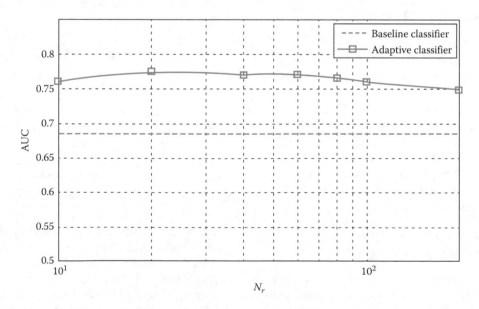

Figure 3.7   Classification performance achieved by the baseline and case-adaptive classifiers.

However, so far, CADx has not yet been introduced clinically. One difficulty in implementing CADx clinically is that a CADx classifier is often criticized for being a *black box* approach in its decision. When presented with a numerical value, such as the likelihood of malignancy, but without additional supporting evidence, it may be difficult for a radiologist to incorporate optimally this number into his or her decision. Thus, despite study results that suggest the potential benefit of CADx for clinical use, it is yet to be tested clinically.

As an alternative aid, image retrieval has been studied as a CADx tool in recent years. We conjecture that by integrating a retrieval system with the CADx classifier, the retrieved images could serve as supporting evidence to the CADx classifier, which may facilitate the interpretation of the likelihood of malignancy by the radiologists.

ACKNOWLEDGMENT

This work was supported in part by NIH grant EB009905.

REFERENCES

Alto, H., J. Desautels, and R. Rangayyan. 2005. Content-based retrieval and analysis of mammographic masses. *J. Electron. Imaging.* 14:023016.

American Cancer Society (ACS). 2014. *Cancer Facts and Figures.* American Cancer Society, Atlanta.

Andrieu, C., N.D. Freitas, A. Doucet, and M.I. Jordan. 2003. An introduction to MCMC for machine learning. *Machi. Learn.* 50:5–43.

Astley, S.M. 2004. Computer-based detection and prompting of mammographic abnormalities. *Br. J. Radiol.* 77:S194–S200.

Baker, J., P. Kornguth, J. Lo, M. Williford, and C. Floyd. 1995. Breast cancer: Prediction with artificial neural network based on BI-RADS standardized lexicon. *Radiology* 196(3):817–822.

Baker, S. and P. Pinsky. 2001. A proposed design and analysis for comparing digital and analog mammography: Special receiver operating characteristic methods for cancer screening. *J. Am. Stat. Assoc.*, 96:421–428.

Bazzani, A., A. Bevilacqua, D. Bollini, R. Brancaccio, R. Campanini, N. Lanconelli, A. Riccardi, and D. Romani. 2001. An SVM classifier to separate false signals from microcalcifications in digital mammograms. *Phys. Med. Biol.* 46:1651–1663.

Bilska-Wolak, A. and E. Floyd. 2002. Development and evaluation of a case-based reasoning classifier for prediction of breast biopsy outcome with BI-RADS™ lexicon. *Med. Phys.* 29:2090.

Birdwell, R.L., P. Bandodkar, and D.M. Ikeda. 2005. Computer-aided detection with screening mammography in a university hospital setting. *Radiology* 236:451–457.

Bishop, C.M. 2006. *Pattern Recognition and Machine Learning.* Springer, New York.

Bocchi, L., G. Coppini et al. 2004. Detection of single and clustered microcalcifications in mammograms using fractals models and neural networks. *Med. Eng. Phys.* 26(4):303–312.

Bocchi, L.G. and J. Nori. 2007. Shape analysis of microcalcifications using radon transform. *Med. Eng. Phys.* 29(6):691–698.

Brem, R.F., J.W. Hoffmeister, G. Zisman, M.P. DeSimio, and S.K. Rogers. 2005. A computer-aided detection system for the evaluation of breast cancer by mammographic appearance and lesion size. *Am. J. Roentgenol.* 184:893–896.

Bunch, P.C., J.F. Hamilton et al. 1978. A free-response approach to the measurement and characterization of radiographic-observer performance. *J. Appl. Eng.* 4:166–171.

Burhenne, L.J., S.A. Wood et al. 2000. Potential contribution of computer-aided detection to the sensitivity of screening mammography. *Radiology* 215:554–562.

Burnside, E.S., J. Davis et al. 2009. Probabilistic computer model developed from clinical data in national mammography database format to classify mammographic findings. *Radiology* 251(3):663–672.

Caputo B., T.E. La, S. Bouattour, G.E. Gigante. 2002. A new kernel method for microcalcification detection: Spin Glass-Markov Random Fields. *Studies in Health Technology and Informatics*, 90:30–34.

Casaseca-de-la-Higuera, P., A.J. Ignacio, E. Munoz-Moreno, C. Alberola-Lopez. 2005. A comparative study on microcalcification detection methods with posterior probability estimation based on Gaussian mixture models. *IEEE Engineering in Medicine and Biology Society*, 1:49–54.

Chan, H., B. Sahiner et al. 1998. Computerized analysis of mammographic microcalcifications in morphological and texture feature space. *Med. Phys.* 25:2007–2019.

Chan, H.P., K. Doi et al. 1990. Improvement in radiologists' detection of clustered microcalcifications on mammograms: The potential of computer-aided diagnosis. *Invest. Radiol.* 25:1102–1110.

Chan, H.P., B. Sahiner et al. 1999. Improvement of radiologists' characterization of mammographic masses by using computer-aided diagnosis: An ROC study. *Radiology* 212:817–827.

Chan, H.P., D. Wei, K. Lam, S. Lo, B. Sahiner, M. Helvie, and D. Adler. 1995. Computerized detection and classification of microcalcifications on mammograms. *SPIE* 2434:612–620.

Cheng, H.D., X. Cai, X. Chen, L. Hu, X. Lou. 2003. Computer-aided detection and classification of microcalcifications in mammograms: A survey. *Pattern Recog.* 36:2967–2991.

Chhatwal, J., O. Alagoz, M. Lindstrom, C. Kahn, K. Shaffer, E. Burnside. 2009. A logistic regression model based on the national mammography database format to aid breast cancer diagnosis. *Am. J. Roentgenol.* 192(4):1117–1127.

Cho, H., L. Hadjiiski, B. Sahiner, H.P. Chan, M. Helvie, C. Paramagul, and A. Nees. 2011. Similarity evaluation in a content-based image retrieval (CBIR) CADx system for characterization of breast masses on ultrasound images. *Med. Phys.* 38:1820.

Cupples, T.E., J.E. Cunningham, J.C. Reynolds. 2005. Impact of computer-aided detection in a regional screening mammography program. *Am. J. Roentgenol.* 185:944–950.

Dengler, J., S. Benrens, and H.F. Desaga. 1993. Segmentation of microcalcifications in mammograms. *IEEE Trans. Med. Imag.* 12:664–669.

Descombes, X. and J. Zerubia. 2002. Marked point process in image analysis. *IEEE Signal Proc. Mag.* 19:77–84.

Descombes, X., F. Kruggel, G. Wollny, and H.J. Gertz. 2004. An object-based approach for detecting small brain lesions: Application to Virchow-Robin spaces. *IEEE Trans. Med. Imag.* 23:246–255.

Dhawan, A.P., Y. Chitre et al. 1996. Analysis of mammographic microcalcifications using gray-level image structure features. *IEEE Trans. Med. Imag.* 15(3):246–259.

El-Naqa, I., Y. Yang, M.N. Wernick, and N.P. Galasanos. 2000. Image retrieval based on similarity learning. *International Conference on Image Processing* , Chicago, IL. 13:722–725.

El-Naqa, I., Y. Yang, M.N. Wernick, and N.P. Galasanos. 2002a. Content-based image retrieval for digital mammography. *Intl. Conf. Image Process.* 3:141–144.

El-Naqa, I., Y. Yang et al. 2002b. A support vector machine approach for detection of microcalcifications. *IEEE Trans. Med. Imag.* 21(12):1552–1563.

El-Naqa, I., Y. Yang et al. 2004. A similarity learning approach to content based image retrieval: Application to digital mammography. *IEEE Trans. Med. Imag.* 23:1233–1244.

El-Naqa, I. and Y. Yang. 2005. Techniques in the detection of microcalcification (MC) clusters in digital mammograms. In *Medical Imaging Systems: Technology and Applications*, Edited by Cornelius T. Leondes World Scientific Publishing Co. Pvt. Ltd, 4:15–36.

Elmore, J.G., M.B. Barton, V.M. Moceri, S. Polk, P.J. Arena, and S.W. Fletcher. 1998. Ten-year risk of false positive screening mammograms and clinical breast examinations. *N Engl. J. Med.* 338:1089–1096.

Elter, M. and A. Horsch. 2009. CADx of mammographic masses and clustered microcalcifications: A review. *Med. Phys.* 36:2052–2068.

Floyd, C.E., J. Lo, and G.D. Tourassi. 2000. Case-based reasoning computer algorithm that uses mammographic findings for breast biopsy decisions. *Am. J. Roentgenol.* 175(5):1347–1352.

Freer, T.W. and M.J. Ulissey. 2001. Screening mammography with computer-aided detection: Prospective study of 12,860 patients in a community breast center. *Radiology* 220:781–786.

Gang, D. and S.T. Acton. 2005. Object identification by marked point process. In *39th Asilomar Conference on Signals, Systems and Computers*, Pacific Grove, CA. 294–297.

Grayer, C.J. and J. Moeller. 1994. Simulation procedures and likelihood inference for spatial point processes. *Scand. J. Stat.* 21:359–373.

Gupta, S., P.E. Chyn, and M.K. Markey. 2006. Breast cancer cadx based on bi-rads descriptors from two mammographic views. *Med. Phys.* 33(6):1810–1817.

Gur, D., J.H. Sumkin et al. 2004. Changes in breast cancer detection and mammography recall rates after the introduction of a computer-aided detection system. *J. Natl. Cancer Inst.* 96:185–190.

Gurcan, M.N., H.P. Chan et al. 2002. Optimal neural network architecture selection: Improvement in computerized detection of microcalcifications. *Acad. Radiol.* 9(4):420–429.

Gurcan, M.N., Y. Yardimci, A.E. Cetin, R. Ansari. 1997. Detection of microcalcifications in mammograms using higher order statistics. *IEEE Signal Processing Letters*, 4(8):213–216.

Guyon, I. and A. Elisseeff. 2003. An introduction to variable and feature selection. *J. Mach. Learn. Res.* 3:1157–1182.

Hadjiiski, L., H.P. Chan et al. 2004. Improvement in radiologists' characterization of malignant and benign breast masses on serial mammograms with computer-aided diagnosis: An ROC study. *Radiology* 233:255–265.

Haralick, R., K. Shanmugam, and I. Dinstein. 1973. Textural features for image classification. *IEEE Trans. Systems, Man Cyber.* 3:610–621.

Heath, M., K. Bowyer, D. Kopans, R. Moore, and W.P. Kegelmeyer. 2001. The digital database for screening mammography. *The Fifth International Workshop on Digital Mammography*, Toronto, Canada. 212–218.

Holt, A., I. Bichindaritz, R. Schmidt, and P. Perner. 2005. Medical applications in case-based reasoning. *Knowl. Eng. Rev.* 20:289–292.

Horsch, K., M.L. Giger, C.J. Vyborny, L. Lan, E.B. Mendelson, and R.E. Hendrick. 2006. Classification of breast lesions with multimodality computer-aided diagnosis: Observer study results on an independent clinical data set. *Radiology* 240:357–368.

Huo, Z., M.L. Giger, C.J. Vyborny, and C.E. Metz. 2002. Breast cancer: Effectiveness of computer-aided diagnosis observer study with independent database of mammograms. *Radiology* 224:560–568.

Jiang, Y., R.M. Nishikawa, E.E. Wolverton, C.E. Metz, M.L. Giger, R.A. Schmidt, and C.J. Vyborny. 1996. Malignant and benign clustered microcalcifications: Automated feature analysis and classification. *Radiology* 198:671–678.

Jiang, Y., R.M. Nishikawa, M.L. Giger, K. Doi, R. Schmidt, and C. Vyborny. 1992. Method of extracting signal area and signal thickness of microcalcifications from digital mammograms. *Proc. SPIE.* 1778:28–36.

Jiang, Y., R.M. Nishikawa, R.A. Schmidt, C.E. Metz, M.L. Giger, and K. Doi. 1999. Improving breast cancer diagnosis with computer-aided diagnosis. *Acad. Radiol.* 6:22–33.

Jing, H. and Y. Yang. 2009. Detection of clustered microcalcifications using spatial point process modeling. *Intl. Symp. Biomed. Imaging.* 81–84.

Jing, H. and Y. Yang. 2010. Case-adaptive classification based on image retrieval for computer-aided diagnosis. *IEEE International Conference on Image Processing*, Hong Kong. 4333–4336.

Jing, H., Y. Yang, and R.M. Nishikawa. 2011. Detection of clustered microcalcifications using spatial point process modeling. *Phys. Med. Biol.* 56:1–17.

Joshua, J., M.D. Fenton et al. 2007. Influence of computer-aided detection on performance of screening mammography. *N. Engl. J. Med.* 356:1399–1409.

Kallergi, M. 2004. Computer-aided diagnosis of mammographic microcalcification clusters. *Med. Phys.* 31:314–326.

Kallergi, M., G.M. Carney, and J. Garviria. 1999. Evaluating the performance of detection algorithms in digital mammography. *Med. Phys.* 26(2):267–275.

Karssemeijer, N. 1992. Stochastic model for automated detection of calcifications in digital mammograms. *Image Vision Comput.* 10:369–375.

Kegelmeyer, W.P. Jr., J.M. Pruneda, P.D. Bourland, A. Hillis, M.W. Riggs, and M.L. Nipper. 1994. Computer-aided mammographic screening for spiculated lesions. *Radiology* 191:331–337.

Kolb, T.M., J. Lichy, and J.H. Newhouse. 2002. Comparison of the performance of screening mammography, physical examination, and breast US and evaluation of factors that influence them: An analysis of 27,825 patient evaluations. *Radiology* 225:165–175.

Li, H., K.J. Liu, and S. Lo. 1997. Fractal modeling and segmentation for the enhancement of microcalcifications in digital mammograms. *IEEE Trans. Med. Imag.* 16:785–798.

Linguraru, M.G., K. Marias et al. 2006. A biologically inspired algorithm for microcalcification cluster detection. *Med. Image. Anal.* 10(6):850–862.

Lo, J.Y., M.A. Gavrielides, M.K. Markey, and J.L. Jesneck. 2003. Computer-aided classification of breast microcalcification clusters: Merging of features from image processing and radiologists. *Proc. SPIE—Int. Soc. Opt. Eng.* (USA), 5032:882–889.

Lo, J., M.K. Markey, J. Baker, and C. Floyd. 2002. Cross-institutional evaluation of BI-RADS predictive model for mammographic diagnosis of breast cancer. *Am. J. Roentgenol.* 178(2):457–463.

Markopoulos, C., E. Kouskos, K. Koufopoulos, V. Kyriakou, and J. Gogas. 2001. Use of artificial neural networks (computer analysis) in the diagnosis of microcalcifications on mammography. *Eur. J. Radiol.* 39(1):60–65.

Mazurowski, M.A., P.A. Habas, J.M. Zurada, and G.D. Tourassi. 2008. Decision optimization of case-based computer-aided decision systems using genetic algorithms with application to mammography. *Phys. Med. Biol.* 53(4):895–908.

Mcloughlin, K.J., P.J. Bones, and N. Karssemeijer. 2004. Noise equalization for detection of microcalcification clusters in direct digital mammogram images. *IEEE Trans. Med. Imag.* 23(3):313–320.

Metz, C. 2008. ROC analysis in medical imaging: A tutorial review of the literature. *Radiol. Phys. Technol.* 1:2–12.

Metz, C., B. Herman, and J. Shen. 1998. Maximum-likelihood estimation of ROC curves from continuously-distributed data. *Stat. Med.* 17:1033–1053.

Morrow, W.M., R.B. Paranjape, R.M. Rangayyan, and J.E.L. Desautels. 1992. Region-based contrast enhancement of mammograms. *IEEE Trans. Med. Imag.* 11:392–406.

MØller, J. and R.P. Waagepetersen. 2006. Modern statistic for spatial point processes. *Nordic Conference on Mathematical Statistics*, Rebild, Denmark.

Muller, H., N. Michoux, D. Bandon, and A. Geissbuhler. 2004. A review of content-based image retrieval system in medical applications-clinical benefits and future directions. *Int. J. Med. Informat.* 73:1–23.

Muramatsu, C., Q. Li, R. Schmidt, J. Shiraishi, K. Suzuki, G. Newstead, and K. Doi. 2007. Investigation of similarity measures for selection of similar images for breast lesions on mammograms. *Med. Phys.* 34:23–38.

Mushlin, A.I., R.W. Kouides, and D.E. Shapiro. 1998. Estimating the accuracy of screening mammography: A meta-analysis. *Am. J. Prev. Med.* 14:143–153.

Nakayama, R., H. Abe, J. Shiraishi, and K. Doi. 2009. Potential usefulness of similar images in the differential diagnosis of clustered microcalcifications on mammograms. *Radiology* 253:625–631.

Netsch, T. 1996. A scale-space approach for the detection of clustered microcalcifications in digital mammograms. In *Digital Mammography, Proceedings of the 3rd International Workshop on Digital Mammography*, Chicago, IL. 301–306.

Nishikawa, R.M. 2007. Current status and future directions of computer-aided diagnosis in mammography. *Comput. Med. Imag. Graph.* 31:224–235.

Nishikawa, R.M., M.L. Giger et al. 1995. Computer-aided detection of clustered microcalcifications on digital mammograms. *Med. Biol. Eng. Comput.* 33:174–178.

Oh, J., Y. Yang, and I. El-Naqa. 2010. Adaptive learning for relevance feedback: Application to digital mammography. *Med. Phys.* 37:4432.

Papadopoulos, A., D.I. Fotiadis, and A. Likas. 2005. Characterization of clustered microcalcifications in digitized mammograms using neural networks and support vector machines. *Artif. Intell. Med.* 34:141–150.

Peng, Y., B. Yao et al. 2006. Knowledge-discovery incorporated evolutionary search for microcalcification detection in breast cancer diagnosis. *Artif. Intell. Med.* 37(1):43–53.

Qian, W., F. Mao et al. 2002. An improved method of region grouping for microcalcification detection in digital mammograms. *Comput. Med. Imag. Graph* 26(6):361–368.

Rahman, M., T. Want, and B. Desai. 2004. Medical image retrieval and registration: Towards computer assisted diagnostic approach. In *Proceedings of IDEAS Workshop on Medical Information Systems: The Digital Hospital*, Beijing, China. 78–89.

Rangayyan, R.M., J.A. Fabio, and J.L. Desautels. 2007. A review of computer-aided diagnosis of breast cancer: Toward the detection of subtle signs. *J. Franklin Inst.* 344:312–348.

Sajda, P., C. Spence et al. 2002. Learning contextual relationships in mammograms using a hierarchical pyramid neural network. *IEEE Trans. Med. Imag.* 21(3):239–250.

Salfity, M.F., R.M. Nishikawa, Y. Jiang, and J. Papaioannou. 2003. The use of a priori information in the detection of mammographic microcalcifications to improve their classification. *Med. Phys.* 30:823–831.

Sampat, M.P., M.K. Markey, and A.C. Bovik. 2005. Computer-aided detection and diagnosis in mammography. Chap. 10.4, *Handbook of Image & Video Processing*, 2nd ed., Elsevier Academic Press.

Shen, L., R. Rangayyan, and J. Desautels. 1994. Application of shape analysis to mammographic calcifications. *IEEE TMI.* 13:263–274.

Singh, S., V. Kumar et al. 2006. SVM based system for classification of Microcalcifications in digital mammograms. *Conference Proceedings of IEEE Engineering in Medicine Biology and Society* 1:4747–4750.

Soltanian-Zadeh, H., F. Rafiee-Rad, and S. Pourabdollah-Nejad. 2004. Comparison of multiwavelet, wavelet, Haralick, and shape features for microcalcification classification in mammograms. *Pattern Recog.* 37:1973–1986.

Strickland, R.N. and H.L. Hahn. 1996. Wavelet transforms for detecting microcalcifications in mammograms. *IEEE Trans. Med. Imag.* 15:218–229.

Strickland, R.N. and H.L. Hahn. 1997. Wavelet transforms methods for object detection and recovery. *IEEE Trans. Image Proc.* 6:724–735.

Stoica, R., X. Descombes, and J. Zerubia. 2004. A Gibbs process for road extraction from remotely sensed images. *Int. J. Comput. Vis.* 57:2004.

Tan, A., D.H. Freeman, Jr., J.S. Goodwin, and J.L. Freeman. 2006. Variation in false-positive rates of mammography reading among 1067 radiologists: A population-based assessment. *Breast Cancer Res. Treat.* 100:309–318.

Tay, P. and Y. Ma. 2010. A novel microcalcification shape metric to classify regions of interests. *IEEE Southwest Symposium on Image Analysis & Interpretation*, Austin, TX. 201–204.

Thiele, D.L., C. Kimme-Smith, T.D. Johnson, M. McCombs, and L. Bassett. 1996. Using tissue texture surrounding calcification clusters to predict benign vs malignant outcomes. *Med. Phys.* 23(4):549–555.

Urbain, J.L. 2005. Breast cancer screening, diagnostic accuracy and health care policies. *Can. Med. Assoc. J.* 172:210–211.

Veldkamp, W. and N. Karssemeijer. 2000. Noise of local contrast in mammograms. *IEEE Trans. Med. Imag.* 19:731–738.

Wei, L., Y. Yang et al. 2005. Relevance vector machine for automatic detection of clustered microcalcifications. *IEEE Trans. Med. Imag.* 24(10):1278–1285.

Wei, L., Y. Yang, R.M. Nishikawa, and Y. Jiang. 2005. A study on several machine-learning methods for classification of malignant and benign clustered microcalcifications. *IEEE Trans. Med. Imag.*, 24(3):371–380.

Wei, L., Y. Yang, R.M. Nishikawa, and Y. Jiang. 2006. Learning of perceptual similarity from expert readers for mammogram retrieval. *IEEE International Symposium on Biomedical Imaging*, Arlington, VA. 1356–1359.

Wei, L., Y. Yang, and R.M. Nishikawa. 2009. Microcalcification classification assisted by content-based image retrieval for breast cancer diagnosis. *Pattern Recog.* 42:1126–1132.

Wu, Y., M. Giger, K. Doi, C. Vyborny, R. Schmidt, and C. Metz. 1993. Artificial neural networks in mammography: Application to decision making in the diagnosis of breast cancer. *Radiology* 187(1):81–87.

Yoshida, H., K. Doi, and R.M. Nishikawa. 1994. Automated detection of clustered microcalcifications. In *Digital Mammograms Using Wavelet Transform Techniques. Medical Imaging*. Bellingham, WA: SPIE, pp. 868–886.

Yu, S. and L. Guan. 2000. A CAD system for the automatic detection of clustered microcalcifications in digitized mammogram films. *IEEE Trans. Med. Imag.* 19:115–126.

Zhang, P., B. Verma, and K. Kumar. 2004. A neural-genetic algorithm for feature selection and breast abnormality classification in digital mammography. *IEEE International Joint Conference on Neural Networks (IJCNN)*.

Zheng, B., 2009. Computer-aided Diagnosis in mammography using CBIR approaches: current status and future perspective. *Algorithms*, 2(2):828–849.

Zheng, B., A. Lu et al. 2006. A method to improve visual similarity of breast masses for an interactive computer-aided diagnosis environment. *Med. Phys.* 33:111–117.

Zweig, M.H. and G. Campbell. 1993. Receiver-operating characteristic (ROC) plots: A fundamental evaluation tool in clinical medicine. *Clin. Chem.* 39(8):561–577.

Chapter 4

Detection and Diagnosis of Breast Mass in Digital Tomosynthesis

Heang-Ping Chan

CONTENTS

4.1 INTRODUCTION

Breast cancer is the most prevalent cancer and ranks second as a cause of cancer death among American women (American Cancer Society, 2011). Despite the recent controversial recommendations by the U.S. Preventive Services Task Force (2009), considerable evidences continue to indicate that early diagnosis and treatment resulting from mammographic screening significantly improve the chance of survival for patients with breast cancer (Hendrick and Helvie, 2011; Mook et al., 2011; Tabár et al., 2011; van Schoor et al., 2011). Although mammography has a high sensitivity for the detection of breast cancers when compared to other diagnostic modalities, studies indicate that radiologists' sensitivities vary over a wide range (Breast Cancer Surveillance Consortium, 2009; Elmore et al., 2009). A major problem in screening mammography is the limited sensitivity in dense breasts (Mandelson et al., 2000; Pediconi et al., 2009) due to the reduced conspicuity of lesions obscured by overlapping dense fibroglandular tissue. Another problem in screening is the high recall rate (Schell et al., 2007). Many of these recalls are caused by overlapping tissue mimicking a lesion. Finally, the specificity of screening mammography for differentiating lesions as malignant and benign is

very low. In the United States, the positive predictive value of recommended biopsies ranges from about 15% to 30% (Rosenberg et al., 2006). Recall and benign biopsies not only cause patient anxiety, but also increase health care costs.

A potential approach to reducing missed cancer is to include ultrasound (US) scans in the screening exams of dense breasts. US scanning is time consuming and relatively operator dependent. It may be used only as an adjunct to mammography for a selected patient population. Automated breast US is under development but has not reached consistent image quality for routine clinical use. Breast magnetic resonance will be too expensive and has relatively low specificity, limiting its use to high-risk patients and diagnostic purposes.

The advent of high-resolution digital detectors has enabled the development of new techniques for reducing overlapping breast structures such as digital breast tomosynthesis (DBT) (Niklason et al., 1997), breast computed tomography (breast CT) (Boone et al., 2001; Chen and Ning, 2002), and stereomammography (Goodsitt et al., 2000, 2002; Getty et al., 2001; Chan et al., 2003). These techniques provide image information in the third dimension, which can not only reduce the camouflaging effects of overlapping tissue but also improve the assessment of lesion characteristics, thus facilitating the differentiation of normal tissue from cancerous lesions even in fatty breasts (Rafferty et al., 2002; Chan et al., 2003; Helvie et al., 2008). Breast CT is a true 3D imaging modality and does not use compression during exposure. However, the availability of breast CT system is limited at present, and only a few studies have been performed to evaluate its image quality, radiation dose, and lesion detectability (Lindfors et al., 2010; O'Connell et al., 2010).

Pilot clinical studies using prototype DBT systems have been conducted to compare DBTs with mammography in breast cancer detection. Promising initial results have prompted full-field digital mammography (FFDM) system manufacturers to develop DBT systems, and one has obtained FDA approval for using DBT in conjunction with FFDM in screening. Important issues related to image quality and visibility of microcalcifications, protocols for integrating DBT into screening (e.g., as a stand-alone modality replacing both views of FFDM, used in parallel with FFDM by replacing one view, or as an adjunct by adding one or two DBT views to two-view FFDM, etc.), and the associated system design parameters, patient exposure, and radiologists' reading time are still at early stages of investigation. Poplack et al. (2007) compared the image quality of diagnostic film mammograms to DBT and evaluated the effect of adding DBT to FFDM screening on the recall rate in 98 women. They found that the recall rate could be reduced by 40% with the addition of DBT, and the DBT image quality was equivalent or superior to the diagnostic mammogram in 89% of the cases, but the conspicuity of microcalcifications was inferior in 8 of the 14 cases. Smith et al. (2008) performed an observer study using 316 cases and 12 observers to compare lesion detection on FFDM to that on combined FFDM and DBT. They found that the combined FFDM and DBT reading improved the area under the receiver operating characteristic (ROC) curve (AUC) for all radiologists and the mean recall rate decreased by about 39%. However, this improvement was gained at the cost of doubling the dose. Gur et al. (2009) conducted an observer study to compare two-view FFDM alone to two-view DBT alone and FFDM (two-view) + DBT (two-view). They found that DBT alone can reduce recall rate by about 10% while FFDM + DBT could reduce recall rate by 30% without a conclusive change in sensitivity due to the small number of cancers in their study. In the verified truth table (Table 1) of their paper, it appears that three benign MC clusters that were seen in FFDM were not visible in DBT, whereas six benign masses not seen in FFDM were seen in DBT. Gennaro et al. (2010) performed an ROC study to compare lesion detection and characterization in two-view FFDM with that in single mediolateral oblique (MLO)-view DBT acquired at the same dose as standard screen-film mammography in 376 breasts. They found that the proportions of lesions classified by radiologists with

DBT conspicuity higher than or equal to that of FFDM were more prevalent than the proportions of lesions rated otherwise. They also demonstrated that clinical performance of DBT in one view is noninferior to FFDM in two views.

Helvie et al. (2008) evaluated two-view DBT for subjects that were recommended for the biopsy of breast masses. They found four T1 invasive cancers (size 5–8 mm) by DBT not diagnosed by conventional breast imaging or physical examination in a series of 190 consecutive subjects who were recommended for biopsy of other lesions in the same breast. Two of these were found in Breast Imaging–Reporting and Data System density 1 and 2 breasts. They also conducted a number of observer studies to compare lesion visibility in DBT with that in mammograms. In a comparison of 30 consecutive mass cases, Helvie et al. (2007) found that the number of masses seen and the mass margin visibility were significantly better in DBT, and the likelihood of malignancy assessment was more accurate in DBT. In a study of 92 breasts with biopsy-proven MC clusters, Helvie et al. (2009) found that, using maximum intensity projection in 1 cm thick slabs, by view, 97% of the malignant and 96% of the benign MC clusters were visible in DBT, and by case, 100% were visible.

One of the major concerns of bringing DBT into clinical practice is the large number of reconstructed slices for each breast that need to be read by radiologists. Even at 1 mm slice thickness, the number of slices per view of the breast will range from about 30 to over 80. Although the correlation between adjacent slices and the less complex background makes it much more efficient in reading each slice than reading a regular mammogram, an initial study showed that the time required for the interpretation of a DBT case was still substantially longer than that for mammograms (Gur et al., 2009). With the increase in radiologists' workload, the chance for oversight of subtle lesions may increase. Computer-assisted reading may therefore play an important role in DBT.

Computer-aided detection (CADe) in screening mammography has been introduced into clinical use for over 10 years. Studies to date shows that CADe can improve radiologists' lesion detection sensitivity in retrospective studies (Chan et al., 1990; WarrenBurhenne et al., 2000; Brem et al., 2003; Destounis et al., 2004) and in prospective clinical trials (Freer and Ulissey, 2001; Bandodkar et al., 2002; Helvie et al., 2004; Birdwell et al., 2005; Cupples et al., 2005; Khoo et al., 2005; Dean and Ilvento, 2006; Morton et al., 2006; Gilbert et al., 2008; Gromet, 2008; James et al., 2010), but moderately increase recall rate due to its recommended use as a second reader. The majority of prospective clinical trials in screening mammography reported an increase in cancer detection sensitivity ranging from 5% to 19%, accompanied by an increase in recall rate from 6% to 31%. Gur et al. (2004) found that CADe had no significant effect on the radiologists in their academic setting when they averaged the results from both low-volume and high-volume radiologists.

Further analysis of Gur's data by Feig et al. (2004) indicated that the 17 low-volume radiologists in Gur's study achieved an increase in the sensitivity of 19.7%, similar to those reported in other studies. In another prospective study, Gromet (2008) compared nine experienced radiologists' first reading of 112,413 cases without CADe followed by a double read by a general radiologist, and a single reading of 118,808 cases with CADe. It was found that CADe increased breast cancer detection sensitivity by 11% with only a 3.9% increase in the recall rate. The improvement in sensitivity was comparable to double reading, while the increase in recall rate was significantly lower, demonstrating that single reading with CADe is a viable alternative to double reading. Gilbert et al. (2008) compared single reading with CADe to double reading in a prospective randomized trial for over 28,000 cases in three mammography screening centers and found that single reading with CADe was similar to double reading in cancer detection sensitivity with a significant increase in recall rate in one of the three centers. Fenton et al. (2011) estimated the change in sensitivity, specificity, breast cancer detection rate, and recall rates, among measures, after the implementation of CADe in 25 community screening facilities, together with another 65 screening facilities never implemented CADe as reference. They reported that the sensitivity for the detection of ductal carcinomas in situ (DCIS) increased, while that for invasive cancers decreased with CADe, although neither reached statistical significance. If radiologists use CADe as a second reader as approved by FDA, the sensitivity of cancer detection should never decrease, that is, even if the CADe system is totally useless, the radiologists should have detected as many cancers as they would without CADe if they read the mammograms in the same way as they should as the sole reader. The fact that their computer-aided readings seem to track the performance of the CADe systems, which generally have higher sensitivity for microcalcifications (more likely DCIS) and lower sensitivity for masses (more likely invasive cancer) than radiologists, raised a strong concern that the participating radiologists might have overrelied on the CADe system and did not maintain their vigilance in the first read. Or worse, as stated by Fenton et al. (2011), some community radiologists may use CADe in a *nonstandardized idiosyncratic* fashion; for example, they may decide not to recall women because of the absence of CADe marks on otherwise suspicious lesions. Similar observation was also reported by Taplin et al. (2006). These studies demonstrate that improper use of CADe could cause serious problems, similar to the improper use of other well-intended medical devices or drugs. User training and certain safeguard to assure proper use of CADe in the clinic are essential in order to realize the true potential of CADe.

Other than studies with possible misuse of CADe, most studies indicate that CADe in screening mammography can generally improve radiologists' sensitivity in lesion detection, but the extent of the influence will depend on the performance of the CADe system, the level of experience of the radiologist, and, most importantly, how the radiologist makes use of the CADe information. Since DBT is a new modality, whether radiologists' experience in the interpretation of mammograms without or with CADe can be directly transferred to DBT is still unknown. Further studies will be needed to evaluate the impact of CADe in DBT when CADe systems for DBT become available.

4.2 IMAGING CHARACTERISTICS OF BREAST TOMOSYNTHESIS

The principle of tomosynthesis is the same as conventional tomography, but digital imaging allows the reconstruction of slices at any depths from a single scan, resulting in much lower dose and higher image quality. The trajectory of the x-ray source in tomosynthesis can take on many forms, but a linear path or an arc about a fulcrum is most commonly used because of the relatively simple mechanical design. At present, all DBT systems take the latter approach. A stationary DBT system that uses a carbon nanotube-based multibeam field emission X-ray source in a linear array is under development (Qian et al., 2009). If successful, multibeam X-ray source will eliminate the mechanical motion and may provide faster image acquisition for tomosynthesis imaging.

A schematic of a typical mechanical scanning DBT system is shown in Figure 4.1. DBT is similar to mammography such that the breast is imaged under compression. A sequence of projection views (PVs) is acquired by the digital detector as the X-ray source is rotated to different angular positions about a fulcrum over a finite angular range (referred to as the tomo angle in the following). The detector may be stationary or moving synchronously in the opposite

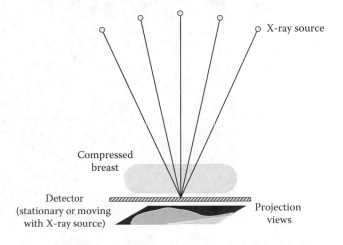

Figure 4.1 A schematic of a digital breast tomosynthesis system.

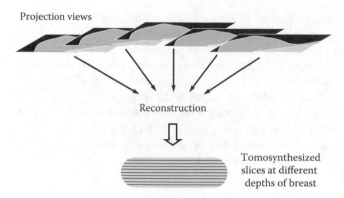

Figure 4.2   Tomosynthesis reconstruction to produce image slices.

direction to the X-ray source to acquire a PV at each angular position. The X-ray source may be moved continuously or in a step-and-shoot fashion during image acquisition. With a proper tomosynthesis reconstruction algorithm, tomographic slices focused at any depth can be generated from the PVs (Figure 4.2). Because of the wide dynamic range and the linear response of the digital detector, each PV can be acquired with a fraction of the exposure used for a regular mammogram. The total dose required for DBT may be kept at essentially the same as that of a regular mammogram.

DBT image quality depends on the angular range of the tomographic scan, the number and the distribution of PVs, and reconstruction algorithms. Reconstruction methods including shift-and-add, tuned aperture computed tomography, maximum likelihood-convex (ML-convex) algorithm, matrix inversion tomosynthesis, filtered backprojection

(FBP), and simultaneous algebraic reconstruction technique (SART) have been investigated (Niklason et al., 1997; Suryanarayanan et al., 2001; Dobbins and Godfrey, 2003; Wu et al., 2003; Zhang et al., 2006), and studies to improve the reconstruction methods and artifact reduction techniques are ongoing (Zhang et al., 2007, 2009; Sidky et al., 2009; Lu et al., 2010). DBT images are usually reconstructed in slices parallel to the detector plane. The spatial resolution on the reconstructed DBT slices can approach that of the digital detector if the geometry of the scanning system is accurately known and patient motion is kept at a minimum. However, some degree of blurring is inevitable due to the reconstruction from multiple PVs with different X-ray incident angles and oblique incidence of the X-ray beam to the detector, especially at large projection angles (Mainprize et al., 2006). Because of the lack of PVs at large projection angles, the spatial resolution in the direction perpendicular to the detector plane (the depth or z-direction) is poor. The depth resolution is mainly determined by the tomographic angle; the larger the angle, the higher the depth resolution and the less the interplane artifact. The reconstruction method can affect the interplane artifact to a certain extent, but tomosynthesis cannot provide true 3D information due to the lack of sampling over a wide angular range.

Figure 4.3 shows an example of a DBT volume containing a mass reconstructed by SART with 1 mm slice interval to demonstrate the resolution in the three perpendicular planes. Figure 4.4 shows another example of a DBT volume that contained a cluster of microcalcifications. Both scans were obtained with a DBT system that acquired 21 PVs at an

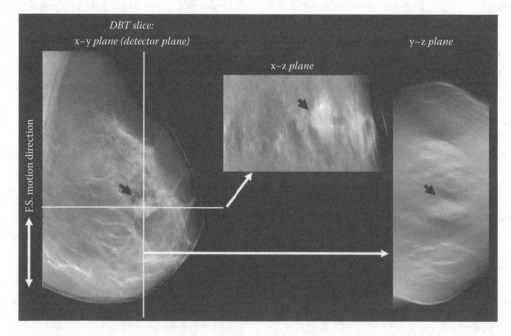

Figure 4.3   Example of a DBT reconstructed volume and the three cross-sectional planes intersecting the mass. The x–y plane is parallel to the detector.

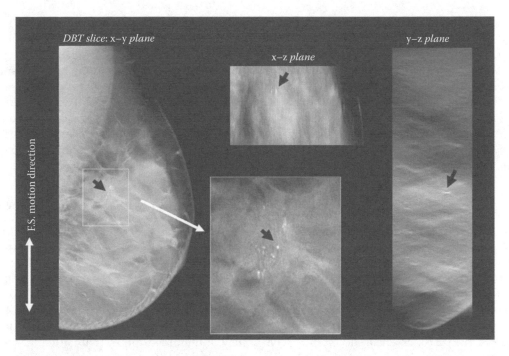

Figure 4.4 Example of a DBT reconstructed volume and the three cross-sectional planes intersecting a microcalcification. The x–y plane is parallel to the detector.

angular increment of 3° over a tomo angle of 60°. The dense calcification is sharp on the x–y plane, but its shadow extends a few slices above and below the in-focus plane. The mass has lobulated margin clearly seen on the detector (x–y) plane, but is blurry, especially in the z direction, on the x–z or y–z plane. The density of the mass extends to much greater distance in the z-direction than is expected from its diameter seen on the x–y plane. The limited resolution in the z-direction makes it difficult to perform accurate segmentation or volumetric analysis of lesions or glandular tissue in DBT volume. The texture patterns on the x–z and y–z planes are also different from that on the x–y plane. Feature extraction on the x–z and y–z planes may result in inaccurate representation of the lesion characteristics. Despite the limitations, the reduction of tissue overlap on the x–y planes has been shown to be useful in lesion detection and characterization (Helvie et al., 2007, 2008, 2009).

Zhao and Zhao (2008) and Zhao et al. (2009) developed a 3D linear model for DBT to study the effects of imaging parameters and the FBP reconstruction filter on the noise power spectrum and modulation transfer function and detective quantum efficiency of a prototype DBT system. Sechopoulos and Ghetti (2009) developed a computer model that included breast structured noise background to study the relationship between the acquisition geometry and an image quality factor, which accounted for both the in-plane contrast-to-noise ratio (CNR) and the artifact spread function (ASF), defined as the normalized CNR as a function of distance in the depth direction from the focal plane of an object of interest. They found that, under the conditions in their study

(5 cm thick breast, 3 mm spherical mass, 0.4 x 0.4 x 0.4 mm³ calcification, ML-expectation-maximization reconstruction, and limited total dose), the image quality factor improved with increasing tomo angle, while the number of PVs had a threshold value beyond which the ASF did not improve further. Zhang et al. (2008) and Lu et al. (2011) performed preliminary phantom studies and compared reconstruction image quality for DBT scans by selecting six subsets of 11 PVs including different tomo angles and uniform or nonuniform angular increments from the original DBT scans that acquired 21 PVs at 3° increments over a 60° angular range. It was shown that DBT acquired with a large angular range or, for an equal angular range, with a large fraction of PVs at large angles yielded superior ASF with smaller full width half maximum (FWHM) in the z-direction. PV distributions with a narrow angular range or a large fraction of PVs at small angles had stronger interplane artifacts. In the x–y focal planes, the effect of PV distributions on spatial blurring depended on the directions. In the x-direction (perpendicular to the chest wall), the difference in the spatial blurring among the different PV distributions is negligibly small. In the y-direction (x-ray source motion), the PV distributions with a narrow angular range or a large fraction of PVs at small angles had less blurring. In addition, PV distributions with a narrow angular range or a large fraction of PVs at small angles yielded slightly higher CNR than those with a wide angular range for small objects such as subtle microcalcifications; however, PV distributions had no obvious effect on CNR for relatively large high-contrast objects such

as dense calcifications. In general, PV distributions affect the image quality of DBT. The relative importance of the impact depends on the characteristics of the signal and the direction relative to the tomographic scan. For a given number of PVs, the angular range and the distribution of the PVs affect the degree of in-plane and interplane blurring in opposite ways. The design of the scan parameters of tomosynthesis systems would require proper consideration of the characteristics of the signals of interest and the potential trade-off of the image quality of different types of signals.

4.3 COMPUTER-AIDED DETECTION AND DIAGNOSIS METHODS IN BREAST TOMOSYNTHESIS

In DBT, two sets of images are available for analysis: one set contains the PVs acquired at different angles and the other contains the reconstructed DBT slices that constitute the breast volume. An example showing a conventional mammogram, one of the PVs in a DBT scan and a slice from a reconstructed DBT volume, is shown in Figure 4.5. Computerized lesion detection or characterization can be performed in many different ways and may be loosely grouped into three main approaches. One approach is to perform image analysis in the individual 2D PV images and then combine the information from the multiple PVs. The second approach is to combine the information in the PVs first by tomosynthesis reconstruction and then perform image analysis in the reconstructed slices or in the 3D volume. The third approach is to perform the 2D and 3D approaches in parallel and then combine the information from the two approaches, or

performing image analyses on the PVs, DBT slices, or the 3D volume at different processing steps in combination. Since there are numerous alternative computer-vision techniques that can be used in performing the different processes in a CADe system, such as prescreening, feature extraction, and feature classification, specific techniques for these processes will not be described here. Rather, we will discuss some general approaches and point out the differences and similarities between CADe in DBT and regular mammograms that may serve as a guide for future developments.

4.3.1 Analysis of Projection View Images

In this approach, image analysis is performed directly on the PV images. The information extracted from the detected lesion candidates on the PV images is then combined in 3D using the known geometry of the DBT system, as illustrated in Figure 4.6. This approach has the advantage of being independent of the reconstruction method. In addition, an individual PV is basically a regular mammogram so that computer-vision techniques developed for 2D mammograms may be applicable to PV images. However, the signal-to-noise ratio (SNR) in a PV is much lower than in a regular mammogram due to the much lower dose used for PV acquisition so that the previous methods will have to be adapted to the noisy images (see Figure 4.5a and b). Because of the low SNR, the signals may be difficult to detect without including a large number of false positives (FPs), and some weak signals may be rendered undetectable in the noisy background. The subsequent integration of information from the multiple PVs is an important step in reducing FPs. The lesion

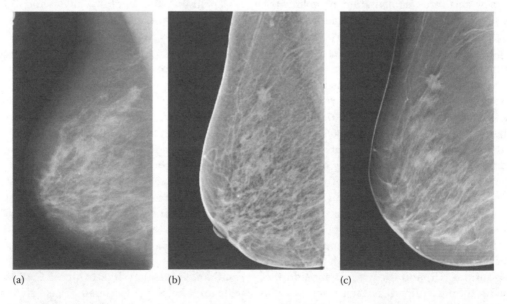

(a)   (b)   (c)

Figure 4.5   (a) An MLO mammogram of a breast with a spiculated mass. (b) The central projection view mammogram from a DBT scan of 21 PVs at 3° increment. (c) A slice intersecting the spiculated mass after SART reconstruction of the DBT.

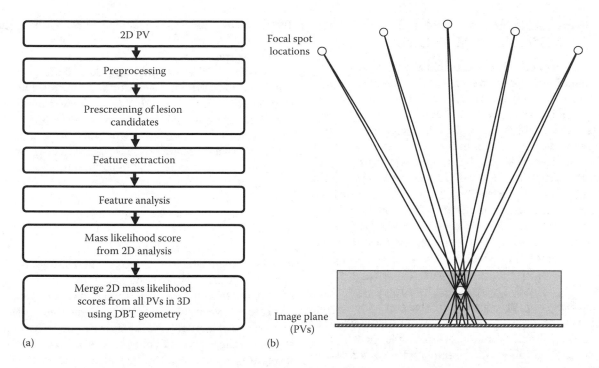

Figure 4.6   Illustration of a 2D lesion detection approach in DBT. (a) Lesion detection is first performed on individual PVs. Each PV is processed to identify lesion candidates. (b) The correspondence of the lesion candidates detected on different PVs is determined by using the geometric information of the DBT system. The information extracted from the corresponding lesion candidates can then be combined in the 3D breast volume.

candidates detected on different PVs that correspond to the same lesion in the breast volume can be determined by ray-tracing back to the breast volume using the known geometry of the DBT system. A true lesion is more likely to be detected in a larger number of PVs, while the locations of FPs will be relatively random on different PVs. The rays from corresponding true lesions on PVs would converge at a location when they are traced back to the breast volume. One the other hand, the rays from FPs that occur randomly on different PVs would not converge except for intersecting by chance. The number of rays from different PVs that intersect at the same location by chance is generally small unless too many lesion candidates are kept. FPs from a focal density in the breast may lead to lesion candidates on a larger number of PVs the rays of which would converge, similar to those of a true lesion. Further differentiation of focal density from true lesion would have to rely on feature analysis.

The features extracted from the candidates on different PVs can be merged if their rays converge in the 3D volume, indicating that they may correspond to the same object. Many different methods can be used for merging the feature values. As an example, the features of a given candidate extracted from a PV may be first merged by a trained classifier or decision rules into a score that may represent the *likelihood* that the candidate is a true lesion. The term *likelihood* here may or may not be interpreted in a strict statistical sense, depending on how the score is derived. The 2D mass likelihood scores from different PVs can then be further merged in 3D following the ray paths. Another way of merging the features from the corresponding candidates may be first combining the individual features from different PVs in 3D and then combining the merged features into an overall mass likelihood score. The merging of features or 2D mass likelihood scores from different PVs can also be performed in different manners. For example, the values may be weighted by the path lengths and then summed for each voxel. Since the feature values or the 2D mass likelihood scores do not follow a physical model like the X-ray attenuation coefficients, the process is not as well-defined as backprojection so that the weighting factors may be designed differently.

Because of the correlation and the larger number of rays converging to the same location for a true lesion that is detected on different PV images, the merged mass likelihood score or features of a true lesion will tend to amplify in comparison to those of FPs. The merged mass likelihood score of a true mass will have a better chance to be distinguishable from FPs and noise than the scores or features on the individual PVs. The combination of multiple PV information based on DBT geometry therefore is an important step for FP reduction in a CADe system for DBT.

4.3.2 Analysis of Reconstructed DBT Slices or DBT Volume

Instead of utilizing the correlation between features of true lesions from different PVs, this approach takes advantage of the highly precise image reconstruction technique in combining the spatial information of all breast tissue structures in 3D before image analysis. The SNR in the reconstructed slices is increased compared to that in the individual PVs because the quantum noise is reduced by integration of rays from the PVs, and the structured noise is reduced by separating the overlapping tissue to different depths. Image processing can then be performed directly in the 3D volume or alternatively in the individual DBT slices, and the extracted information is subsequently combined using the spatial relationship among the slices as shown in Figure 4.7a and b, respectively. In practice, these two approaches may be mixed at different stages of processing in the CADe system. For example, prescreening and segmentation of lesion candidates may be performed in the 3D volume across the slices. This has the advantage that a segmented object that spans multiple slices will be connected and continuous after segmentation, whereas prescreening and segmentation performed on individual slices will require additional processing techniques and criteria to identify objects on different slices that belong to the same 3D object. In the latter case, because of noise and irregularity, the segmented objects from adjacent slices may not be connected over the object area or objects in some slices may not be detected and segmented even if they belong to the same true lesion. Alternatively, FPs from different slices may be connected to be a 3D object or FPs in some slices may be connected to a true object in other slices. These variabilities may cause additional errors in the identification of lesion candidates in 3D and feature extraction.

Segmentation of a spiculated malignant mass and a well-circumscribed benign mass in the DBT volume is demonstrated in the examples in Figures 4.8 and 4.9, respectively.

The segmentation was performed in a volume of interest containing the mass by 3D clustering over the voxels to obtain an approximate mass region, which was then used to initialize a 3D active contour (AC) model to refine the segmentation of the mass boundary. Figures 4.8c and 4.9c show that the mass boundaries in the x–z plane and the y–z plane are not well defined, regardless of whether the mass was well circumscribed or not. The spiculations of the spiculated mass are not visible in these planes. The top and bottom of the mass cast long shadows beyond its size without clear boundaries due to the interplane blurring in the z-direction. These characteristics of objects in DBT volume will impose constraints in the design of segmentation methods and will limit the segmentation accuracy and the subsequent feature analysis. Similar problems will occur for the differentiation of malignant and benign masses in a computer-aided diagnosis system or for the differentiation of true and false masses identified in a CADe system.

Feature extraction from the segmented objects may be performed in the 3D volume or on the individual slices that form the segmented object. As shown in the examples in Figures 4.8 and 4.9, the spatial resolution of the reconstructed DBT volume in the z-direction perpendicular to the detector plane (or DBT slice) is low due to the limited-angle tomographic data. The texture of the breast tissue in the x–z and the y–z planes is distorted. Spatial information extracted in the z-direction contains large uncertainty, and texture analysis on planes other than the x–y plane can be misleading. These limitations should be taken into consideration in the design of feature analysis techniques. Some features may be analyzed on individual DBT slices, which are then merged into features for the object. Other features may be better extracted for the object as a whole. The different types of features may then be combined with a trained classifier or other unsupervised methods to differentiate true and false lesions.

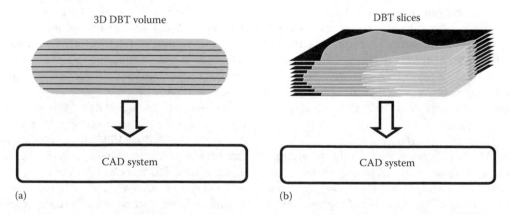

3D DBT volume

DBT slices

CAD system

CAD system

(a)

(b)

Figure 4.7 Illustration of two alternative 3D approaches to lesion detection in DBT. (a) Image analysis is performed in the reconstructed breast volume. (b) Image analysis is performed in the individual DBT slices and then combined in the 3D volume. The two alternatives may be mixed or interchanged at different stages.

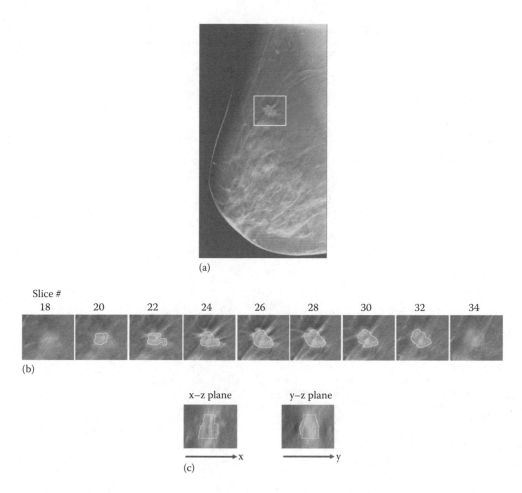

Figure 4.8   Segmentation of a spiculated malignant mass from a volume of interest in a reconstructed DBT breast volume. Segmentation was performed with 3D clustering and 3D active contour model. (a) A DBT slice (x–y plane) in MLO view intersecting approximately the center of the mass. (b) Segmented mass boundary superimposed on the DBT slices. (c) Segmented mass boundary shown on an x–z plane and on a y–z plane intersecting approximately the central region of the mass. The X-ray source scanned in the y-direction.

A disadvantage of this approach is that the performance of the CADe system may depend to some extent on the reconstruction technique used in addition to the DBT image acquisition parameters. Retraining of some of the image processing techniques may be needed if the reconstruction technique is changed. However, previous studies indicated that it may not take extensive effort to adapt a CADe system developed for one modality to another (e.g., film mammogram to digital mammogram) if the system is designed properly.

4.3.3   Combined Approach

The information content in the set of PV images or the DBT slices is basically the same because the latter is derived from the same set of PV images. Postprocessing does not create new information but helps only to bring out the information already recorded in the images. However, the 2D and 3D processing analyze the information in different ways; the extracted information may represent different characteristics of the lesions. If the features or information extracted from the corresponding object in the two approaches are combined, it may provide complementary information to improve the overall detection accuracy. Figure 4.10 illustrates the combined approach, in which the 3D approach can perform image analysis in either the DBT volume, the DBT slices, or a mixture of both as described earlier although only the DBT volume is shown.

Information fusion is a key step to take advantage of the available 2D and 3D information effectively. The corresponding objects from the two approaches can usually be identified by their spatial locations in the breast volume. Different methods for information fusion can be developed. A classifier can be trained to merge the set of features extracted for each object by the two approaches. Alternatively, the features in each approach can first be merged with a classifier into a mass likelihood score. The 2D and 3D mass likelihood scores can then be combined by another trained classifier or other unsupervised methods.

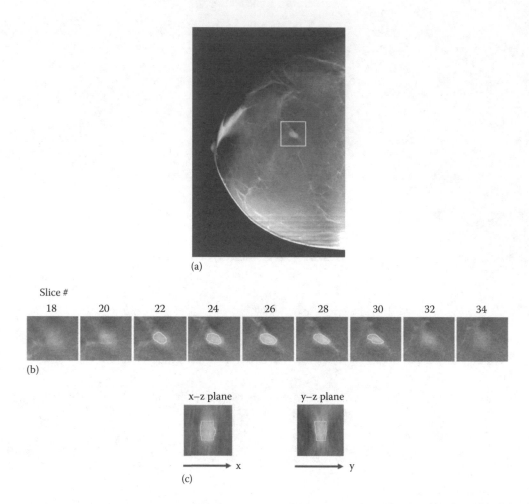

Figure 4.9 Segmentation of a well-circumscribed benign mass from a volume of interest in a reconstructed DBT breast volume. Segmentation was performed with 3D clustering and 3D active contour model. (a) A DBT slice (x–y plane) in CC view intersecting approximately the center of the mass. (b) Segmented mass boundary superimposed on the DBT slices. (c) Segmented mass boundary shown on an x–z plane and on a y–z plane intersecting approximately the central region of the mass. The X-ray source scanned in the y-direction.

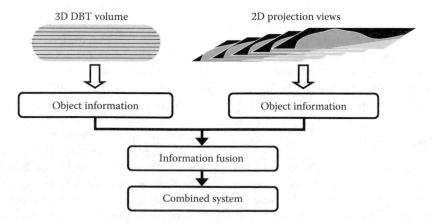

Figure 4.10 Illustration of a combined 3D and 2D approach in which the object information or features extracted from the corresponding objects detected in the 2D or 3D approaches are merged and used to differentiate true and false lesions.

4.3.4 Computer-Aided Diagnosis of Masses in Breast Tomosynthesis

Image analysis for computer-aided classification of malignant and benign lesions in DBT is similar to the feature extraction and classification steps in CADe. The difference is that the purpose of classification is to differentiate malignant and benign lesions, rather than true lesions and FPs. Therefore, the various approaches for image analysis described earlier are generally applicable to computer-aided diagnosis systems.

An example of the classification of malignant and benign masses in DBT is discussed here to demonstrate some differences and similarities between performing segmentation and feature extraction on the reconstructed DBT slices and on the PV images. In this study, the human subjects were recruited with IRB approval and informed consent. Imaging was performed with a prototype DBT system that had a flat panel CsI/a:Si detector with a pixel pitch of 0.1 mm × 0.1 mm and acquired 11 PVs in 5° increments over a 50° tomo angle. All DBT scans were performed in the MLO view. The DBTs were reconstructed using SART at a pixel size of 0.1 mm × 0.1 mm and a slice interval of 1 mm. Experienced radiologists identified 107 masses (56 malignant, 51 benign) in the dataset.

The 2D approach to image analysis on the DBT slices or the PV images is similar to that for the regular mammograms. An automated mass classification system developed for the classification of malignant and benign masses on digitized screen-film mammograms was directly applied to the DBT slices or the PVs without retraining the parameters except that feature selection was performed in each extracted feature space. For each mass, an ROI enclosing the mass was extracted from each of the DBT slices (or the PVs) and used as input to the mass classification system. The image analysis process consists of several steps: segmentation of the mass within the ROI, feature extraction from the segmented mass, and feature classification. The details of the methods can be found in the literature (Chan et al., 1995; Sahiner et al., 1998, 2001) and are briefly described here.

Background correction (Chan et al., 1995) was first performed on the ROI to reduce the low-frequency intensity variation in the image. An adaptive k-means clustering algorithm (Sahiner et al., 1996) was applied to the background-corrected ROI to segment the pixels into two classes: the mass and the surrounding tissue using the original gray-level image and its median-filtered image as components of a feature vector for each pixel. The clustering algorithm estimated whether a pixel would belong to the mass class or the background class based on the ratio of the Euclidean distances from the pixel to the mass

and the background cluster centers in the feature space. Figures 4.11 and 4.12 show examples of the original image and segmentation with clustering for a spiculated mass on DBT slices and PVs, respectively. The segmented object by clustering was used as the initial contour for a 2D AC model. The initial contour was iteratively deformed to push the contour toward the mass boundary by minimization of a cost function containing internal and external force terms. The AC model was trained to segment the body of the mass without the potential spiculations (row 3 of Figures 4.11 and 4.12).

After AC segmentation, spiculation analysis was performed over a band of pixels surrounding the mass boundary to form a spiculation likelihood map (row 4 of Figures 4.11 and 4.12). The approximately radial line structures with high pixel values in the spiculation likelihood map indicated the possible locations of spiculations along the mass border. Spiculation features were extracted from the spiculation likelihood map and used to classify a mass as being spiculated or nonspiculated. Examples of the segmented masses with the detected spiculations are shown in the last row of Figures 4.11 and 4.12 for the DBT slices and PVs, respectively.

In addition to the spiculation features, morphological and texture features were extracted from the segmented mass in the ROI to describe the size and shape of the mass and the texture in the surrounding breast tissue. Each mass was therefore characterized by multiple sets of features, each set obtained from an individual image from either the DBT slices or the PVs. The different sets of features could be combined in many ways. The following comparison demonstrates the difference in classification performance between DBT slices and PVs by simply averaging the corresponding features extracted from multiple images of the same type. A linear discriminant analysis classifier was designed using a two-loop leave-one-case-out feature selection and classification procedure in each of the feature spaces for either the DBT slice or the PV approach. The classification performance was evaluated as the area under the ROC curve (A_z) for the test cases from the two-loop leave-one-case-out procedure.

As discussed earlier, the top and the bottom of the mass in the DBT volume cannot be clearly delineated. The features of the mass would become more and more distorted on slices further away from the central plane of the mass, especially for spiculated masses because the spiculations would intersect the DBT slices at increasingly large oblique angles and also overlap with the interplane shadow of the mass body. It is not known how many slices should be used for the analysis of the mass features. The dependence of A_z on the number of slices or PVs over which the corresponding features were averaged is

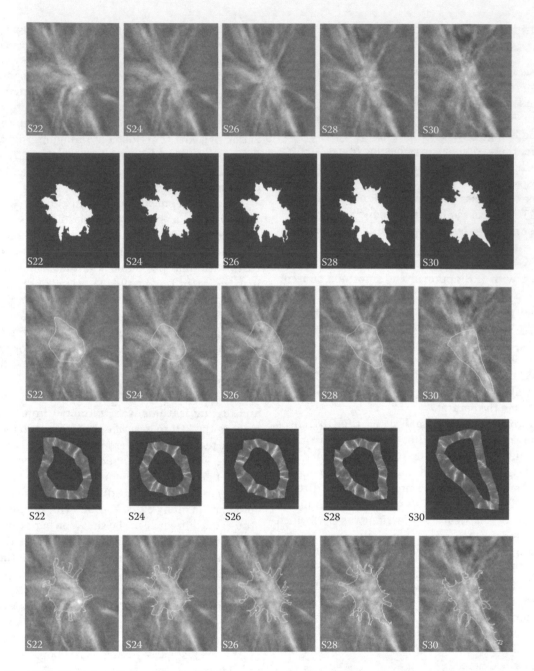

Figure 4.11 Five DBT slices of a spiculated mass. S26 is the central slice identified by an experienced radiologist. Row 1: DBT slices. Row 2: binary images obtained by adaptive k-means clustering. Row 3: mass boundaries segmented by the AC method. Row 4: spiculation likelihood map. Row 5: segmented mass boundary and spiculations.

shown in Figure 4.13. The classification performance was relatively constant over the range of 3–9 slices ($A_z = 0.92$–0.93) and fell off when more slices were included in the feature averaging. The central slice was quite efficient in capturing the image information. Although its A_z was about 0.02 lower than the highest value, the difference did not achieve statistical significance. For classification using the PVs, there was an increasing trend of A_z from

0.79 at 1 PV to 0.84 at 9 PVs and fell off slightly to 0.83 when the features were averaged over all 11 PVs.

This study demonstrates the feasibility of adapting computer-vision techniques developed for 2D mammograms to DBT slices and PVs. The classification performance was reasonable even without retraining except for feature selection, and retraining would likely improve the performance. The results that the features extracted

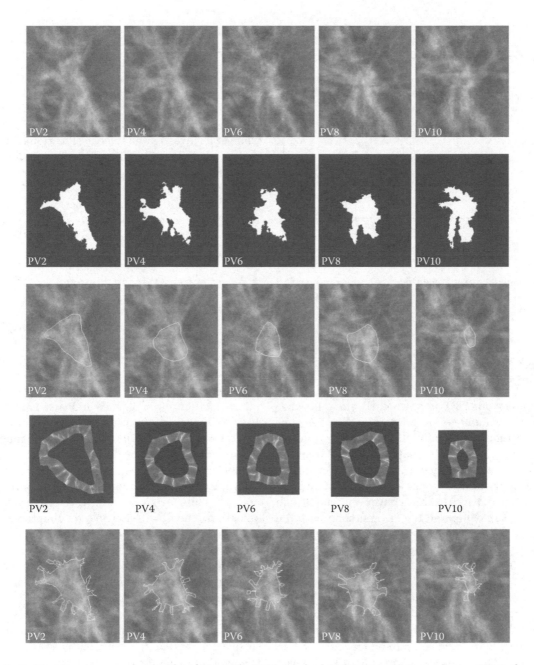

Figure 4.12   Projection view images of a spiculated mass. The DBT scan had 11 PVs, but only 5 are shown. PV6 is the central PV at a projection angle of 0°. Row 1: PVs. Row 2: binary images obtained by adaptive k-means clustering. Row 3: mass boundaries segmented by the AC method. Row 4: spiculation likelihood map. Row 5: segmented mass boundary and spiculations.

from the DBT slices were significantly more effective than those from the PVs may be attributed to the accurate fusion of the information in the individual PVs by the tomosynthesis reconstruction process. Reconstruction essentially averages the photons along all rays that intersect a given voxel from all PVs, thus reducing the random noise and enhances the correlated structures in the DBT slices, which facilitate image analysis and

efficient utilization of the information content. In the PV approach, the image features are extracted from very noisy images, each of which utilizes only a small fraction of the total dose. The subsequent fusion of information by averaging the features extracted from the individual PVs is relatively global and cannot recover the information that may have been masked by the noise in the feature extraction process.

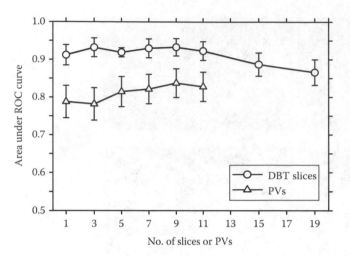

Figure 4.13 Dependence of classification performance (A_z) to differentiate malignant and benign masses on the number of DBT slices or PVs over which the corresponding features were averaged.

4.4 CURRENT STATE OF CADe FOR MASSES IN DBT

CADe development for DBT is at an early stage because few datasets are available to date. Several research groups have been investigating CADe methods for lesion detection in DBT using relatively small datasets. For mass detection, Chan et al. developed a CADe system using 3D gradient field analysis and image segmentation in DBT volume reconstructed by the ML-convex method (Chan et al., 2004b, 2005a), compared the 3D approach with the 2D approach of detecting the masses on individual PVs, and the combined 2D and 3D approach for mass detection (Chan et al., 2004a, 2007a, 2008a), compared mass detection accuracy for SART and ML-convex reconstruction with different number of iterations (Chan et al., 2005b), compared the detection accuracy for different number of PVs and dose (Chan et al., 2008b), evaluated FP reduction method (Wei et al., 2008), and compared mass detection in DBT and regular mammograms (Chan et al., 2009). Reiser et al. compared mass detection in DBT using 2D and 3D radial gradient index segmentation (Reiser et al., 2004b) and evaluated mass detection performance obtained by applying radial gradient filtering to the reconstructed DBT slices or 3D volume (Reiser et al., 2004a, 2005) or by directly processing the PV images (Reiser et al., 2004c, 2006). Peters et al. developed mass segmentation methods on PV images to be applied to detection (Peters et al., 2006, 2007). Jerebko et al. applied CADe algorithms developed for regular mammograms to PVs (Jerebko et al., 2007). Singh et al. performed prescreening of mass candidates on PVs, estimated the candidate locations in the reconstructed volume

from the PV locations, and then performed image analysis on the DBT slices (Singh et al., 2007, 2008a,b,c). van Schie et al. applied a CADe system trained for mass detection on mammograms to DBT slabs and studied the effect of slab size on detection performance (van Schie et al., 2010).

Very few studies have been conducted for computerized lesion characterization in DBT to date. For mass lesions, Chan et al. investigated the classification of malignant and benign masses on DBT slices (Chan et al., 2007b) and compared mass classification accuracy when feature analysis was performed on the DBT slices and the PV images (Chan et al., 2008c, 2010). Palma et al. performed mass segmentation on PV images using level sets and merged the extracted information from all PVs for the classification of spiculated and circumscribed masses (Palma et al., 2008).

4.5 FUTURE DIRECTIONS

DBT is an emerging technology that holds the promise of bringing major advances to breast imaging. CADe is expected to be a useful adjunct to DBT. CADe development in DBT is still at its early stage. Very limited studies have been conducted for the development of CADe for masses, and even fewer studies have been reported for microcalcifications. Studies indicated that mass detection and characterization may be improved in DBT, but the visibility of microcalcifications may be reduced because of the separation of microcalcifications in a cluster into different slices, increased noise associated with multiple low-dose PV acquisitions, and potential blurring and artifacts arising from the tomosynthesis reconstruction. The discussion in this chapter has focused in CADe for masses. However, computer-assisted reading for clustered microcalcifications will play an equally, if not more, important role in DBT. The various approaches and the considerations of the technical factors for CADe development discussed here for masses will be similar for microcalcifications.

Although the development of CADe for DBT is similar to that for regular mammography in principle, the additional 3D information and the flexibility of using different approaches pose greater challenges as well as opportunities for designing computerized lesion detection and characterization algorithms. Many different computer-vision techniques can be designed at each step of each approach. The studies to date indicate that many variables may affect the image quality and thus the accuracy of computerized detection or diagnosis (e.g., 2D detection on PVs or reconstructed slices, 3D detection in reconstructed volumes, or combination of 2D and 3D approaches at different stages of the CADe system). The best combination of techniques and parameters not only will depend on the approach taken, but also may depend on the DBT acquisition parameters such as the tomo angle, the number of PVs, the distribution of the PVs over the tomo scan range (e.g., uniform or nonuniform angular increments) and on the reconstruction methods that may affect the spatial resolution, interplane artifacts, contrast, and noise properties of the structures in the reconstructed volume. Previous studies have explored only very limited variables and image analysis methods for CADe in DBT. It will be challenging to find the optimal combinations of computer-vision techniques for each CADe task that can fully exploit the image information in DBT. The development of CADe methods that may be more robust against the many variables is an important area of investigation. DBT in combination with effective CADe has the potential to become the modality of choice for breast cancer screening and diagnosis in the near future.

ACKNOWLEDGMENTS

The work in digital breast tomosynthesis conducted at the University of Michigan was supported in part by USPHS grants R01 CA151443, R33 CA120234 and R01 CA 91713, and from the efforts of many current and former members of the CAD Research Laboratory and many of our clinical colleagues in the Department of Radiology.

REFERENCES

American Cancer Society (2011). Cancer Facts & Figures 2011. www.cancer.org. Accessed on 2011.

Bandodkar, P., R. L. Birdwell, and D. M. Ikeda. 2002. Computer aided detection (CAD) with screening mammography in an academic institution: Preliminary findings. *Radiology* 225(P): 458.

Birdwell, R. L., P. Bandodkar, and D. M. Ikeda. 2005. Computer-aided detection with screening mammography in a university hospital setting. *Radiology* 236: 451–457.

Boone, J. M., T. R. Nelson, K. K. Lindfors, and J. A. Seibert. 2001. Dedicated breast CT: Radiation dose and image quality evaluation. *Radiology* 221: 657–667.

Breast Cancer Surveillance Consortium. 2009. Performance benchmarks for screening mammography. http://breastscreening.cancer.gov/data/benchmarks/screening/. Last update: 2009, accessed on 2011.

Brem, R. F., J. K. Baum, M. Lechner et al. 2003. Improvement in sensitivity of screening mammography with computer-aided detection: A multi-institutional trial. *American Journal of Roentgenology* 181: 687–693.

Chan, H.-P., K. Doi, C. J. Vyborny et al. 1990. Improvement in radiologists' detection of clustered microcalcifications on mammograms. The potential of computer-aided diagnosis. *Investigative Radiology* 25: 1102–1110.

Chan, H.-P., M. M. Goodsitt, L. M. Hadjiiski et al. 2003. Effects of magnification and zooming on depth perception in digital stereomammography: An observer performance study. *Physics in Medicine and Biology* 48: 3721–3734.

Chan, H.-P., D. Wei, M. A. Helvie et al. 1995. Computer-aided classification of mammographic masses and normal tissue: Linear discriminant analysis in texture feature space. *Physics in Medicine and Biology* 40: 857–876.

Chan, H.-P., J. Wei, B. Sahiner, L. M. Hadjiiski, and M. A. Helvie. 2009. Comparison of computerized mass detection in digital breast tomosynthesis (DBT) mammograms and conventional mammograms. *Proceedings of SPIE* 7260: 0S1–0S7.

Chan, H.-P., J. Wei, B. Sahiner et al. 2004a. Computer-aided detection on digital breast tomosynthesis (DBT) mammograms—Comparison of two approaches. In: *RSNA Program Book*, RSNA, Oak Brook, IL, p. 447.

Chan, H.-P., J. Wei, B. Sahiner et al. 2004b. Computerized detection of masses on digital tomosynthesis mammograms—A preliminary study. In: *Proceedings of the 7th International Workshop on Digital Mammography (IWDM'2004)*, Chapel Hill, NC, pp. 199–202.

Chan, H.-P., J. Wei, B. Sahiner et al. 2005a. Computer-aided detection system for breast masses on digital tomosynthesis mammograms—Preliminary experience. *Radiology* 237: 1075–1080.

Chan, H.-P., J. Wei, T. Wu et al. 2005b. Computer-aided detection on digital breast tomosynthesis (DBT) mammograms: Dependence on image quality of reconstruction. In: *RSNA Program Book*, RSNA, Oak Brook, IL, p. 269.

Chan, H.-P., J. Wei, Y. Zhang et al. 2007a. Computer-aided detection of masses in digital tomosynthesis mammography: Combination of 3D and 2D detection information. *Proceedings of SPIE* 6514: 161–166.

Chan, H.-P., J. Wei, Y. H. Zhang et al. 2008a. Computer-aided detection of masses in digital tomosynthesis mammography: Comparison of three approaches. *Medical Physics* 35: 4087–4095.

Chan, H.-P., J. Wei, Y. H. Zhang et al. 2008b. Detection of masses in digital breast tomosynthesis mammography: Effects of the number of projection views and dose. In: *Proceedings of the 9th International Workshop on Digital Mammography (IWDM'2008)*, LNCS 5116, Springer-Verlag. Berlin, Heidelberg, pp. 279–285.

Chan, H.-P., Y. T. Wu, B. Sahiner et al. 2007b. Digital breast tomosynthesis mammography: Computerized classification of malignant and benign masses. *Medical Physics* 34: 2645.

Chan, H.-P., Y. T. Wu, B. Sahiner et al. 2008c. Digital tomosynthesis mammography: Comparison of mass classification using 3D slices and 2D projection views. *Proceedings of SPIE* 6915: 6915061–6915066.

Chan, H.-P., Y. T. Wu, B. Sahiner et al. 2010. Characterization of masses in digital breast tomosynthesis: Comparison of machine learning in projection views and reconstructed slices. *Medical Physics* 37: 3576–3586.

Chen, B. and R. Ning. 2002. Cone-beam volume CT breast imaging: Feasibility study. *Medical Physics* 29: 755–770.

Cupples, T. E., J. E. Cunningham, and J. C. Reynolds. 2005. Impact of computer-aided detection in a regional screening mammography program. *American Journal of Roentgenology* 185: 944–950.

Dean, J. C. and C. C. Ilvento. 2006. Improved cancer detection using computer-aided detection with diagnostic and screening mammography: Prospective study of 104 cancers. *American Journal of Roentgenology* 187: 20–28.

Destounis, S. V., P. DiNitto, W. Logan-Young et al. 2004. Can computer-aided detection with double reading of screening mammograms help decrease the false-negative rate? Initial experience. *Radiology* 232: 578–584.

Dobbins, J. T. and D. J. Godfrey. 2003. Digital x-ray tomosynthesis: Current state of the art and clinical potential. *Physics in Medicine and Biology* 48: R65–R106.

Elmore, J. G., S. L. Jackson, L. Abraham et al. 2009. Variability in interpretive performance at screening mammography and radiologists' characteristics associated with accuracy. *Radiology* 253: 641–651.

Feig, S. A., E. A. Sickles, W. P. Evans, and M. N. Linver. 2004. Re: Changes in breast cancer detection and mammography recall rates after the introduction of a computer-aided detection system. *Journal of the National Cancer Institute* 96: 1260–1261.

Fenton, J. J., L. Abraham, S. H. Taplin et al. 2011. Effectiveness of computer-aided detection in community mammography practice. *Journal of the National Cancer Institute* 103: 1152–1161.

Freer, T. W. and M. J. Ulissey. 2001. Screening mammography with computer-aided detection: Prospective study of 12,860 patients in a community breast center. *Radiology* 220: 781–786.

Gennaro, G., A. Toledano, C. di Maggio et al. 2010. Digital breast tomosynthesis versus digital mammography: A clinical performance study. *European Radiology* 20: 1545–1553.

Getty, D. J., R. M. Pickett, and C. J. D'Orsi. 2001. Stereoscopic digital mammography: Improving detection and diagnosis of breast cancer. In: H. U. Lemke, M. W. Vannier, K. Inamura, A. G. Farman, and K. Doi (eds.). *International Congress Series*, June 27–30, 2001, Vol. 1230. Berlin, Germany, pp. 506–511 (Elsevier, Amsterdam, the Netherlands).

Gilbert, F. J., S. M. Astley, M. G. C. Gillan et al. 2008. Single reading with computer-aided detection for screening mammography. *The New England Journal of Medicine* 359: 1675–1684.

Goodsitt, M. M., H.-P. Chan, K. L. Darner, and L. M. Hadjiiski. 2002. The effects of stereo shift angle, geometric magnification and display zoom on depth measurements in digital stereomammography. *Medical Physics* 29: 2725–2734.

Goodsitt, M. M., H.-P. Chan, and L. M. Hadjiiski. 2000. Stereomammography: Evaluation of depth perception using a virtual 3D cursor. *Medical Physics* 27: 1305–1310.

Gromet, M. 2008. Comparison of computer-aided detection to double reading of screening mammograms: Review of 231,221 mammograms. *American Journal of Roentgenology* 190: 854–859.

Gur, D., G. S. Abrams, D. M. Chough et al. 2009. Digital breast tomosynthesis: Observer performance study. *American Journal of Roentgenology* 193: 586–591.

Gur, D., J. H. Sumkin, H. E. Rockette et al. 2004. Changes in breast cancer detection and mammography recall rates after the introduction of a computer-aided detection system. *Journal of the National Cancer Institute* 96: 185–190.

Helvie, M. A., H.-P. Chan, L. M. Hadjiiski et al. 2009. Digital breast tomosynthesis mammography: Successful assessment of benign and malignant microcalcifications. In: *RSNA Program Book*, RSNA, Oak Brook, IL, p. 389.

Helvie, M. A., L. M. Hadjiiski, E. Makariou et al. 2004. Sensitivity of noncommercial computer-aided detection system for mammographic breast cancer detection—A pilot clinical trial. *Radiology* 231: 208–214.

Helvie, M. A., M. A. Roubidoux, L. M. Hadjiiski et al. 2007. Tomosynthesis mammography vs conventional mammography: Comparison of breast masses detection and characterization. In: *RSNA Program Book*, RSNA, Oak Brook, IL, p. 381.

Helvie, M. A., M. A. Roubidoux, L. M. Hadjiiski et al. 2008. Research digital tomosynthesis mammography: Detection of t1 invasive breast carcinomas not diagnosed by conventional breast imaging or physical exam. In: *RSNA Program Book*, RSNA, Oak Brook, IL, p. 468.

Hendrick, R. E. and M. A. Helvie. 2011. United states preventive services task force screening mammography recommendations: Science ignored. *American Journal of Roentgenology* 196: W112–W116.

James, J. J., F. J. Gilbert, M. G. Wallis et al. 2010. Mammographic features of breast cancers at single reading with computer-aided detection and at double reading in a large multicenter prospective trial of computer-aided detection: CADET II. *Radiology* 256: 379–386.

Jerebko, A., Y. Quan, N. Merlet et al. 2007. Feasibility study of breast tomosynthesis CAD system. *Proceedings of SPIE* 6514: 141–148.

Khoo, L. A. L., P. Taylor, and R. M. Given-Wilson. 2005. Computer-aided detection in the united kingdom national breast screening programme: Prospective study. *Radiology* 237: 444–449.

Lindfors, K. K., J. M. Boone, M. S. Newell, and C. J. D'Orsi. 2010. Dedicated breast computed tomography: The optimal cross-sectional imaging solution? *Radiologic Clinics of North America* 48: 1043–1054.

Lu, Y., H.-P. Chan, J. Wei et al. 2011. Image quality of microcalcifications in digital breast tomosynthesis: Effects of projection-view distributions. *Medical Physics* 38: 5703–5712.

Lu, Y., H.-P. Chan, J. Wei, and L. M. Hadjiiski. 2010. Selective-diffusion regularization for enhancement of microcalcifications in digital breast tomosynthesis reconstruction. *Medical Physics* 37: 6003–6014.

Mainprize, J. G., A. K. Bloomquist, M. P. Kempston, and M. J. Yaffe. 2006. Resolution at oblique incidence angles of a flat panel imager for breast tomosynthesis. *Medical Physics* 33: 3159–3164.

Mandelson, M. T., N. Oestreicher, P. L. Porter et al. 2000. Breast density as a predictor of mammographic detection: Comparison of interval- and screen-detected cancers. *Journal of the National Cancer Institute* 92: 1081–1087.

Mook, S., L. J. Van't Veer, E. J. Rutgers et al. 2011. Independent prognostic value of screen detection in invasive breast cancer. *Journal of the National Cancer Institute* 103: 585–597.

Morton, M. J., D. H. Whaley, K. R. Brandt, and K. K. Amrami. 2006. Screening mammograms: Interpretation with computer-aided detection—Prospective evaluation. *Radiology* 239: 375–383.

Niklason, L. T., B. T. Christian, L. E. Niklason et al. 1997. Digital tomosynthesis in breast imaging. *Radiology* 205: 399–406.

O'Connell, A., D. L. Conover, Y. Zhang et al. 2010. Cone-beam CT for breast imaging: Radiation dose, breast coverage, and image quality. *American Journal of Roentgenology* 195: 496–509.

Palma, G. J., G. Peters, S. Muller, and I. Bloch. 2008. Masses classification using fuzzy active contours and fuzzy decision trees. *Proceedings of SPIE* 6915: 0901–0911.

Pediconi, F., C. Catalano, A. Roselli et al. 2009. The challenge of imaging dense breast parenchyma is magnetic resonance mammography the technique of choice? A comparative study with x-ray mammography and whole-breast ultrasound. *Investigative Radiology* 44: 412–421.

Peters, G., S. Muller, S. Bernard, R. Iordache, and I. Bloch. 2006. Reconstruction-independent 3D CAD for mass detection in digital breast tomosynthesis using fuzzy particles. *Proceedings of SPIE* 6144: Z1441.

Peters, G., S. Muller, B. Grosjean, S. Bernard, and I. Bloch. 2007. A hybrid active contour model for mass detection in digital breast tomosynthesis. *Proceedings of SPIE* 6514: V1–V11.

Poplack, S. P., T. D. Tosteson, C. A. Kogel, and H. M. Nagy. 2007. Digital breast tomosynthesis: Initial experience in 98 women with abnormal digital screening mammography. *American Journal of Roentgenology* 189: 616–623.

Qian, X., R. Rajaram, X. Calderon-Colon et al. 2009. Design and characterization of a spatially distributed multibeam field emission x-ray source for stationary digital breast tomosynthesis. *Medical Physics* 36: 4389–4399.

Rafferty, E. A., D. Georgian-Smith, D. B. Kopans et al. 2002. Comparison of full-field digital tomosynthesis with two view conventional film screen mammography in the prediction of lesion malignancy. *Radiology* 225(P): 268.

Reiser, I., R. M. Nishikawa, M. L. Giger et al. 2004a. Computerized detection of mammographic masses in digital breast tomosynthesis images using radial gradient index filtering. *International Congress Series* 1268: 1352.

Reiser, I., R. M. Nishikawa, M. L. Giger et al. 2004b. Computerized detection of mass lesions in digital breast tomosynthesis images using two- and three dimensional radial gradient index segmentation. *Technology in Cancer Research and Treatment* 3: 437–441.

Reiser, I., R. M. Nishikawa, M. L. Giger et al. 2005. A multi-scale 3D radial gradient filter for computerized mass detection in digital tomosynthesis breast images. *International Congress Series* 1281: 1058–1062.

Reiser, I., R. M. Nishikawa, M. L. Giger et al. 2006. Computerized mass detection for digital breast tomosynthesis directly from the projection images. *Medical Physics* 33: 482–491.

Reiser, I., E. Y. Sidky, M. L. Giger et al. 2004c. A reconstruction-independent method for computerized mass detection in digital tomosynthesis images of the breast. *Proceedings of SPIE* 5370: 833–838.

Rosenberg, R. D., B. C. Yankaskas, L. A. Abraham et al. 2006. Performance benchmarks for screening mammography. *Radiology* 241: 55–66.

Sahiner, B., H.-P. Chan, N. Petrick, M. A. Helvie, and M. M. Goodsitt. 1998. Computerized characterization of masses on mammograms: The rubber band straightening transform and texture analysis. *Medical Physics* 25: 516–526.

Sahiner, B., H.-P. Chan, N. Petrick, M. A. Helvie, and L. M. Hadjiiski. 2001. Improvement of mammographic mass characterization using spiculation measures and morphological features. *Medical Physics* 28: 1455–1465.

Sahiner, B., H.-P. Chan, N. Petrick et al. 1996. Image feature selection by a genetic algorithm: Application to classification of mass and normal breast tissue on mammograms. *Medical Physics* 23: 1671–1684.

Schell, M. J., B. C. Yankaskas, R. Ballard-Barbash et al. 2007. Evidence-based target recall rates for screening mammography. *Radiology* 243: 681–689.

Sechopoulos, I. and C. Ghetti. 2009. Optimization of the acquisition geometry in digital tomosynthesis of the breast. *Medical Physics* 36: 1199–1207.

Sidky, E. Y., X. Pan, I. Reiser et al. 2009. Enhanced imaging of microcalcifications in digital breast tomosynthesis through improved image-reconstruction algorithms. *Medical Physics* 36: 4920–4932.

Singh, S., G. D. Tourassi, J. A. Baker, E. Samei, and J. Y. Lo. 2008a. Automated breast mass detection in 3D reconstructed tomosynthesis volumes: A featureless approach. *Medical Physics* 35: 3626–3636.

Singh, S., G. D. Tourassi, A. S. Chawla et al. 2008b. Computer aided detection of breast masses in tomosynthesis reconstructed volumes using information-theoretic similarity measures. *Proceedings of SPIE* 6915: 6915051–6915058.

Singh, S., G. D. Tourassi, and J. Y. Lo. 2007. Breast mass detection in tomosynthesis projection images using information-theoretic similarity measures. *Proceedings of SPIE* 6514: 6514151–6514158.

Singh, S., G. D. Tourassi, and J. Y. Lo. 2008c. Effect of similarity metrics and ROI sizes in featureless computer aided detection of breast masses in tomosynthesis. *IWDM 2008—Lecture Notes in Computer Science* 5116: 286–291.

Smith, A. P., E. A. Rafferty, and L. Niklason. 2008. Clinical performance of breast tomosynthesis as a function of radiologist experience level. *IWDM 2008—Lecture Notes in Computer Science* 5116: 61–66.

Suryanarayanan, S., A. Karellas, S. Vedantham et al. 2001. Evaluation of linear and nonlinear tomosynthetic reconstruction methods in digital mammography. *Academic Radiology* 8: 219–224.

Tabár, L., B. Vitak, T. H.-H. Chen et al. June 28, 2011. Swedish two-county trial: Impact of mammographic screening on breast cancer mortality during 3 decades. *Radiology* 260: 658–663 (electronic online).

Taplin, S. H., C. M. Rutter, and C. D. Lehman. 2006. Testing the effect of computer-assisted detection on interpretive performance in screening mammography. *American Journal of Roentgenology* 187: 1475–1482.

U.S. Preventive Services Task Force. 2009. Screening for breast cancer: U.S. Preventive Services Task Force recommendation statement. *Annals of Internal Medicine* 151: 716–726.

van Schie, G., M. G. Wallis, K. Leifland et al. 2010. The effect of slab size on mass detection performance of a screen-film CAD system in reconstructed tomosynthesis volumes. In: *Proceedings of the 10th International Workshop on Digital Mammography (IWDM'2010)*, Girona, Spain, pp. 497–504.

van Schoor, G., S. M. Moss, J. D. M. Otten et al. 2011. Increasingly strong reduction in breast cancer mortality due to screening. *British Journal of Cancer* 104: 910–914.

Warren Burhenne, L. J., S. A. Wood, C. J. D'Orsi et al. 2000. Potential contribution of computer-aided detection to the sensitivity of screening mammography. *Radiology* 215: 554–562.

Wei, J., H.-P. Chan, Y. Zhang et al. 2008. Classification of breast masses and normal tissues in digital tomosynthesis mammography. *Proceedings of SPIE* 6915: 6915081–6915086.

Wu, T., A. Stewart, M. Stanton et al. 2003. Tomographic mammography using a limited number of low-dose cone-beam projection images. *Medical Physics* 30: 365–380.

Zhang, Y., H.-P. Chan, B. Sahiner et al. 2006. A comparative study of limited-angle cone-beam reconstruction methods for breast tomosynthesis. *Medical Physics* 33: 3781–3795.

Zhang, Y., H.-P. Chan, B. Sahiner et al. 2007. Application of boundary detection information in breast tomosynthesis reconstruction. *Medical Physics* 34: 3603–3613.

Zhang, Y., H.-P. Chan, M. M. Goodsitt et al. 2008. Investigation of different PV distributions in digital tomosynthesis mammography (DTM). In: *Proceedings of the 9th International Workshop on Digital Mammography* (*IWDM'2008*), Tucson, AZ, pp. 593–600.

Zhang, Y., H.-P. Chan, B. Sahiner et al. 2009. Artifact reduction methods for truncated projections in iterative breast tomosynthesis reconstruction. *Journal of Computer Assisted Tomography* 33: 426–435.

Zhao, B. and W. Zhao. 2008. Three-dimensional linear system analysis for breast tomosynthesis. *Medical Physics* 35: 5219–5232.

Zhao, B., J. Zhou, Y. H. Hu et al. 2009. Experimental validation of a three-dimensional linear system model for breast tomosynthesis. *Medical Physics* 36: 240–251.

Chapter 5

Assessment of Breast Density

Sir Michael Brady, Ralph Highnam, and Nico Karssemeijer

CONTENTS

5.1 INTRODUCTION

The World Health Organization reports that "Breast cancer is the most common cancer in women worldwide, comprising 16% of all female cancers. It is estimated that 519,000 women died in 2004 due to breast cancer, and although breast cancer is thought to be a disease of the developed world, a majority (69%) of all breast cancer deaths occurs in developing countries" (ACS 2010, WHO 2011). According to the National Cancer Institute (NCI 2011), in the United States, approximately 1 woman in 8 will be diagnosed with breast cancer at some point during their lives, and the website notes that "on 1st January 2008… 2,632,005 women [are] alive who had a history of cancer of the breast." The WHO further asserts that "The incidence of breast cancer is increasing in the developing world due to increase(d) life expectancy, increase(d) urbanization and adoption of western lifestyles." Evidently, the threat of breast cancer is a major concern for women around the world; it is a significant cause of mortality and a major contributor to healthcare costs.

Early diagnosis improves prognosis, and this can be augmented in association with appropriate therapy, for example, drugs such as tamoxifen (Nolvadex®). Based on this observation, many countries, including most European countries, Australia, and New Zealand, now have government-funded, population-based screening programs in which asymptomatic women within a certain age range (e.g., 50–75 in the United Kingdom) are invited every 2 or 3 years to have a mammogram (x-ray image of the tightly compressed breast). In the United States, even without the centralized screening programs, there are still 8,700 breast imaging centers staffed by just 2,500 specialist mammography radiologists, augmented by 15,000 general radiologists, who use mammography to screen 43 million women each year. Currently, every screening program is based on mammography since it optimizes the trade-off between sensitivity, specificity, and cost, including the time to image the woman. Screening is proven to save lives. For example, the UK Breast Screening Programme reports that "For every 400 women screened regularly by the NHS Breast Screening Programme over a 10 year period, one woman fewer will die from breast cancer than would have died without screening." The current NHS Breast Screening Programme saves an estimated 1400 lives each year in England (BSP61 2006). However, mammographic screening is far from perfect: only 20% of all diagnosed breast cancers are caught by screening. Of the cancers that are present at screening, 20% are missed, and 50%–80% of biopsies find only benign disease. Why is this so?

Refer to Figure 5.1, which shows two mammograms (of the same breast, on the same day). These 2D images are projections of the breast after it has been squeezed tightly between two compression plates. The bright tissue in the interior of the breast is referred to as dense or fibroglandular, and is composed primarily of glandular aggregates and fibrocollagenous stroma. The darker areas, for example, near the periphery of the breast, indicate regions that are primarily fat. The bright triangle at top right is the pectoral muscle. There is a skin fold at the top of both breasts. If one were to look at the mammogram of a young woman, it would typically appear uniformly white. The first thing to notice is that the images are quite complex, certainly relative to most images analyzed in computer vision research. They have complex textures, few sharp intensity changes, and the objects of interest—microcalcifications and masses—often have low contrasts to their backgrounds. However, there is a more fundamental problem with such images, and this is exemplified by the mammograms in Figure 5.1. The two mammograms appear quite different, even though the tissue contents are the same. This is because the two radiographers (technologists) who took the images chose different machine settings. This is analogous to the reason why (in the predigital era) two photographs of the same scene could appear very different as the time of exposure, film speed, and aperture setting were changed.

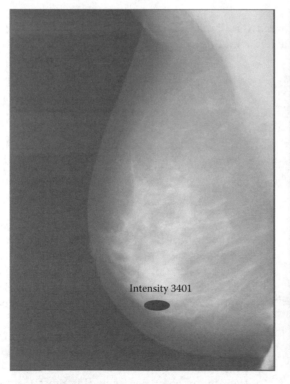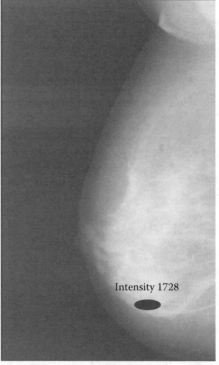

Intensity 3401

Intensity 1728

Figure 5.1 Two mammograms. The bright tissue in the interior of the breast is referred to as fibroglandular and is composed primarily of glandular aggregates and fibrocollagenous stroma. The darker areas, for example, near the periphery of the breast are primarily fat. The bright triangle at top right is the pectoral muscle. There is a skin fold at the top of both breasts. The two mammograms were taken on the same day, with imaging settings chosen by two radiographers (technologists) and reported by two different radiologists. In fact, the images are of the same breast. The points indicated on the images correspond to the same tissue location, but the brightness of the one on the left is approximately double that on the right.

Intensity differences usually occur because fat attenuates X-rays much less than fibroglandular tissue, so much so that a radiologist can often *infer* the contents of the breast from the intensity distribution within the image. However, the two images in Figure 5.1, in which the intensity distributions are so different and yet the breast contents are the same, sound a cautionary warning against such inferences. Typically, abnormal tissue such as tumors and fibroadenomas attenuates X-rays to an extent that is roughly equal to fibroglandular tissue, so much so that they are collectively known as *dense* tissue. This is why it is often difficult to detect abnormalities in mammograms and why such abnormalities may be missed—particularly in mammograms that contain a great deal of *dense* tissue where the detection of cancers can be as low as 48% compared to 98% for very fatty breasts. For a long time, it was widely believed that all women had dense breasts until the menopause, after which much of the dense tissue transforms into fat, a complex biochemical process known as involution. The precise details of this process are still not completely understood, though it is evident that the major changes in hormonal production vs. demand play a key role. This observation about the menopause is the reason many screening programs started at age 50, that is, *after menopause* where X-ray is more effective due to less dense tissue. However, as we show later, it is now far from certain that there is a sharp drop in density at any age, and it appears more likely that a women's breast density peaks early on and then slowly decreases to age 65 or so—this is the information that automated breast density solutions are now providing by being run over hundreds of thousands of images.

We noted earlier that dense tissue can hide cancers, and this means that detection of such cancers might be delayed, worsening the prognosis for the woman. However, and again for reasons that are still not completely understood, it has become clear over the past two decades that a woman whose breasts are substantially more dense than her (suitably defined) peer group is actually at greater risk of eventually developing breast cancer, even if, at the time of imaging, there is no tumor present. In short, such a woman suffers a double whammy: first, she is at greater risk of developing breast cancer; and second, if she does, the tumor will be harder to detect. In fact, there have been suggestions of a triple whammy: if a tumor develops in a dense breast, not only is it harder to detect, and not only is there increased risk of the woman developing such a tumor, but it seems that the tumor that does develop will be one of the more aggressive phenotypes. The distinction between difficulty in *detecting* cancers in dense breasts and the increased risk of developing breast cancer has been stressed, for example, by Boyd et al. (2007). Clearly, breast density is an important aspect of assessing a breast, for determining the clinical management of the individual woman and for assessing a woman's risk of developing breast cancer. The next section reviews briefly some of the evidence implicating

breast density, then Sections 5.3 and 5.4 outline the challenge of measuring breast density from a single mammogram and describe a recent method developed by the authors. We sketch recent progress in estimating breast density from intrinsically 3D imaging modalities—computed tomography (CT), MRI, and ultrasound—in Section 5.5. Finally, we draw a number of conclusions, and look forward, in Section 5.6.

5.2 RECOGNITION OF THE IMPORTANCE OF BREAST DENSITY

Recognition of the importance of breast density for both breast cancer detection and for breast cancer risk assessment developed steadily, but until recently rather slowly. It may be that this reflects the fact that interest in breast density arose in two different strands of research, whose findings have now converged. A consequence is that breast density will from now on play an increasingly important role in patient management. The two strands of research referred to earlier have been radiology, with its intrinsic concentration on the management of the individual woman, and epidemiology, with its emphasis on population statistical analysis. Recently, Norman Boyd and colleagues published a comprehensive and lucid review of breast density, primarily its relationship to breast cancer risk prediction (Boyd et al. 2010, 2011). They highlight, among numerous other issues, an apparent paradox:

> The average percent mammographic density in the population decreases with increasing age, which seems paradoxical given that breast cancer incidence increases with age. This apparent paradox may be explained by a model of breast cancer incidence proposed by Pike et al. (1983). The Pike model is based on the concept that "breast tissue exposure," rather than chronological age, is the relevant measure for describing the incidence of breast cancer. Breast tissue exposure refers to exposure of breast tissue to hormones and growth factors, and to the effects that menarche, pregnancy, and menopause have on these exposures and on the susceptibility of breast tissue to carcinogens.
>
> Boyd et al. (2010, p. 1227)

They briefly summarize the Pike model (Figure 5.2) and then conclude that "Percent mammographic density may thus reflect the cumulative exposure of breast stroma and epithelium to hormones and growth factors" (Boyd et al. 2010, p. 1227).

There have been several subsequent models to predict 5-year, 10-year, and lifetime risk of a woman getting breast cancer. For example, Dr. Mitchell Gail of the Biostatistics Branch of NCI's Division of Cancer Epidemiology and Genetics developed a statistical model (Gail et al. 1989, Palomares et al. 2006), which "uses a woman's own personal medical history (number of previous breast biopsies and the presence of atypical hyperplasia in any previous

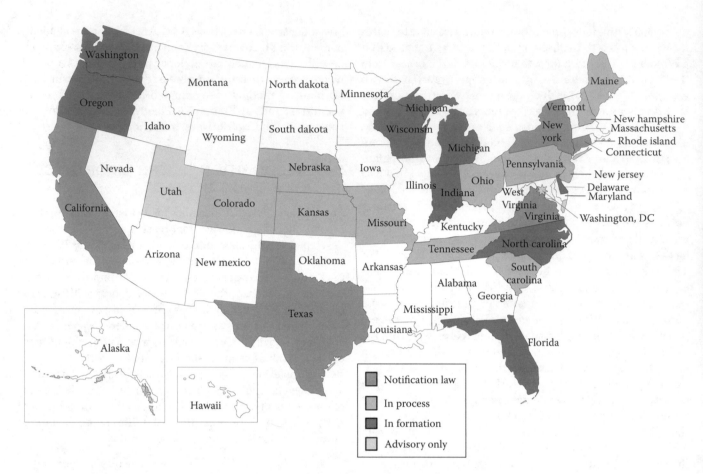

Figure 5.2 The (fluid) state of legislation requiring a woman to be told her breast density following breast imaging, as of January 2013. (Image courtesy of G. Kolb.)

breast biopsy specimen), her own reproductive history (age at the start of menstruation and age at the first live birth of a child), and the history of breast cancer among her first-degree relatives (mother, sisters, daughters) to estimate her risk of developing invasive breast cancer over specific periods of time." This quotation is taken from the National Cancer Institute website: http://www.cancer.gov/bcrisk-tool/, which is an implementation of the Gail model and is accessed up to 30,000 times a month, an indicator of the importance that clinicians and women increasingly attach to assessing the risk of developing cancer. Because of the difficulties in measuring breast density accurately, it is not included in the Gail model or the other models we mention later; however, Boyd et al. (2010) notes that breast density "is more strongly associated with breast cancer risk than the other variables included in the Gail model."

One alternative to the Gail model is the Tyrer–Cuzick model (also called the IBIS [International Breast Cancer Intervention Study] Breast Cancer Risk Evaluation Tool) (Tyrer et al. 2004). The Tyrer–Cuzick model includes not only extensive family history information but also

benign breast disease and endogenous estrogen exposure. It aims to infer differences in breast cancer risk on the basis of increased breast density (strictly, atypical hyperplasia). There have been several published comparisons of the Gail and Tyrer–Cuzick models. For example, in a recent retrospective study of the Mayo Benign Breast Disease cohort, Boughey et al. (2010) conclude that "the Tyrer–Cuzick model significantly overpredicts the risk of breast cancer development at 10 years in women with atypical hyperplasia, and that it is not able to accurately classify women into higher and lower risk groups. Neither the Tyrer–Cuzick model nor the Gail model predict individual risk in women with atypia better than chance alone." Conversely, the two models were also discussed by Professor Jennifer A. Harvey in a lecture on a "radiologist's perspective on adding risk assessment to mammography exams" delivered at the Workshop on Breast Density, San Francisco, CA, June 2011. Reporting results from the High Risk Clinic at the University of Virginia, she noted that the accuracy of the Gail model was 0.48, while that of Tyrer–Cuzick was 0.81. A new model incorporating density is likely to be far more accurate if it can be estimated reliably enough.

The importance of breast density to cancer risk was first noted by Wolfe in 1976 in two seminal papers (Wolfe 1976a,b) in which he proposed a stratification of breast density patterns into four classes: N1 (very little dense tissue, predominately fat), P1 and P2 (prominent ductal patterns in *less than one-fourth or more than one-fourth*, respectively), and DY (extensive dense tissue). He noted that a woman whose breasts were assigned to class DY was substantially more likely to develop breast cancer than a woman assigned to class N1. The concept of *substantially more likely* is often quantified using odds ratios, as we describe later. Seven years after Wolfe's papers, the American College of Radiology published its Breast Imaging Reporting and Data System (BI-RADS). This also requires the radiologist to assign a breast to one of four classes. The initial BI-RADS breast density categories were descriptive and subject to widely varying interpretation.

Recognizing this, the American College of Radiology (2003) subsequently issued quantitative definitions of the four mammographic density categories in 2003, namely, <25%, 25%–50%, 51%–75%, and >75%. This has become the standard for radiological reporting around the world. Nevertheless, Nicholson et al. (2006) compared percent mammographic densities (as estimated using CUMULUS) with radiologist-assigned BI-RADS mammographic density categories as defined by the 2003 quantitative measures. They note that "200 consecutive negative analog screening mammograms were assigned BI-RADS mammographic density categories independently by three radiologists blinded to the other readers' density assignment." They found that while "the percent mammographic density ranges for fatty and extremely dense breasts correlated well with BI-RADS definitions," this was by far less the case for scattered and heterogeneously dense categories. They conclude that "scattered fibroglandular densities and heterogeneously dense categories have broad percent mammographic density ranges and may not function well in breast cancer risk models."

Though Wolfe's insight and the subsequent BI-RADS classification have proven to be highly influential in clinical practice, note the intrinsically perceptual nature of the classifications that are problematic given the variations in brightness distributions illustrated in Figure 5.1. As per the N1/DY comparison in Wolfe's classification, a woman whose breasts are assigned to BI-RADS class 4 is substantially more likely to develop breast cancer than a woman whose breasts are assigned to BI-RADS class 1. Generally, radiologists have little difficulty assigning a breast to class 1 to class 4, but the intermediate classes are often problematic. Unsurprisingly, there is substantial inter- and intraradiologist disagreement (reportedly as high as 35%). Note also that radiologists whose legal liability is reduced if they declare a breast above BI-RADS class 1 (as then a disclaimer is usually put into the patient's letter) tend to avoid using the BI-RADS class 1 too frequently.

Other stratifications have been proposed, including the six-category classification used by Boyd in his work on breast cancer risk (see Boyd et al. 2010 and the references therein). This assigns breasts to one of six equal sextiles according to the analysis using the CUMULUS program, described in the next section. Note that this also implicitly assumes that the population is not heavily skewed, which is a reasonable assumption for populations of the sizes studied by Boyd and colleagues.

The *substantially* increased risk of developing breast cancer is typically calculated in terms of an odds ratio. Consider two populations 1, 2 that are to be compared, for example, BI-RADS class 1 vs. BI-RADS class 4, and suppose that the probability of a woman in population 1 subsequently developing breast cancer is p_1 and in population 2 is p_2. Then, the odds ratio of population 2 relative to population 1 is

$$\frac{p_2/(1-p_2)}{p_1/(1-p_1)}$$

An odds ratio that is greater than 1 quantifies the additional risk of belong to population 2 relative to population 1. We would expect that the odds ratio for a woman in BI-RADS class 4 relative to a woman in BI-RADS class 1 would be greater than 1, indeed greater than the odds ratio of BI-RADS 3 relative to BI-RADS 1. Note that the odds ratio calculations have to be applied with care. If, for example, $p_2 \approx 1$ (i.e., almost all women in that class go on to develop breast cancer), then $(1-p_2) \approx 0$, whereas it may be that for class 1 $p_1 \approx 0.5$ (i.e., almost as many women go on to develop breast cancer as do not), then the odds ratio approaches infinity. Of course, this extreme situation does not arise in practice, but it does stress the need for there to be sufficient numbers of women in each population who do and do not subsequently develop breast cancer; otherwise, the estimation of the probabilities from the specific sample of the population may be poor. Of course, fundamental to any such application of odds ratios is the *correct assignment* of women to the classes. Unfortunately, as we have noted, inter- and intraradiologist assignment of BI-RADS classifications is highly variable. Unsurprisingly, a considerable range of odds ratios have been reported in the literature ranging from 6 to 2 for dense (e.g., BI-RADS 4) to fatty (e.g., BI-RADS 1). If a *typical* population has approximately equal numbers of breasts in each BI-RADS class, then it is understandable why the four classes are used, approximately equally, even for a highly skewed population, as noted in the previous paragraph.

Recently, breast density has been given new impetus as a result of legislation, particularly, though not only, in the United States that requires that following a mammogram, women be told their breast density. At the time of writing, this is a fluid situation, though as Figure 5.2 shows, legislation has already been passed in Connecticut, New York, Virginia, Texas, and California. In total, these five states account for over 30% of women in the Unites States. Note that there is (at time of writing) an additional 11 states where legislation is in process, and a further 8 where it is not currently mandated but is advisory. Elsewhere, the Netherlands is well advanced toward mandating a breast density measure after a mammogram, and the United Kingdom, Australia, and New Zealand are framing similar policies. An important practical implication of such legislation is that density can then be used to justify follow-on images (ultrasound, MRI), which insurance companies must pay for.

Evidently, breast density is important for assessing the risk of developing breast cancer, and for patient management, not least in determining those women who should have additional complementary images in order to detect cancer, monitor the progression of a (suspected or proven) cancer, and/or evaluate responses to therapy. However, not least because of the inter- and intra-radiologist disagreement in a density class to a breast, there is increasing interest in computer-based measurements. However, for routine clinical use, such measurements need to be quantitative, repeatable, accurate, relate to numbers that radiologists are familiar with, can be deployed routinely, not disrupt clinical workflow, and not be overly slow. These are substantial challenges, and progress toward achieving them is discussed in the next section.

5.3 MEASURING BREAST DENSITY FROM IMAGES

The most widely used computer-based method to aid the quantitative estimation of breast density was the CUMULUS method, originally developed by Yaffe et al. (Byng et al. 1994), but see Boyd et al. (2010) for a contemporary display and outline description. The user is invited to select a brightness threshold that captures the area of dense tissue in the breast most effectively. The area of this region is divided by the estimated area of the breast (in general, a nontrivial problem to automate) and expressed as a percentage. These percentages then form the basis for the six-category classification referred to in the previous section. Other researchers, for example, have re-implemented substantially the same method (Shepherd et al. 2011). Though CUMULUS has become the basis for comparison for subsequent methods, such area-based measures are

intrinsically subjective, and there is substantial inter- and intraobserver variability (Martin 2006, Nicholson et al. 2006), despite extensive training to use the software. Also, such methods require additional decision time by skilled users. As a result, although the results generated by trained users in research environments are encouraging, the applicability of such methods in the real world is at best problematic. Unfortunately, to date at least, the automation of area-based density measures, to the point where they can be incorporated into clinical workflow, has proven to be difficult, primarily due to differences in imaging parameters making the image brighter or darker or affecting the contrast (recall Figure 5.1), hence appearing more or less dense; and to textural similarities between very fatty and very dense breasts.

A mammogram is a 2D image of the compressed 3D breast, and so CUMULUS measures the amount of dense tissue from a projection. However, the *amount* of dense tissue is intrinsically volumetric, a 3D measure (Kontos 2010). As a trivial (possibly unrealistic) example, which aims to make the point, consider a breast in which there is single thin sheet of dense tissue that lies parallel to the compression plates. An algorithm based on thresholding a 2D image, such as CUMULUS, would report BI-RADS 4, whereas the likelihood that the breast should be classified as BI-RADS 1. (Of course, this would be picked up immediately in the MLO image.) Nevertheless, this highlights the fact that the amount of dense breast tissue is a question that pertains fundamentally to the *volume* of dense tissue in the breast. This immediately poses the question whether a 3D measurement can be computed from a single mammogram.

There have been three classes of methods developed for analyzing mammograms to date, and they are described in the following sections: (1) *absolute* physics methods, typified by standardized mammogram form (SMF) (Highnam and Brady 1999, Highnam et al. 2006); (2) use of a calibration device; and (3) the *relative* physics model developed by Highnam et al. (2010).

5.3.1 Absolute Physics Models of Image Acquisition

Figure 5.1 reminds us that a mammographic image is a result of the breast contents, in particular dense tissue, *and* the choice of image settings chosen by the technician (radiographer). Over the past 20 years, there has been a succession of mathematical and/or computational methods devised aimed at eliminating (most of) the image formation choices, to yield an approximation to the density information, in effect a 3D representation of the breast. The first of these was the h_{int} approach developed by Highnam and Brady (1999), also known as *standardized mammogram form—SMF* (Highnam et al. 2006). We use h_{int} and SMF interchangeably in the following very brief outline of how it works. Note that the method was originally developed for film-screen mammography, but was subsequently adapted to *for processing* digital mammograms.

Alternative models have been proposed, most notably that of van Engeland (2006): we return to it in Section 5.3.3.

Refer to Figure 5.3. The SMF method begins with an equation that models the flow of X-ray photons from the tube to the imager. In particular, it models the energy $E^{imp}(\mathbf{x})$ that is

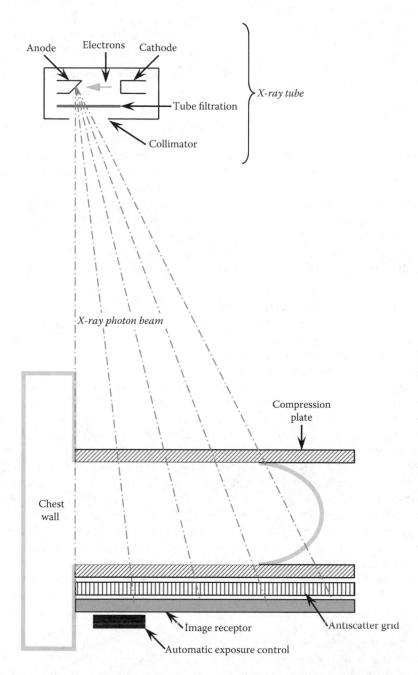

Figure 5.3 The components of a typical mammography unit, shown here taking a CC exposure. The upper part is the x-ray tube, from which the emerging photons are filtered and collimated. The photon beam passes through the upper compression plate (shown here as rigid and horizontal), though there is increasing use of compression plates that angle to conform more closely to the shape of the breast as it lies on the lower plate. The compression plates are generally made of a composite material such as PMMA. An antiscatter grid reduces the angle over which photons arrive to expose a particular imaging element (digital or analog film). The exposure control aims to reduce automatically the dose of x-rays imparted to the breast. The breast is typically compressed to a force of 130–150 N.

imparted to the detector where **x** denotes the pixel location in the image:

$$E^{\text{imp}}(\mathbf{x}) = \phi(V_t, \mathbf{x}) A_p t_s$$

$$\int_0^{E_{\max}} N_0^{\text{rel}}(V_t, \varepsilon) G(\varepsilon) D(\varepsilon) \exp^{-\mu_{\text{lucite}}(\varepsilon) h_{\text{plate}}} \exp^{-h\mu(\varepsilon)} d\varepsilon$$

$$(5.1)$$

where

ϕ denotes the X-ray photon fluence

V_t is the voltage of the X-ray tube

A_p is the area of a pixel location on the X-ray detector

t_s is the exposure time

$N_0^{\text{rel}}(\varepsilon)$ is the relative number of X-ray photons incident upon the compression plates and breast at the particular energy ε

$G(\varepsilon)$ models the effect of the antiscatter grid

$D(\varepsilon)$ models the detector (either a directly digital detector or a film-screen combination)

$h\mu(\varepsilon)$ is the linear X-ray attenuation coefficient in the (primary) column defined by the X-ray tube to pixel location **x**

Note that this equation defines the *primary* fluence to the detector and ignores scatter. Though it is beyond the scope of this chapter, there have been a number of models developed for the scatter component, ranging in complexity from a convolution with the primary image to a component that varies from pixel to pixel in the image (Highnam and Brady 1999, Tromans 2010, Tromans et al. 2012b). The latter is computationally much more expensive but is more accurate. Note also that in Equation 5.1, we use linear attenuation coefficients, which are a function of the energy. However, we have subsequently, for example, in the *Volpara*™ system (Section 5.4), used effective attenuation coefficients, which also depend on the breast thickness.

The fundamental assumption of SMF is that, so far as mammography is concerned, the overwhelming majority of tissue within the breast is either fat or *interesting* (which implicitly assumes that adipose tissue is of no interest clinically, a reasonable assumption in the case of the breast, though not in the case of the stomach or liver!). Interesting tissue comprises stromal, glandular, and abnormal (benign or malignant) tissues. The justification for combining these various tissues into a single *interesting* class is that they cannot (currently) be differentiated on the basis of their x-ray attenuation rates (for the imaging conditions of mammography, it is an open question whether or not they can be distinguished in dual/multiple energy x-ray imaging that is increasingly made possible by novel detectors such as those based on silicon drift detectors). Note that the SMF model assumes that if microcalcifications are present, they are in such small quantities that they do not

affect the overall estimate. Microcalcification detection methods based on SMF have been developed, for example, Yam et al. (1999) and Linguraru et al. (2001). It has been explored for multimodal breast image registration (Marias et al. 2006).

Suppose that the compressed thickness of the breast, that is, the separation between the compression plates, is H (cm), then the SMF model seeks to estimate, for each pixel **x** in the image, the amount of interesting tissue $h_{\text{int}}(\mathbf{x})$ and the amount of fat tissue $h_{\text{fat}}(\mathbf{x})$ so that

$$0 \le h_{\text{int}}(\mathbf{x}), \quad h_{\text{fat}}(\mathbf{x}) \le H; \quad h_{\text{int}}(\mathbf{x}) + h_{\text{fat}}(\mathbf{x}) = H$$

SMF assumes that the separation H is known. This is (reasonably) accurately recorded in the DICOM header for digital mammograms; however, it was often not available for film-screen mammography. Nevertheless, it can be estimated to reasonable accuracy even in the latter case (Highnam et al. 2006).

As a consequence of the SMF assumption, there are two attenuation coefficients $\mu_{\text{int}}(\varepsilon)$, $\mu_{\text{fat}}(\varepsilon)$ whose values are assumed to be known. The linear x-ray attenuation coefficient in Equation 5.1 then satisfies (for each pixel **x**—which for clarity is omitted in the following set of equations) as follows:

$$h\mu(\varepsilon) = h_{\text{int}}\mu_{\text{int}}(\varepsilon) + h_{\text{fat}}\mu_{\text{fat}}(\varepsilon)$$

$$= h_{\text{int}}\mu_{\text{int}}(\varepsilon) + (H - h_{\text{int}})\mu_{\text{fat}}(\varepsilon)$$

$$= h_{\text{int}}(\mu_{\text{int}}(\varepsilon) - \mu_{\text{fat}}(\varepsilon)) + H\mu_{\text{fat}}(\varepsilon) \quad (5.2)$$

Suppose that we can estimate $h\mu(\varepsilon)$, then the only unknown is h_{int} and so it can be solved for. In the SMF implementations to date, digital or film screen, the energy imparted $E^{\text{imp}}(\mathbf{x})$ is mapped to intensity (the details for film screen are sketched in Highnam et al. (2006)). Highnam and Brady (1999) demonstrate if sufficient calibration data are available, then it is possible to map from the observed intensity value at pixel **x** to an observed value $E_{\text{obs}}^{\text{imp}}(\mathbf{x})$. From Equations 5.1 and 5.2, there is then just one unknown, namely, $h_{\text{int}}(\mathbf{x})$ whose value can be varied until the left-hand side of Equation 5.1 equates to the observed value $E_{\text{obs}}^{\text{imp}}(\mathbf{x})$. This, in essence, is how the SMF estimation processes work. Note again that Equation 5.2 uses linear attenuation coefficients; we have subsequently used effective attenuation coefficients.

What results is a surface of interesting tissue thicknesses $\{h_{\text{int}}(\mathbf{x}) : \text{pixels } \mathbf{x}\}$, where h_{int} is measured in centimeters, and so mammography becomes quantitative. Now, assuming that the breast region B can be segmented accurately, we can in principle *measure* the amount of breast density by summing the values $\sum_{\mathbf{x} \in B} h_{\text{int}}(\mathbf{x})$. To date, however, the correlation between the (volumetric) amount of breast density measured this way and breast cancer risk has been quite variable (McCormack 2007). The fundamental reasons why this is so seem to be as follows: (1) as is always the case in science, a number of simplifying assumptions have to made to make the model mathematically tractable (parallel beam, convolution scatter model, etc.) and (2) the $h_{int}(\mathbf{x})$ values are sensitive (in the sense of a Taylor's series expansion) to inaccuracies in the physics data on which the SMF model depends. One stream of research subsequent to that presented in Highnam and Brady (1999) has aimed to remove most, if not all of those simplifying assumptions. A recent example of this trend is Tromans et al. (2012a,b).

This section may be summarized as follows: there is good news and bad news about the *explicit* absolute physics models developed to date. The good news is that despite the inevitable simplifying assumptions, if sufficient calibration data are available with sufficient accuracy, then SMF gives remarkably accurate $h_{int}(\mathbf{x})$ values. This has been the basis for novel algorithms to detect microcalcifications (Yam et al. 1999, Linguraru et al. 2001), 3D reconstruction from CC and MLO views of the breast (Yam et al. 2001), temporal matching of mammograms (2006), and grid/cloud-based analysis of mammograms (Gilbert et al. 2004). The bad news is the limited availability of comprehensive accurate calibration data. Is there an alternative approach?

5.3.2 3D from 2D Using a Calibration Device

An alternative to *explicit* modeling is to develop one that is *implicit*. A familiar example of this is a lookup table or, in the case of neural networks, learned associations. In the case of mammography, the challenge is to devise a method that allows estimation of a function:

$$\hat{h}(\mathbf{x}) = f\left(I_{obs}(\mathbf{x}) \,|\, \mathbf{p}\right)$$

where

$\hat{h}(\mathbf{x})$ is the amount of dense tissue in the column of the breast corresponding to the pixel $\mathbf{x}$ (the notation aims to stress the correspondence $\hat{h}(\mathbf{x}) \approx h_{int}(\mathbf{x})$)

$I_{obs}(\mathbf{x})$ is the intensity observed at the pixel $\mathbf{x}$

$\mathbf{p}$ is the *unknown* set of calibration parameters

Generally, the (unknown) function f is approximated by using a suitable *calibration object* that is placed next to the breast during imaging, so that it does not occlude any identifying labels on the mammogram. The calibration object has known geometry, say, for the sake of illustration, that it comprises a step wedge, whose steps have heights $\{h_i | i = 1,...,n\}$. Each step will correspond to a set of pixels, whose observed intensities may (e.g.) be averaged, establishing, for the unknown parameter values, a set of correspondences:

$$\{I_i \Leftrightarrow h_i \,|\, i = 1,...,n\}$$

Now, given an observed intensity, $I_{obs}(\mathbf{x})$; the set of correspondences is used to *infer* most likely $\hat{h}(x)$. Generally, this is done by interpolation from the set of correspondences. Evidently, it is straightforward to modify this method to work with any calibration object geometry. A number of variations on this theme have been proposed. The first was developed by Pawluczyk et al. (2003), see also Mawdsley et al. (2009), and led to the development of CUMULUS V, the volumetric version of the originally 2D CUMULUS.

Though the method is straightforward in concept, there are a number of issues that have to be addressed in practice. First, the geometry of the calibration object needs to be considered carefully. Sticking with a step wedge, for illustration, if the step heights are too small, then the difference in heights between successive steps can give rise to intensity differences that are swamped by noise, rendering the estimation uncertain. Conversely, if they are too large, then the interpolation can be problematic, since the relationship between height and intensity is unlikely to be linear. Finally, the object needs to span the vast majority of heights expected in practice, since although interpolation is mathematically sound and gives accurate results in many cases, extrapolation is not. A second issue concerns the material of which the object is made. For example, while several authors have used lucite, Diffey et al. (2006) used aluminum. An alternative calibration object was proposed by Shepherd et al. (2005).

The good news about the use of calibration objects in this way is that it can be shown to lead to highly accurate modeling, see, for example, Mawdsley et al. (2009) and Shepherd et al. (2011). Alonzo-Proulx et al. (2010) further demonstrate good correspondence with breast CT data. This suggests that they be used as a *gold standard* in research studies, for example, to evaluate explicit methods that work directly from the image (such as those outlined in Sections 5.3.1 and 5.3.3). However, the bad news is that there are a number of significant challenges to their use in routine clinical environments where breast density measurements are required, for example, for determining whether or not a screened woman should have additional images taken. Among these challenges are (1) that retrospective images used to gauge changes to breast density almost certainly would not have the calibration object in view—for example, Shepherd (2011) reports that 40% of cases in their study could not be treated for this reason; (2) the need to remove the calibration object when imaging large breasts; (3) the potential for parts of the calibration object to be occluded by the breast; (4) overlap between the calibration object and the labels attached to the film (in the case of film-screen mammography—happily, less of a problem with digital mammography); and (5) the additional time needed to place the calibration object interferes with workflow and lengthens the acquisition time.

Is there an alternative to the absolute physics approach that does not have the practical limitations of using calibration objects?

5.3.3 Relative Physics Model of Image Acquisition

Recently, Highnam et al. (2010) combined a number of features of the SMF model described in Section 5.3.1 with those of the method proposed by van Engeland et al. (2006). The revised model, which we call Volpara*, begins by finding an area of the breast that corresponds entirely to fatty tissue and is used to define a reference intensity value I_{fat}. From this, the thickness of dense tissue $h_d(\mathbf{x})$ at each pixel $\mathbf{x}$ is measured according to the method proposed by van Engeland et al.:

$$h_d(\mathbf{x}) = \frac{\ln\left(I_{obs}(\mathbf{x})/I_{fat}\right)}{\mu_{fat} - \mu_{dense}} \tag{5.3}$$

This equation assumes that the observed intensity value $I_{obs}(\mathbf{x})$ is related linearly to the energy $E^{imp}(\mathbf{x})$ imparted to the x-ray detector, an assumption that generally holds for all direct digital images. The two constants in the denominator of Equation 5.3 are the effective x-ray linear attenuation coefficients for fat and dense tissue at the particular target, filter, tube voltage, and recorded breast thickness combination. Strictly, following the previous sections, we should write $\mu_{fat/dense}(\mathbf{p}, H)$ but for clarity, we omit this extra notation; nevertheless, to be precise, we should write $h_d(\mathbf{x}|\mathbf{p}, H)$. Crucially, unlike the sensitivity of measurements $h_{int}(\mathbf{x})$ to errors in the estimations of $\mathbf{p}$ that were noted in Section 5.3.1, the formulation in Equation 5.3 is intrinsically robust to errors in time of exposure, detector gain, and other multiplicative variations, since those values appear both in the reference level and in the actual pixel values, so cancel out.

As ever, the devil is in the detail.† In this case, as noted by Highnam and Brady (1999) and McCormack et al. (2007), the difficulty lies in finding an area of the breast that is entirely fat, especially when the breast in question is very dense (which is the category of highest risk and thus of greatest interest). Highnam et al. (2010) overcome this difficulty, while retaining a relative physics model approach by (1) using the phase congruency model of early image analysis (Kovesi 1999), which not only is invariant to imaging conditions but also enables a wide range of intensity changes (not just step changes in intensity) to be detected, and (2) an iterative approach to finding the fatty uncompressed breast edge as documented in Highnam and Brady (1999) along with realistic, relative, breast edge models (Highnam and Brady 1999, van Engeland 2006). With an accurate breast edge found, in practice, one can always find I_{fat}.

The performance of our new breast edge detection algorithm, and thus the robustness of finding I_{fat} (see the previous section) on some very dense breasts, is illustrated in Figure 5.4, where we show the inner and outer limits of the uncompressed fatty breast edge within which we search for I_{fat}. Critically, note that the inner limit of the determined breast edge does not overlay any dense tissue.

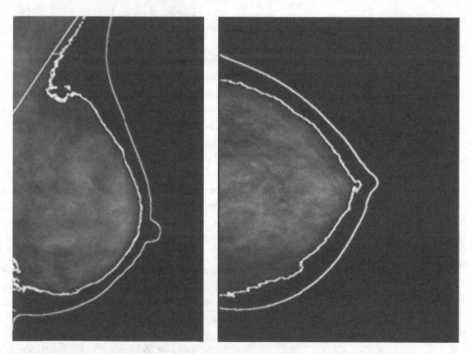

Figure 5.4 Illustration of segmentation of the inner and outer breast boundaries for the case of a dense breast.

* VolparaTM is the name of a product developed by Matakina Ltd., a company founded by Ralph Highnam, Sir Michael Brady, Nico Karssemeijer, Martin Yaffe, and John Hood.

† This graphic phrase has a fascinating history, see "the devil is in the detail."

Recalling that Equation 5.1 refers to primary fluence, it is necessary to include a scatter removal process. There are several such reported in the literature. The one used in Volpara is a modified version of the algorithm reported in van Engeland (2006). A second consideration in increasing practice is the use of compression plates that are deliberately not parallel (see the legend to Figure 5.3). Recently, an enhanced version of Volpara beyond that reported in Highnam et al. (2010) has been developed and made available commercially and which accommodates almost all nonparallel compression plates without relying upon the DICOM header.

The volume of dense tissue is computed as the sum $\sum_{x \in Image} h_d(x)$ over the entire image, while the volume of the breast is determined by multiplying the area of the breast by the recorded breast thickness H; the breast density is then the ratio of the two. Evidently, errors in recorded breast thickness remain important; we return to this issue later, where we demonstrate Volpara's robustness. The commercial version of Volpara received FDA 510(K) clearance in October 2010 and, at the time of writing, is installed in over 200 hospital centers in 30 countries.

5.4 EXPERIMENTS ON MEASURING BREAST DENSITY USING RELATIVE PHYSICS MODEL

In this section, to give a better appreciation of the current situation regarding quantitative assessment of breast density from a single mammogram, we review some of the clinical trial data using Volpara over the past 2 years. At the outset, we wish to make two things clear. First, the authors are all founders (together with Professor Martin Yaffe) of Matakina Ltd., which has developed Volpara. Though we have attempted to present the following evidence entirely factually, we want the reader to be aware of our involvement with Matakina Ltd. Second, Hologic Ltd. offers a rival product Quantra™ and could, presumably, provide similar evidence. Our point in this section is *not* to advocate Volpara, rather to establish the current level of performance of *clinically available commercial* analysis software. For those to whom it is of interest, the results presented in this section are for version 1.3.1 of Volpara, but will be referred to as commercial analysis software.

In the following, we present the results of a series of studies:

1. A phantom study, which aimed at assessing the absolute value of the volumetric density, and its repeatability as the parameters governing the imaging of the phantom are changed.
2. A study in which the extent to which the volumetric density estimate assessed remains invariant over images taken using different X-ray detectors.

3. The results of a trial that compares volumetric density against BI-RADS readings (Highnam et al. 2012).
4. A comparison of volumetric densities for the same woman imaged 1 year apart on different manufacturer's mammography units, namely, a GE mammography unit and a Hologic unit (in some cases first GE, some cases first Hologic).
5. Anticipating Section 5.5, results of a trial comparing volumetric density estimated by commercial software with that estimated from the corresponding MRI volume.

To conclude the section, we present the results of two further studies:

6. Comparison of the results of volumetric density estimated by commercial software with those reported in a reader study by Kopans (2003).
7. Studies on the change in breast density in a population over a number of years.

5.4.1 Phantom Study

First, we report results of a phantom study. We estimate breast density using commercial software on a set of five images of a test phantom acquired with different imaging combinations, kindly supplied by the University of Toronto. Each image had five *plugs* inserted (labeled A–E) with different densities, and the average error between actual and estimated densities is 1.11%. See Table 5.1.

5.4.2 Different X-Ray Detectors

We analyzed the results over a set of different detectors. Table 5.2 shows the median breast density for each detector, along with the Pearson correlation coefficient for L/R and CC/MLO along with numbers of images. This demonstrates that we achieve consistent results across detectors. We note the exception of the PM34_05 detector, that is, the detector on which we have collected the images of young women who have been imaged prior to having breast MRI, thus the high breast density.

Next, to investigate the robustness of the results to imaging conditions, we edited the mAs in an image (MoMo, 29 kVp) by ±20% and then again ran commercial software, as shown in Table 5.3. As that table shows, we found identical results that we also obtained when multiplying the pixel values in the image by various factors to simulate variations in detector gain such as you might expect between detectors, over time, and between manufacturers.

For further demonstration, we introduced extra noise into a set of images by randomly adding or subtracting up to 5% and 10% of the pixel value and found that, as expected, noise has limited effect apart from at low breast density. See Table 5.4.

TABLE 5.1   PHANTOM DATA

Toronto Plug Phantoms

Image	A	B	C	D	E	Imaging Factors
Actual plug densities						
#1	0.0	25.0	25.0	12.5	25.0	MoMo26
						76 mAs
#2	0.0	25.0	25.0	12.5	25.0	MoMo28
						51 mAs
#3	0.0	20.0	20.0	10.0	20.0	MoMo26
						110 mAs
#4	0.0	16.7	16.7	8.3	16.7	MoRh26
						155 mAs
#5	12.5	37.5	37.5	25.0	37.5	MoMo28
						55 mAs
Estimated plug densities						
#1	0.43	23.9	24.3	9.9	23.0	
#2	0.16	23.8	24.0	9.7	22.9	
#3	0.41	20.1	20.2	8.6	18.0	
#4	0.64	17.8	18.0	7.8	15.8	
#5	13.6	39.2	39.2	25.2	37.6	

TABLE 5.2   COMPARISONS ACROSS DETECTORS

	Median	PCC L/R	PCC CC/MLO	# Images
All	8.8	0.923	0.915	2217
PM54_01	8.9	0.930	0.908	937
PM460_2	7.8	0.914	0.878	290
PM34_05	16.1	0.915	0.931	104
PM079_04	8.0	0.911	0.916	881

TABLE 5.3   EFFECT OF ERRORS IN MAS ON COMMERCIAL SOFTWARE TOOL

	−20% (80 mAs)	0% (100 mAs)	+20% (120 mAs)
Volume of dense tissue (cm³)	114	114	114
Volume of breast (cm³)	575	575	575
Breast density (%)	19.8	19.8	19.8

As noted earlier, breast thickness's major influence is in the breast volume, but it is also present to a lesser degree in the dense tissue volume when we work out the effective energy. Fortunately, whereas previous implementations (Highnam and Brady 1999) had seen these two factors act

TABLE 5.4   EFFECT OF VARYING LEVEL OF RANDOM NOISE ON COMMERCIAL SOFTWARE TOOL

Breast Density Results Running On

Original Image (%)	Original Image ± 5% Random Noise (%)	Original Image ± 10% Random Noise (%)
2.3	3.4	5.1
12.4	12.5	13.5
19.6	19.7	17.1
28.1	28.2	28.2

TABLE 5.5   EFFECT OF ERRORS IN BREAST THICKNESS ON THE COMMERCIAL SOFTWARE TOOL

	Variation in Breast Thickness (H)				
H (mm)	−20%	−10%	0%	+10%	+20%
86	2.5%	2.4%	2.3%	2.2%	2.1%
32	15.1%	13.6%	12.4%	11.4%	10.6%
20	23.7%	21.4%	19.6%	18.0%	16.8%
40	33.6%	30.5%	28.1%	26.2%	24.4%

in different ways so as to amplify the errors, commercial software's implementation has the factors acting in the same way—so, if breast thickness rises, then both breast volume rises and the volume of dense tissue rises so that the overall ratio does not vary widely. Table 5.5 shows the results from the commercial software over four different images when the breast thickness was varied by 20% up and down. Clearly, breast thickness errors will inevitably introduce small errors into the breast density measurement, but thanks to quality requirements in the field, they should rarely exceed 10%, and so, as can be seen, the resulting estimate of breast density remains remarkably accurate. Furthermore, because breast thickness is almost always underestimated by the x-ray machine, the woman's density assessment will rise, not lower, and thus the woman will never be treated in a lower density and thus risk category.

5.4.3   Volumetric Density vs. BI-RADS

Having presented the results of phantom studies, we now transition to clinical studies. First, recalling the interrater variations reported in Section 5.2, we next present results showing the correlation between volumetric density and the BI-RADS score assessed by an experienced radiologist. Figure 5.5 is reproduced from Highnam et al. (2012).

In Figure 5.5, the average breast density is depicted by the middle line in each of the blue boxes, as is the inter quartile range (25%–75% of the data and the outliers).

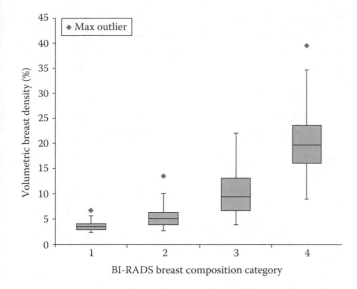

Figure 5.5   Comparison of BI-RADS rating of a mammogram (abscissa) compared with volumetric density (ordinate), as estimated by a commercial software tool.

5.4.4   Volumetric Density on Different Manufacturer's Mammography Units

As a woman moves through her screening lifetime, she will likely be imaged on several different X-ray machines; it is thus important that any method to estimate volumetric density should give very similar results on each machine. Figure 5.6 shows the results of a trial in which 84 women were imaged 1 year on GE and 1 year on Hologic, sometimes GE first, sometimes Hologic first. The results of estimating volumetric density using a commercial software tool are shown in Figure 5.6. This study was carried out at the Elizabeth Wende Breast Clinic by Dr. Stamatia Destounis.

The volumetric density estimated by the commercial software tool is determined using the DICOM *For Processing* data, so theoretically, it should be independent of the image processing applied by the individual manufacturer. That proves to be the case: the correlation between the two sets of values is 0.91. Note that one would not expect perfect correlation as the images were taken 1 year apart.

5.4.5   Comparison of Volumetric Density Estimated Using Commercial Software with That Estimated from MRI

Anticipating Section 5.5, we next compare the volumetric density estimated using commercial software with that estimated using MRI, which is often touted as *ground truth*. Figure 5.7 shows the results of a comparison done at the University of Utrecht Medical Centre. The figure shows the results for 44 women. The MRI values involved a radiologist manually thresholding each individual slice of the MRI volume into fibroglandular and fat. Summation over the slices gives the volume of fibroglandular tissue reported in the figure. The correlation between the volumetric density and MRI is 0.93.

5.4.6   Kopans's Reader Study

In his seminal book *Breast Imaging* (2007), D. Kopans published a graph showing how many women at each age group had a BI-RADS 3 or 4 breast vs. a 1 or 2 breast, based on review by human readers of 3000 patients at Massachusetts General Hospital. We replicated Kopans's work at the University of Toronto on 15,000 patient datasets. The percentage densities measured using commercial software were then grouped into BI-RADS 1 and 2 vs. 3 and 4. The result is shown in Figure 5.8 and closely resembles the figure in Kopans's book.

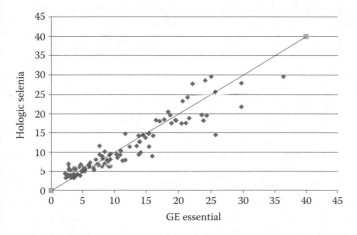

Figure 5.6   Comparison of percentage densities estimated using a commercial software tool for 84 women imaged using either a GE or Hologic mammography unit 1 year, the other the following year.

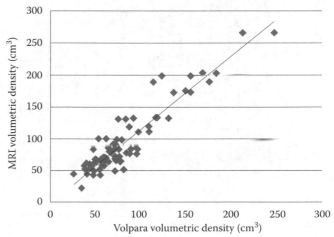

Figure 5.7   Comparison of volumetric density (in cm³) estimated using a commercial software tool (abscissa) and MRI (ordinate).

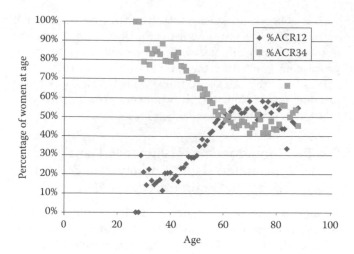

Figure 5.8 Volumetric density grade, estimated using a commercial software tool (ordinate) vs. age of the woman (abscissa). The study was inspired by Kopans's (2007) similar study using human readers.

5.4.7 Population Breast Density Change over Time

To conclude this section, we return to the theme established at the outset of this chapter: the expected change in breast density over time, postmenopause. Figure 5.9 shows the results of one of a number of studies that we have carried out, this one at the University Medical Centre, Utrecht. Fifty

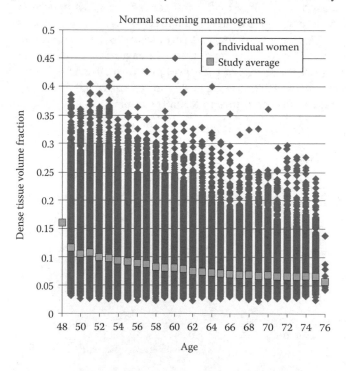

Figure 5.9 Dense tissue volume fraction as a function of age for 50,000 women.

thousand women were imaged on a Hologic Selenia full-field digital mammography unit and the percentage volumetric density plotted against the age of the woman. Evidently, average density decreases with age, as expected.

5.5 DIRECT 3D ESTIMATION OF THE VOLUME OF BREAST DENSITY

So far, this chapter has been concerned with establishing the importance of assessing quantitatively the amount of dense tissue in the (postmenopausal) breast, both as a major risk factor for developing breast cancer and as a stratification criterion for further imaging. The focus has been entirely on mammography for reasons of sensitivity and specificity, but largely for reasons of cost and the ubiquity of mammography, which is almost always the first port of call in imaging the breast. Evidently, a mammogram is a single 2D image of the projected breast, and while we have described techniques to estimate the (3D) volume of dense tissue in the breast from a mammogram, and while such techniques are remarkably performance imaging methods that are intrinsically 3D will always inspire greater confidence even if—at this stage in the evolution of imaging—they are costly in terms of time, money, and even radiation dose.

There is increasing interest in direct 3D imaging of the breast. The methods that have been explored most fully to date are CT, MRI, and ultrasound, though a range of other methods including optical tomography and microwave imaging have also been experimented with (primarily, at this point, on phantoms). This section briefly summarizes the current situation, but the reader should be aware that this is a field that is evolving rapidly, for several reasons. First, each of the imaging modalities discussed in this section is becoming ever more affordable, delivering results ever more rapidly. Second, the limitations of mammographic imaging, primarily of dense breasts, are becoming of increasing concern (see Section 5.1). Finally, radiation dose accumulates, and so there is both inevitable reluctance to image the breast mammographically *too often* (how often is a contentious issue that is beyond the scope of this chapter) and a desire to embrace imaging modalities, particularly MRI, which do not involve ionizing radiation.

5.5.1 Breast CT

Of course, CT is a 3D X-ray-based imaging technology, and so it does involve ionizing radiation, and so imaging has to be optimized while restricting the dose imparted to the breast to the level equivalent to a craniocaudal (CC) plus a mediolateral oblique (MLO) image (typically both are taken in mammography). This is increasingly possible by using low-noise fast X-ray detectors and using cone-beam CT.

Breast CT has been pioneered at the University of California, Davis, by Professor John M. Boone and his colleagues (Boone et al. 2006a,b, Lindfors et al. 2008). Two recent variants are presented by McKinley et al. (2012) and Shah et al. (2012).

In the device developed by Boone and colleagues, the patient lies prone on a table with the breast pendant through an aperture (a similar arrangement is used for breast MRI). As in conventional (cone-beam) CT, an x-ray tube and detector, on diametrically opposite sides of the breast, rotate through 360° acquiring a set of projection images at different orientations. These images are then reconstructed using any of the many well-known tomographic reconstruction algorithms. The result is a volume (array) whose voxels have sizes ranging between 0.21 and 0.41 mm in the coronal plane and between 0.25 and 0.41 mm in the sagittal plane. A number of preliminary clinical trials using breast CT devices have been reported (see the references in the previous paragraph). In addition, Alonzo-Proulx et al. (2010) have done a comparison of breast volumes estimated using Boone's CT device, and the CUMULUS V mammography device described earlier reported encouraging correlation between the assessments (differences typically around 9%).

5.5.2   Breast MRI

Breast imaging was one of the first clinical applications of MRI, see, for example, Heywang-Koebrunner (1989) and the references therein. Naturally, early work in breast MRI concerned the detection of tumors. It was quickly realized that the intrinsic relaxation parameters T_1, T_2^* did not, in many cases, enable reliable detection, and so contrast agents were used. To date, though there have been numerous experiments with agents such as iron oxide, the contrast agents approved for clinical use are chelates of lanthanides, most notably gadolinium. The relative large Gd-based molecules can traverse, but are slowed by the leaky microvasculature constructed by a (relatively mature) tumor. Initial work compared the MRI volumes taken pre- and postcontrast agent bolus injection. Subsequent work, for example, Hayton et al. (1997) and the references therein, took advantage of the increasing speed at which volumes of the breast could be sampled and began to model the pharmacokinetics (PK) of contrast agent take-up. Currently, it is possible to acquire entire breast volumes every few (typically 5) seconds, greatly improving the numerical fitting of such PK models. Contrast uptake curves, one per voxel, are typically classified into a small number of cases, such as no take-up, steady increase throughout the sampling period, normal, and significantly enhanced (generally corresponding to regions of angiogenesis). An example of such classification is given in Chen et al. (2010a,b).

However, our interest in this chapter is breast density not tumor detection. There has been increasing interest in the estimation of the volume of breast density based on MRI—indeed, a comparison with MRI as *ground truth* was required by the FDA in approving Hologic's *Quantra* product and Matakina's *Volpara* described earlier.

Early work on estimating the volume of breast density using MRI has been done by Graham et al. (1996), Schnall (2003), Klifa et al. (2010), and Brown et al. (2000). More generally, there has naturally been interest in classifying tissue in MRI images into a range of types: fat, muscle, fibroglandular, and *others* (e.g., bone, air). The pulse sequences used to make such a classification depend on the region of the body for which the tissue classification is to be done. More precisely, it depends upon the extent to which fatty tissue and other types share the same voxel—the partial volume problem. In the stomach, for example, this occurs to a significant extent, and so techniques such as Dixon's two-point method have been developed. As explained, for example, by Dahlqvist Leinhard et al. (2008), "Dixon imaging is performed by acquiring two separate images: one where the signals from fat and water are 180° out of phase ($I1 = w - f$) and one where they are in phase ($I2 = w + f$). Ideally, water and fat can then be obtained as the sum and difference of these images, respectively, and the total fat content in any region of interest can then easily be calculated." In practice, the situation is not nearly so straightforward, and so the authors propose a method to improve the basic method.

Generally, however, methods to segment fat from fibroglandular tissue in the breast have not been nearly so sophisticated. Consider, for example, the MARIBS project (Brown et al. 2000, Leach et al. 2005, Thompson et al. 2009) in which (to quote Thompson et al. 2009)

> the study population was taken from women who participated in the MARIBS study [4,5], in which 837 asymptomatic women aged 31 to 49 years thought to be at high genetic risk of breast cancer (carriers of *BRCA1*, *BRCA2* or *TP53* mutations, their first degree relatives, or untested women with a strong family history of breast and/or ovarian cancer, or a family history suggestive of Li-Fraumeni syndrome; estimated annual risk of breast cancer ≥ 0.9%) consented, of whom 741 attended for MRI and/or X-ray mammography (XRM) in at least one year.

The MARIBS project developed a novel method to analyze dense tissue on the basis of MRI, detailed in Khazen et al. (2008). A precontrast T_1-weighted image is taken and then corrected (for coil uniformity) using the proton density image. Finally, the water-containing tissues were segmented interactively. A software tool, MRIBview, was developed to determine the volume of nonfat tissue and the percentage of dense tissue.

Some authors have noted that the breast skin is often counted as part of the dense tissue, and so methods have been developed to segment out the skin, for example, using a classification technique based on fuzzy C-means clustering (Nie et al. 2010a,b).

5.5.3 Breast Ultrasound

A number of screening studies have demonstrated high sensitivity of ultrasound for breast cancer, particularly for aggressive forms of cancer (Berg et al. 2008), who reported on the ACRIN (American College of Radiology Imaging Network) 6666 trial. While the sensitivity of mammography for such women can be as low as 30%–48%, ultrasound screening was shown to increase sensitivity to 77.5%. This result was relevant for a large fraction of the population, where more than half were younger than 50 and one-third of those who were older than 50 had dense breast tissue. More recently, it has been shown that in combination with mammography, detection rates are doubled in dense breasts (Kelly et al. 2010). Similar findings are reported by Steenbergen and Weigert (2011). The introduction of 3D Automated Breast Ultrasound volume scanning has reduced the time for imaging and lessened the dependence on experienced radiologists. However, the assessment of breast ultrasound images remains a challenging task, not least for image analysis algorithms. This is certain to be the subject of intensive research effort over the next few years, for example, in the EU ASSURE project.

5.6 DISCUSSION

It is increasingly important to provide quantitative, repeatable, and, ideally, automatic measurements of the amount of dense tissue in the breast. Given the ubiquity of mammography, not least as the basis for screening, and as a first port of call for breast imaging, this implies that such a measurement

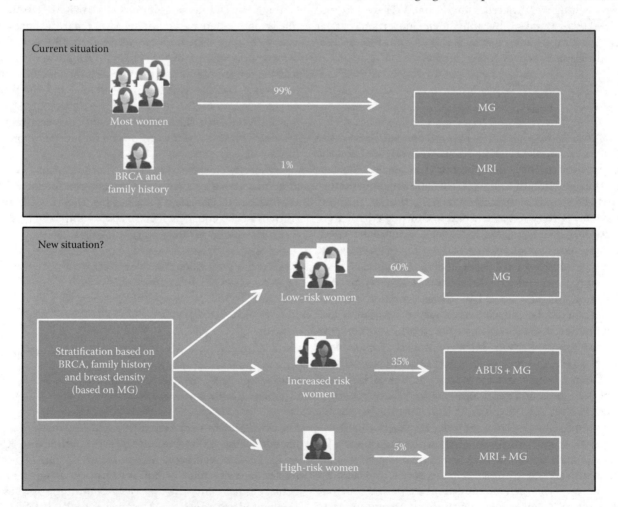

Figure 5.10   Schematic of current screening and screening the future based on risk.

be based in the first instance on the woman's mammograms. The original motivation, based on a number of epidemiological studies and radiological observations, was to provide a woman with an assessment of her risk of developing breast cancer. Reporting standards such as BI-RADS continue to be used widely and have contributed a great deal to radiological assessment of mammograms, but such assessments are neither quantitative nor automatic, and a number of studies have shown that they are not repeatable either.

We have described a number of encouraging steps toward the estimation of the *volume* of breast tissue from a single mammogram (or from a CC–MLO pair). As well, we have sketched recent progress toward estimating breast density from intrinsically 3D imaging modalities: CT, MRI, and ultrasound. It is likely that the coming years will see continued and rapid progress on all of these fronts. As well, it is likely that there will be increasing interest in image fusion: the integration of information from a set of images of different modalities.

To realize this opportunity will require taking account of the very different breast postures in at least the last three cases. This in turn poses some very difficult—and currently unsolved—nonrigid image registration problems, which, if they are to be constrained to converge to a sensible transformation, will require the deployment of biomechanical models of breast tissue that will probably need to be at least hyperelastic. Again, once breast density measurements are readily available, there will immediately be interest in comparing such measurements over time, between the left and right breasts, and across views. The application of the breast density measurements enshrined in Volpara to tomosynthesis reconstruction has not escaped our attention.

It is appropriate to close with Figure 5.10, which forms the basis for the recently started EU ASSURE project. The top panel shows that currently breast imaging is almost entirely based on mammography, a few women at high risk qualifying for an MRI. The lower panel envisages a personalized imaging workflow, in which mammography is used to stratify women for additional imaging, if such imaging is deemed necessary. An early step toward clinical deployment of such a workflow can be seen in Highnam et al. (2012).

ACKNOWLEDGMENTS

Sir Michael Brady, Ralph Highnam, Nico Karssemeijer, and Martin Yaffe are shareholders in Matakina Ltd. Sir Michael Brady acknowledges support from the UK Engineering and Physical Sciences Research Council, the UK Technology Strategy Board, and Cancer Research UK. The graphic reproduced in section was developed by G. Kolb, who gave permission for its use here.

REFERENCES

ACR (American College of Radiology). 2003. *Breast Imaging Reporting and Data System* (*BI-RADS*), 3rd edn. American College of Radiology, Reston, VA.

ACS (American Cancer Society). 2010. Breast Cancer Facts & Figures 2009–2010. https://www.google.co.uk/#q=american+cancer+society+breast+cancer+facts+and+figures+2010

Alonzo-Proulx O, Packard N, Boone JM, Al-Mayah A, Brock KK, Shen SZ, and Yaffe MJ. 2010. Validation of a method for measuring the volumetric breast density from digital mammograms. *Phys. Med. Biol.* 55:3027–3044.

Berg WA, Zhang Z, Lehrer D et al. 2008. Combined screening with ultrasound and mammography vs mammography alone in women at elevated risk of breast cancer. *J. Am. Med. Assoc.* 303(15):1482.

Boone JM, Kwan AL, Yang K, Burkett GW, Lindfors KK, and Nelson TR. 2006b. Computed tomography for imaging the breast. *J. Mammary Gland Biol. Neoplasia* 11:103–111.

Boone JM, Nelson TR, Kwan AL, and Yang K. 2006a. Computed tomography of the breast: Design, fabrication, characterization, and initial clinical testing. *Med. Phys.* 33:2185.

Boughey JC, Hartmann LC, Anderson SS, Degnim AC, Vierkant RA, Reynolds CA, Frost MH, and Pankratz VS. August 1, 2010. Evaluation of the Tyrer–Cuzick (International Breast Cancer Intervention Study) model for breast cancer risk prediction in women with atypical hyperplasia. *J. Clin. Oncol.* 28(22):3591–3596.

Boyd N, Guo H, Martin L, Sun L, Stone J, Fishell E, Jong R, Hislop G, Chiarelli A, Minkin S, and Yaffe M. 2007. Mammographic density and the risk and detection of breast cancer. *New Engl. J. Med.* 356(3):227–236.

Boyd NF, Martin LJ, Bronskill M, Yaffe MJ, Duric N, and Minkin S. 2010. Breast tissue composition and susceptibility to breast cancer. *J. Natl. Cancer Inst.* 102:1224–1237.

Boyd NF, Martin LJ, Yaffe MJ, and Minkin S. 2011. Mammographic density and breast cancer risk: Current understanding and future prospects. *Breast Cancer Res.* 13:223.

Brown J, Buckley D et al. 2000. Magnetic resonance imaging screening in women at genetic risk of breast cancer: Imaging and analysis protocol for the UK multicentre study. UK MRI Breast Screening Study Advisory Group. *Magn. Reson. Imaging* 18:765–776.

BSP61 (NHS Breast Screening Programme, Report 61). 2006. Screening for breast cancer in England: Past and future. Accessed on February 2006. Available at: http://www.cancerscreening.nhs.uk/breastscreen/publications/nhsbsp61.pdf.

Byng JW, Boyd NF, Fishell E, Jong RA, and Yaffe MJ. 1994. The quantitative analysis of mammographic densities. *Phys. Med. Biol.* 39:1629.

Chen W, Giger ML, Newstead GM, Bick U, Sanaz SA, Li H, and Lan I. 2010b. Computerized assessment of breast lesion malignancy using DCE-MRI: Robustness study on two independent clinical datasets from two manufacturers. *Acad. Radiol.* 17:822–829.

Chen W, Metz CE, Giger ML, and Drukker K. 2010a. A novel hybrid linear/nonlinear classifier for two-class classification: Theory, algorithm, and applications. *IEEE Trans. Med. Imaging* 29:428–441.

Dahlqvist Leinhard O, Johansson A, Rydell J, Smedby Ö, Nyström F, Lundberg P, and Borga M. 2008. Quantitative abdominal fat estimation using MRI. In: *Proc. of 19th ICPR*, Tampa, FL, pp. 361–364.

Diffey J, Hufton A, and Astley S. 2006. A new step-wedge for volumetric measurement of mammographic density. In: *International Workshop on Digital Mammography 2006. Lecture Notes in Computer Science*, Vol. 4046. Springer, Berlin, Germany, pp. 131–136.

Gail MH, Brinton LA, Byar DP et al. 1989. Projecting individualized probabilities of developing breast cancer for white females who are being examined annually. *J. Natl. Cancer Inst.* 81(24):1879–1886.

Gilbert F, Lloyd S, Jirotka M, Gavaghan D, Simpson A, Highnam R, Bowles T et al. 2004. eDiaMoND: The UK's Digital Mammography National Database. In: *7th International Workshop of Digital Mammography*, June 18–21, 2004, Chapel Hill, NC, pp. 231–236.

Graham SJ, Bronskill MJ, Byng JW et al. 1996. Quantitative correlation of breast tissue parameters using MR and x-ray mammography. *Br. J. Cancer* 73(2):162–168.

Hayton PM, Moore N, Brady M, and Tarassenko L. 1997. Model-based registration of contrast-enhanced dynamic MR breast images. *Med. Image Anal.* 1(3):1–18.

Heywang-Koebrunner SH, Wolf A, Pruss E, Hilbertz T, Eiermann W, and Permanetter W. 1989. MR imaging of the breast with Gd-DTPA: Use and limitations. *Radiology* 171:95–103.

Highnam R and Brady M. 1999. *Mammographic Image Analysis*. Kluwer Academic, the Netherlands.

Highnam R, Brady M et al. 2010. Robust breast composition measurement—Volpara™. In: *Digital Mammography. Lecture Notes in Computer Science*, Vol. 6136. Girona, Spain, Springer, pp. 342–349.

Highnam R, Pan X, Warren R, Jeffreys M, Davey Smith G, and Brady M. 2006. Breast composition measurements using retrospective standard mammogram form (SMF). *Phys. Med. Biol.* 51:2695–2713.

Highnam R, Sauber N, Destounis S, Harvey J, and McDonald D. 2012. Breast density into clinical practice. In: *Proc. of IWDM'12*, Philadelphia, PA, pp. 466–473.

Kelly KM, Dean J, Scott Comulada W, and Lee S-J. March 2010. Breast cancer detection using automated whole breast ultrasound and mammography in radiographically dense breasts. *Eur. Radiol.* 20(3):734–742.

Khazen M, Warren RM, Boggis CR, Bryant EC, Reed S, Warsi I, Pointon LJ et al. 2008. A pilot study of compositional analysis of the breast and estimation of breast mammographic density using three-dimensional T1-weighted magnetic resonance imaging. *Cancer Epidemiol. Biomark. Prev.* 17:2268–2274.

Klifa C, Carballido-Gamio J, Wilmes L, Laprie A, Shepherd J, Gibbs J, Fan B, Noworolski S, and Hylton N. January 2010. Magnetic resonance imaging for secondary assessment of breast density in a high-risk cohort. *Magn. Reson. Imaging* 28(1):8–15.

Klifa C, Partridge S, Lu Y, and Hylton N. 2003. Quantification of breast tissue texture from magnetic resonance imaging data. *Int. Soc. Magn. Reson. Med.* (Toronto).

Kontos D, Bakic PR, Acciavatti RJ, Conant EF, and Maidment AD. 2010. A comparative study of volumetric and area-based breast density estimation in digital mammography: Results from a screening population. In: *Digital Mammography. Lecture Notes in Computer Science*, Vol. 6136, pp. 378–385.

Kopans D. 2003. *Breast Imaging*. Lippincott Williams & Wilkins, Philadelphia, PA.

Kovesi P, Videre. 1999. Image features from phase congruency. *J. Comput. Vision Res.* 1(3):1–26.

Leach MO, Boggis CR, Dixon AK, Easton DF, Eeles RA, Evans DG, Gilbert FJ et al. 2005. Screening with magnetic resonance imaging and mammography of a UK population at high familial risk of breast cancer: A prospective multicentre cohort study (MARIBS). *Lancet* 365:1769–1778.

Lindfors KK, Boone JM, Nelson TR, Yang K, Kwan AL, and Miller DF. 2008. Dedicated breast CT: Initial clinical experience. *Radiology* 246:725–733.

Linguraru MG, Brady M, and Yam M. 2001. Filtering h_{int} images for the detection of microcalcifications. In: W. Niessen and M. Viergever (eds.), *Medical Image Computing and Computer-Assisted Intervention. Lecture Notes in Computer Science*, Vol. 2208. Springer-Verlag, Berlin, Germany, pp. 629–636.

Marias K, Behrenbruch CP, Parbhoo S, Sefalian A, and Brady M. 2006. A registration framework for the comparison of mammogram sequences. *IEEE Trans. Med. Imaging* 24(6):782–790.

Martin KE, Helvie MA, Zhou C, Roubidoux MA, Bailey JE, Paramagul C, Blane CE, Klein KA, Sonnad SS and Chan HP. 2006. Mammographic density measured with quantitative computer-aided method: Comparison with radiologists' estimates and BI-RADS categories. *Radiology* 240(3):656.

Mawdsley GE, Tyson AH, Peressotti CL, Jong RA, and Yaffe MJ. 2009. Accurate estimation of compressed breast thickness in mammography. *Med. Phys.* 36:577–586.

McCormack V, Highnam R, Perry N, and dos Santos Silva I. 2007. Comparison of a new and existing method of mammographic density measurement. *Cancer Epidemiol. Biomark. Prev.* 16(16):1148–1154.

McKinley RL, Tornai MP, Tuttle LA, Steed D, and Kuzmiak CM. 2012. Development and initial demonstration of a low-dose dedicated fully 3D breast CT system. In: *Proc. of IWDM'12*, Philadelphia, PA, pp. 442–449.

NCI. 2011. http://seer.cancer.gov/statfacts/html/breast.html.

Nicholson B, LoRusso A et al. 2006. Accuracy of assigned BIRADS breast density category definitions. *Acad. Radiol.* 13(9):1143–1149.

Nie K, Chang D, Chen J-H, Hsu C-C, Nalcioglu O, and Su M-Y. January 2010b. Quantitative analysis of breast parenchymal patterns using 3D fibroglandular tissues segmented based on MRI. *Med. Phys.* 37(1):217–226.

Nie K, Chang D, Chen J-H, Shih T-C, Hsu C-C, Nalcioglu O, and Su M-Y. January 2010a. Impact of skin removal on quantitative measurement of breast density using MRI. *Med. Phys.* 37(1):227–233.

Palomares MR, Machia JRB, Lehman CD, Daling JR, and McTiernan A. 2006. Mammographic density correlation with Gail model breast cancer risk estimates and component risk factors. *Cancer Epidemiol. Biomark. Prev.* 15:1324–1330.

Pawluczyk O, Augustine BJ, Yaffe MJ, Rico D, Yang J, Mawdsley GE, and Boyd NF. 2003. A volumetric method for estimation of breast density on digitized screen-film mammograms. *Med. Phys.* 30:352–364.

Pike MC, Krailo MD, Henderson BE, Casagrande JT, and Hoel DG. 1983. "Hormonal" risk factors, "breast tissue age" and the age-incidence of breast cancer. *Nature* 303(5920):767–770.

Schnall M. 2003. Breast MR imaging. *Radiol. Clin. North Am.* 41(1):43–50.

Shah JP, Mann SD, Polemi AM, Tornai MP, McKinley RL, Zentai G, Richmond M, and Partain L. 2012. Initial evaluation of a newly developed high resolution CT imager for dedicated breast CT. In: *Proc. of IWDM'12*, Philadelphia, PA, pp. 85–94.

Shepherd JA, Herve L, Landau J, Fan B, Kerlikowske K, Cummings SR. 2005. Novel use of single x-ray absorptiometry for measuring breast density. *Technol. Cancer Res. Treat.* 4:173–182.

Shepherd JA, Kerlikowske K et al. 2011. Volume of mammographic density and risk of breast density. *Cancer Epidemiol. Biomark. Prev.* 20:1473–1482 (Published Online May 1, 24).

Steenbergen S and Weigert J. 2011. The Connecticut experiment: The role of ultrasound in the screening of dense breasts. *Radiol. Soc. North Am.*

Thompson DJ, Leach MO, Kwan-Lim G, Gayther SA, Ramus SJ, Warsi I, Lennard F et al. for The UK study of MRI screening for breast cancer in women at high risk (MARIBS). 2009. Assessing the usefulness of a novel MRI-based breast density estimation algorithm in a cohort of women at high genetic risk of breast cancer: The UK MARIBS study. *Breast Cancer Res.* 11:R80.

Tromans CE, Cocker MR, and Brady SM. 2012a. Quantification and normalization of x-ray mammograms. *Phys. Med. Biol.* 57:6519–6540.

Tromans CE, Cocker MR, and Brady SM. 2012b. A model of primary and scattered photon fluence for mammographic x-ray image quantification. *Phys. Med. Biol.* 57:6541–6570.

Tromans CE, Diffey J, and Brady M. 2010. Investigating the replacement of the physical anti-scatter grid with digital image processing. In: *Digital Mammography. Lecture Notes in Computer Science*, Vol. 6136. Girona, Spain, Springer, pp. 205–212.

Tyrer J, Duffy SW, and Cuzick J. 2004. A breast cancer prediction model incorporating familial and personal risk factors. *Stat. Med.* 23:1111–1130.

van Engeland S, Snoeren P, Huisman H, Boetes C, and Karssemeijer N. March 2006. Volumetric breast density estimation from full-field digital mammograms. *IEEE Trans. Med. Imaging* 25(3):273–282.

WHO. 2011. http://www.who.int/cancer/detection/breastcancer/en/index1.html, http://www.who.int/cancer/detection/breast cancer/en/.

Wolfe JN. 1976a. Risk for breast cancer development determined by mammographic parenchymal pattern. *Cancer* 37(5):2486–2492.

Wolfe JN. 1976b. Breast patterns as an index of risk for developing breast cancer. *Am. J. Roentgenol.* 126(6):1130–1137.

Yam M, Brady M, Highnam R, Behrenbruch CP, English RE, and Kita Y. 2001. Three-dimensional reconstruction of microcalcification clusters from two mammographic views. *IEEE Trans. Med. Imaging* 20(6):479–489.

Yam M, Highnam R et al. 1999. Detecting calcifications using the h_{int} representation. In: *Proceedings of the 13th International Conference on Computer-Assisted Radiology and Surgery*, Paris, France, pp. 373–377, June 1999.

Chapter 6

Case-Based CAD Systems in Breast Imaging

Georgia D. Tourassi and Maciej A. Mazurowski

CONTENTS

6.1 INTRODUCTION

Knowledge-based systems (KBS) is a general term used to describe artificial intelligence techniques that rely on domain-specific knowledge to solve a new problem within that domain. The ultimate role of knowledge-based systems is to *support human decision-making, learning, and action* [1]. In that respect, all breast imaging CAD systems developed for detection, diagnosis, risk assessment, prognosis and other applications are essentially different examples of KBS technology. What differentiate these CAD systems are mainly the application domain (determined by the imaging modality and the clinical task of interest) and the methodologies used to represent the domain-specific knowledge and make inferences.

By far, the dominant methodologies employed in breast imaging CAD are neural networks, support vector machines, and decision trees [2]. These are all machine learning techniques that model domain knowledge into a generalized function. The function is learned from existing cases with known ground truth (i.e., labeled images). Through a supervised learning process, the knowledge is extracted from the available cases and condensed into a succinct model (e.g., a set of rules in a decision tree or the weight parameters of a multi-layered neural network). The model function is applied to future unknown cases (i.e., unlabeled images) to make an intelligent inference regarding their most probable labels.

One of the less explored machine learning methodologies in breast imaging CAD is instance-based learning, more commonly known as case-based reasoning (CBR) [3]. In contrast to learning methods that construct an explicit model of the domain knowledge from the example cases, CBR systems (also known as case-based systems) simply store the examples as they become available. In that respect, case-based systems are not real learners, but procrastinating inference engines. When presented with a query case, a case-based system reviews the stored examples, assesses the query's relatedness to them, and determines the most probable query label accordingly. Case-based CAD systems in medical imaging are related to another popular technology, content-based image retrieval (CBIR) [4]. Given a query image, case-based CAD systems operate initially as CBIR systems to identify similar example images according to the low-level visual content of the images. However, case-based CAD systems go one step further. They subsequently apply an inference algorithm to provide a high-level semantic interpretation for the query using the retrieved examples.

According to the reviewed literature and our personal experience, there are no clear winners among the various CAD methodologies with respect to performance (at least for detection and diagnosis applications in breast imaging). There are however some key advantages for the case-based CAD systems when it comes to flexibility and clinical relevance. First, case-based systems are adaptive. Since they do not go through a learning process to determine the explicit knowledge domain model, they avoid the retraining bottleneck of the learning-based methodologies. New knowledge (i.e., new learning examples) can be easily stored in a case-based system and it becomes immediately available for future use as soon as it is captured. Second, due to their case-centric reasoning approach, case-based systems offer solutions that are easily interpretable. However, these advantages often come at a cost of high computation and memory/storage requirements, which should not be underestimated in medical applications that involve storage and analysis of large images such as mammograms.

Regardless of whether "reasoning by remembering" is superior to "reasoning by modeling," there is increased interest in case-based CAD systems, not only in breast imaging but also in radiology in general [5–7]. The interest is driven by how well these systems can relate to the modern radiology practice. First, case-based systems emulate the pragmatic "learn from experience" approach that radiologists employ in order to interpret a new imaging study. Radiologists tend to recall former studies similar to the current one in question. In other words, their knowledge base does not consist simply of sets of rules but also of cases they have encountered before in their clinical practice. Furthermore, case-based CAD systems give an additional advantage to the radiologist; the ability to enhance his own knowledge base by tapping into the system's knowledge base—a great resource that can retain significantly more cases than any given radiologist could experience directly in his lifetime. Last but not least, case-based CAD systems operate with the underlying assumption that similar problems should have similar solutions. Even though this assumption is not always true, it is a fundamental principle of the modern evidence-based medicine paradigm.

This chapter provides an overview of case-based CAD technology developed thus far in the breast imaging domain. Since the technology is still in its infancy compared to the commercially available learning-based CAD, the chapter draws attention to the unique methodological aspects of the technology, highlights key challenges for the specific application domain, and reviews state-of-the-art research on these topics.

6.2 THE CASE-BASED CAD SYSTEM FRAMEWORK

6.2.1 The General Architecture

The typical case-based system consists of four key components: (1) a case base, (2) an algorithm for pairwise similarity assessment, (3) an intelligent search algorithm, and (4) a decision algorithm. The domain knowledge is captured in the case base in the form of prior cases with known ground truth (i.e., labeled cases). When a new query arrives for evaluation, the system searches for similar cases in the case base using brute force (exhaustive search) or a more sophisticated search approach to reduce the computational burden. Then, based on those similarity assessments, the decision algorithm is applied to provide a prediction regarding the label (or class) of the query case.

Figure 6.1 shows an illustration of a general case-based classifier. Note that the general framework is applicable to either whole images or specific image regions. What differs between "whole image" vs. "region only" systems is how the cases (i.e., whole images or image regions) are represented and compared. With full images, case-based systems must typically incorporate sophisticated similarity algorithms that take into account the spatial organization of multiple signs of interest that may be present in the full image (e.g., microcalcifications, masses, lymph nodes in a mammogram). In contrast, comparing image regions is less demanding since the comparison is typically done with a specific sign of interest. A small region is extracted centered on the sign of interest (e.g., a suspicious mass-looking structure in a mammogram) and analyzed further to make a location-specific inference. Spatial organization of additional structures that maybe present in the region is not typically a concern.

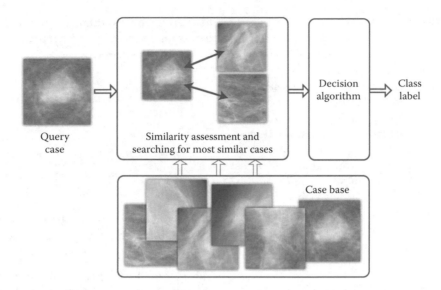

Figure 6.1 The general architecture of a case-based classifier.

6.2.2 The Key Components

6.2.2.1 Case Base

The case base is simply a database of previously collected cases that serve as examples of different classes. The number and type of classes depend on the clinical task at hand (e.g., detection, differential diagnosis). Given that the case base contains all prior knowledge used for problem solving, it is a crucial component for case-based systems.

For image applications, previous cases can be stored as raw image data or in the form of feature vectors. The latter is certainly the most computationally efficient way to store medical images. It is also the most common way of representing objects for classification problems in general within the machine learning discipline. Each case has a form of $x = \langle x^{(1)},..., x^{(N)} \rangle$ where is $x^{(i)}$, for $i = 1,..., N$ are the features. The features are descriptions of the cases. Examples of popular features for breast imaging case-based CAD systems include morphological and textural descriptors of breast lesions as well as general descriptors of breast parenchyma. Such features can be extracted using automatic computer-based methods (computer vision) or visually by a human expert. Non-image features such as patient-specific clinical findings maybe included if they are considered important. As with learning-based CAD systems, identifying the best features to represent prior knowledge is one of the most critical steps. For medical imaging applications, a lot of background research work is required to find features that are not only useful for the specific application but also behave robustly under different environments (e.g., for different image acquisition protocols).

Another way of storing cases is in the form of entire images. While the feature vectors described before are typically small (e.g., 10–50 numbers), the entire images are sizable (e.g., a 512×512 pixels region of interest = 262,144 numbers). This imposes higher storage requirements. It also requires more elaborate similarity measures that are tolerant to the noise present in the medical images. On the positive side, this approach does not require any feature extraction which might be time consuming as well as very sensitive to image acquisition parameters as mentioned before.

The general recommendation from the CBIR community is to pursue the necessary abstraction level for image representation so that unnecessary image information is disregarded [8]. This process certainly helps with noise tolerance as well as with speeding up the pairwise image similarity assessment step. However, achieving the optimal level of abstraction can be a time-consuming process, heavily dependent on image preprocessing steps such as filtering and segmentation. Particularly in breast imaging, feature extraction requires often lesion segmentation. This is a demanding task and segmentation algorithms fail more often than CAD designers are willing to admit. Extracting features from poorly segmented images is one of the most common ways to compromise the performance of an otherwise competent case-based CAD system.

Regardless of the approach followed for case representation, building a comprehensive case base is important to the success of a case-based classifier. In Section 6.4.1 we discuss the problem of optimal case base construction in detail with respect to case-based CAD systems in breast imaging.

6.2.2.2 Similarity Assessment

Similarity is central to the retrieval step of a case-based CAD system. The literature is rich of publications on the topic of similarity. An insightful discussion on the philosophical and computational aspects of similarity as it pertains to case-based reasoning and pattern recognition can be found in [9]. The following is a brief introduction on how similarity has been approached in the medical imaging domain. Please note that for the rest of the chapter the terms similarity and distance (or dissimilarity) are used as the two different sides of the same coin.

A variety of measures have been proposed for assessment of similarity (or distance) between two cases. These measures differ depending on the representation of the cases [7]. For images, similarity measures can be generally divided into the following groups:

1. Feature-based measures
2. Pixel-based measures
3. Structure-based measures

For feature-based representation, by far the most popular distance measure is the Euclidean distance:

$$d(x,y) = \sqrt{\sum_{i=1}^{N} (x_i - y_i)^2} \tag{6.1}$$

However, other distance measures operating on feature vectors can be used such as the Manhattan distance, Minkowsky distance, or Mahalanobis distance [10]. One of the most comprehensive studies on feature-based image similarity measures can be found in [11]. As with feature selection, determining the best feature-based similarity measure is an empirical process.

Pixel-based similarity measures operate on the raw image data. In that respect, they are *featureless* since they do not impose any level of image abstraction. The most popular featureless image similarity measure is the cross-correlation coefficient, a common choice in medical image registration [10]. Some of the limitations of the correlation-based measures are their lack of robustness with multi-modality images and with images that differ substantially in their intensity scale [11]. Nevertheless, they are easy to compute and studies have shown that they can be quite effective in content-based medical image retrieval applications [10], including in breast imaging [12]. Some really interesting choices that overcome the limitations of correlation-like similarity measures come from information theory. These are based on the concept of entropy [13]. Entropy is considered a measure of the uncertainty or complexity in an image, captured by the dispersion of the probability distribution of the image intensity levels. Information theoretic measures essentially compare the

histograms of two images X and Y. The two most popular measures are mutual information (MI) and the Kullback–Leibler divergence (KL):

$$MI(X,Y) = \sum_{i=1}^{N} \sum_{i=1}^{N} p(x,y) \log_2 \frac{p(x,y)}{p(x)p(y)} \tag{6.2}$$

$$D_{KL}(X,Y) = \sum_{i=1}^{N} p(x) \log \left[\frac{p(x)}{p(y)} \right] \tag{6.3}$$

where
$p(x)$ and $p(y)$ are the probability distributions of the pixel values within image X and Y, respectively
$p(x,y)$ is their joint probability distribution [10]

The marginal and joint probability functions are usually estimated using the histogram approach [14] with an empirically determined number of histogram bins i. The main difference between these two measures is that KL focuses only on corresponding histogram bins (i.e., bin-by-bin measure) but MI incorporates information for non-corresponding bins (i.e., cross-bin measure). Note also that MI is a symmetric similarity measure but KL is a non-symmetric dissimilarity measure. For CBIR applications, a symmetric version is required and there have been various ways proposed to achieve that. A more detailed list of information-theoretic measures for application to breast imaging can be found in [15].

There are several other histogram-based (dis)similarity measures that are quite popular among the CBIR community. For example, the χ^2 distance measure is a commonly used bin-by-bin measure while the Earth Mover's Distance is one of the newer cross-bin measures [10]. The latter is based on the amount of effort it takes to convert image X to another image Y. Although histogram-based measures have been successful in a wide range of applications, they have their own limitations. First, they are computationally expensive to calculate for real-time application (particularly the cross-bin measures such as MI). Second, the arbitrariness of histogram binning is considered undesirable. Determining the optimal number of histograms bins in a mathematically disciplined manner is an active area of research with several rules and methods proposed (e.g., Refs. [16–19]).

Structure-based similarity measures are appropriate to compare global images which contain multiple interesting structures and for which the spatial relationship of these structures is important. Various techniques such as point-based and graph-based methods have been proposed thus far and many more are continuously introduced (e.g., Refs. [20–26]).

The CBIR literature is rich with studies proposing new image similarity measures for specific domains and image representations. In our view, clinical images pose unique challenges compared to other application domains. The performance expectations are much higher with respect to the visual and diagnostic relevance of the retrieved cases. As such, identifying suitable similarity measures requires rigorous analysis with careful fine-tuning or even creative fusion of several different techniques. Related research in the breast imaging domain is discussed in more detail later.

6.2.2.3 Search Engine

The initial goal of a case-based CAD system is to identify effectively and efficiently images similar to the query case. Effectiveness is measured by the quality of the decision made regarding the query case. Efficiency is measured by how fast the system performs this step. Clearly, the similarity measure is the key factor that affects both effectiveness and efficiency. But there is usually a trade-off involved. Sophisticated similarity measures may produce case-based CAD systems with high effectiveness but they are more often than not computationally demanding which can severely compromise the system's efficiency. This is particularly true for applications in radiology where accommodation of continuously growing case bases and real-time use of the technology are strict requirements.

When efficiency becomes an issue, having a system perform an exhaustive search to find relevant cases in the case base becomes computationally burdensome. Furthermore, blind storing of new knowledge cases may result in redundancies that do not necessarily improve diagnostic performance. Intelligent search algorithms can be introduced to improve the system's efficiency during the retrieval stage without compromising the system's overall effectiveness [27]. For dissimilarity measures that are true distance metrics (i.e., satisfy the triangle inequality), there is wide range of algorithms proposed to reduce the number of pairwise dissimilarity calculations needed for effective case retrieval [28–31]. However, often the most effective similarity measures do not behave as typical metrics. In these scenarios, clustering techniques offer a competitive alternative [32,33]. First, the case base is clustered in several groups of highly related cases. Then, for each cluster a prototype case is selected as the representative cluster case. For example, if the clustering is done using feature-based case representation, then the centroid of the feature vectors that belong to a cluster can be selected as the prototype case for the specific cluster. Initially, a query case is compared only with the prototype cases to identify the most relevant cluster(s) to the query. Then, the query is compared in more detail with only the cases that belong to those relevant clusters. Although the above are two general approaches, customized solutions that meet the specific needs of a particular application domain are quite common.

6.2.2.4 Decision Engine

After the similarity assessment step is complete, a decision needs to be made regarding the query case. The decision algorithm returns a class label or a continuous value (e.g., probability of the query case belonging to a certain class) that can be used to assign such label.

The simplest decision algorithm for case-based classifiers is to assign to the query case the label of its nearest neighbor (i.e., of the case in the case base that has the smallest distance/highest similarity to the query). Such rule however is very sensitive to noisy cases in the case base. To account for this drawback, a majority rule can be used where the label assigned to the query case is the most common label of its k nearest neighbors. Similarly, an average of the labels represented as integers (e.g., 0 = negative class, 1 = positive class) for the k nearest neighbors can be used as the decision variable. To further take into account the differences in distances to the query case among the nearest neighbors, one can use the following formula:

$$f(x_q) = \frac{\sum_{i=1}^{k} w_i v(x_i)}{\sum_{i=1}^{k} w_i} \qquad (6.4)$$

where

$$w_i = \frac{1}{d(x_q, x_i)^2} \qquad (6.5)$$

where

x_q is the query case

$f(x_q)$ is the value of the decision function for the query case

$x_i, i = 1, ..., k$ are the k nearest neighbors of x_q

w_i is the weight of the case x_i

$v(x_i)$ is the label of x_i (e.g., 0 or 1)

$d(x_q, x_i)$ is the distance between the query case x_q and a case base example x_i

This decision function assigns a higher weight in making the decision to the cases x_i that are closer to the query case. As one can see from Equation 6.5, the weight decreases with the squared distance from the query case. Other functions could be applied instead, such as a Gaussian kernel. The classifiers discussed above are called k-nearest neighbor (k-NN) classifiers since they rely on the labels of the k nearest neighbors of the query case. The value of k is a design choice and is typically small (e.g., $k = 3$).

As with search algorithms, customized decision algorithms are also quite common. For example, in a case-based system developed for discrimination between true masses and normal parenchyma from raw image data [34], the authors used simply the sum of similarities $s(x_q, x_k)$ of the query case x_q to the k most similar case base mass examples x_k:

$$f\left(x_q\right) = \sum_{i=1}^{k} s\left(x_q, x_k\right) \qquad (6.6)$$

The same application investigated also a decision algorithm that is based on the difference between the average similarity of the query case x_q to the k closest mass cases x_k and the k closest normal cases x_j:

$$f\left(x_q\right) = \frac{1}{k}\sum_{i=1}^{k} s\left(x_q, x_i\right) - \frac{1}{k}\sum_{j=1}^{k} s\left(x_q, x_j\right) \qquad (6.7)$$

The purpose of that comparison was to determine whether the system requires explicit knowledge of both abnormal and normal examples or whether knowledge of abnormal examples is sufficient. This question is actually tied to the more general issue of case base composition, which is addressed in detail later.

This is only a general description of possible choices for the decision algorithm component of a case-based system. For the most part, choosing a decision algorithm is a trial-and-error process.

6.3 CASE-BASED CAD APPLICATIONS IN BREAST IMAGING

As discussed in Section 6.1, case-based CAD systems are developed with a very narrowly defined application domain in mind. The breast CAD literature has several heavily customized systems. By far, most publications target detection and diagnosis of breast lesions in mammograms. This section reviews those publications. The review is organized based on the clinical task. It is not intended to be an exhaustive review of all published studies, but rather a review highlighting the variety of case-based CAD implementations.

6.3.1 Detection

Chang et al. presented one of the earlier applications of case-based classification for breast cancer detection [35]. Specifically, the authors developed a case-based CAD scheme for the discrimination of true masses from normal (yet suspicious looking) breast parenchyma. The analysis involved regions of interest (not full mammograms), feature-based representation, and a decision algorithm that relied on the query's average similarity with the k nearest example *mass* cases only. The system showed decent classification performance but not as good as the one achieved by a rule-based CAD system published earlier by the same group. The authors attributed the inferior performance

partly to the lack of negative (normal) examples in their case base. In a follow-up study [36], the authors reported that the addition of negative examples in the case base improved the classification performance of their system.

Tourassi et al. also confirmed the importance of building a case base with both normal and abnormal examples for their own featureless case-based CAD system and the same region-based clinical task [34]. Singh et al. used the same system successfully for application in breast tomosynthesis [37]. The same group later extended the system for breast mass screening in full mammograms and tomosynthesis slices [38].

6.3.2 Diagnosis

There are several studies on the use of a case-based classifier for the discrimination between malignant and benign lesions. In 2005, Alto et al. presented such a system for mammographic masses. The authors used feature-based case representation of breast masses [39]. The features spanned a wide range of shape, textural, and edge-sharpness descriptors. The similarity and decision algorithms were rather basic, Euclidean distance and majority vote based on the $k = 5, 7$ most similar cases. Using 57 biopsy-proven breast lesions and cross-validation, the authors observed very high classification accuracy of 96.5% using only one mass shape and one edge-sharpness feature.

El-Naqa et al. presented a case-based CAD system for the diagnostic classification of microcalcifications in mammograms [40]. Instead of applying one of the many popular similarity measures discussed in the previous section, the authors employed machine learning technique such as neural networks and support vector machines to learn a similarity measure that is consistent with human perception. Later, the authors improved upon their system with a more sophisticated decision algorithm; namely an adaptive support vector machine that incorporates local information [41].

Case-based systems have been also applied for the diagnostic characterization of breast lesions in sonograms. Kuo et al. presented such system [42]. The system relied on three texture features, a weighted Euclidean distance dissimilarity measure, and a decision algorithm similar to that shown in Section 6.2.2.4, where the class label of a retrieved case is assigned an importance weight according to its retrieval rank. The authors reported 94.44% sensitivity and 90.84% specificity. Huang et al. presented a similar system relying on different texture features with a very impressive ROC performance ranging from $A_z = 0.91$ to 0.98 across four different ultrasonic systems [43]. Cho et al. [44] presented their own case-based system for breast mass characterization. The authors explored two different retrieval implementations. The first one used traditional feature-based distance measures such Euclidean distance and cosine distance.

The second approach used classifiers such as a Bayesian neural network and linear discriminant analysis to synthesize the image features into a classification score. Similar cases were retrieved based on the similarity of their classification scores (not their feature-based similarity). The authors reported the best ROC performance ($A_z = 0.87$) for a system that uses the Bayesian neural network as the similarity algorithm and a k-NN classifier as the decision algorithm.

6.3.3 Other Applications

Other than detection and diagnosis, the next most common breast imaging application of case-based classifiers is the automatic classification of breast parenchymal density in mammograms according to the BI-RADS lexicon. In 2007, Kinoshita et al. [45] presented such system using an elaborate feature-based representation of mammograms. The features included shape, texture, Radon transform, moments, histogram, and granulometry descriptors. The authors implemented an unsupervised learning approach (Kohonen's self-organizing map) to assess the feature-based similarity between a query case and the case base examples. Using large database of 1088 mammograms and a leave-one-out sampling scheme, the authors reported that on average 79%–86% of the top 25% retrieved cases were related to the query in terms of their respective BI-RADS density ratings. For this study, the authors assumed that if a retrieved case had a BI-RADS density rating within ± 1 category from the querys, then it is a relevant retrieval.

In 2011, de Oliveira et al. presented a different case-based system for the same problem [46]. Their system also used feature-based representation of the mammographic cases and a singular value decomposition technique to determine a reduced set of useful image features. Then, the authors employed support vector machines to assess case similarity and a 1-NN classifier for decision making. The authors reported 82% average precision based on a 10-fold cross validation scheme.

6.4 HOT TOPICS

There are some fundamental questions that are of high interest among case-based CAD researchers. This section discusses those "hot topics" and highlights related research in the context of breast imaging.

6.4.1 Which Cases Should Be Included in the Case Base?

When constructing a case-based classifier, one is presented with a set (T) of learning examples. The question arises of whether all cases from T should be included in the case base

or only some of them could suffice. If only a few selected cases are enough, which ones should they be? We will discuss these and related issues in this section. But first, we will try to put the main question in the proper statistical context.

A common knowledge in machine learning is that when training pattern classifiers, the more cases we use for training, the better classifier we are going to end up with [47]. This is a very intuitive result: the more information about the classification problem we have, the better we can perform in solving the problem. The same applies to case-based classifiers: the more cases are included in the case base, the better the resulting performance of the classifier. However, this regularity assumes that the added cases are drawn from the underlying distributions randomly, that is, the probability of certain types of cases (in terms of features) being included in the training is the same as the probability of these cases occurring in general.

Nevertheless, if we knew which cases should be included in the case base, the situation might look different. We could avoid including misleading cases and focus on those that are the most useful for best classification of future cases. Consider the following example of a simple classification problem from Figure 6.2. A simulated dataset with two variables ($x = \langle x_1, x_2 \rangle$) was used for this example. Each class had a Gaussian underlying distribution with diagonal covariance matrix. Development (1,000) and testing (10,000) cases were sampled randomly from the underlying Gaussian distributions. Red crosses are used to illustrate positive training cases and green circles to illustrate negative training cases. For this problem, it can be shown that two cases (those shown in yellow squares) are enough to determine a nearest-neighbor (k-NN) classifier that performs nearly as well as the ideal observer for this problem. The value of the function $f(x)$ generated by a k-NN with the two selected cases is illustrated by the contour lines (brighter area means area where $f(x)$ is higher). The ROC performance of this k-NN classifier is $A_z = 0.895$ while the ideal observer's ROC performance for this problem (calculated based on explicit knowledge of the underlying distributions) is $A_z = 0.9$.

This simple example demonstrates that when the "right" cases are selected for inclusion in the case base, a dramatically reduced number of cases can be selected (i.e., most of the cases can me dismissed from future participation in the decision making process) while still obtaining a close to ideal classification performance on the test set.

The potential for dramatic reduction of the case base through intelligent selection of example cases without loss in performance is well documented in the machine learning literature [48–54]. The benefits of including only few carefully selected cases in the case base of a classifier are threefold. First, fewer cases mean lower storage requirements. This is particularly important in systems

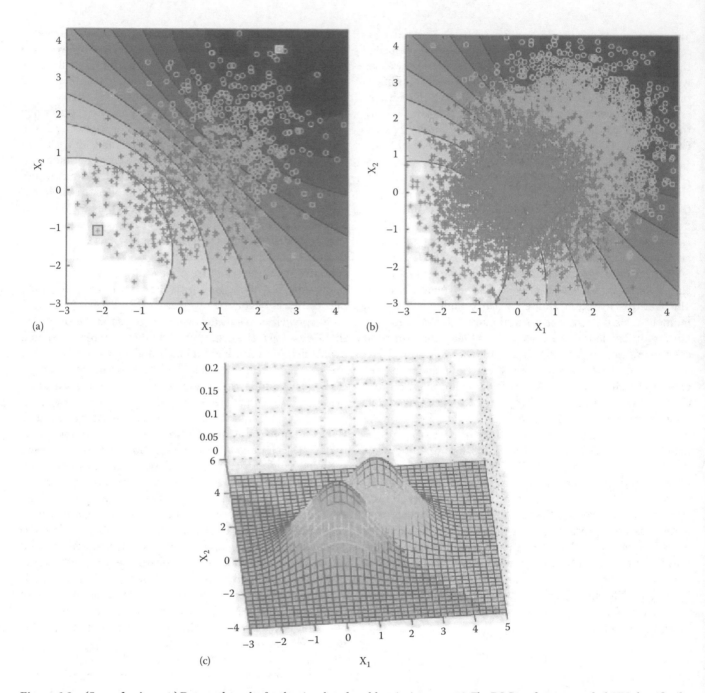

Figure 6.2   (See color insert.) Data and results for the simulated problem in Argument 3. The ROC performance of a k-NN classifier for this problem was $A_z = 0.895$ while the optimal performance for this problem is $A_z = 0.90$. (a) Cases from development set (red crosses—positive, green circles—negative, yellow squares—selected by RMHC) and values of the k-NN classifier function based on two cases (contour plot in the background). (b) Cases from test set (red crosses—positive, green circles—negative, yellow squares—selected by RMHC) and values of the k-NN classifier function based on two cases (contour plot in the background). (c) Probability density function for positive (red) and negative (red) classes.

that store cases in the form of entire images, not simply as feature vectors. Second, reduction of the case base size translates into lower time complexity of the decision algorithm (i.e., faster classifier). By eliminating redundant learning examples, the retrieval process is reduced to a few strategic comparisons between the query case and the most useful example cases. Again, this benefit is particularly important for systems such as the one in [34] where time consuming measures are applied to assess pairwise similarity. Finally, intelligent selection could potentially lead to better system performance by removing the noisy examples. Arguably, the latter is the most important benefit in the context of CAD systems where typically effectiveness (i.e., classification performance) outweighs efficiency (i.e., decision time).

Still, the question remains: how to select the "right" cases for inclusion in the case base. Multiple algorithms have been proposed for this task within the machine learning literature (for a comprehensive review on the topic see Ref. [48]). While based on different rationales, these algorithms generally utilize the entire available learning dataset T to construct a smaller set S that will serve as the case base of the constructed system.

In a recent study, Mazurowski et al. [55] performed a comparative analysis of seven previously proposed case reduction algorithms for case selection as well as random selection for three classification datasets: (1) an artificially generated dataset based on Gaussian probability distributions, (2) a dataset for a breast cancer diagnosis problem based on BI-RADS features, and (3) a dataset for a breast cancer detection problem using computer-extracted image features. The conclusions of that study were as follows. First, it was confirmed that a dramatic reduction of the database size is possible (to <3% of the original size for all three analyzed datasets) while maintaining or improving the classification performance. Second, a fairly simple selection algorithm called random mutation hill climbing [53] performed the best among all compared algorithms. Third, the study established that even though a small subset S can be selected from the available set T of cases available for training without loss in performance, it is still very important that a large set T is initially available since the entire set T is used in the selection process. Specifically, the authors reported that when more cases are available to select from (i.e., the size of T is larger) the resulting classifier based on the selected subset S has generally better performance.

Finally, in the same study, the authors compared the performance of the "intelligent" algorithms to a simple random selection. This topic has not been addressed enough both in the machine learning and the CAD literature. Specifically, imagine a situation that a proposed selection algorithm A selected m cases and the resulting system that is based on those cases achieved testing performance P. We believe that it is of importance to know what would be the performance of the system if the m instances were selected randomly. We will call such performance P_B (for baseline). If the performance of the proposed system P is in average lower than P_B (with similar variability), then there is no good reason to use the algorithm A unless a good claim can be made showing that there is some additional benefit for using the selection algorithm A. Such claim is typically nearly impossible to make for real-world applications where performance is the most important

evaluation criterion followed by computational efficiency of the resulting system. The comparison described above is virtually not existent in the literature on case selection. Mazurowski et al. addressed this issue in their own study and they observed that actually some of the algorithms previously proposed in the literature can perform notably worse than random selection [55].

Although supported in the machine learning community, purposely reducing the case base size seems counter-intuitive in the clinical context. For example, Park et al. observed also that elimination of detrimental examples from the case base significantly improved the performance of their own case-based CAD system [56]. However, in a later study, the same authors questioned the concept of dramatic case base reduction because their selection approach appeared to impact negatively their CAD system's performance on subtle cases [57]. It is important to point out that the above studies are consistent about the following finding. Having access to a large comprehensive database is a very important starting point. As shown in [55], the larger a case base is, the more effective intelligent reduction algorithms are. Whether all cases should be reserved for the decision making step is a different question. If the role of the case-based CAD system is to provide a reliable decision in an efficient manner, then intelligent reduction of the case base is very useful. If providing visual justification is also an important aspect of the system, then case base reduction may not be a good strategy since it limits the variety of similar cases available for retrieval and visualization.

6.4.2 What Is the Most Effective Way to Assess Similarity?

By far the most commonly used method in assessing case similarity in breast imaging applications is the one that uses feature-based case representation. Even though feature-based techniques are computationally desirable, they require substantial background work to determine a concise set of useful features. Furthermore, feature extraction builds upon image segmentation, a challenging task in breast imaging applications. Regardless of these constraints, feature-based similarity measures are reportedly more effective than pixel-based ones. Wang et al. [58] compared Euclidean distance, mutual information, and Pearson's correlation coefficient with respect to their case-based CAD system that relied on a k-NN decision algorithm. The authors reported a dramatically superior ROC performance (for discriminating true masses and false positive regions detected by another CAD scheme) when their system used Euclidean distance ($A_z = 0.89$) compared to the other two pixel-based methods ($A_z = 0.61$ for mutual information and $A_z = 0.70$ for Pearson's correlation coefficient). The authors observed that pixel-based methods were very sensitive to the size of the suspected mass relative to the size of the extracted region of interest (ROI). When the ROI size was adaptively adjusted relative to the suspected mass, the ROC performance of both pixel-based similarity measures improved significantly ($A_z = 0.72$ for mutual information and $A_z = 0.79$ for Pearson's correlation coefficient).

The effect of the ROI size on pixel-based similarity measures is expected, as reported earlier by Tourassi et al. [59] with respect to their own CAD system that relies on mutual information. Since mass sizes vary substantially, using a fixed-size ROI introduces a potential limitation. When two ROIs are compared, it is unclear how much the parenchymal background contributes in the calculated similarity measure. This could deteriorate CAD performance in extreme cases, namely when a small mass is present in the ROI or when a large mass extends beyond the fixed-size ROI. The authors investigated the effect of ROI size based on two datasets of ROIs (Dataset 1: mass vs. randomly chosen normal ROIs and Dataset 2: mass vs. false positive ROIs) and three fixed ROI sizes. The authors reported a statistically significant decline of the performance as the ROI size increased in both datasets. Detailed analysis for masses stratified in three size groups (i.e., small, medium, large) confirmed that the smaller the size of the suspected mass, the smaller the ROI size should be to ensure optimal CAD performance. The authors investigated also a multi-size fusion analysis using a linear model. In other words, for each query location, multiple size ROIs were extracted and analyzed by their case-based CAD system. Then, these individual decisions were merged with a linear discriminant model. This approach achieved a significant improvement for both datasets. An even better improvement was observed for a "customize-and-resize" approach in which a custom size ROI is extracted around the suspected lesion to ensure that the ROI captures the full lesion with the lowest possible contribution of background parenchyma. Even though the customized approach was shown to be superior, it requires reliable visual or computer assessment of the lesion's boundary. The advantage of the multi-size approach is its independence from such step. The approach is though computationally more demanding since each suspicious location must be analyzed at several different ROI sizes.

Undoubtedly, the debate between feature-based and pixel-based similarity measures is very interesting. When executed carefully, feature-based representation appears to be superior. However, its robustness across different imaging databases can be easily compromised since the numerical values of the features can change dramatically based on the image acquisition device and the preprocessing algorithms. Also, feature selection depends on the clinical question, which must be defined very narrowly. For example, different image features are important for first-stage screening of a full mammogram than for second-stage false-positive reduction. Case-based CAD systems with pixel-based similarity measures can be more versatile. In their studies, Tourassi et al. have shown that their information-theoretic CAD system remains robust across different classifications tasks or modalities [15,34,37,38].

Actually, Tourassi et al. investigated the topic of multiplatform translation in detail in [60]. They performed a series of experiments where they evaluated the ability of their case-based CAD system to transfer knowledge across different platforms (i.e., screen-film mammograms digitized using different digitizers, full-field digital mammograms, and breast tomosynthesis). The authors reported remarkable performance robustness for their system.

6.4.3 What about Perceptual Similarity?

One of the ongoing challenges in CBIR research is the semantic gap, which refers to the gap between the low-level feature content of two images and the high-level concepts that a human searches for and perceives when comparing two images [61]. Many common image similarity measures that are successfully used in case-based CAD systems cannot capture as well perceptual similarity, particularly in the clinical domain. This can be a serious limitation if the intended role of the CAD system is to provide not only an opinion but also a visual justification by displaying visually similar cases.

There is a lot of research activity in developing image similarity measures that can bridge the semantic gap for breast imaging applications. The techniques span a wide range from machine learning, to relevance feedback, to more customized methods (e.g., Refs. [44,60,62–68]). Given that visual similarity is a highly subjective concept [69], more studies are needed to determine the robustness of these measures for a wide range of cases and observers. Regardless of challenges addressing the semantic gap, there are studies in breast imaging suggesting that visualization of similar cases is helpful. For example, in 2006, Horsh et al. reported that their multimodality CAD system improves the radiologists' accuracy in assessing the likelihood of malignancy of breast masses [70]. Their system provided not only a numerical opinion regarding a query's probability of malignancy but also pictorial justification with similar cases. However, the incremental value of the pictorial justification component of their system was not explicitly assessed. Nakayama et al. reported dramatic improvement in the radiologists' ability to distinguish between malignant and benign microcalcifications if they were shown similar known examples as the one in question [71]. The study though did not compare whether providing simply a CAD opinion could be as effective.

Based on the existing literature, the fundamental question remains unanswered. Is a perceptual similarity measure necessary in a case-based CAD system? While intuitively important for visualization of similar case base examples, perceptual similarity might be of less importance if classification accuracy is what matters the most. Image similarity measures that are more consistent with human perception may not be the best choice for case-based classification. This was clearly the case in [44]. Although this conclusion can easily vary depending on the specific system and clinical application, the topic certainly deserves further exploration. To the best of our knowledge, there are no studies comparing directly the clinical benefit of a conventional CAD system vs. one that is enhanced with presentation of similar cases as a means of explaining the CAD decision. Therefore, the incremental value of pictorial explanation has not been proven yet.

6.4.4   Optimizing the Case Base Search

Finding relevant case base examples in a computationally efficient way is very important for real-time use and thus clinical acceptance of case-based CAD systems. Solutions to this challenge depend on the specifics of the particular system such as case base representation, similarity measure, and case base size. In [72], the authors used a case indexing method to quickly eliminate a large portion of the case base from further consideration. Their system was developed for regional interrogation of screening mammograms to determine whether a particular location depicts a true mass or normal parenchyma. Because their system employed the computationally demanding mutual information as the similarity measure, the authors used a case indexing method to quickly eliminate a large portion of the case base from further consideration. Entropy-based indexing was a logical choice, since calculating the image entropy is not only fast but also a necessary step to derive the MI of two images. The indexing scheme was evaluated for two different problems (mass detection and false-positive reduction) and in two different capacities: (1) as a search mechanism to sort through the case base and (2) as a selection mechanism to build a smaller, concise case base that is easier to maintain but still effective. There were two important findings in that study. First, entropy-based indexing is an effective strategy to identify fast a subset of case base examples that are most relevant (i.e., with similar complexity) to a given query. Only this subset could be analyzed in more detail using MI for optimized performance. Second, a selective entropy-based deposit strategy where only high entropy cases (i.e., the ones with the highest information content) are stored in the case base sustains the detection performance of the CAD system while trimming its case base. Overall, the entropy-based indexing scheme reduced the computational cost of their system by 55%–80% while maintaining its diagnostic performance.

A similar indexing strategy was used in [73] for their feature-based case-based CAD system. Their system was also developed for false-positive reduction in a mass detection CAD scheme. A single indexing feature (fractal dimension) was applied as a prescreening tool to disregard case base examples that had substantially different fractal signature than the query case. By performing elaborate similarity comparisons only between the query and case base examples with similar texture, the authors were able to achieve similar ROC performance with higher computational efficiency than without the indexing method.

6.4.5   Optimizing the Decision Algorithm

Although the majority of case-based CAD research appears to be more focused on the similarity assessment algorithm, various heuristics could be applied in effort to improve the decision function as well. In this section, we will focus on selected research on this topic.

Mazurowski et al. explored an optimization strategy based on the assumption that the examples stored in a case base are not necessarily of equal importance [74]. Specifically, some cases might be more representative and similarity of the query case to such case should be more important than to cases that are less representative of their class or even misleading. Therefore, they proposed a decision algorithm that assigns a different importance weight to each stored case that is not dependent on the query. They formalized the task of assigning these weights as an optimization problem where the objective function is the performance of the resulting case-based system. Then they solved this optimization problem using genetic algorithms. The optimized decision function allowed for statistically significant improvement of the classifier performance from $A_z = 0.86 \pm 0.03$ to 0.91 ± 0.02. In a different study, the same authors investigated ensemble techniques to improve upon the decision algorithm [75]. Their ensemble technique concept is illustrated in Figure 6.3. Specifically, they evaluated two general ways of constructing sub-classifiers by resampling the available case base: random division and random selection. Furthermore, they proposed two adaptively incremental techniques that determine the number of the ensemble subclassifiers automatically rather than by trial-and-error as typical ensemble techniques do. The ensemble components were fused linearly. The authors reported that the ensemble techniques provide a statistically significant improvement in performance to the original system (from $A_z = 0.86 \pm 0.01$ to 0.91 ± 0.01).

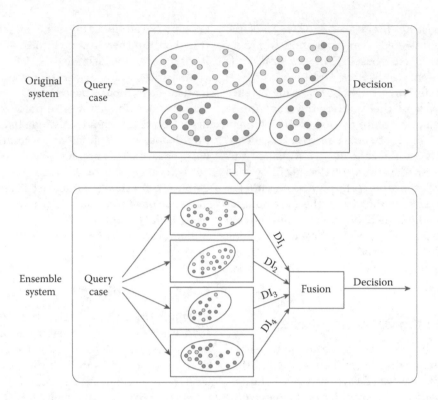

Figure 6.3   Ensemble-based decision algorithm for a case-based CAD system.

6.5 CONCLUDING REMARKS

To date the breast imaging CAD literature does not provide evidence of superior performance for case-based CAD over conventional CAD systems. It is our belief though that case-based CAD research will continue. Its direct relevance to evidence-based radiology is the main drive. Furthermore, since imaging technology advances at a rapid rate, being able to update accordingly the knowledge base is crucial in radiology. Case-based systems can handle this challenge since new up-to-date cases can be continuously added in the case base without disrupting system operation. Still, the fundamental question is whether case-based CAD systems can deliver more effective use of the knowledge than conventional CAD systems in terms of improving the performance of radiologists. Scientific advancements in the hot topics highlighted in the previous section and clinical evaluation studies will need to follow to provide the answer.

ACKNOWLEDGMENTS

This chapter has been co-authored by UT-Battelle, LLC, under Contract No. DE-AC05-00OR22725 with the U.S. Department of Energy. The United States Government retains and the publisher, by accepting the article for publication, acknowledges that the United States Government retains a non-exclusive, paid-up, irrevocable, world-wide license to publish or reproduce the published form of this manuscript, or allow others to do so, for United States Government purposes.

REFERENCES

1. Akerkar R, Sajja P. *Knowledge-Based Systems*. Jones & Bartlett Publishers, Sudbury, MA, 2009.
2. Giger ML, Chan HP, Boone J. Anniversary paper: History and status of CAD and quantitative image analysis: The role of medical physics and AAPM. *Medical Physics* 2008; 35(12):5799–5820.
3. Bichindaritz I, Marling C. Case-based reasoning in the health sciences: What's next? *Artificial Intelligence in Medicine* 2006; 36:127–135.
4. Muller H, Michoux N, Bandon D, Geissbuhler A. A review of content-based image retrieval systems in medical applications—Clinical benefits and future directions. *International Journal of Medical Informatics* 2004; 73(1):1–23.
5. Smeulders AWM, Worring M, Santini S, Gupta A, Jain R. Content-based image retrieval at the end of the early years. *IEEE Transactions on Pattern Analysis and Machine Intelligence* 2000; 22:1349–1380.
6. Müller H, Rosset A, Garcia A, Vallée J-P, Geissbuhler A. Benefits of content-based visual data access in radiology. *Radiographics* 2005; 25:849–858.

7. Vannier MW, Summers RM. Sharing images. *Radiology* 2003; 228:23–25.

8. Perner P. Why case-based reasoning is attractive for image interpretation? In: *Case-Based Reasoning Research and Development*, Aha D, Watson I (Eds.), Vancouver, BC, Canada. *Lecture Notes in Computer Science*, Vol. 2080, 2001, pp. 27–44.

9. Richter MM. Similarity. In: *Case-Based Reasoning on Signals and Images*, Perner P (Ed.), Springer Verlag, 2007, pp. 25–90.

10. Mitchell HB. Image similarity measures. In: *Image Fusion*, Springer, Berlin, Heidelberg, 2010, pp. 167–185.

11. Santini S, Jain R. Similarity measures. *IEEE Transactions on Pattern Recognition and Machine Intelligence* 1999; 21:871–883.

12. Filev P, Hadjiiski LM, Sahiner B, Chan HP, Helvie MA. Comparison of similarity measures for the task of template matching of masses on serial mammograms. *Medical Physics* 2005; 32:515–529.

13. Cover TM, Thomas JA. *Elements of Information Theory*. Wiley, New York, NY, 1991.

14. Maes F, Collignon A, Vandermeulen D, Marchal G, Suetens P. Multi-modal image registration by maximization of mutual information. *IEEE Transactions on Medical Imaging* 1997; 16:87–198.

15. Tourassi GD, Harrawood B, Singh S, Lo JY, Floyd CE. Evaluation of information-theoretic similarity measures for content-based retrieval and detection of masses in mammograms. *Medical Physics* 2007; 34:140–150.

16. Sturges HA. The choice of a class interval. *Journal of American Statistical Association* 1926; 21:65–66.

17. Scott DW. On optimal and data-based histograms. *Biometrika* 1979; 66:605–610.

18. Wand MP. Data-based choice of histogram bin width. *The American Statistician* 1997; 51:59–60.

19. Pluim JPW, Maintz JBA, Viergever MA. Mutual-information-based registration of medical images: A survey. *IEEE Transactions on Medical Imaging* 2003; 22:986–1004.

20. Wang YN. Principles and applications of structural image matching. *Journal of Photogrammetry and Remote Sensing* 1998; 53:154–165.

21. Petrakis EGM. Design and evaluation of spatial similarity approaches for image retrieval. *Image and Vision Computing* 2002; 20:59–76.

22. Lee AJT, Chiu HP. 2D Z-String: A new spatial knowledge representation for image databases. *Pattern Recognition Letters* 2003; 24:3015–3026.

23. Lee SY, Hsu FJ. Spatial reasoning and similarity retrieval of images using 2D C-string knowledge representation. *Pattern Recognition* 1992; 25:305–318.

24. Sciascio ED, Mongiello M, Donini FM, Allegretti I. Retrieval by spatial similarity: An algorithm and a comparative evaluation. *Pattern Recognition* 2004; 25:1633–1645.

25. Gudivada VN. θR-String: A geometry-based representation for efficient and effective retrieval of images by spatial similarity. *IEEE Transactions on Knowledge and Data Engineering* 1998; 10:504–512.

26. Zhou XM, Ang CH, Ling TW. Image retrieval based on object's orientation spatial relationship. *Pattern Recognition Letters* 2001; 22:469–477.

27. Lu G. Techniques and data structures for efficient multimedia retrieval based on similarity. *IEEE Transactions on Multimedia* 2002; 4:372–384.

28. Baeza-Yates R, Cunto W, Manber U, Wu S. Proximity matching using fixed-queries trees. In: *Combinatorial Pattern Matching*. Springer, Berlin, Heidelberg, 1994, pp. 198–212.

29. Barros J, French J, Martin W, Kelley P, Cannon M. Using the triangle inequality to reduce the number of comparisons required for similarity-based retrieval. *Proceedings of SPIE Storage and Retrieval for Still Image and Video Databases* 1996; 2670:392–403.

30. Berman AP, Shapiro LG. Efficient image retrieval with multiple distance measures. *Proceedings of SPIE Storage and Retrieval for Image and Video Databases* 1997; 3022:12–21.

31. Berman AP, Shapiro LG. Triangle-inequality based pruning algorithms with triangle tries. *Proceedings of SPIE Storage and Retrieval for Image and Video Databases* 1999; 3656:356–365.

32. Jain AK. Data clustering: 50 years beyond k-means. In: *Proceedings of the International Conference in Pattern Recognition (ICPR)*, Vol. 31, Istanbul, Turkey, 2010, pp. 651–666.

33. Prabhakar S, Agrawal D, Abbadi AE. Data clustering for efficient range and similarity searching. *Proceedings of SPIE Multimedia Storage and Archiving System III* 1998; 3527:419–430.

34. Tourassi GD, Vargas-Voracek R, David M. Catarious J, Carey E. Floyd J. Computer-assisted detection of mammographic masses: A template matching scheme based on mutual information. *Medical Physics* 2003; 30:2123–2130.

35. Chang Y-H, Hardesty LA, Hakim CM, Chang TS, Zheng B, Good WF, Gur D. Knowledge-based computer-aided mass detection on digitized mammograms: A preliminary assessment. *Medical Physics* 2001; 28:455–461.

36. Chang Y-H, Wang X, Hardesty LA, Hakim CM, Zheng B, Good WF, Gur D. Incorporation of negative regions in a knowledge-based computer-aided detection scheme. *Proceedings of SPIE Medical Image* 2002; 4684:726–732.

37. Singh S, Tourassi GD, Baker JA, Samei E, Lo JY. Automated breast mass detection in 3D reconstructed tomosynthesis volumes: A featureless approach. *Medical Physics* 2008; 35:3626–3636.

38. Mazurowski MA, Lo JY, Harrawood B, Tourassi GD. Mutual information-based template matching scheme for detection of breast masses: From mammography to digital breast tomosynthesis. *Journal of Biomedical Informatics* 2011; 44:815–822.

39. Alto H, Rangayyan RM, Desautels JEL. Content-based retrieval and analysis of mammographic masses. *Journal of Electronic Imaging* 2005; 14(2):1–17.

40. El-Naqa I, Yang Y, Galatsanos NP, Nishikawa RM, Wernick MN. A similarity learning approach to content based image retrieval: Application to digital mammography. *IEEE Transactions on Medical Imaging* 2004; 23:1233–1244.

41. Wei L, Yang Y, Nishikawa R. Microcalcification classification assisted by content-based image retrieval for breast cancer diagnosis. *Pattern Recognition* 2009; 42:1126–1132.

42. Kuo W-J, Chang R-F, Lee CC, Moon WK, Chen DR. Retrieval technique for the diagnosis of solid breast tumors on sonogram. *Ultrasound in Medicine and Biology* 2002; 28:903–909.

43. Huang YL et al. Image retrieval with principal component analysis for breast cancer diagnosis on various ultrasonic systems. *Ultrasound in Obstetrics and Gynecology* 2005; 26(5):558–566.

44. Cho H-C et al. Similarity evaluation in a content-based image retrieval (CBIR) CADx system for characterization of breast masses on ultrasound images. *Medical Physics* 2011; 38:1820–1831.

45. Kinoshita SK, de Azevedo-Marques PM, Pereira RR, Rodrigues J, Rangayyan R. Content-based retrieval of mammograms using visual features related to breast density patterns. *Journal of Digital Imaging* 2007; 20:172–190.

46. de Oliveira JEE, Araujo A, Deserno TM. Content-based image retrieval applied to BI-RADS tissue classification in screening mammography. *World Journal of Radiology* 2011; 3:24–31.

47. Raudys SJ, Jain AK. Small sample size effects in statistical pattern recognition: Recommendations for practitioners. *IEEE Transactions on Pattern Analysis and Machine Intelligence* 1991; 13:252–264.

48. Wilson R, Martinez TR. Reduction techniques for instance-based learning algorithms. *Machine Learning* 2000; 38:257–286.

49. Grochowski M, Jankowski N. Comparison of instance selection algorithms II. Results and comments. *Lecture Notes in Computer Science* 2004; 3070:580–585.

50. Brighton H. Advances in instance selection for instance-based learning algorithms. *Data Mining in Knowledge and Discovery* 2002; 6:153–172.

51. Cano JR, Herrera F, Lozano M. Using evolutionary algorithms as instance selection for data reduction in KDD: An experimental study. *IEEE Transactions on Evolutionary Computation* 2003; 7:561–575.

52. de Haro-Garcia A, Garcia-Pedrajas N. A divide-and-conquer recursive approach for scaling up instance selection algorithms. *Data Mining in Knowledge and Discovery* 2009; 18(3):392–418.

53. Skalak DB. Prototype and feature selection by sampling and random mutation hill climbing algorithm. In: *Proceedings of the 11th International Conference on Machine Learning*, New Brunswick, NJ, 1994, pp. 293–301.

54. Li Y, Shiu SCK, Pal SK, Liu JNK. A rough set-based case-based reasoner for text categorization. *International Journal of Approximate Reasoning* 2006; 41:229–255.

55. Mazurowski MA, Malof JM, Tourassi GD. Comparative analysis of instance selection algorithms for instance-based classifiers in the context of medical decision support. *Physics in Medicine and Biology* 2011; 56(2):473–489.

56. Park SC et al. Optimization of reference library used in content-based medical image retrieval scheme. *Medical Physics* 2007; 34:4331–4339.

57. Wang XH, Park SC, Zheng B. Assessment of performance and reliability of computer-aided detection scheme using content-based image retrieval approach and limited reference database. *Journal of Digital Imaging* 2011; 4(2):352–359.

58. Wang XH, Park SC, Zheng B. Improving performance of content-based image retrieval schemes in searching for similar breast mass regions: An assessment. *Physics in Medicine and Biology* 2009; 54:949–961.

59. Ike R, Harrawood B, Tourassi GD. Effect of ROI size on the performance of an information-theoretic CAD system in mammography: Multisize analysis fusion. *Proceedings SPIE Conference on Medical Imaging* 2008; 6915:691527.

60. Tourassi GD, Sharma AC, Singh S, Saunders RS, Lo JY, Samei E, Harrawood B. Knowledge transfer across breast cancer screening modalities: A pilot study using an information theoretic CADe system for mass detection. In: *International Workshop on Digital Mammography*, Tucson, AZ, July 25–28, 2008, pp. 292–298.

61. Datta R, Joshi D, Li J, Wang JZ. Image retrieval: Ideas, influences, and trends of the new age. *ACM Computing Surveys* 2008; 40:34–94.

62. Sklansky J, Tao EY, Bazargan M, Ornes CJ, Murchison RC, Teklehaimanot S. Computer-aided, case-based diagnosis of mammographic regions of interest containing microcalcifications. *Academic Radiology* 2000; 7:395–405.

63. Muramatsu C, Li Q, Suzuki K, Schmidt RA, Shiraishi J, Newstead GM, Doi K. Investigation of psychophysical measure for evaluation of similar images for mammographic masses: Preliminary results. *Medical Physics* 2005; 32:2295–2304.

64. Muramatsu C, Li Q, Schmidt RA, Suzuki K, Shiraishi J, Newstead GM, Doi K. Experimental determination of subjective similarity for pairs of clustered microcalcifications on mammograms: Observer study results. *Medical Physics* 2006; 33:3460–3468.

65. Zheng B, Lu A, Hardesty LA, Sumkin JH, Hakim CM, Ganott MA, Gur D. A method to improve visual similarity of breast masses for an interactive computer-aided diagnosis environment. *Medical Physics* 2006; 33:111–117.

66. de Azevedo-Marques PM, Rosa NA, Traina AJM, Traina C, Kinoshita SK, Rangayyan RM. Reducing the semantic gap in content-based image retrieval in mammography with relevance feedback and inclusion of expert knowledge. *International Journal of Computer-Assisted Radiology and Surgery* 2008; 3:123–130.

67. Oh JH, El-Naqa I, Yang Y. Adaptive learning for relevance feedback: Application to digital mammography. *Medical Physics* 2010; 37:4432–4444.

68. Nakayama R, Abe H, Shiraishi J, Doi K. Evaluation of objective similarity measures for selecting similar images of mammographic lesions. *Journal of Digital Imaging* 2010; 24:75–85.

69. Sahiner B, Hadjiiski L, Chan HP, Cui J, Paramagul C, Nees A, Helvie M. Inter- and intra-observer variability in radiologists' assessment of mass similarity on mammograms. *Proceedings SPIE Conference on Medical Imaging* 2009; 7263:726315.

70. Horsch K, Giger ML, Vyborny CJ, Lan L, Mendelson EB, Hendrick E. Classification of breast lesions with multimodality computer-aided diagnosis: Observer study results on an independent clinical data set. *Radiology* 2006; 240:357–368.

71. Nakayama R, Abe H, Shiraishi J, Doi K. Potential usefulness of similar images in the differential diagnosis of clustered microcalcifications on mammograms. *Radiology* 2009; 253:625–631.

72. Tourassi GD, Harrawood B, Singh S, Lo JY. Information-theoretic CAD system in mammography: Entropy-based indexing for computational efficiency and robust performance. *Medical Physics* 2007; 34:3193–3204.

73. Park SC, Wang X, Zheng B. Assessment of performance improvement in content-based medical image retrieval schemes using fractal dimension. *Academic Radiology* 2009; 16:1171–1178.

74. Mazurowski MA, Zurada JM, Tourassi GD. Database decomposition of a knowledge-based CAD system in mammography: An ensemble approach to improve detection. *Proceedings SPIE Conference on Medical Imaging* 2008; 6915:69151K.

75. Mazurowski MA, Habas PA, Zurada JM, Tourassi GD. Decision optimization of case-based computer-aided decision systems using genetic algorithms with application to mammography. *Physics in Medicine and Biology* 2008; 53:895–908.

Chapter 7

Multimodality CAD Systems for Breast Cancer

Karen Drukker and Charlene A. Sennett

CONTENTS

7.1 INTRODUCTION

Since the initial development in the mid-1980s of computer-aided detection (CADe) and computer-aided diagnosis (CADx) methods, progress in this area of research has been tremendous. This has culminated in quite a few commercially available CADe systems (such as ImageChecker® by Hologic and SecondLook Digital® by iCAD) and a wealth of scientific literature. Many, if not most, of the scientifically developed computer-aided detection and diagnosis (CAD) methods have not yet reached the stage of commercialization, however. Quite a few reviews and book chapters have already been devoted to CAD in breast imaging (e.g., Hadjiiski et al. 2006; Giger et al. 2008), but with the advent of new imaging technologies and the increased clinical use of multimodality imaging, many exciting opportunities have emerged for the development of novel CAD methods with the ultimate long-term goal of improving patient care. Moreover, CAD is being extended to quantitative imaging analysis for prognosis (Bhooshan et al. 2010; Madabhushi et al. 2011), risk assessment (Li et al. 2004; Sickles 2007) (see Chapter 5), and evaluation of the response to therapy (Shi et al. 2009).

The first CAD methods for breast imaging were developed for mammography and involved digitization of the screen films before further analysis. The aim was to alert radiologists to the location of potential abnormalities visible on mammograms. Even when using only a single imaging modality, radiologists are often confronted with large amounts of data to be processed, for example, when interpreting screening mammograms or analyzing 4D magnetic resonance imaging (MRI) data (three spatial dimensions in addition to time). This can lead to reader fatigue and interpretation errors. In many breast imaging centers, multimodality imaging has become the norm and is aimed at increasing specificity (fewer unnecessary biopsies), increasing sensitivity (detecting more cancer cases), and disease staging. With the incorporation of multimodality imaging approaches in clinical practice, the need for efficient information processing has expanded steadily, burdening radiologists more than ever and creating opportunities for computerized analysis to become part of clinical decision making. The development of multimodality CAD methods for breast imaging is still relatively new, and while generally the potential of a multimodality approach is recognized, relatively few publications have addressed this topic. This chapter will provide an overview of multimodality approaches for CAD in breast imaging. First, however, we will briefly describe the current status and some of the emerging breast imaging modalities that in the future may inspire—and increase the need for—the development of novel multimodality CAD approaches.

7.2 RECENT DEVELOPMENTS IN BREAST IMAGING

X-ray mammography, either film screen of full-field digital mammography (FFDM), is still the main screening method for breast cancer in the general population (Hinz et al. 2011).

While most people agree that annual screening mammograms have decreased mortality by about 30% (Tabar et al. 2003), the technique is far from perfect with an adjusted sensitivity of 89% in entirely fatty breasts and 62.9% in extremely dense breasts. Likewise, adjusted specificity is 96.9% in entirely fatty breasts, but only 89.1% in extremely dense breasts (Carney et al. 2003). For these reasons, other imaging modalities have gained acceptance as adjuncts to mammography (Karellas and Vedantham 2008), most notably ultrasound (US) (Berg et al. 2008; Corsetti et al. 2011; Youk et al. 2011) and MRI. Each imaging modality has its strengths and weaknesses. For example, X-ray mammography is known to have lower sensitivity for women with dense breast tissue (Carney et al. 2003; Evans et al. 2007; Taylor et al. 2011), handheld US is by definition operator dependent, and MRI is costly. To date, the screening protocol for women at high risk at many institutions includes the use of X-ray mammography, US, and MRI (Boetes 2011a; Dhar et al. 2011; Feig 2011; Houssami and Ciatto 2011; Hutton et al. 2011; Le-Petross et al. 2011). Moreover, it has become general practice to include US in the clinical workup of patients for whom a screening or diagnostic mammogram raises suspicion of breast cancer or is inconclusive (Zanello et al. 2011), thus increasing the specificity over the use of mammography alone. Breast MRI has been invaluable in the evaluation of breast diseases. Diagnostic breast MRI is indicated in the staging of breast cancer, the postoperative assessment of histological positive margins, the assessment of women with known metastatic axillary lymphadenopathy and a negative mammogram and breast US, the assessment of response to neoadjuvant chemotherapy, the evaluation of the integrity of silicone implants, and the evaluation of ambiguous clinical or imaging findings (Levin 2008). In 2007, the American Cancer Society (ACS) published guidelines for the performance of screening breast MRI including BRCA mutation, untested first-degree relative of a BRCA carrier, calculated lifetime risk of 20%–25% or greater, chest radiation between the ages of 10 and 30, and certain genetic syndromes (Saslow et al. 2007). The sensitivity of MRI is generally superior to that of X-ray mammography as is its specificity for the latest technology (Boetes 2011b). To further improve diagnostic accuracy, *second-look* US is often performed to provide additional information for findings on breast MRI (Linda et al. 2008; Destounis et al. 2009; Abe et al. 2010; Carbognin et al. 2010; Trop et al. 2010; Candelaria and Fornage 2011; Luciani et al. 2011). The high cost of MRI and use of a contrast agent (in the case of dynamic contrast-enhanced MRI [DCE-MRI]), however, are drawbacks for the implementation as a general screening modality. In fact, the ACS guidelines specifically state that MRI is not indicated as a screening modality in women at average risk of developing breast cancer. All three modalities—mammography, US, and MRI—are also valuable for the assessment of response to neoadjuvant therapy (Schlossbauer et al. 2010).

Quite a few new breast imaging techniques are being developed, some of which arguably have potential as a screening modality. Most of these modalities, however, may not ever—or at least not any time soon—be suitable for the screening of the general population, but may be valuable for the evaluation of women at high risk of developing breast cancer.

One of the most promising recent developments is dedicated breast computed tomography (CT), which has been under simultaneous development in several groups (Prionas et al. 2010; Sechopoulos et al. 2010; Diekmann 2011; Huang et al. 2011; Kalender et al. 2012; Weigel et al. 2011). The dose of an exam is roughly the same as that for a routine four-view screening mammogram (Sechopoulos et al. 2010), making it a viable potential alternative to mammography in that respect. Moreover, it does not suffer from one of mammography's main drawbacks where overlapping normal parenchymal tissue can obscure lesions, which makes it a promising approach for women with dense breasts. Downsides of breast CT are the expected cost and large amount of image data that need to be analyzed by radiologists. The latter, however, makes it an ideal candidate for the use of CAD methods, whether single modality or multimodality. Tomosynthesis is another X-ray-based breast imaging modality that avoids the problem of normal breast tissue obscuring lesions through its semi-3D nature (Svane et al. 2011).

In breast US, recent developments include 3D US (both handheld and automated full breast [Wohrle et al. 2010; Chang et al. 2011a,b]) and elastography (Weismann et al. 2011). Automated full-breast US may have future potential as a screening modality, since it is reproducible, whereas the handheld techniques generally are not (Berg et al. 2006). Advantages are that 3D US involves no ionizing radiation, is relatively low cost, and requires no or little breast compression. Disadvantages are the long acquisition time (minutes) with respect to mammography and a more limited ability to image microcalcifications modality and its relatively low sensitivity with respect to MRI.

Elastography is based on the theory that benign and malignant breast lesions have different tissue firmness with benign lesions being less firm (i.e., softer) than malignant lesions (i.e., stiffer) when compared to surrounding normal tissue. In the United States, the degree of tissue deformation is displayed as a color array rather than a specific numerical value. Several US vendors have FDA-approved software packages currently available for clinical use that utilize either strain wave or shear wave technology for calculating tissue stiffness. Burnside et al. in a study published in radiology found that the integration of elastography with conventional US imaging improved the differentiation between benign and malignant solid masses, although operator dependence was still a limitation of the technique

(Burnside et al. 2007). In the future, elastography may increase the specificity of breast US and decrease the number of false-positive US-guided core biopsy procedures.

DCE-MRI has become quite widely used as part of high-risk screening protocols and staging of known cancer cases. The T1-weighted images (pre- and post-contrast T1 source and subtraction images) and associated dynamic time intensity curves are most frequently used in patient assessment. More recently, however, T2-weighted images (which do not involve a contrast agent) have become part of the analysis (Baltzer et al. 2011). Another promising technique currently under development that exhibits extraordinary image quality and does not involve the use of a contrast agent is high spectral and spatial (HiSS) MRI (Fan et al. 2006; Medved et al. 2006, 2009, 2010), but the long acquisition times with respect to DCE-MRI are a drawback.

Breast-specific gamma imaging (BSGI) is another relatively new imaging modality using a radiotracer and a specialized gamma camera to detect gamma rays emitted by breast tissue. Normal breast tissue has a low background level of radioactivity, while malignant lesions have a level of radioactivity (Goldsmith et al. 2010; Pinker et al. 2010; Moadel 2011). Studies have shown BSGI to have a sensitivity of 96% and a specificity of 60% in small clinical studies (Brem et al. 2008; Kessler et al. 2011). BSGI may have utility in screening, especially in high-risk women with dense breast tissue. The use of a radiotracer, however, is a serious drawback. Studies are currently underway, however, to minimize the dose, while maintaining diagnostic accuracy (Hendrick 2010). Another breast imaging modality that relies on radioactivity is dedicated positron emission mammography (PEM), which has recently become commercially available and has shown promise as an adjunct modality (Narayanan et al. 2011). PEM provides 3D images of the breast and axilla, albeit at low spatial resolution. The need for a radioactive tracer, patient fasting, and long total acquisition times (on the order of hours) currently limit its use to a small segment of the patient population, for example, for the staging of breast cancer patients and for the assessment of response to therapy.

7.3 CURRENT CLINICAL MULTIMODALITY VIEWING SYSTEMS FOR BREAST IMAGING

Although mammography is considered the gold standard for breast cancer screening, the introduction and advancement of new technologies have made a multimodality approach to breast imaging a clinical reality. In the breast imaging arena, viewing systems are needed that will incorporate all of the needed data referable to breast disease and display all of the available patient images, with cross-referencing of imaging findings and incorporation of all pertinent CAD features. As the pace of development of medical science increases and moves toward the delivery of personalized medicine with emphasis on drug discovery, molecular biology of breast cancer, and image-based clinical trials, it is likely that no single imaging modality will be able to provide all the information required. Unfortunately, most interpretations of these studies occur on stand-alone, vendor-specific, modality-specific review workstations, with selected images pushed to them for interpretation. Difficulties frequently arise when viewing images from different vendors such as imperfect auto-sizing/auto-processing (Figure 7.1). In addition, generally only one application can be viewed at a time, which seriously hampers the workflow (Figure 7.2). Multiple other problems exist as well such as the frequent inability to upload and review studies obtained from other clinics for referred patients, the mismatch in exam dates for the studies from a different clinic that actually were successfully uploaded (i.e., the date indicated is not the actual date of service but rather the date of the image upload), and the poor resolution of digitized analog mammograms uploaded onto workstations for comparison to digitally acquired mammograms.

In order to function optimally, radiologists need fully integrated workspaces that are linked to the general archive system, have the ability to scale images from different acquisition units with variable pixel pitches, and set comparable window and level parameters for viewing. This would allow for a reasonable comparison of current and prior examinations. *Change from previous* is the hallmark sign of a potential developing breast cancer. The current setup in the clinical viewing area, however, is far from ideal, and the pandemonium of images now being presented seriously jeopardizes the screening endeavor.

Also needed is a seamless integration of multimodality breast CAD data, with the goal of integrating the benefits of computer artificial intelligence into the clinical workflow. Evaluations have already been performed on three levels—computer performance, robustness evaluation, and effect of systems on radiologists' performances in observer studies. Methods are now under development for all three common breast imaging modalities—mammography, US, and MRI—requiring only the radiologist's indication of the lesion, with all the subsequent steps being automated.

Despite the obvious need for an exam-based data archiving and retrieval system, as implemented in a picture archiving and communication system (PACS), the actual use of the data in decision making requires a completely different organization. Clinicians use and combine data that are stored and retrieved separately in PACS. Oncologists (especially surgeons), for example, are concerned with the location and character of specific masses, clustered microcalcifications, and architectural distortions.

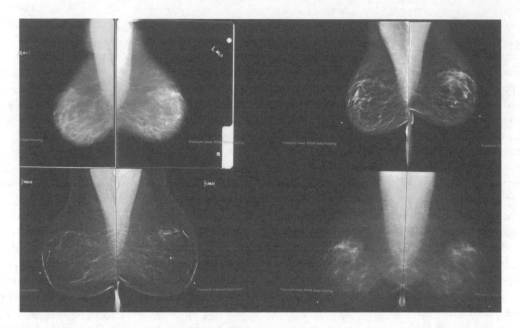

Figure 7.1   Viewing images from different vendors on a single workstation results in imperfect autosizing and autoprocessing. Top left: Digitized analog images. Top right: Digital images acquired at 50 µm per pixel. Bottom left: Digital images acquired at 70 µm per pixel. Bottom right: Digital images acquired at 100 µm per pixel.

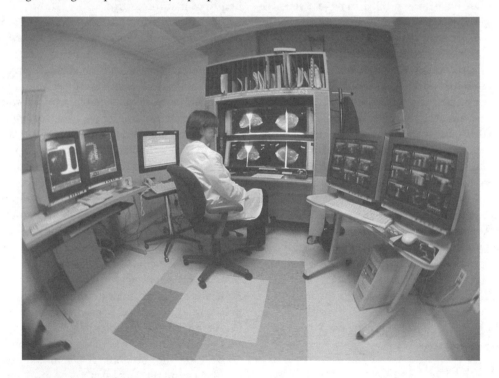

Figure 7.2   Currently, a radiologist needs multiple-modality-specific, vendor-specific workstations in order to manage a breast imaging clinic.

They must extirpate lesions with clear margins as determined histologically by pathologists. Each imaging encounter (for mammography, US, or MRI) is accessed separately on PACS, while the radiologist or surgeon uses them together. Radiation oncologists are concerned with local (e.g., MammoSite brachytherapy) and regional structures including the breast itself and lymphatic drainage network. Dosimetry and treatment planning as well as treatment delivery use morphologic information gathered from CT simulation (stored separately from all other images).

Medical oncologists are concerned with breast target lesions as well as local and regional lymph nodes, as well as metastases. This, again, is an example of how information from multiple exams stored in different locations needs to be combined in the clinical decision-making process: evaluation of treatment response is based on serial evaluation of lesions, so the change between exams is more important than any single isolated study.

In general, for all of these and related applications (such as biopsy), organization of image datasets according to specific identifiable lesions and related structures (such as lymph nodes) over time is much more important than the current timelines in PACS systems. Breast imaging is unique in its dedication to assembling lifelong data on specific lesions in patients, as well as screening surveys of the whole breast. Unfortunately, no commercially available integrated workstations are available, and the current image archiving systems and most workstations do a relatively poor job of managing data regarding individual lesions across modalities and over time, leading to built-in inefficiency and propensity for errors. Multimodality CAD systems integrated into multimodality workstations would aid the radiologist in processing this vast amount of information.

7.4   STAND-ALONE PERFORMANCE OF MULTIMODALITY BREAST CAD

The development of CAD algorithms for breast imaging has been an active research area for quite some time, but most systems to date have been based on information from a single imaging modality. A comprehensive review paper on breast CAD by Ayer et al. (2010) emphasizes the need for future CAD systems to incorporate information from all possible sources when making recommendations to radiologists. Just as the radiologist takes into account information from different sources (imaging modalities and other patient information), so can—and probably should—the computer. Indeed, the increasing use in clinical practice of US as an adjunct to mammography sparked interest in the development of multimodality CAD algorithms (Horsch et al. 2002a,b; Hong et al. 2004). Here, we will discuss papers published to date in peer-reviewed journals. A limitation shared by all studies discussed in this section is that they consider only the performance of a CAD scheme itself, not the impact such a system may (or may not) have on the decision-making process of a radiologist in clinical practice.

One of the first peer-reviewed papers on multimodality breast CAD was published in 2005 (Drukker et al. 2005).The authors investigated the performance of a CADx scheme for the distinction between benign and malignant breast masses based on computer-extracted (and computer-selected) features from mammography alone, from US alone,

and from a combination of the two (Figure 7.3). This investigation employed a relatively small dataset of 100 lesions (cases)—of which 40 were cancerous. The CADx scheme was completely automated apart from the indication of lesion centers, that is, seed points, by a radiologist. The seed points together with the image data formed the input to the CADx scheme that consisted of a preprocessing stage, computerized lesion segmentation (Horsch et al. 2001), feature extraction, feature selection, and classification for malignancy. For each physical lesion, multiple images (views) were available for each modality. Lesion features obtained from different views were combined before further by-lesion analysis in three different ways: (1) by averaging features obtained from different views, (2) by obtaining the minimum value, and (3) by obtaining the maximum value. The authors used stepwise feature selection in a leave-one-case-out protocol and subsequently used the selected features in classifier training and testing in a leave-one-case-out analysis. Performance was assessed by the area under the ROC curve (AUC). The study used a limited number of features as input to feature selection. These features were chosen based on past experience, and there were five features for mammography (Giger et al. 2000, pp. 915–1004) and four features for US (Horsch et al. 2002a,b). Note, however, that the mean, minimum, and maximum values of each feature were included in the lesion-based feature selection process, which effectively increased the overall number of possible choices. The inclusion of features selected from both modalities in the CADx scheme (without increasing the total number of features selected) boosted the AUC from 0.77 and 0.88 for mammography and US alone, respectively, to 0.92 for the combined mammography plus US system. This increase in performance was statistically significant (p-value <0.05). Thus, this study showed promise that a CADx system combining features from multiple imaging modalities may be more powerful than one using features from a single modality. Some limitations of this study, however, were its relatively small database size, the limited number of features included in the feature selection, and the potential for database bias by performing feature selection (albeit in a leave-one-case-out scenario) and classifier/testing on the same set.

A different, and slightly more recent, study also investigated the combination of lesion characteristics from mammography and sonography in a CADx scheme (Jesneck et al. 2007). Here, radiologists assigned mammographic and sonographic Breast Imaging and Reporting Data System (BI-RADS®) descriptors (D'Orsi et al. 2003)—plus a few additional descriptors such as patient age—to a large number of lesions. These descriptors were subsequently used as input features to a CADx scheme for the task of distinguishing biopsy-proven solid benign lesions from malignancies. This study employed a different approach than the one described

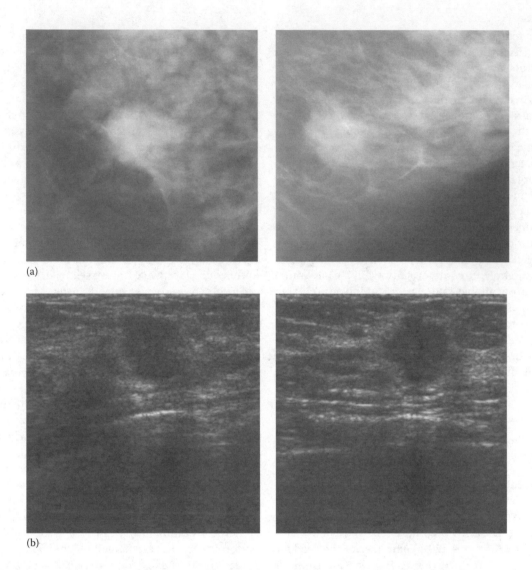

Figure 7.3   Example of mammographic (a) and sonographic (b) views of the same (malignant) lesion. (Reprinted from Drukker, K. et al., *Acad. Radiol.*, 12, 970, 2005. With permission.)

in the previous paragraph, in that the features input to the CADx scheme were not computer extracted but determined by experienced radiologists. An additional three features were obtained from the clinical patient history. Moreover, this study did not attempt to assess differences in performance for single-modality CADx versus multimodality CADx and assess only the potential of multimodality CADx. The employed dataset was substantial and consisted of 803 lesions, of which the pathology was proven by biopsy in all instances, including 296 breast cancers. Since the dataset was sufficiently large, the authors employed a train, validate, and retest approach to avoid pitfalls of classifier overtraining. Here, the 303 most recently imaged lesions formed the retest set, which was used only in the final assessment of classifier performance, not in fine-tuning or feature selection. The performance of two commonly used classifiers was compared: linear discriminant analysis (LDA) and an artificial neural network (ANN). Both classifiers obtained respectable performance on the retest set with identical AUC values of 0.92 (0.01 standard error). The partial AUCs at 90% sensitivity were also very similar at 0.54 (0.08) and 0.55 (0.08) for the LDA and ANN classifiers, respectively. The authors failed to find any statistically significant differences in performance for the AUC values of the two classifiers, and also differences in the specificity, positive predictive value, and negative predictive value (all at 98% sensitivity) failed to reach statistical significance. While this study demonstrated promising performance of the two classifiers for the task of distinguishing between benign and malignant breast lesions as well as agreement with radiologist assessment scores, it did not shed any light on whether multimodality is better than single modality when it comes to CADx.

Moreover, in this retrospective study, the participating radiologists knew that their input to the CADx system had no effect on patient care, which may have biased their BI-RADS scoring. Since this CADx scheme was based on the input of somewhat subjective BI-RADS descriptors assessed by radiologists, the objectivity of this CADx scheme may be brought into question more than for a more objective CADx scheme based on computer-extracted features. Note, however, that subjectivity plays a role in the assessment of the performance of—and impact of—*all* CAD systems in observer studies (see next section) since there are no medical or legal consequences to the retrospective decisions of the participating radiologists. Retrospective studies are an essential part of CAD performance assessment in spite of these shortcomings.

Unlike the two studies discussed earlier, which combined information from mammography and sonography, Yuan et al. (2010) recently investigated a multimodality breast CADx scheme for mammography and DCE-MRI. Their work used three datasets: (1) a set of 432 lesions imaged with FFDM (255 malignant, 177 benign), (2) a set of 476 lesions imaged with DCE-MRI (347 malignant, 129 benign), and (3) a multimodality set of 213 lesions imaged with both FFDM and DCE-MRI (168 malignant, 45 benign). The components of the CADx scheme were based on previously published work for single-modality FFDM (Li et al. 2008) and DCE-MRI CADx (Chen et al. 2006b), respectively. Stepwise feature selection was performed within each dataset in a leave-one-case-out scenario. The most frequently selected features were used as input to a Bayesian neural network in another leave-one-case-out training and testing protocol for the task of discriminating between cancers and benign breast lesions using *the same* dataset as for feature selection. The classification performance in terms of AUC value for the multimodality dataset improved from 0.74 (0.04 standard error) and 0.78 (0.04) for FFDM alone and DCE-MRI alone, respectively, to 0.87 (0.03) for the multimodality approach (Figure 7.4). The improvement in performance was statistically significant (p-value < 0.05). In the multimodality analysis, three features were selected and used for subsequent classification. Of these features, two were dynamic features from DCE-MRI (peak location and curve shape index) and one was from FFDM (spiculation), illustrating the synergy from combining morphology from FFDM and kinetics from DCE-MRI. One should note that the reported AUC values for the single-modality schemes were substantially lower than what is usually reported. This may have been due to the difficulty of the dataset and/or high cancer prevalence.

Apart from the task of cancer classification discussed earlier, there are other tasks for which a multimodality approach is ideally suited, such as for the staging of breast cancer and generally for the identification of corresponding findings on image data from different modalities.

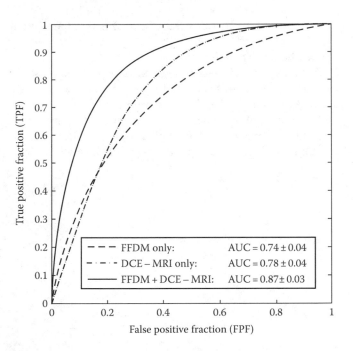

Figure 7.4 ROC curves for the task of distinguishing benign from malignant breast lesions for a stand-alone CADx scheme based on full-field digital mammography (FFDM) alone, DCE-MRI alone, and a combination of the two modalities. The improvement in performance when combining FFDM and MRI was statistically significant. (Reprinted from Yuan, Y. et al., *Acad. Radiol.*, 17, 1158, 2010. With permission.)

Since lymph node status has a substantial effect on patient prognosis, treatment, and outcome, it is important to know whether a cancer has metastasized to the lymph nodes in patients newly diagnosed with cancer. For this purpose, lymph nodes are routinely assessed with US and increasingly frequently with breast MRI. If lymph nodes appear in the least suspicious, biopsy is performed. Hence, the evaluation of axillary lymph nodes is essential in the staging of breast cancer. Breast MRI is frequently part of the workup of a breast cancer patient, while most biopsies (both lesion and lymph node biopsies) are performed under US guidance. It is hence important to be able to correlate what is seen on an MRI with that on US. The development of multimodality CAD for the staging of breast cancer is in its infancy, and a pilot study was recently published by Meinel et al. (2010). The aim was to assess whether it was possible to correlate axillary lymph nodes imaged on breast MRI with those seen on breast US. The ultimate goal of CAD for prognosis is to provide a preoperative noninvasive method for improved staging of breast cancer, thereby improving diagnostic accuracy and reducing the number of unnecessary biopsies. The pilot study was performed with an extremely small dataset of only 16 lymph nodes. For this set, it appeared that the shortest Euclidean distance could be used to identify the same lymph node on US and MRI. Since the dataset was so small, no solid conclusions could be drawn about any imaging characteristics of the lymph nodes on either modality or the relationship between the two.

A more extensive—although still preliminary—study on correlating lesions seen in different modalities was performed by Yuan (2010). Many patients present with multiple findings along with the main lesion of interest. For example, many women have breast cysts—which are usually of no consequence and are generally easily identified on US—which may present as indeterminate or even suspicious on mammography. It is then important to correlate the US findings with those on mammography. The authors investigated whether it was possible to identify lesions seen on mammography as the same as, or as different from, those seen on breast MRI for patients with multiple lesions (Figure 7.5). Moreover, the investigation proposed a protocol to incorporate *lesion correspondence scores* into multimodality CADx. Since the breast is deformable,

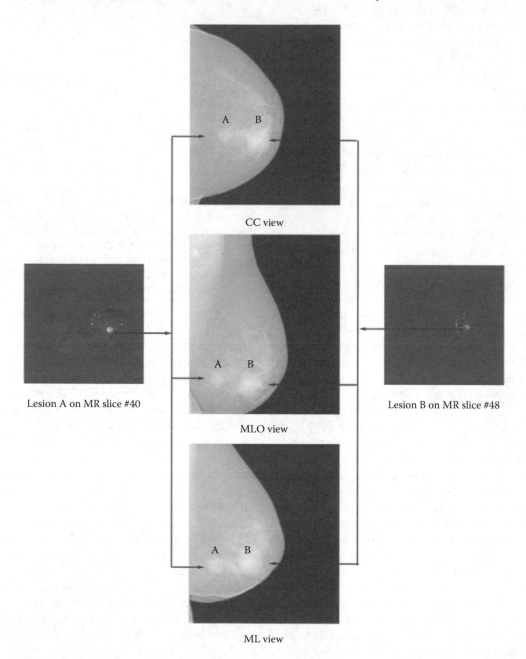

Lesion A on MR slice #40

CC view

MLO view

Lesion B on MR slice #48

ML view

Figure 7.5   Example of the correlation of lesions between imaging modalities in patients with multiple lesions imaged with mammography and DCE-MRI. (Reprinted from Yuan, Y., Correlative analysis of breast lesions full-field digital mammography and magnetic resonance imaging, PhD thesis, University of Chicago, Chicago, IL, 2010. With permission.)

the use of image registration to identify corresponding lesions seen on different views obtained with the same imaging modality is often quite challenging for patients with multiple abnormalities. The use of different imaging modalities further complicates matters since one also has to take into account that patient positioning is frequently different for each modality (e.g., prone for MRI, upright for mammography, and supine for US [Figure 7.6]), hampering image registration. Hence, the authors calculated feature-based *correspondence scores* as an estimate of the probability of being the same lesion. This was done based on individual lesion features extracted from each modality and also based on a combination of individual-feature scores into a multifeature score after performing stepwise selection in a two-stage leave-one-case-out protocol.

Note that for the correspondence scores, the task of interest was the distinction between corresponding and noncorresponding lesion pairs. The features could be divided into three categories: morphological, texture, and geometric (such as the distance from the nipple). The multifeature composite correspondence score was used in a preliminary application to assess whether it had the ability to improve multimodality CADx performance for the task of distinguishing between benign and malignant breast lesions. The database was of moderate size, and the number of lesion pairs to be investigated differed for each combination of views (e.g., mammography MLO versus MRI). The number of pairs ranged from 77 noncorresponding lesion pairs (on mammography MLO versus MRI) to 243 corresponding lesion pairs (mammography CC versus MRI). It was

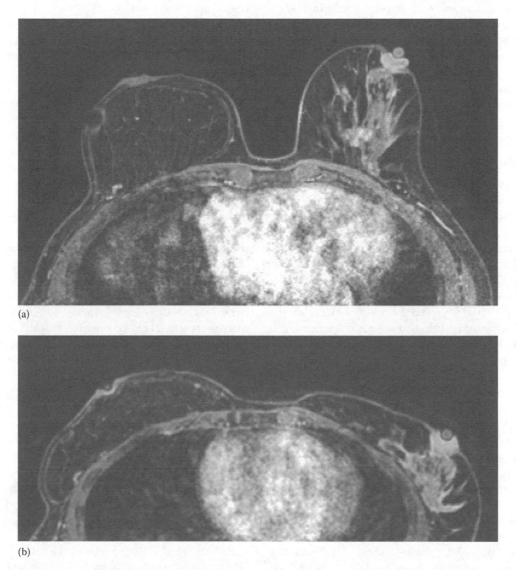

(a)

(b)

Figure 7.6 Conventional prone (a) and nonconventional supine (b) positions demonstrating the difficulty in verifying lesion concordance in the different positions used in different imaging modalities. (Image courtesy of G.M. Newstead.)

found that a multifeature composite *correspondence score* performed significantly better than any of the individual-feature *correspondence scores* for the task of distinguishing between corresponding and noncorresponding lesion pairs. The best performance for the task of identifying corresponding lesion pairs was observed for the lesion correlation between mammography MLO and breast MRI with an AUC value of 0.86 (standard error 0.03) for the multifeature composite correspondence score and 0.75 (0.03) for the best-performing single-feature correspondence score. When the composite correspondence score was incorporated into a multimodality CADx scheme for cancer classification, a trend toward a modest increase in classification performance could be observed with the best cancer classification performance reaching an AUC of 0.84 (0.03). This paper demonstrated an interesting pilot study, but due to the modest sizes of the datasets combined with the use of a dual-stage method, database bias may have been an issue. When the *correspondence scores* were incorporated into a multimodality CADx scheme, differences in cancer classification performance failed to reach statistical significance.

7.5 OBSERVER STUDY PERFORMANCE OF MULTIMODALITY CAD

After a CAD scheme has been found promising in stand-alone performance analyses, the next logical step is usually to perform an observer study mimicking its clinical use. These retrospective studies are essential in the evaluation of CAD schemes. Obviously, it first has to be proven that there will be no patient harm (and hopefully a benefit) before considering incorporating a CAD scheme in clinical decision making.

In 2006, Horsch et al. published a study in radiology (Horsch et al. 2006) that assessed the effect of a multimodality breast CADx system on the classification performance of radiologists. For that purpose, a CADx scheme and a user interface were developed in which a computer assessment was given for mammographically and sonographically imaged lesions. For each physical lesion imaged with both mammography and US, the CADx scheme estimated and displayed the probability of malignancy (PM) and provided several pictorial outputs in the form of a reference atlas and histograms. The output probabilities of malignancy were provided separately for each modality and *not* merged into a by-lesion PM. Ten observers participated in the study, of whom five were expert breast radiologists and five were fellows with 1 year of training in breast imaging. The computer mammographic and sonographic classifiers were trained on different relatively large databases consisting of lesions imaged by each modality, respectively. The dataset used in the observer study was an independent dataset of 97 lesions, so the lesions were unknown to

both the computer classifiers and to the observers. Before beginning the study, observers received information on the stand-alone performance of the CADx classifiers, as well as training on 18 lesions (cases), which were not part of the test set. For each lesion, observers were asked to estimate the PM and to give a recommendation for follow-up (biopsy versus imaging follow-up) under two conditions: (1) before seeing any computer output (unaided) and (2) after seeing the computer output (aided). The authors performed a detailed case-by-case analysis of the changes in PM and follow-up recommendation as well as more general ROC analysis ([partial] AUC, sensitivity, and specificity). Paired t-tests were used to assess statistical significance of the average performance of the observers. The performance of the observers improved overall after taking into account the computer output with the AUC of the expert radiologists increasing from 0.87 to 0.91, and the AUC of the fellows increasing from 0.88 to 0.93. Both increases in performance were statistically significant within the statistical analysis used. Encouraging trends were observed in that, on average, for malignant lesions, the observers correctly altered their clinical workup recommendation from follow-up to biopsy more frequently than vice versa. For benign lesions, the (favorable) reversed trend was observed. There were several limitations in this study. A first limitation was that the study assessed only the effect of the multimodality CADx workstation without assessing whether the improvement in observer performance could have been achieved solely by using a single-modality CADx workstation. A second limitation was that only biopsy-proven lesions were included in the study, while in clinical practice, the majority of imaged lesions are not referred to biopsy. Hence, this study does not reflect if and how the use of this multimodality CADx station would alter clinical assessment of these lesions, that is, if it would result in more unnecessary biopsies for a dataset more representative of clinical practice. Note, however, that in order to maintain statistical power for a reasonable study design, it is frequently necessary to *enrich* a dataset with more cancer cases to higher cancer prevalence than seen in clinical practice. A third limitation was the choice of statistical analysis for the determination of statistical significance. If a similar study would be performed today, it would be highly advisable to use a more rigorous statistical analysis such as multi-case multi-reader (MRMC) ROC analysis (Roe and Metz 1997; Wagner et al. 2002). The dual-modality CADx scheme described here has recently been extended to triple modality (mammography, US, and MRI) and presented at the conference of the Radiological Society of North America (Giger et al. 2010).

Sahiner et al. (2009) performed a retrospective observer study using mammography and 3D whole breast US. As in the study by Horsch et al. (2006) (described earlier), the aim was to investigate the effect of CADx on the radiologists' performance in discriminating between benign and malignant breast masses. Here, the features extracted from mammography and US were merged by an LDA classifier into a single multimodality estimate of the PM. The latter was in contrast to the Horsch study, where the probabilities of malignancy were calculated and provided separately for each modality. Ten experienced radiologists participated in this study and provided probabilities of malignancy along with BI-RADS assessments, where it was assumed that categories 4 and 5 implied a recommendation for biopsy, while lesions assigned to other categories were not recommended for biopsy. The dataset was rather small consisting of image data of 67 biopsied breast masses (32 benign and 35 malignant). There were three subsequent reading modes: (1) mammography alone (unaided), (2) 3D US after mammography (unaided), and (3) multimodality CADx after modes 1 and 2 (aided). So, radiologists first gave their impression based on mammography alone, then reassessed after viewing the 3D US data, and reassessed again after taking into account the CADx output. To assess performance, the probabilities of malignancy estimated by the radiologists were used in ROC analysis, and the biopsy/follow-up categories were used to determine sensitivity and specificity. The authors assessed the impact of changing from reading mode 1 (mammography) to reading mode 2 (mammography plus US) and from reading mode 2 to reading mode 3 (mammography plus US plus CADx) both for individual radiologists and for all radiologists overall. The latter was done within an MRMC ROC framework (Roe and Metz 1997). An interesting result of this study was that the increase in radiologist performance was the largest when going from reading mode 1 (interpretation based on mammography alone) to mode 2 (combination of mammography and 3D US), with average AUCs of 0.87 and 0.93 for the two reading modes, respectively. While the impact of the CADx on the radiologists' performance was also positive, this effect was smaller bringing the *final* average AUC to 0.95. It should also be noted that the AUCs of the observers in reading mode 2 already appeared higher than that of the multimodality CADx system that had an average AUC of 0.91. However, the fact that a CADx system with a performance comparable to—or even a bit lower than—that of the observers can have a positive impact on radiologists' performance has been shown in other studies as well (Horsch et al. 2004). Because of the small dataset size, however, most differences in performance failed to reach statistical significance. The statistical analysis included ROC analysis within an MRMC framework, but in other aspects, this study had similar drawbacks as the study of Horsch et al. (2006) (no comparison of single-modality versus multimodality CADx, small dataset, and inclusion of lesions of biopsy-proven pathology only).

Note that, as expected for all observer studies, the discussed retrospective ROC studies may not give a completely realistic picture and cannot be directly translated into an expected CADx performance in clinical practice. As mentioned before, however, this type of study is an important step toward conducting more realistic (and more costly) clinical trials.

7.6 FUTURE OF MULTIMODALITY CAD: CLINICAL DECISION SUPPORT SYSTEMS

The development of computer-aided quantification and analysis of breast lesions, with a view to providing clinical decision support systems to optimize radiologist interpretation of breast examinations, is underway (Figure 7.7). These systems will be developed for the interpretation of not only standard mammography, US, and DCE-MRI, but also for advanced MRI acquisitions such as diffusion (Iacconi and Giannelli 2011; Ueguchi et al. 2011), spectroscopy (Belkic and Belkic 2011), T2* (Baltzer et al. 2011), and HiSS images (Fan et al. 2006; Medved et al. 2006, 2009, 2010) of the breast. Extension of these methods to be included in a novel intelligent workstation, with merging results from computer vision analysis and visualization methods (CAVA), is an important clinical goal. Analyses of the breast images to assist the radiologist could be combined with analyses of the clinical image data relative to a standardized database of known cases on a known system and that of the parametric image data. Pilot studies have shown that automated analysis of MRI breast lesions can predict, to a relatively high level of performance, the PM (Chen et al. 2006a,b). New investigations also suggest that for cancerous cases, the estimated prognosis (relative to invasive versus noninvasive, lymph node involvement, and tumor grade) and an estimated probability of response after neoadjuvant chemotherapy can be estimated (Bhooshan et al. 2010).

No manufacturers currently provide a commercially available fully integrated breast workstation for use in the clinical domain. Ideally, such systems will not only integrate mammography, US, and MRI images with CAD but also incorporate all clinical data including patient history, pathology, and a complete BI-RADS reporting system with a single-click user system. The final product would be fully integrated with PACS systems and would assemble data on patient-specific lesions over time as well as provide screening surveys of the whole breast leading to more efficient and accurate detection, diagnosis, and management of breast disease.

The development of advanced multimodality decision support systems is within reach, but as illustrated by the research discussed here, much work remains to be done before these systems can become clinical reality.

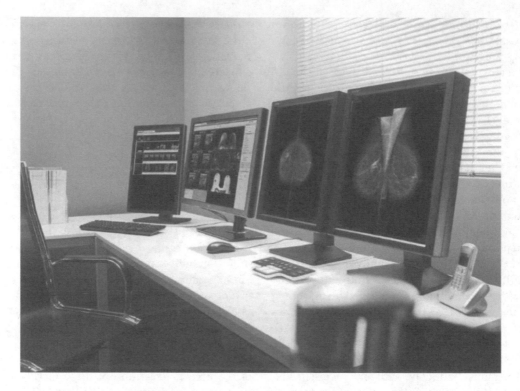

Figure 7.7 The dual-modality CADx. A multimodality clinical decision support system for breast imaging (not yet integrated with CAD). (Courtesy of Philips HealthCare US Division, Andover, MA.)

REFERENCES

Abe, H., R. A. Schmidt, R. N. Shah, A. Shimauchi, K. Kulkarni, C. A. Sennett and G. M. Newstead. 2010. MR-directed ("Second-Look") ultrasound examination for breast lesions detected initially on MRI: MR and sonographic findings, *American Journal of Roentgenology* 194: 370–377.

Ayer, T., M. U. Ayvaci, Z. X. Liu, O. Alagoz and E. S. Burnside. 2010. Computer-aided diagnostic models in breast cancer screening, *Imaging in Medicine* 2: 313–323.

Baltzer, P. A., M. Dietzel and W. A. Kaiser. 2011. Nonmass lesions in magnetic resonance imaging of the breast: Additional t2-weighted images improve diagnostic accuracy, *Journal of Computer Assisted Tomography* 35: 361–366.

Belkic, K. and D. Belkic. 2011. Possibilities for improved early breast cancer detection by Pade-optimized magnetic resonance spectroscopy, *The Israel Medical Association Journal* 13: 236–243.

Berg, W. A., J. D. Blume, J. B. Cormack and E. B. Mendelson. 2006. Operator dependence of physician-performed whole-breast US: Lesion detection and characterization, *Radiology* 239: 355–365.

Berg, W. A., J. D. Blume, J. B. Cormack, E. B. Mendelson, D. Lehrer, M. Bohm-Velez, E. D. Pisano et al., ACRIN 6666 Investigators. 2008. Combined screening with ultrasound and mammography vs mammography alone in women at elevated risk of breast cancer, *The Journal of the American Medical Association* 299: 2151–2163.

Bhooshan, N., M. L. Giger, S. A. Jansen, H. Li, L. Lan and G. M. Newstead. 2010. Cancerous breast lesions on dynamic contrast-enhanced MR images: Computerized characterization for image-based prognostic markers, *Radiology* 254: 680–690.

Boetes, C. 2011. Update on screening breast MRI in high-risk women, *Obstetrics and Gynecology Clinics of North America* 38: 149–158, viii–ix.

Brem, R. F., A. C. Floerke, J. A. Rapelyea, C. Teal, T. Kelly and V. Mathur. 2008. Breast-specific gamma imaging as an adjunct imaging modality for the diagnosis of breast cancer, *Radiology* 247: 651–657.

Burnside, E. S., T. J. Hall, A. M. Sommer, G. K. Hesley, G. A. Sisney, W. E. Svensson, J. P. Fine, J. Jiang and N. J. Hangiandreou. 2007. Differentiating benign from malignant solid breast masses with US strain imaging, *Radiology* 245: 401–410.

Candelaria, R. and B. D. Fornage. 2011. Second-look US examination of MR-detected breast lesions, *Journal of Clinical Ultrasound* 39: 115–121.

Carbognin, G., V. Girardi, C. Calciolari, A. Brandalise, F. Bonetti, A. Russo and R. Pozzi Mucelli. 2010. Utility of second-look ultrasound in the management of incidental enhancing lesions detected by breast MR imaging, *La Radiologia Medica* 115: 1234–1245.

Carney, P. A., D. L. Miglioretti, B. C. Yankaskas, K. Kerlikowske, R. Rosenberg, C. M. Rutter, B. M. Geller et al. 2003. Individual and combined effects of age, breast density, and hormone replacement therapy use on the accuracy of screening mammography, *Annals of Internal Medicine* 138: 168–175.

Chang, J. M., W. K. Moon, N. Cho, J. S. Park and S. J. Kim. 2011a. Breast cancers initially detected by hand-held ultrasound: Detection performance of radiologists using automated breast ultrasound data, *Acta Radiologica (Stockholm, Sweden: 1987)* 52: 8–14.

Chang, J. M., W. K. Moon, N. Cho, J. S. Park and S. J. Kim. 2011b. Radiologists' performance in the detection of benign and malignant masses with 3D automated breast ultrasound (ABUS), *European Journal of Radiology* 78: 99–103.

Chen, W., M. L. Giger and U. Bick. 2006a. A fuzzy c-means (FCM)-based approach for computerized segmentation of breast lesions in dynamic contrast-enhanced MR images, *Academic Radiology* 13: 63–72.

Chen, W., M. L. Giger, U. Bick and G. M. Newstead. 2006b. Automatic identification and classification of characteristic kinetic curves of breast lesions on DCE-MRI, *Medical Physics* 33: 2878–2887.

Corsetti, V., N. Houssami, M. Ghirardi, A. Ferrari, M. Speziani, S. Bellarosa, G. Remida, C. Gasparotti, E. Galligioni and S. Ciatto. 2011. Evidence of the effect of adjunct ultrasound screening in women with mammography-negative dense breasts: Interval breast cancers at 1 year follow-up, *European Journal of Cancer (Oxford, England: 1990)* 47: 1021–1026.

Destounis, S., A. Arieno, P. A. Somerville, P. J. Seifert, P. Murphy, R. Morgan, M. Skolny, S. Hanson and W. Young. 2009. Community-based practice experience of unsuspected breast magnetic resonance imaging abnormalities evaluated with second-look sonography, *Journal of Ultrasound in Medicine: Official Journal of the American Institute of Ultrasound in Medicine* 28: 1337–1346.

Dhar, S. U., H. P. Cooper, T. Wang, B. Parks, S. A. Staggs, S. Hilsenbeck and S. E. Plon. 2011. Significant differences among physician specialties in management recommendations of BRCA1 mutation carriers, *Breast Cancer Research and Treatment* 128: 221–227.

Diekmann, F. 2011. Contrast-enhanced dedicated breast CT, *Radiology* 258: 650 (author reply 650–651).

D'Orsi, C. J., E. B. Mendelson and D. M. Ikeda. 2003. *Breast Imaging Reporting and Data System: ACR BI-RADS—Breast Imaging Atlas*. American College of Radiology, Reston, VA.

Drukker, K., K. Horsch and M. L. Giger. 2005. Multimodality computerized diagnosis of breast lesions using mammography and sonography, *Academic Radiology* 12: 970–979.

Evans, A. J., E. Kutt, C. Record, M. Waller, L. Bobrow and S. Moss. 2007. Radiological and pathological findings of interval cancers in a multi-centre, randomized, controlled trial of mammographic screening in women from age 40–41 years, *Clinical Radiology* 62: 348–352.

Fan, X., H. Abe, M. Medved, S. Foxley, S. Arkani, M. A. Zamora, O. I. Olopade, G. M. Newstead and G. S. Karczmar. 2006. Fat suppression with spectrally selective inversion vs. high spectral and spatial resolution MRI of breast lesions: Qualitative and quantitative comparisons, *Journal of Magnetic Resonance Imaging* 24: 1311–1315.

Feig, S. 2011. Comparison of costs and benefits of breast cancer screening with mammography, ultrasonography, and MRI, *Obstetrics and Gynecology Clinics of North America* 38: 179–196, ix.

Giger, M. L., H. P. Chan and J. Boone. 2008. Anniversary Paper: History and status of CAD and quantitative image analysis: The role of medical physics and AAPM, *Medical Physics* 35: 5799–5820.

Giger, M. L., K. Drukker, L. Lan, R. Tomek, H. Li, N. Bhooshan, G. Newstead, Y. Yuan, A. Jamieson, L. Pesce, J. Bancroft-Brown, K. Horsch, C. Sennett and M. Chinander. 2010. Image-based biomarkers for breast cancer diagnosis, prognosis, and response to therapy. In *Quantitative Imaging Reading Room of the Future, RSNA*.

Giger, M. L., Z. Huo, M. A. Kupinski and C. J. Vyborny. 2000. Computer-aided diagnosis in mammography. In *Handbook of Medical Imaging*, M. Sonka and J. M. Fitzpatrick (eds.). The Society of Photo-Optical Instrumentation Engineers, Bellingham, WA, pp. 915–1004.

Goldsmith, S. J., W. Parsons, M. J. Guiberteau, L. H. Stern, L. Lanzkowsky, J. Weigert, T. F. Heston, E. Jones, J. Buscombe, M. G. Stabin and Society of Nuclear Medicine. 2010. SNM practice guideline for breast scintigraphy with breast-specific gamma-cameras 1.0, *Journal of Nuclear Medicine Technology* 38: 219–224.

Hadjiiski, L., B. Sahiner and H. P. Chan. 2006. Advances in computer-aided diagnosis for breast cancer, *Current Opinion in Obstetrics and Gynecology* 18: 64–70.

Hendrick, R. E. 2010. Radiation doses and cancer risks from breast imaging studies, *Radiology* 257: 246–253.

Hinz, E. K., R. Kudesia, R. Rolston, T. A. Caputo and M. J. Worley Jr. 2011. Physician knowledge of and adherence to the revised breast cancer screening guidelines by the United States Preventive Services Task Force, *American Journal of Obstetrics and Gynecology* 205: 201.e1–e5.

Hong, A. S., J. A. Baker, J. Y. Lo, J. L. Nicholas and M. S. Soo. 2004. Computer-aided classification of breast masses using mammogram, ultrasound, and clinical inputs, *American Journal of Roentgenology* 182: 33.

Horsch, K., M. L. Giger, L. A. Venta and C. J. Vyborny. 2001. Automatic segmentation of breast lesions on ultrasound, *Medical Physics* 28: 1652–1659.

Horsch, K., M. L. Giger, L. A. Venta and C. J. Vyborny. 2002a. Computerized diagnosis of breast lesions on ultrasound, *Medical Physics* 29: 157–164.

Horsch, K., M. L. Giger, C. J. Vyborny, L. Lan, E. B. Mendelson and R. E. Hendrick. 2006. Classification of breast lesions with multimodality computer-aided diagnosis: Observer study results on an independent clinical data set, *Radiology* 240: 357–368.

Horsch, K., M. L. Giger, C. J. Vyborny and L. A. Venta. 2004. Performance of computer-aided diagnosis in the interpretation of lesions on breast sonography, *Academic Radiology* 11: 272–280.

Horsch, K. J., M. L. Giger, Z. Huo, C. J. Vyborny, L. Lan and E. Hendrick. 2002b. Pre-clinical evaluation of multimodality CAD for breast cancer diagnosis, *presented at the annual meeting of the Radiologic Society of North America 2002*.

Houssami, N. and S. Ciatto. 2011. The evolving role of new imaging methods in breast screening, *Preventive Medicine* 53: 123–126.

Huang, S. Y., J. M. Boone, K. Yang, N. J. Packard, S. E. McKenney, N. D. Prionas, K. K. Lindfors and M. J. Yaffe. 2011. The characterization of breast anatomical metrics using dedicated breast CT, *Medical Physics* 38: 2180–2191.

Hutton, J., L. G. Walker, F. J. Gilbert, D. G. Evans, R. Eeles, G. E. Kwan-Lim, D. Thompson, L. J. Pointon, D. M. Sharp, M. O. Leach and UK Study Group for MRI Screening in Women at High Risk Study. 2011. Psychological impact and acceptability of magnetic resonance imaging and x-ray mammography: The MARIBS study, *British Journal of Cancer* 104: 578–586.

Iacconi, C. and M. Giannelli. 2011. Can diffusion-weighted MR imaging be used as a biomarker for predicting response to neoadjuvant chemotherapy in patients with locally advanced breast cancer? *Radiology* 259: 303–304.

Jesneck, J. L., J. Y. Lo and J. A. Baker. 2007. Breast mass lesions: Computer-aided diagnosis models with mammographic and sonographic descriptors, *Radiology* 244: 390–398.

Kalender, W. A., M. Beister, J. M. Boone, D. Kolditz, S. V. Vollmar and M. C. Weigel. 2012. High-resolution spiral CT of the breast at very low dose: Concept and feasibility considerations, *European Radiology* 22: 1–8.

Karellas, A. and S. Vedantham. 2008. Breast cancer imaging: A perspective for the next decade, *Medical Physics* 35: 4878–4897.

Kessler, R., J. B. Sutcliffe, L. Bell, Y. C. Bradley, S. Anderson and K. P. Banks. 2011. Negative predictive value of breast-specific gamma imaging in low suspicion breast lesions: A potential means for reducing benign biopsies, *The Breast Journal* 17: 319–321.

Le-Petross, H. T., G. J. Whitman, D. P. Atchley, Y. Yuan, A. Gutierrez-Barrera, G. N. Hortobagyi, J. K. Litton and B. K. Arun. 2011. Effectiveness of alternating mammography and magnetic resonance imaging for screening women with deleterious BRCA mutations at high risk of breast cancer, *Cancer* 117: 3900–3907.

Levin, E. 2008. Diagnostic applications of breast MRI, *Seminars in Breast Disease* 76–87.

Li, H., M. L. Giger, Z. Huo, O. I. Olopade, L. Lan, B. L. Weber and I. Bonta. 2004. Computerized analysis of mammographic parenchymal patterns for assessing breast cancer risk: Effect of ROI size and location, *Medical Physics* 31: 549–555.

Li, H., M. L. Giger, Y. D. Yuan, W. J. Chen, K. Horsch, L. Lan, A. R. Jamieson, C. A. Sennett and S. A. Jansen. 2008. Evaluation of computer-aided diagnosis on a large clinical full-field digital mammographic dataset, *Academic Radiology* 15: 1437–1445.

Linda, A., C. Zuiani, V. Londero and M. Bazzocchi. 2008. Outcome of initially only magnetic resonance mammography-detected findings with and without correlate at second-look sonography: Distribution according to patient history of breast cancer and lesion size, *Breast (Edinburgh, Scotland)* 17: 51–57.

Luciani, M. L., F. Pediconi, M. Telesca, F. Vasselli, V. Casali, E. Miglio, R. Passariello and C. Catalano. 2011. Incidental enhancing lesions found on preoperative breast MRI: Management and role of second-look ultrasound, *La Radiologia Medica* 116: 886–904.

Madabhushi, A., S. Agner, A. Basavanhally, S. Doyle and G. Lee. 2011. Computer-aided prognosis: Predicting patient and disease outcome via quantitative fusion of multi-scale, multi-modal data, *Computerized Medical Imaging and Graphics: The Official Journal of the Computerized Medical Imaging Society* 35: 506–514.

Medved, M., G. M. Newstead, H. Abe, O. I. Olopade, A. Shimauchi, M. A. Zamora and G. S. Karczmar. 2010. Clinical implementation of a multislice high spectral and spatial resolution-based MRI sequence to achieve unilateral full-breast coverage, *Magnetic Resonance Imaging* 28: 16–21.

Medved, M., G. M. Newstead, H. Abe, M. A. Zamora, O. I. Olopade and G. S. Karczmar. 2006. High spectral and spatial resolution MRI of breast lesions: Preliminary clinical experience, *American Journal of Roentgenology* 186: 30–37.

Medved, M., G. M. Newstead, X. Fan, Y. P. Du, O. I. Olopade, A. Shimauchi, M. A. Zamora and G. S. Karczmar. 2009. Fourier component imaging of water resonance in the human breast provides markers for malignancy, *Physics in Medicine and Biology* 54: 5767–5779.

Meinel, L. A., H. Abe, M. Bergtholdt, J. Ecanow, R. Schmidt and G. Newstead. 2010. Multi-modality morphological correlation of axillary lymph nodes, *International Journal of Computer Assisted Radiology and Surgery* 5: 343–350.

Moadel, R. M. 2011. Breast cancer imaging devices, *Seminars in Nuclear Medicine* 41: 229–241.

Narayanan, D., K. S. Madsen, J. E. Kalinyak and W. A. Berg. 2011. Interpretation of positron emission mammography and MRI by experienced breast imaging radiologists: Performance and observer reproducibility, *American Journal of Roentgenology* 196: 971–981.

Pinker, K., P. Brader, G. Karanikas, K. El-Rabadi, W. Bogner, S. Gruber, M. Reisegger, S. Trattnig and T. H. Helbich. 2010. Functional and molecular imaging of breast tumors, *Der Radiologe* 50: 1030–1038.

Prionas, N. D., K. K. Lindfors, S. Ray, S. Y. Huang, L. A. Beckett, W. L. Monsky and J. M. Boone. 2010. Contrast-enhanced dedicated breast CT: Initial clinical experience, *Radiology* 256: 714–723.

Roe, C. A. and C. E. Metz. 1997. The Dorfman-Berbaum-Metz method for statistical analysis of multi-reader, multi-modality ROC data: Validation by computer simulation, *Academic Radiology* 4: 298–303.

Sahiner, B., H. P. Chan, L. M. Hadjiiski, M. A. Roubidoux, C. Paramagul, J. E. Bailey, A. V. Nees et al. 2009. Multi-modality CADx: ROC study of the effect on radiologists' accuracy in characterizing breast masses on mammograms and 3D ultrasound images, *Academic Radiology* 16: 810–818.

Saslow, D., C. Boetes, W. Burke, S. Harms, M. O. Leach, C. D. Lehman, E. Morris et al., American Cancer Society Breast Cancer Advisory Group. 2007. American Cancer Society guidelines for breast screening with MRI as an adjunct to mammography, *CA: A Cancer Journal for Clinicians* 57: 75–89.

Schlossbauer, T., M. Reiser and K. Hellerhoff. 2010. Importance of mammography, sonography and MRI for surveillance of neoadjuvant chemotherapy for locally advanced breast cancer, *Der Radiologe* 50: 1008–1013.

Sechopoulos, I., S. S. Feng and C. J. D'Orsi. 2010. Dosimetric characterization of a dedicated breast computed tomography clinical prototype, *Medical Physics* 37: 4110–4120.

Shi, J., B. Sahiner, H. P. Chan, C. Paramagul, L. M. Hadjiiski, M. Helvie and T. Chenevert. 2009. Treatment response assessment of breast masses on dynamic contrast-enhanced magnetic resonance scans using fuzzy c-means clustering and level set segmentation, *Medical Physics* 36: 5052–5063.

Sickles, E. A. 2007. Wolfe mammographic parenchymal patterns and breast cancer risk, *American Journal of Roentgenology* 188: 301–303.

Svane, G., E. Azavedo, K. Lindman, M. Urech, J. Nilsson, N. Weber, L. Lindqvist and C. Ullberg. 2011. Clinical experience of photon counting breast tomosynthesis: Comparison with traditional mammography, *Acta Radiologica (Stockholm, Sweden: 1987)* 52: 134–142.

Tabar, L., M. F. Yen, B. Vitak, H. H. Tony Chen, R. A. Smith and S. W. Duffy. 2003. Mammography service screening and mortality in breast cancer patients: 20-year follow-up before and after introduction of screening, *Lancet* 361: 1405–1410.

Taylor, L., S. Basro, J. P. Apffelstaedt and K. Baatjes. 2011. Time for a re-evaluation of mammography in the young? Results of an audit of mammography in women younger than 40 in a resource restricted environment, *Breast Cancer Research and Treatment* 129: 99–106.

Trop, I., M. Labelle, J. David, M. H. Mayrand and L. Lalonde. 2010. Second-look targeted studies after breast magnetic resonance imaging: Practical tips to improve lesion identification, *Current Problems in Diagnostic Radiology* 39: 200–211.

Ueguchi, T., S. Yamada, N. Mihara, Y. Koyama, H. Sumikawa and N. Tomiyama. 2011. Breast diffusion-weighted MRI: Comparison of tetrahedral versus orthogonal diffusion sensitization for detection and localization of mass lesions, *Journal of Magnetic Resonance Imaging: JMRI* 33: 1375–1381.

Wagner, R. F., S. V. Beiden, G. Campbell, C. E. Metz and W. M. Sacks. 2002. Assessment of medical imaging and computer-assist systems: Lessons from recent experience, *Academic Radiology* 9: 1264–1277.

Weigel, M., S. V. Vollmar and W. A. Kalender. 2011. Spectral optimization for dedicated breast CT, *Medical Physics* 38: 114–124.

Weismann, C., C. Mayr, H. Egger and A. Auer. 2011. Breast sonography—2D, 3D, 4D ultrasound or elastography? *Breast Care (Basel, Switzerland)* 6: 98–103.

Wohrle, N. K., K. Hellerhoff, M. Notohamiprodjo, M. F. Reiser and D. A. Clevert. 2010. Automated breast volume scanner (ABVS): A new approach for breast imaging, *Der Radiologe* 50: 973–981.

Youk, J. H., E. K. Kim, M. J. Kim, J. Y. Kwak and E. J. Son. 2011. Performance of hand-held whole-breast ultrasound based on BI-RADS in women with mammographically negative dense breast, *European Radiology* 21: 667–675.

Yuan, Y. 2010. Correlative analysis of breast lesions full-field digital mammography and magnetic resonance imaging, PhD thesis. University of Chicago, Chicago, IL.

Yuan, Y., M. L. Giger, H. Li, N. Bhooshan and C. A. Sennett. 2010. Multimodality computer-aided breast cancer diagnosis with FFDM and DCE-MRI, *Academic Radiology* 17: 1158–1167.

Zanello, P. A., A. F. Robim, T. M. Oliveira, J. Elias Junior, J. M. Andrade, C. R. Monteiro, J. M. Sarmento Filho, H. H. Carrara and V. F. Muglia. 2011. Breast ultrasound diagnostic performance and outcomes for mass lesions using Breast Imaging Reporting and Data System category 0 mammogram, *Clinics (Sao Paulo, Brazil)* 66: 443–448.

Computer-Aided Detection and Diagnosis in Chest and Abdominal Imaging

Chapter 8

Detection of Lung Nodules in Chest Radiography

Bram van Ginneken

CONTENTS

8.1 INTRODUCTION

In 1963, Gwilym S. Lodwick published the first paper on computer-aided diagnosis of pulmonary nodules in chest radiographs (CXRs) (Lodwick et al., 1963). He described a system with over 50 features for a given nodule that described the lesion's location, size, shape, and texture together with global features of the case at hand. These data could be punched in a tabulator card for a machine prediction of the significance of the finding. Lodwick wrote that "The built-in capacity to retain vast numbers of facts, to accept instruction from the physician to compare new facts with its stored information, to report the result of such comparison in the form of statistical probability, and to carry out these functions with great speed and accuracy makes the usefulness

of the computer most obvious." Lodwick was a true pioneer of computer-aided diagnosis and coined the phrase for the first time in 1966 (Lodwick, 1966). The first paper to outline a complete computerized detection scheme was published by Ballard and Sklansky (1976), a result of the PhD work of Dana Ballard, who later published an authoritative textbook on computer vision (Ballard and Brown, 1982). This classic text is now available online (Ballard and Brown, 1982) and features many examples of image processing applied to CXRs.

In the 1980s, several research groups started to work on nodule detection in CXRs. There are several reasons that, taken together, make this a very worthwhile CAD application. First of all, the incidence and mortality rate of lung cancer are high; lung cancer is by far the most deadly cancer worldwide.

Second, chest radiography is the most common radiological exam. Third, it is easy to miss a lung nodule on a CXR. Many studies have shown that a high percentage of missed nodules were visible in retrospect (Muhm et al., 1983; Quekel et al., 1999). Missed lung cancer is, in fact, the second most common cause of malpractice suits addressed at radiologists in the United States. In most of these cases, the alleged error occurred because findings were missed on CXRs (White et al., 1999; Pinto and Brunese, 2010). In 2001, the first product for lung nodule detection in CXRs, Rapidscreen by Deus Technologies, Rockville, MD, received US Food and Drug Administration marketing approval. Currently, several companies have products on the market for this CAD task.

A lung nodule is a round solid lesion with a density close to that of water. The nodule may be in contact with the chest wall or with pulmonary vessels, but it is typically largely surrounded by lung parenchyma that consists of over 80% of radiolucent air. Thus, it shows up white on a radiograph with a darker surrounding. Clinical guidelines (MacMahon et al., 2005) say that a nodule is not actionable if its effective diameter is below 4 or 5 mm. The resolution of CXRs is much smaller, at least 0.25 mm. Then, why is it so hard to see nodules on CXRs? The answer is that CXRs are projection images, and the contrast between the radiodense nodule and its surrounding radiolucent lung parenchyma drowns in the signal of the superimposed structures. This is illustrated in Figure 8.1.

This effect of superimposed structures impeding the view and detectability of nodules has been called *anatomical noise* to emphasize that it is different from radiographic noise, or

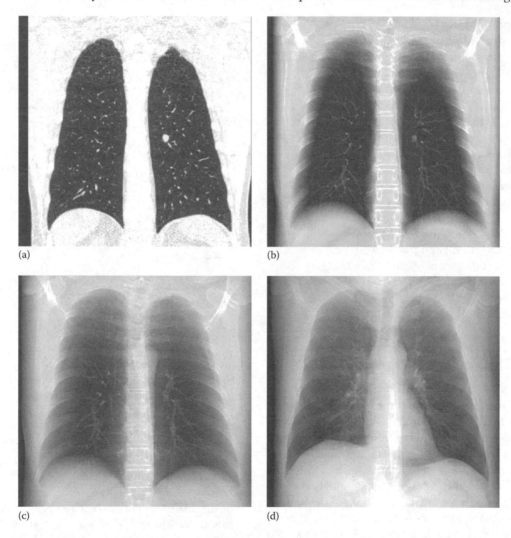

(a)   (b)

(c)   (d)

Figure 8.1 The vanishing nodule. (a) Shows a coronal slice of a CT scan with a nodule in the left lung that is immediately evident. (b) Shows the average of 35 mm of CT sections. The nodule is still clearly visible, surrounded by the shadows of vessels in its vicinity. (c) Shows an average of 70 mm around the nodule. Now it is already difficult to discern the nodule because large pulmonary vessels are nearby. (d) Shows all CT slices averaged, a simulated radiograph. The nodule is now completely obscured by the heart and the pulmonary vessels.

mottle, that is related to the imaging process. Anatomical noise is the main reason why nodules are so hard to detect. Samei et al. (2003) found that "local anatomic variations surrounding and overlying a subtle lung nodule on a chest radiograph that are created by the projection of anatomic features in the thorax, such as ribs and pulmonary vessels, can greatly influence the detection of nodules." A European trial (Håkansson et al., 2005) concluded about the detection of a lung nodule with a size in the order of 10 mm: (1) this is largely dependent on its location in the chest, (2) system noise has a minor impact on the detectability at the dose levels used today, (3) the disturbance of the anatomical noise is larger than that of the system noise but smaller than that of the anatomical background, and (4) the anatomical background acts as noise to a large extent and is the major component affecting the detectability.

To improve nodule detectability, various innovations have been introduced, such as digital image enhancement, dual-energy subtraction, image processing–based subtraction of bony anatomy, temporal subtraction, and contralateral subtraction. These techniques all aim at increasing the conspicuity of a lesion by reducing the impact of anatomic noise. CAD takes a different approach and attempts to explicitly point the reader to suspicious areas in a CXR. If it would have been shown convincingly that the performance of CAD is comparable to that of an expert radiologist, it might be acceptable that computers read the images stand-alone for the presence of nodules. Currently, this is not the case yet (we will discuss the state of the art in Section 8.3), and CAD is aimed to be used as an aid to the reader. The digital techniques listed earlier can be useful for both radiologists and CAD algorithms and will be discussed in Section 8.4.

In addition to research prototypes described in literature, there are currently two FDA-approved systems available on the market (OnGuard; Riverain Medical, Miamisburg, OH and IQQA-Chest, EDDA Technology, Inc., Princeton Junction, NJ). Other commercial systems are Truedia (Mitsubishi Space Software, Tokyo, Japan) (Kakeda et al., 2004) and Syngo CXR CAD (Siemens HealthCare, Malvern, PA).*

We have decided to not discuss research on attempts to differentiate benign and malignant nodules on CXR, akin to the pioneering work of Lodwick et al. (1963) and Lodwick (1966). One reason is that this area has received relatively little attention. More importantly, clinical workup with CT of pulmonary nodules detected with radiography is standard practice nowadays and recommended for diagnosis and for follow-up and growth assessment. Even telling if a nodule is calcified is difficult with plain chest radiography (Berger et al., 2001). This chapter is therefore organized as follows.

We start with a description of the components of a CXR nodule detection system. We do not aim for a complete review of all literature on the topic. For this, the reader is referred to the various papers or other surveys (van Ginneken et al., 2001). Then, we briefly review the state of the art of the field from the perspective of an algorithm developer. For an excellent review of the performance of nodule CAD system from a clinical perspective, we refer the reader to de Boo et al. (2009). Next, we discuss various opportunities for further improving nodule CAD, and we draw conclusions.

8.2 ANATOMY OF A NODULE DETECTION SYSTEM

The pipeline for most nodule detection systems for chest radiography is similar to the general pipeline for CAD systems aimed at focal lesions. The following steps can be distinguished:

- Preprocessing of the CXR
- Segmentation of the unobscured lung fields
- Candidate detection
- Candidate segmentation
- Feature computation and classification

In the remainder of this section, we discuss each step and briefly describe how different authors have addressed each step.

8.2.1 Preprocessing of the Chest Radiograph

Giger et al. (1988) proposed a difference-image technique for the initial preprocessing step. Variants of this technique have been used in other works. The main idea is to produce two images, one in which nodular structures are enhanced and the other in which they are suppressed but other structures are preserved. Subsequently, subtracting the second from the first image yields an image in which only nodule-like structures are visible. Giger et al. (1988) used three spherical filters of 6, 9, and 12 mm diameter and pointed out that this small set of filters would not be ideal for all nodules. For the nodule suppressing image, a large median filter was used. Other authors (Carreira et al., 1998; Keserci and Yoshida, 2002) have used variants of such an approach.

Enhancing nodules and suppressing background structures is a very direct preprocessing technique, immediately targeting the end goal of the CAD pipeline. Other authors have focused more on generic enhancement and equalization. A large number of acquisition techniques exist for radiography, and settings such as the kV of the x-ray beam have a large influence on the appearance of structures in the image. Many manufacturers produce equipment and often

---

* These systems are listed in the Buyer's Guide of Aunt Minnie (http://www.auntminnie.com) under Computer-Aided Detection & Reading.

postprocess the (digital) data with proprietary algorithms (one example of such a technique is described in Dippel et al. (2002)). As a result, a set of CXRs taken from different institutions will show a lot of variation. One could attempt to equalize the images in a preprocessing step.

The approach taken by various authors (Penedo et al., 1998; Schilham et al., 2006; Hardie et al., 2008) is to locally equalize the distribution of pixel values. This can be done by locally (in a sliding window, or in a Gaussian region around each pixel) constructing a histogram or computing the mean and standard deviation and equalizing the histogram or subtracting the mean and dividing by the standard deviation. A myriad of more elaborate variations of such techniques are conceivable, for example, performing such operations in different energy bands. The hope is that after this normalization procedure, images look locally more alike, which is important as subsequent steps will compare data extracted from local regions in training images to local region in test images, and if these images show structural differences, this may decrease the effectiveness of such steps.

8.2.2 Segmentation of the Unobscured Lung Fields

Most CAD algorithms specifically reduce the area of the image in which they will look for nodule candidates by segmenting the unobscured lung fields. A large number of methods have been proposed to do this. Earlier work tended to use rule-based approaches, and recent methods predominantly rely on supervised methods. A good overview of lung segmentation methods can be found in van Ginneken et al. (2001). Comparisons of several methods can be found in van Ginneken and ter Haar Romeny (2000) and more recently in van Ginneken et al. (2006). In the latter study, three widely used supervised methods, namely, active shape models (Cootes et al., 1995), active appearance models (Cootes et al., 2001) and pixel classification, and combinations thereof, are compared on the publicly available JSRT database (Shiraishi et al., 2000). On the SCR website (2014), manual outlines of the lung fields can be downloaded for all images in the JSRT database, and results of many segmentation methods can be compared. Seghers et al. (2007) published a generic 2D segmentation method that is an elegant variation of active shape models and dynamic programming and that has obtained the best results on the SCR data set. This is probably the best lung field segmentation technique to date.

8.2.3 Candidate Detection

With a preprocessed image and the lung fields as search area available, the next step is to find possible nodules. This candidate selection step should have a high sensitivity; anything that is not picked up at this stage will never be detected. Specificity is not so important; in subsequent steps, false positives (FPs) will be reduced.

If the preprocessing step was already squarely aimed at enhancing nodules and suppressing other structures, the procedure to obtain nodule candidates can be a simple thresholding operation. This was the approach taken in Giger et al. (1988), but it was observed that many of the FP candidates had a different size and noncircular shape, especially when the threshold was varied. Therefore, a few tests that involved the size and circularity of the thresholded regions at different threshold steps were added. This approach of adding a few simple rules, inspired by key observations in a small set of training images, is typical for many CAD schemes.

Ballard and Sklansky (1976) used a Hough transform to locate circular bright objects. Schilham et al. (2006) used a multiscale blob detection to find nodule candidates. This is a widely used scale-space technique (Lindeberg, 1998). One employs a blob detector that finds roughly circular structures of a given scale; in this work, the Laplacian was used. Mathematically, it can be shown how to weigh the output of detectors of different scales so that they become comparable. With this weighting formula, one can run the detector at many scales and take the output at the scale of maximum response. Schilham et al. (2006) show that the local normalization preprocessing is necessary to reduce the number of false responses of the blob detector at edge- and ridge-like structures. Hardie et al. (2008) uses a convergence index filter. These filters quantify how many pixels in the neighborhood of a central pixel have a gradient pointing toward that pixel. As nodules are spherical and brighter than their surroundings, there should be many pixels roughly located at the radius distance of the center of the nodule, with an intensity gradient vector pointing toward the center. There exist many variations of such filters. The one employed by Hardie et al. (2008) does not take the magnitude of the gradient into account. This potentially increases robustness as the gradient orientation is largely invariant to monotonic gray-level transformations. Similar techniques have been used in mammography CAD (Karssemeijer, 1999).

The techniques described so far rely on simple rules or sensible geometric reasoning. On the other end of the spectrum, one could treat the problem of which pixels belong to a nodule as a standard supervised classification task. This is the approach taken by Penedo et al. (1998). They slide a window over the lung pixels and enter the pixel values in the window into an artificial neural network trained to fire on nodule pixels. In the second stage, more complex features are used for classification. Using pixel classification for candidate detection is common in CAD, and, for example, also used in mammography, in combination with the earlier-mentioned gradient orientation features (te Brake et al., 2000).

8.2.4 Candidate Segmentation

In some systems, the candidate selection steps yield carefully segmented candidates, but in most cases, only a rough outline of the potential lesion is obtained, and subsequent analysis could benefit from a more precise delineation of the lesion. Note that segmentation of a projected 3D structure is hardly possible and the segmentation does not typically serve a clinical purpose as such; it might at best give a rough indication of the nodule's size and volume. The most important use of candidate segmentation step in a nodule CAD system is in subsequent feature computation.

Many techniques for segmentation have been applied. Schilham et al. (2006) use a ray-shooting technique from the candidate center of mass that tries to identify edges. The resulting segmentation is improved by angular smoothing of the ray lengths. Hardie et al. (2008) employ an adaptive threshold on the preprocessed locally normalized image. The threshold varies with the distance to the nodule center, and morphological processing is applied. Chen et al. (2011) applied a watershed transformation and clustering process. In one of the earliest publications on the topic, Sklansky and Ballard (1973) already used dynamic programming, and this step was also applied in the complete CAD system from Ballard and Sklansky (1976). This technique is widely used in other areas, for example, mammography CAD (Timp and Karssemeijer, 2004).

How important accurate segmentation is for the overall CAD performance likely depends on how sensitive the feature computations in the next stage are to slight variations in the segmentation. For example, some schemes define a narrow band around the segmented border of a candidate lesion and extract statistics from that band. A small displacement of the segmentation border can now greatly affect the feature values. In Schilham et al. (2006), the authors found no improvement when adding a specific segmentation stage to the overall CAD scheme.

8.2.5 Feature Computation and Classification

The goal of the next stage is to characterize the candidates in more detail and use a statistical classifier to estimate how likely it is that the candidate constitutes a real nodule and not an FP such as a rib crossing or a vessel. Every publication uses a different set of features. For most systems, local features, derived from the intensity information in the candidate and its immediate surroundings, are most important. Often, a few of these features have already been computed in the candidate stage. The segmentation can be used to compute features averaged over the region inside or outside the candidate (such as the average intensity and standard deviation) or in a band around the candidate border. The segmentation can also be used

to derive shape features. Spatial features can be added to let a classifier treat nodules at different positions within the lung in a different way. Examples of spatial features are the position within a local coordinate system typically determined by the lung segmentation, such as a bounding box around the lung or a position relative to the center of gravity of the lung, or the distance to the chest wall. One can also employ pixel-based processing of the patch around a nodule candidate to derive features from Penedo et al. (1998) and Suzuki et al. (2005). For a detailed description of all the features, the reader is referred to the individual papers on the topic.

Once the candidates are described by a feature vector, each candidate can be thought of as a point in feature space. This feature space has a dimension that is identical to the number of features. This places the CAD problem squarely within the well-established domain of pattern classification, also known as machine learning. A function needs to be defined that maps each position in the feature space to a likelihood that that position represents a nodule and not an FP. A wide variety of well-established techniques exist (Duda et al., 2001) to produce such a mapping. Ballard and Sklansky (1976) used a nearest neighbor classifier, and so did Schilham et al. (2006), but in this study, feature selection techniques were also investigated. Other studies used decision trees, neural networks, and various linear classifiers. It is quite common to carry out the classification in multiple stages. If the early stages use only features that are simple to compute and simple classifiers and subsequent stages use more complex features and complex classification techniques, a lot of computation time can be saved because for most nodule candidates, the complex features and complex classification procedures do not need to be carried out.

8.3 CURRENT PERFORMANCE OF COMPUTERIZED LUNG NODULE DETECTION

It is extremely difficult to evaluate CAD. The commercial CAD systems for nodule detection in CXRs are meant to be used as a second reader. Therefore, most clinical papers that have investigated the potential of CAD describe the results of observer studies. Here, a set of cases is presented to one or, preferably, more readers, and the readers typically indicate locations of potential nodules and supply a degree of suspiciousness for each location. They do this in a session with and without the help of CAD, and CAD is deemed useful when the readers aided by CAD achieve a higher sensitivity at a fixed level of specificity, or vice versa. There are many potential pitfalls in such studies, and a detailed discussion of those is outside the scope of this chapter. An excellent discussion and an overview through 2009 of observer studies for x-ray nodule CAD can be found in de Boo et al. (2009). Recently, more studies have appeared that show for various commercial CAD systems that they have potential (Moore et al., 2011; Xu et al., 2011) or that they do not have a positive effect on reader performance (de Hoop et al., 2010; de Boo et al., 2011).

From the perspective of a CAD developer, results from observer studies have great limitations. A major drawback is that only one CAD system is tested at a time, and different studies use different data sets and different readers. The studies therefore do not reveal information about the relative performance of various CAD systems. One learns much more if CAD stand-alone performance is measured for different systems on the same database in the same manner. Recently, such studies have been performed for CAD for the first time aimed at nodule detection in computed tomography (CT) scans (van Ginneken et al., 2010) and red lesion detection in retinal images (Niemeijer et al., 2010). Applying multiple CAD systems to the same database also allows one to evaluate the potential of combining CAD systems. This may lead to dramatic increases in performance (Niemeijer et al., 2011).

The JSRT database (Shiraishi et al., 2000) is the only publicly available database with CXRs with and without a proven lung nodule. The database contains 247 posterior–anterior (PA) CXRs. It is an excellent research resource, and the main limitation of the database is that all images are analog. They were digitized to 12 bits, scanned at a resolution of 2048 × 2048 pixels. The database contains 93 normal cases and 154 x-ray images with a proven lung nodule (100 malignant ones). Normal cases were confirmed to be normal by follow-up or CT. All nodules were proven by CT. Diameters and positions of all nodules are provided for. The nodule diameters range from 5 to 60 mm (median = 15 mm); they are located throughout the lungs (also behind the heart and under the diaphragm) and are subdivided in five groups from obvious to very subtle. Shiraishi et al. (2000) provide receiver operating characteristic (ROC) curves of 30 radiologists on the JSRT database and averaged curves per subtlety category.

In several studies, the JSRT database has been used for training and evaluation. However, the exact process used for evaluation is different from study to study, and this makes it hard to compare the results. For example, several studies have excluded cases where nodules were located behind the heart or the diaphragm. Moreover, when constructing statistics of a CAD experiment, it is necessary to define when a CAD marker *hits* a lesion. Lenient hit rules can boost CAD performance substantially. Li et al. (2010) reported that when using a lenient rule compared to a more strict but entirely reasonable hit rule, sensitivity for a commercial nodule detection algorithm applied to a data set of 34 radiologist-missed cancers went up by 24%. It is therefore essential for a meaningful comparison that not only the same data, but also the same evaluation procedure is used for all systems.

That said, the results reported in the literature on the JSRT database do give an indication of the state of the art of academic and commercial nodule detection algorithms. At 2.0 and 4.0 FPs per image, Schilham et al. (2006) reported 51% and 67% sensitivity, respectively; at these operating points, Hardie et al. (2008) reported 57% and 71% sensitivity. Other papers reported sensitivity at higher FP rates, for example, 60% at 4.3 FPs per image. Recently, Samulski (2011) published the FROC curve of OnGuard 5.0 (Riverain Medical, Miamisburg, OH) on the JSRT database. This software achieved a sensitivity of 76% at only 1.0 FP per image. This indicates that this commercial system performs well ahead of academic systems. Meziane et al. (2012) provided data of four versions of this commercial system on the same database and reported a significant reduction in the average number of FPs per image for each version with comparable or slightly better sensitivity.

Data from de Hoop et al. (2010), however, indicate that expert radiologists perform still substantially better than CAD stand-alone. In this observer study, 46 individuals with 49 CT-detected and histologically proven lung cancers and 65 patients without nodules at CT were included. The CAD (OnGuard 5.0; Riverain Medical, Miamisburg, OH) stand-alone sensitivity was 61% (30 of 49), with on average 2.4 FP annotations per image. Sensitivity of two radiologists was similar at 63% (the same for both readers), however, with 0.25 and 0.22 FP marking per image. This indicates that there is still quite a gap to bridge between humans and CAD. In this study also, no benefit was found for humans when using CAD because the researchers conclude, "observers were unable to sufficiently differentiate true-positive from false-positive CAD marks."

8.4   HOW TO IMPROVE

In this section, we discuss a number of ways to further improve on CAD performance. Some of these suggestions have already been researched quite extensively; others have hardly received attention.

8.4.1   False-Positive Reduction

The most obvious way to improve an existing CAD system is to inspect the most common errors that are made and to try to design better features, tailored at avoiding these mistakes, or additional classification layers in the CAD pipeline. For example, Meziane et al. (2012) determined that the most common causes for FPs with four versions of a commercial CAD system were vessels and rib crossings. Only in the last version, which had less FPs, also fibrosis became an important category. This indicates that dedicated algorithms or features aimed at detecting vessels, posterior and anterior ribs, and fibrotic lesions have a potential to improve nodule CAD.

In most cases, nodule CAD systems can be improved directly by training them with far more examples. Many systems have been trained with the JSRT database. This was an excellent resource and a highly laudable initiative, but the JSRT database is film based and has a relative small number of nodule cases. A new large publicly available database of digital CXRs with proven nodules could provide an enormous impetus to the field. The LIDC database for chest CT scans (Armato et al., 2004) that has recently been extended is a great example of such a resource for chest CT nodule detection.

8.4.2 What about the Lateral?

Lateral views of the chest are commonly obtained together with frontal views (also called posterior–anterior or PA views) in many medical centers and clinical institutions. Although it is rare for radiologists to detect a nodule only from the lateral film (Quekel et al., 1999), it seems reasonable to use a lateral view when available in a CAD scheme. In mammography, where multiple views are typically available, many CAD schemes take advantage of more than one views, explicitly linking findings (van Engeland and Karssemeijer, 2007; Velikova et al., 2009; Wei et al., 2009). The only study on chest radiography was published by Shiraishi et al. (2007) where a CAD system for nodule detection on lateral CXRs was presented. The frontal image was also analyzed with a CAD system, and the authors showed that some nodules were detected only on the lateral film. No explicit linking of findings was attempted. The authors stated that they "believe that the lateral view would not be the primary one for the detection of lung nodules on chest radiographs. Instead, we should use the CAD scheme for lateral views as a supporting tool in addition to the results obtained with the CAD scheme for PA views."

8.4.3 Where to Look?

Most nodule CAD systems analyze only on the unobscured lung fields in standard PA. This area can be defined as those parts of a CXR that contain lungs not obscured by either diaphragm, mediastinum, or heart. An alternative would be to consider the total project area, that is, any pixel of the image for which the radiation has passed through the lungs. However, this total projected area is difficult to determine from a CXR because of the density of the overlying diaphragm, heart, and mediastinum. It was estimated (Chotas and Ravin, 1994) that on average, 26% of the lung volume and 43% of the total projected area are obscured by one of these structures.

Figure 8.2 gives an impression how much projected lung field is missed if only the unobscured lung fields are taken into account. van Ginneken et al. (2008) describe a method to automatically estimate this information from a single PA CXR or from the combination of a PA and a lateral image (in the latter case, the estimation is more accurate). It should be possible to determine with reasonable accuracy and extended zone around the unobscured lung fields where lung, and thus nodules, could be located. Radiologists are more likely to miss nodules that are obscured by the heart or mediastinum or are located below the diaphragm, so CAD support for these regions could be of extra value. I am not aware of any study that has specifically analyzed the effect of CAD for the detection of nodules in those areas.

8.4.4 Suppression of Overlying Normal Anatomy

Three techniques to remove normal anatomy are discussed.

8.4.4.1 Bone Suppression

It is well known that a high kilovoltage can be used in chest radiography to make the bony structures more transparent. With the advent digital radiography, dual-energy imaging became a practical possibility. There are two main techniques for producing dual-energy images. The topic and the effect of dual-energy imaging on detectability of lesions in CXRs have been reviewed in MacMahon et al. (2008). Dual-energy imaging results in a bone image and a soft tissue image. Some centers routinely apply dual-energy imaging, and those users believe that this does not noticeably increase interpretation time, though it does reduce interpretation errors (MacMahon et al., 2008). The vast majority of imaging centers, however, does not. Li et al. (2008) have shown in a reader study with six radiologists that the average area under the ROC curve for nodule detection improved when soft tissue images obtained from dual-energy imaging were provided in addition to the standard frontal view.

If only a regular radiograph is available, one could attempt to simulate a soft tissue image using a software algorithm. Several groups have worked on this topic (Loog et al., 2006; Suzuki et al., 2006; Hogeweg et al., 2010), and recently, commercial software to produce soft tissue images has become available. Figure 8.3 shows an example of how SoftView (Riverain Medical, Miamisburg, OH) can enhance the appearance of a subtle nodule. In a large reader study, Freedman et al. (2011) recently showed that the use of SoftView images increased radiologists' detection rate of lung cancers and benign nodules at a fixed, albeit rather low specificity (this is to be expected as the more conspicuous nodules can be detected equally well without rib suppression).

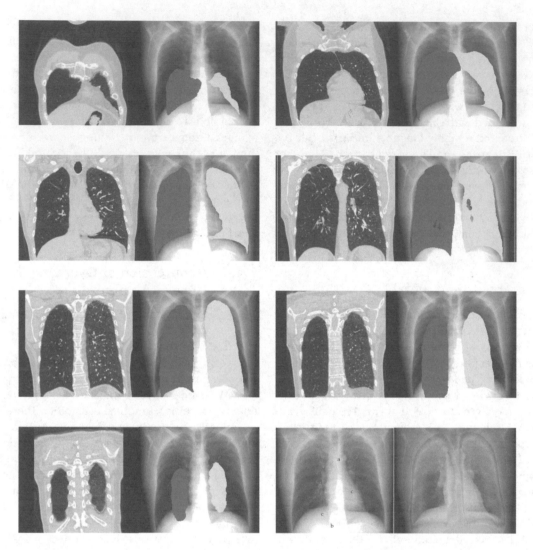

Figure 8.2   (See color insert.) Where are the lungs? Seven equally spaced coronal slices are shown with the lungs superimposed on the radiograph simulated from the CT data. It is evident that the unobscured lung fields do not account for all of the lung volume. In the bottom-right image, a color-coding is shown indicating how much lung is behind each pixel in the projection image. In the bottom right figure, the areas indicated with labels a, b, c, d correspond approximately to the depth of 3 cm, 5 cm, 10 cm, and 20 cm, respectively.

If the application of an image processing algorithm to remove rib shadows and other bony structures can help human experts in the detection of nodules, it is reasonable to assume that CAD systems could also benefit from such techniques. They could be applied as preprocessing steps, and (additional) features could be extracted from the bony structure suppressed images. Interestingly, Balkman et al. (2010) showed that the direct application of a commercial nodule detection CAD program (OnGuard 3.0, Riverain Medical, Miamisburg, OH) to soft tissue images obtained with dual-energy imaging improved performance compared to applying the same CAD system, unaltered, with identical settings to the corresponding standard PA images.

Figure 8.3 shows an example of a rib suppressed image produced by the commercial SoftView algorithm. A subtle nodule is more clearly visible in the processed image. Figure 8.4 shows the effect of suppressing five ribs using the technique described in Hogeweg et al. (2010). This algorithm works by considering profiles perpendicular to a rib border and constructing a statistical model from these profiles using principal component analysis. This model is fitted to the input profiles and subtracted. As a result, only the structures that only occasionally disturb the profiles, such as vessel crossing the rib, are preserved. Hogeweg et al. (2010) demonstrated that this suppression technique improved the performance of a CAD system to detect subtle interstitial abnormalities, but it was not applied to computerized nodule detection.

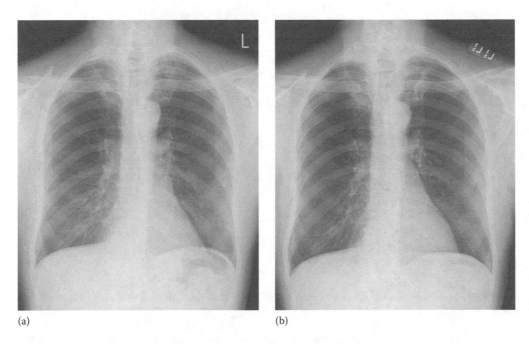

(a)   (b)

Figure 8.3 A chest radiograph (a) with a subtle nodule in the right lung that is enhanced on the SoftView (Riverain Medical, Miamisburg, OH) image (b).

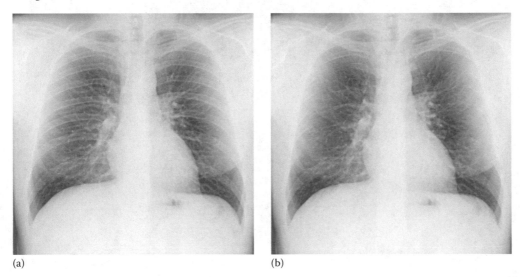

(a)   (b)

Figure 8.4 A chest radiograph (a) in which the central parts of the fifth through ninth rib have been removed (b) with the algorithm from Hogeweg et al. (2010).

8.4.4.2 Temporal Subtraction

Computerized detection of lung nodules in CXRs has generally been studied only for a single radiograph. In clinical practice, when a chest radiography exam of a patent has to be reported on, there is very frequently a previous exam of the same patient available. In this case, the radiologist is concerned with the comparison of a prior image with a current image. The task is therefore not only to detect nodules, but also to detect any interval change. Temporal subtraction has been developed as an aid to facilitate interval change detection.

The prior radiograph is warped so as to match the current image and subtracted from it. Increased and decreased areas of density now show up as black-and-white regions in a grayish image. The warping is a very difficult problem because of the projection that is inherent to radiography; in general, the pulmonary vasculature moves in a different way compared to the bony structures, and it is not possible to warp all these structures with a single deformation field. A practical solution is to apply the previously discussed bone suppression techniques in the context of temporal subtraction to improve

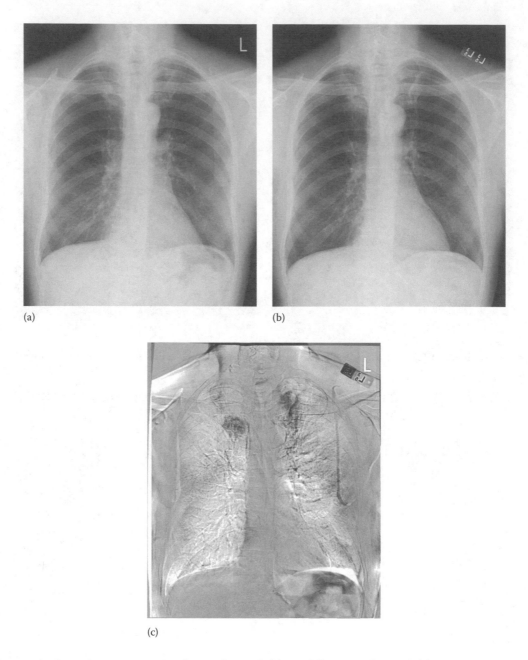

(a)   (b)

(c)

Figure 8.5   Temporal subtraction warps a prior chest radiograph (a) to a follow-up radiograph (b). By subtracting the warped prior from the follow-up case (c), subtle changes can become visible. The two dark areas are new densities that were confirmed by CT. (Case courtesy of Samuel Armato, University of Chicago, Chicago, IL.)

the subtraction results. A review of temporal subtraction is given in MacMahon et al. (2008). An example of the effect of temporal subtraction is given in Figure 8.5.

A temporal subtraction technique was evaluated by Kakeda et al. (2002) where the use of temporal subtraction images improved observer performance for nodule detection for both radiologist and residents. Johkoh et al. (2002) describes an observer study with commercially available software for temporal subtraction (Truedia/XR; Mitsubishi Space Software, Amagasaki, Japan). In this study, only

residents benefited from the use of temporal subtraction. Uozumi et al. (2001) showed that access to a prior radiograph improved radiologists' nodule detection substantially, but showing the two images sequentially was equivalent to providing a temporal subtraction image.

These studies were carried out a decade ago, and temporal subtraction imaging has not gained ground in clinical practice. It is, however, possible that CAD could benefit more from analyzing temporal subtraction images. This research area is still largely not investigated.

A particular interesting new approach is to use images from different patients for subtraction. Aoki et al. (2011) presented a method in which a computer algorithm searched a database of 15,000 normal CXRs, using correlation values between patches in the lung fields, to select a *similar patient* to the one at hand and produce a subtraction image, in a way similar to temporal subtraction. They showed that the subtraction images helped radiologists, especially less experienced readers, in nodule detection. Including true temporal subtraction or subtraction of similar images in a nodule CAD system is in principle rather straightforward; additional features could be computed from the subtraction images.

8.4.4.3 Contralateral Subtraction

One important observation that is nicely illustrated by eye tracking experiments is that radiologists tend to compare the same area in the (a) and (c) lung fields to look for subtle difference that may indicate the presence of subtle lesions. Contralateral subtraction has been investigated as a visualization technique to improve the visibility of lesions on CXRs. The technique is comparable to temporal subtraction, but now, the contralateral lung field is flipped and used for warping and subtraction (Li et al., 2000a,b). The obvious advantage of contralateral subtraction over temporal subtraction is that a prior radiograph of the same patient is not needed. Tsukuda et al. (2002) demonstrated an improvement in the nodule detection performance of radiologist when they had access to a contralateral subtraction image in addition to the PA radiograph alone.

Contextual features derived from contralateral regions have been used to improve mammography CAD (Hupse and Karssemeijer, 2009; Wei et al., 2011). The only study where contralateral subtraction was used to improve lung nodule detection was published by Yoshida (2004). He applied a registration technique based on wavelets to obtain, given a nodule candidate, a corresponding position in the contralateral lung field. The warped contralateral patch was subtracted from the image patch around the nodule candidate, and it was shown that adding features derived from this subtraction image improved candidate classification performance.

8.4.5 Image Enhancement and Equalization

The appearance of CXRs depends on the acquisition parameters, the imaging equipment, and the application of proprietary postprocessing techniques. Several vendors include such processing, which involves sharpening and manipulation of the dense areas in the image to improve visibility of fine structures in these regions. In an interesting study, He et al. (2008) showed that such processing can affect CAD substantially. They applied a commercial CAD system (IQQA-Chest, EDDA Technology, Inc., Princeton Junction, NJ) to

116 radiographs. Three types of multiscale processing (Unique Image Processing Package, Philips Medical Systems) were applied: a standard setting using the default processing parameters of the package and two settings in which high- and low-frequency structures were emphasized. This package is widely used in practice and based on standard multiscale image processing techniques (Stahl et al., 2000; Dippel et al., 2002). Many hospitals store only processed radiographs, and the chosen settings vary between institutions. In the study, CAD performance in terms of area under the ROC curve was 0.70 for the standard images, 0.59 for the high-pass images, and 0.78 for the low-pass images.

This result indicates that it may be crucially important for CAD developers to equalize the images in a preprocessing step to make sure that differences in image characteristics do not affect CAD output. The local normalization processing applied in some CAD systems (Schilham et al., 2006; Hardie et al., 2008) is a step in this direction, but it is plausible that better equalization and preprocessing will lead to further improved CAD.

8.4.6 Learning from Simulations

Even a very large training database will not have examples of all types of nodules located throughout the lung fields, with all possible signs of overprojection. Normal radiographs, on the other hand, are easy to come by, and this raises the question if it would be beneficial to simulate nodules and use these for the training of CAD systems. Simulated lesions have been widely used in observer studies (Samei et al., 1999). Samei et al. (1997) used spherical templates for simulating nodules. Recently, Litjens et al. (2010) have simulated nodules using segmented findings from CT as templates. These CT templates can be scaled and rotated and added at any position in any CXR. The authors show that human observers cannot differentiate between real and simulated lesions. We await studies in which the effect of the addition of simulated training cases on the performance of CAD nodule detection schemes is investigated.

8.4.7 Interactive CAD

Current commercially available CAD systems have been developed to display markers on CXRs on regions that could contain a lung nodule. The rationale for this approach is that these prompts can help to prevent oversight. Several studies have shown that the majority of errors in the detection of nodules are related to *interpretation* of findings and not to incomplete search patterns. In a landmark study from 1975, Kundel and Nodine (1975) showed that most nodules are already detected by radiologists after flashing an image for 0.2 s. Manning et al.

(2004) measured fixations of radiologists while reading radiographs and found that nearly 70% of the missed lesions (i.e., lesions that the radiologist did not report on, not even with a low confidence rating) held a gaze duration of greater than 1 s. This indicates that the interpretation of a detected region (is it a nodule or not?) is difficult, and the actual detection (did I see and consider a region at all?) is less of a problem.

This indicates that clinical application of CAD might better focus on aiding the radiologist in the interpretation of suspect regions. Samulski et al. (2011) performed a study that did exactly that. They compared unaided reading, reading with conventional CAD, CAD stand-alone, and interactive use of CAD, in a study with six nonradiologist readers, the JSRT database (Shiraishi et al., 2000), and the OnGuard 5.0 CAD system (Riverain Medical, Miamisburg, OH). In conventional CAD, prompts were shown around regions deemed suspicious by the software. In the interactive CAD mode, users clicked on suspect regions and obtained a numeric CAD score in the range from 0 to 1. CAD stand-alone performance, computed as mean localization fraction in the FP fraction range from 0 to 1, was 0.391, which was higher than the average of the readers (0.352) unaided. With the conventional CAD, reader performance increased to 0.428. Interactive CAD, however, increased their performance to 0.495.

Although this is a preliminary result, obtained with nonradiologist readers, it indicates that alternative ways of presenting the computer output to readers, which may also include combinations of CAD and processing techniques such as bone suppression and temporal subtraction, are a worthwhile novel direction of research.

8.5 CONCLUDING REMARKS

Nodule detection in chest radiography was the earliest and initially also the most important CAD application. In the last two decades, mammography has become the most important CAD application area, and chest radiography has attracted less attention. In the last decade, only a handful serious papers that describe new nodule detection systems have been published. On the other hand, several commercial systems have been developed the last 5 years, and as far as these can be deduced from a few studies, these systems have been improved substantially but still do not reach the performance of a human expert.

The strong growth in chest CT imaging might be one explanation for the relative lack of interest for nodule detection in radiography. Still, plain chest radiography is by far the most common radiological exam, and despite the increasing numbers of chest CT exams obtained, the number of chest radiography exams is not decreasing (Bhargavan, 2008). Detection of suspicious nodules therefore remains a common task for any radiologist, even if the primary diagnostic question is not cancer related. One could even argue that it is now more important than ever to develop excellent CAD algorithms for this task because low-dose CT is available as a relatively cheap and efficient follow-up test for suspicious findings on chest radiography and because, as some say (Robinson, 1998), the level of expertise of younger radiologists for reading radiographs is decreasing.

There are many possibilities for further improving nodule CAD. This chapter has provided a number of suggestions. Some of these have been studied already or are part of proprietary commercial systems, but many have not been explored in detail yet. The most important open task for the research community would be to construct a large publicly available database of digital radiographs with proven nodules, coupled to a challenge website with an evaluation data set, following the concept of the grand challenges for medical image analysis (Grand-Challenges, 2014) that have been successfully applied to other CAD tasks already. The availability of a large high-quality database would lower the threshold for outsiders to enter this field. Many machine learning researchers are interested in medical applications, but lack access to the data needed to compete with research laboratories and industry that work closely with radiologists. If this is implemented, it is likely that in the coming decade, the performance of computerized detection of nodules in CXRs will greatly improve.

REFERENCES

Aoki, T., N. Oda, Y. Yamashita, K. Yamamoto, and Y. Korogi. Usefulness of computerized method for lung nodule detection on digital chest radiographs using similar subtraction images from different patients. *European Journal of Radiology*, 81:1062–1067, 2011.

Armato, S. G., G. McLennan, M. F. McNitt-Gray, C. R. Meyer, D. Yankelevitz, D. R. Aberle, C. I. Henschke et al. Lung image database consortium: Developing a resource for the medical imaging research community. *Radiology*, 232:739–748, 2004.

Balkman, J. D., S. Mehandru, E. DuPont, R. D. Novak, and R. C. Gilkeson. Dual energy subtraction digital radiography improves performance of a next generation computer-aided detection program. *Journal of Thoracic Imaging*, 25:41–47, 2010.

Ballard, D. H. and C. M. Brown. *Computer Vision*. Prentice-Hall, Englewood Cliffs, NY, 1982.

Ballard, D. H. and J. Sklansky. A ladder-structured decision tree for recognizing tumors in chest radiographs. *IEEE Transactions on Computers*, 20:503–513, 1976.

Berger, W. G., W. K. Erly, E. A. Krupinski, J. R. Standen, and R. G. Stern. The solitary pulmonary nodule on chest radiography: Can we really tell if the nodule is calcified? *American Journal of Roentgenology*, 176:201–204, 2001.

Bhargavan, M. Trends in the utilization of medical procedures that use ionizing radiation. *Health Physics Society*, 95:612–627, 2008.

Carreira, M. J., D. Cabello, M. G. Penedo, and A. Mosquera. Computer-aided diagnoses: Automatic detection of lung nodules. *Medical Physics*, 25:1998–2006, 1998.

Chen, S., K. Suzuki, and H. MacMahon. Development and evaluation of a computer-aided diagnostic scheme for lung nodule detection in chest radiographs by means of two-stage nodule enhancement with support vector classification. *Medical Physics*, 38:1844–1858, 2011.

Chotas, H. G. and C. E. Ravin. Chest radiography: Estimated lung volume and projected area obscured by the heart, mediastinum, and diaphragm. *Radiology*, 193:403–404, 1994.

Cootes, T. F., G. J. Edwards, and C. J. Taylor. Active appearance models. *IEEE Transactions on Pattern Analysis and Machine Intelligence*, 23:681–685, 2001.

Cootes, T. F., C. J. Taylor, D. Cooper, and J. Graham. Active shape models—Their training and application. *Computer Vision and Image Understanding*, 61:38–59, 1995.

de Boo, D. W., M. Prokop, M. Uffmann, B. van Ginneken, and C. M. Schaefer-Prokop. Computer-aided detection (CAD) of lung nodules and small tumours on chest radiographs. *European Journal of Radiology*, 72:218–225, 2009.

de Boo, D. W., M. Uffmann, M. Weber, S. Bipat, E. F. Boorsma, M. J. Scheerder, N. J. Freling, and C. M. Schaefer-Prokop. Computer-aided detection of small pulmonary nodules in chest radiographs an observer study. *Academic Radiology*, 18:1507–1514, 2011.

de Hoop, B., D. W. de Boo, H. A. Gietema, F. van Hoorn, B. Mearadji, L. Schijf, B. van Ginneken, M. Prokop, and C. Schaefer-Prokop. Computer-aided detection of lung cancer on chest radiographs: Effect on observer performance. *Radiology*, 257:532–540, 2010.

Dippel, S., M. Stahl, R. Wiemker, and T. Blaffert. Multiscale contrast enhancement for radiographies: Laplacian pyramid versus fast wavelet transform. *IEEE Transactions on Medical Imaging*, 21:343–353, 2002.

Duda, R. O., P. E. Hart, and D. G. Stork. *Pattern Classification*, 2nd edn. John Wiley and Sons, New York, 2001.

Freedman, M. T., S.-C. Benedict Lo, J. C. Seibel, and C. M. Bromley. Lung nodules: Improved detection with software that suppresses the rib and clavicle on chest radiographs. *Radiology*, 260:265–273, 2011.

Giger, M. L., K. Doi, and H. MacMahon. Image feature analysis and computer-aided diagnosis in digital radiography: Automated detection of nodules in peripheral lung fields. *Medical Physics*, 15:158–166, 1988.

Grand-Challenges. Grand challenges in biomedical image analysis. http://www.grand-challenge.org/ (accessed November 24, 2014).

Håkansson, M., M. Båth, S. Börjesson, S. Kheddache, A. Grahn, M. Ruschin, A. Tingberg, S. Mattsson, and L. G. Månsson. Nodule detection in digital chest radiography: Summary of the RADIUS chest trial. *Radiation Protection Dosimetry*, 114:114–120, 2005.

Hardie, R. C., S. K. Rogers, T. Wilson, and A. Rogers. Performance analysis of a new computer aided detection system for identifying lung nodules on chest radiographs. *Medical Image Analysis*, 12:240–258, 2008.

He, Q., W. He, K. Wang, and D. Ma. Effect of multiscale processing in digital chest radiography on automated detection of lung nodule with a computer assistance system. *Journal of Digital Imaging*, 21:S164–S170, 2008.

Hogeweg, L., C. Mol, P. A. de Jong, and B. van Ginneken. Rib suppression in chest radiographs to improve classification of textural abnormalities. In *Medical Imaging. Proceedings of the SPIE*, 7624:76240Y1–76240y6, 2010.

Hupse, R. and N. Karssemeijer. Use of normal tissue context in computer-aided detection of masses in mammograms. *IEEE Transactions on Medical Imaging*, 28:2033–2041, 2009.

Johkoh, T., T. Kozuka, N. Tomiyama, S. Hamada, O. Honda, N. Mihara, M. Koyama et al. Temporal subtraction for detection of solitary pulmonary nodules on chest radiographs: Evaluation of a commercially available computer-aided diagnosis system. *Radiology*, 223:806–811, 2002.

Kakeda, S., J. Moriya, H. Sato, T. Aoki, H. Watanabe, H. Nakata, N. Oda, S. Katsuragawa, K. Yamamoto, and K. Doi. Improved detection of lung nodules on chest radiographs using a commercial computer-aided diagnosis system. *American Journal of Roentgenology*, 182:505–510, 2004.

Kakeda, S., K. Nakamura, K. Kamada, H. Watanabe, H. Nakata, S. Katsuragawa, and K. Doi. Improved detection of lung nodules by using a temporal subtraction technique. *Radiology*, 224:145–151, 2002.

Karssemeijer, N. Local orientation distribution as a function of spatial scale for detection of masses in mammograms. In *Information Processing in Medical Imaging. Lecture Notes in Computer Science*, 1613:280–293, 1999.

Keserci, B. and H. Yoshida. Computerized detection of pulmonary nodules in chest radiographs based on morphological features and wavelet snake model. *Medical Image Analysis*, 6:431–447, 2002.

Kundel, H. L. and C. F. Nodine. Interpreting chest radiographs without visual search. *Radiology*, 116:527–532, 1975.

Li, F., R. Engelmann, K. Doi, and H. MacMahon. Improved detection of small lung cancers with dual-energy subtraction chest radiography. *American Journal of Roentgenology*, 190:886–891, 2008.

Li, F., R. Engelmann, K. Doi, and H. Macmahon. True detection versus "accidental" detection of small lung cancer by a computer-aided detection (CAD) program on chest radiographs. *Journal of Digital Imaging*, 23:66–72, 2010.

Li, Q., S. Katsuragawa, and K. Doi. Improved contralateral subtraction images by use of elastic matching technique. *Medical Physics*, 27:1934–1942, 2000a.

Li, Q., S. Katsuragawa, T. Ishida, H. Yoshida, S. Tsukuda, H. MacMahon, and K. Doi. Contralateral subtraction: A novel technique for detection of asymmetric abnormalities on digital chest radiographs. *Medical Physics*, 27:47–55, 2000b.

Lindeberg, T. Feature detection with automatic scale selection. *International Journal of Computer Vision*, 30:79–116, 1998.

Litjens, G. J. S., L. Hogeweg, A. M. R. Schilham, P. A. de Jong, M. A. Viergever, and B. van Ginneken. Simulation of nodules and diffuse infiltrates in chest radiographs using CT templates. In *Medical Image Computing and Computer-Assisted Intervention. Lecture Notes in Computer Science*, 6362:396–403, 2010.

Lodwick, G. S. Computer-aided diagnosis in radiology: A research plan. *Investigative Radiology*, 1:72–80, 1966.

Lodwick, G. S., T. E. Keats, and J. P. Dorst. The coding of Roentgen images for computer analysis as applied to lung cancer. *Radiology*, 81:185–200, 1963.

Loog, M., B. van Ginneken, and A. M. R. Schilham. Filter learning: Application to suppression of bony structures from chest radiographs. *Medical Image Analysis*, 10:826–840, 2006.

MacMahon, H., J. H. M. Austin, G. Gamsu, C. J. Herold, J. R. Jett, D. P. Naidich, E. F. Patz, S. J. Swensen, and the Fleischner Society. Guidelines for management of small pulmonary nodules detected on CT scans: A statement from the Fleischner Society. *Radiology*, 237:395–400, 2005.

MacMahon, H., F. Li, R. Engelmann, R. Roberts, and S. Armato. Dual energy subtraction and temporal subtraction chest radiography. *Journal of Thoracic Imaging*, 23:77–85, 2008.

Manning, D. J., S. C. Ethell, and T. Donovan. Detection or decision errors? Missed lung cancer from the posteroanterior chest radiograph. *British Journal of Radiology*, 77:231–235, 2004.

Meziane, M., P. Mazzone, E. Novak, M. L. Lieber, O. Lababede, M. Phillips, and N. A. Obuchowski. A comparison of four versions of a computer-aided detection system for pulmonary nodules on chest radiographs. *Journal of Thoracic Imaging*, 27:58–64, 2012.

Moore, W., J. Ripton-Snyder, G. Wu, and C. Hendler. Sensitivity and specificity of a CAD solution for lung nodule detection on chest radiograph with CTA correlation. *Journal of Digital Imaging*, 24:405–410, 2011.

Muhm, J. R., W. E. Miller, R. S. Fontana, D. R. Sanderson, and M. A. Uhlenhopp. Lung cancer detected during a screening program using four-month chest radiographs. *Radiology*, 148:609–615, 1983.

Niemeijer, M., M. Loog, M. D. Abràmoff, M. A. Viergever, M. Prokop, and B. van Ginneken. On combining computer-aided detection systems. *IEEE Transactions on Medical Imaging*, 30:215–223, 2011.

Niemeijer, M., B. van Ginneken, M. J. Cree, A. Mizutani, G. Quellec, C. I. Sánchez, B. Zhang et al. Retinopathy online challenge: Automatic detection of microaneurysms in digital color fundus photographs. *IEEE Transactions on Medical Imaging*, 29:185–195, 2010.

Penedo, M. G., M. J. Carreira, A. Mosquera, and D. Cabello. Computer-aided diagnosis: A neural-network-based approach to lung nodule detection. *IEEE Transactions on Medical Imaging*, 17:872–880, 1998.

Pinto, A. and L. Brunese. Spectrum of diagnostic errors in radiology. *World Journal of Radiology*, 2:377–383, 2010.

Quekel, L. G., A. G. Kessels, R. Goei, and J. M. van Engelshoven. Miss rate of lung cancer on the chest radiograph in clinical practice. *Chest*, 115:720–724, 1999.

Robinson, A. E. The lateral chest radiograph: Is it doomed to extinction? *Academic Radiology*, 5:322–323, 1998.

Samei, E., M. J. Flynn, and W. R. Eyler. Simulation of subtle lung nodules in projection chest radiography. *Radiology*, 202:117–124, 1997.

Samei, E., M. J. Flynn, and W. R. Eyler. Detection of subtle lung nodules: Relative influence of quantum and anatomic noise on chest radiographs. *Radiology*, 213:727–734, 1999.

Samei, E., M. J. Flynn, E. Peterson, and W. R. Eyler. Subtle lung nodules: Influence of local anatomic variations on detection. *Radiology*, 228:76–84, 2003.

Samulski, M. Computer aided detection as a decision aid in medical screening, PhD thesis, Radboud University, 2011.

Samulski, M. R. M., P. R. Snoeren, B. Platel, B. van Ginneken, L. Hogeweg, C. Schaefer-Prokop, and N. Karssemeijer. Computer-aided detection as a decision assistant in chest radiography. In *Medical Imaging. Proceedings of the SPIE*, 7966:796614-1-796614-6, 2011.

Schilham, A. M. R., B. van Ginneken, and M. Loog. A computer-aided diagnosis system for detection of lung nodules in chest radiographs with an evaluation on a public database. *Medical Image Analysis*, 10:247–258, 2006.

SCR Database. Segmentation in chest radiographs. Image Sciences Institute, Utrecht, the Netherlands. http://www.isi.uu.nl/Research/Databases/SCR/ (accessed November 24, 2014).

Seghers, D., D. Loeckx, F. Maes, D. Vandermeulen, and P. Suetens. Minimal shape and intensity cost path segmentation. *IEEE Transactions on Medical Imaging*, 26:1115–1129, 2007.

Shiraishi, J., S. Katsuragawa, J. Ikezoe, T. Matsumoto, T. Kobayashi, K. Komatsu, M. Matsui, H. Fujita, Y. Kodera, and K. Doi. Development of a digital image database for chest radiographs with and without a lung nodule: Receiver operating characteristic analysis of radiologists' detection of pulmonary nodules. *American Journal of Roentgenology*, 174:71–74, 2000.

Shiraishi, J., F. Li, and K. Doi. Computer-aided diagnosis for improved detection of lung nodules by use of posterior-anterior and lateral chest radiographs. *Academic Radiology*, 14:28–37, 2007.

Sklansky, J. and D. Ballard. Tumor detection in radiographs. *Computers and Biomedical Research*, 6:299–321, 1973.

Stahl, M., T. Aach, and S. Dippel. Digital radiography enhancement by nonlinear multiscale processing. *Medical Physics*, 27:56–65, 2000.

Suzuki, K., H. Abe, H. MacMahon, and K. Doi. Image-processing technique for suppressing ribs in chest radiographs by means of massive training artificial neural network (MTANN). *IEEE Transactions on Medical Imaging*, 25:406–416, 2006.

Suzuki, K., J. Shiraishi, H. Abe, H. MacMahon, and K. Doi. False-positive reduction in computer-aided diagnostic scheme for detecting nodules in chest radiographs by means of massive training artificial neural network. *Academic Radiology*, 12:191–201, 2005 (PMID: 15721596).

te Brake, G. M., N. Karssemeijer, and J. H. Hendriks. An automatic method to discriminate malignant masses from normal tissue in digital mammograms. *Physics in Medicine and Biology*, 45:2843–2857, 2000.

Timp, S. and N. Karssemeijer. A new 2D segmentation method based on dynamic programming applied to computer aided detection in mammography. *Medical Physics*, 31:958–971, 2004.

Tsukuda, S., A. Heshiki, S. Katsuragawa, Q. Li, H. MacMahon, and K. Doi. Detection of lung nodules on digital chest radiographs: Potential usefulness of a new contralateral subtraction technique. *Radiology*, 223:199–203, 2002.

Uozumi, T., K. Nakamura, H. Watanabe, H. Nakata, S. Katsuragawa, and K. Doi. ROC analysis of detection of metastatic pulmonary nodules on digital chest radiographs with temporal subtraction. *Academic Radiology*, 8:871–878, 2001.

van Engeland, S. and N. Karssemeijer. Combining two mammographic projections in a computer aided mass detection method. *Medical Physics*, 34:898–905, 2007.

van Ginneken, B., S. G. Armato, B. de Hoop, S. van de Vorst, T. Duindam, M. Niemeijer, K. Murphy et al. Comparing and combining algorithms for computer-aided detection of pulmonary nodules in computed tomography scans: The ANODE09 study. *Medical Image Analysis*, 14:707–722, 2010.

van Ginneken, B., B. de Hoop, and M. Prokop. Automatic estimation of three-dimensional lung volume from posterior-anterior and lateral chest radiographs. In *Annual Meeting of the Radiological Society of North America*, Chicago, IL, 2008, p. 313.

van Ginneken, B., M. B. Stegmann, and M. Loog. Segmentation of anatomical structures in chest radiographs using supervised methods: A comparative study on a public database. *Medical Image Analysis*, 10:19–40, 2006.

van Ginneken, B. and B. M. ter Haar Romeny. Automatic segmentation of lung fields in chest radiographs. *Medical Physics*, 27:2445–2455, 2000.

van Ginneken, B., B. M. ter Haar Romeny, and M. A. Viergever. Computer-aided diagnosis in chest radiography: A survey. *IEEE Transactions on Medical Imaging*, 20:1228–1241, 2001.

Velikova, M., M. Samulski, P. J. F. Lucas, and N. Karssemeijer. Improved mammographic CAD performance using multiview information: A Bayesian network framework. *Physics in Medicine and Biology*, 54:1131–1147, 2009.

Wei, J., H.-P. Chan, B. Sahiner, C. Zhou, L. M. Hadjiiski, M. A. Roubidoux, and M. A. Helvie. Computer-aided detection of breast masses on mammograms: Dual system approach with two-view analysis. *Medical Physics*, 36:4451–4460, 2009.

Wei, J., H.-P. Chan, C. Zhou, Y. Wu, B. Sahiner, L. M. Hadjiiski, M. A. Roubidoux, and M. A. Helvie. Computer-aided detection of breast masses: Four-view strategy for screening mammography. *Medical Physics*, 38:1867–1876, 2011.

White, C. S., A. I. Salis, and C. A. Meyer. Missed lung cancer on chest radiography and computed tomography: Imaging and medicolegal issues. *Journal of Thoracic Imaging*, 14:63–68, 1999.

Xu, Y., D. Ma, and W. He. Assessing the use of digital radiography and a real-time interactive pulmonary nodule analysis system for large population lung cancer screening. *European Journal of Radiology*, 81:e451-e456, 2011.

Yoshida, H. Local contralateral subtraction based on bilateral symmetry of lung for reduction of false positives in computerized detection of pulmonary nodules. *IEEE Transactions on Biomedical Engineering*, 51:778–789, 2004.

Chapter 9

Detection and Diagnosis of Lung Nodules in Thoracic CT

Qiang Li

CONTENTS

9.1 INTRODUCTION

Lung cancer is the leading cause of cancer-related deaths in the United States; it kills more people than colon cancer, breast cancer, prostate cancer, and pancreatic cancer combined (Jemal et al. 2010). Evidence suggests that early detection of lung cancer may allow for timely therapeutic intervention and thus a favorable prognosis for patients (Flehinger et al. 1992). Patients with clinical stage I lung cancer who underwent surgical resection within 1 month after diagnosis had an estimated 10-year survival rate of 92% (Henschke et al. 2006). Therefore, in the 1970s, screening programs for early detection of lung cancer were carried out with chest radiography and cytologic examination of sputum in the United States (Flehinger et al. 1984; Fontana et al. 1984; Frost et al. 1984) as well as in Europe (Kubik and Polak 1986). As the computed tomography (CT) imaging techniques have advanced, screening with low-dose CT has been performed in the United States (Henschke et al. 1999) and Japan (Sone et al. 1998) since early 1990. The National Lung Screening Trial investigators report that subjects undergoing three annual screening examinations with low-dose CT had a 20% reduction in lung cancer mortality as compared with those screened with annual chest radiography (Aberle et al. 2011).

In a screening program with CT, radiologists must read a large number of images, and they are likely to overlook some lung cancers because of either detection error (failure to detect a cancer) or interpretation error (failure to correctly diagnose a detected cancer) (Li et al. 2002). In such a circumstance, a computer-aided diagnostic (CAD) scheme for detection (also known as CADe) and for diagnosis (CADx) of lung nodules would be particularly useful for the reduction in detection errors and interpretation errors, respectively, because a computerized scheme may detect many cancers missed by radiologists and help radiologists make accurate diagnosis for lung cancer (Armato et al. 2002).

CAD schemes have been developed by many investigators for nodule detection in chest radiography (Lo et al. 1995; Xu et al. 1997; Li et al. 2001; Kakeda et al. 2004; Shiraishi et al. 2006). The typical performance of current detection schemes in chest radiography is a 70% sensitivity with three to five false positives per image. Similarly, CAD schemes for nodule detection in thick-section (≥5 mm slice thickness) CT images have been developed by many investigators (Giger et al. 1994; Armato et al. 1999; Brown et al. 2001; Ko et al. 2001; Lee et al. 2001; Schilham et al. 2006). The typical performance of current CAD schemes in thick-section CT is an 80%–90% sensitivity with one to two false positives per section, which translates into dozens of false positives per CT scan.

In a thin-section CT scan, the section thickness is small, typically less than 2.5 mm. A thin-section CT scan includes hundreds of sections and requires radiologists to put considerable time and effort in image interpretation, which stimulates the development of CAD schemes for the detection and characterization of lung cancer. Since 2000, many investigators have attempted to develop CAD schemes for lung nodule in thin-section CT, which represents one of the newest directions of CAD development in thoracic imaging and is the topic of this review chapter. Reviews on CAD schemes for nodule detection and diagnosis can be found in Reeves and Kostis (2000), Li et al. (2005), Sluimer et al. (2006), Li (2007), and Marten and Engelke (2007).

This chapter reviews only publications concerning CAD schemes for lung nodules in thin-section CT that were published in academic journals and could be searched by use of PubMed (http://www.ncbi.nlm.nih.gov/pubmed). Some other chapters in this book review related topics, including CAD schemes for lung nodules in chest radiography (Chapter 8), measurement of nodule size (Chapter 10), and public lung image database (Chapter 11). PubMed was used to obtain relevant publications with the keywords "computer AND (detection OR diagnosis) AND lung AND nodule," and all relevant publications were manually selected from a total of 577 hits, as of July 1, 2011.

9.2 COMPUTERIZED DETECTION OF LUNG NODULE IN CT

A CADe scheme for nodule detection in CT can be broadly divided into two major components, that is, an image processing component and a feature analysis component. The image processing component generally includes lung segmentation, nodule enhancement, initial nodule identification, and nodule segmentation steps. The inputs to these steps are some forms of images. The purpose of this component is to quickly localize suspicious regions in CT images with a high-detection sensitivity for true nodules and, as a result, with a large number of false positives. The feature analysis component generally consists of feature extraction/selection and object classification steps. The inputs to these steps are some forms of feature lists instead of images. The purpose of the second component is to remove as many false positives as possible while maintaining a high detection sensitivity for nodules by analyzing the features of initial nodule candidates. The following sections describe each of these steps.

9.2.1 Lung Segmentation in CT

Since lung nodules are present only inside the lungs, the segmentation of lungs generally represents the first step in a CADe scheme for nodule detection. Nearly all CADe schemes in CT utilized some forms of thresholding technique to separate lungs from other nonlung structures. Thanks to the large contrast between the lungs and adjacent nonlung structures in CT, a fixed threshold was employed to segment the lungs in most CADe schemes (Paik et al. 2004; Li et al. 2008; Pu et al. 2008; Retico et al. 2008; Golosio et al. 2009; Messay et al. 2010). The fixed threshold was typically empirically determined between −400 and −700 Hounsfield Unit (HU) with the value of −500 HU being the most often selected threshold. The threshold for segmenting the lungs could also be adaptively determined by analyzing the profiles or the histogram of CT image data (Armato et al. 2001; Hu et al. 2001; Zhao et al. 2003; Bae et al. 2005). In addition, other more advanced (and complex) methods were employed to segment the lungs, including fuzzy thresholding (Ye et al. 2009), three-dimensional (3D) region growing (Bellotti et al. 2007), k-means clustering (Ge et al. 2005), and genetic cellular neural networks (Ozekes et al. 2008). Simple thresholding with a fixed threshold, combined with some postprocessing techniques, is typically adequate for the segmentation of lungs in a vast majority of thoracic CT scans without gross lung abnormalities. When gross lung abnormalities such as interstitial diffuse lung diseases do exist, most of the lung segmentation methods aforementioned would not work well; more sophisticated algorithms employing

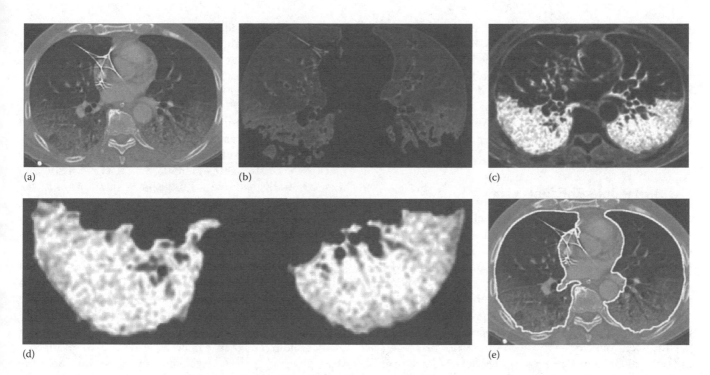

Figure 9.1 (a) Original CT image of lungs with severe interstitial lung disease, (b) initial estimate of the lungs using CT value only, (c) texture feature image, (d) the identified lung regions with severe interstitial lung disease, and (e) the final lung segmentation result obtained by combining the initial estimate (b) and the lung regions with severe disease (d), followed by a postprocessing to fill the holes in the segmented lung regions.

texture information (Sluimer et al. 2005; Wang et al. 2009; Korfiatis et al. 2010) should be able to provide far better lung segmentation results than do the methods aforementioned. Figure 9.1 shows the lung segmentation result with severe interstitial lung disease by use of CT values and texture information together (Wang et al. 2009). The CT value is useful for the segmentation of normal or mildly abnormal lung areas and the texture information for severely abnormal lung areas.

In some slices, the two lungs are attached to each other and should be separated. Armato and Sensakovic (2004) first identified the most anterior point along the cardiac aspect of the lung segmentation region and then searched the anterior junction line from a series of rays (lines) emitting from the most anterior point. Finally, the pixels on the anterior junction line were turned off to force separation of the merged lung region into two distinct regions. Leader et al. (2003) and Messay et al. (2010) first located the narrowest region of the merged lung region in the anterior–posterior direction. A 40-pixel wide window in the medial–lateral (right–left) direction was centered at the narrowest region. The pixels in the window were scanned medial-laterally, and the largest pixel value in each line was identified as the pixel on the junction line. A regression line was fit to the identified pixels and used as the junction line to separate the left and right lungs.

A juxtapleural nodule, which is contiguous with the chest wall, is often excluded from the lungs segmented with the aforementioned lung segmentation methods. In such a case, lung border revision is a key step for lung nodule detection in CT and has significant impact on the performance of CADe schemes. Armato et al. (2001), Bae et al. (2005), Golosio et al. (2009), and Messay et al. (2010) employed morphologic operators such as a rolling ball algorithm to correct such error and to include juxtapleural nodules inside the segmented lungs. Bellotti et al. (2007), Li et al. (2008), and Ye et al. (2009) extracted the lung border first, analyzed the lung border to identify deeply concave portion that represents a missing juxtapleural nodule, and filled the concave portion to include the missing lung nodule. Pu et al. (2008) smoothed the lung boundary using the Jarvis March algorithm that computes the convex hull locally, rather than globally, for identifying the juxtapleural nodules. Armato and Sensakovic (2004) emphasized the importance of lung border revision by showing that, for automated lung nodule detection, 14 of 82 actual nodules (17.1%) were incorrectly excluded from the segmented lung regions prior to the application of lung border revision, whereas only 4 of 82 actual nodules (4.9%) were excluded when the core segmentation method was followed by the lung border revision.

Because of the large contrast between the lung parenchyma and nearby soft tissue, lung segmentation is a relatively straightforward task and, therefore, is typically performed on a 2D slice-by-slice basis. However, Retico et al. (2008) segmented lungs directly in the 3D image space with a fixed threshold. The inclusion of juxtapleural nodules was performed by a 3D morphologic closing operator. Golosio et al. (2009) employed a 3D lung segmentation method that is similar to that of Retico et al. (2008); the major difference is the use of isosurface triangulation for representing all segmented regions including lungs.

9.2.2 Nodule Enhancement

In most CADe schemes, the initial nodule identification technique was applied directly to the original CT images, whereas in some schemes, a nodule enhancement filter was first employed as a preprocessing step prior to the application of the initial identification technique. The application of an effective nodule enhancement filter as a preprocessing step would be advantageous for initial identification of nodules, particularly for nodules with low-contrast ground-glass opacity or those connected to blood vessels. Li et al. (2003b) developed a selective dot-enhancement filter based on Hessian matrix diagonalization for simultaneous enhancement of nodules and suppression of normal anatomic structures such as blood vessels and airway walls, which were the main sources of false positives for nodule detection in CT. Retico et al. (2008) and Ye et al. (2009) also employed this selective dot-enhancement filter for nodule enhancement and initial nodule identification. Figure 9.2 shows a maximum intensity projection (MIP) of an original thin-section CT image with a nodule indicated by an arrow, and an MIP of a nodule-enhanced image by use of the selective dot-enhancement filter. It is apparent that the

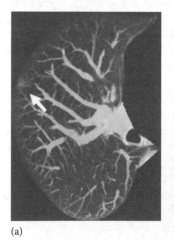 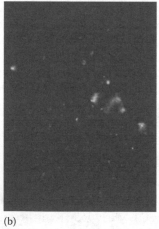

(a)   (b)

Figure 9.2 Maximum intensity projection of a 3D CT original image with a nodule, indicated by an arrow (a), and a nodule-enhanced image (b), in which the nodule was enhanced, and blood vessels were suppressed substantially.

nodule was enhanced significantly and blood vessels were suppressed remarkably in the enhanced image. Therefore, it would be much easier to detect the nodule in the enhanced image than in the original image.

Murphy et al. (2009) and Ye et al. (2009) utilized the volumetric shape-index filter to enhance lung nodules. The filter calculates the shape-index value for each voxel, and different shape-index values represent voxels on five object shapes: 0.0 for cup, 0.25 for rut, 0.5 for saddle, 0.75 for ridge, and 1.0 for cap. The *cap* indicates a nodule-like spherical shape, and the *ridge* indicates a vessel-like shape. In addition to the shape index, Murphy et al. (2009) utilized the curvedness and Ye et al. (2009) employed the dot-enhancement filter developed by Li et al. (2003b) to further improve the performance of initial nodule identification.

Paik et al. (2004) also developed a nodule enhancement filter for initial nodule detection based on the surface normal overlap. The output of their filter for each voxel is a score proportional to the number of surface normals that pass through a neighborhood of the voxel. The filter can enhance nodules because nodules tend to have certain convex regions on their surface, and thus the inward pointing surface normal vectors tend to intersect or nearly intersect within the tissue. Although blood vessels also have convex surfaces, they have a dominant curvature along a single direction, as opposed to high curvatures in two directions as is common on the surface of nodules. Therefore, the score for blood vessels is generally lower than that for nodules. Paik et al. (2004) compared the surface normal overlap with the Hough transform for nodule enhancement, and they found that the surface normal overlap was more robust than the Hough transform for the enhancement of actual nodules that deviated from ideal models of nodule shape.

Bae et al. (2005) developed a CADe scheme for the detection of nodules in three categories: isolated, juxtapleural, and juxtavascular nodules. They employed a morphologic matching filter to enhance nodules only for juxtavascular nodules. The morphologic filters were spherical in shape, with four different kernel sizes (3, 6, 9, and 12 mm in diameter) for identifying nodule candidates ranging from 3 to 30 mm. The morphologic filters were convolved with the 3D image of the vessel group by use of the fast Fourier transform method. Because the morphologic matching filters were isotropic in three dimensions, they would also enhance blood vessels to some extent. Nodule enhancement was not used for the initial identification of isolated and juxtapleural nodules.

9.2.3 Initial Nodule Identification

Thresholding, followed by connected component analysis, is the most common technique for initial nodule identification in thin-section CT, whether or not the nodule enhancement is employed as a preprocessing step. In this technique, the nodule enhancement plays a key role to achieve a high performance level. Paik et al. (2004) reported a sensitivity of 100% with 165 false positives per CT scan by finding the local maxima in the surface normal overlap-enhanced images; Li et al. (2008) identified 98.7% of nodules (151 of 153) with 140 false positives per CT scan by thresholding the selectively enhanced images with a dot-enhancement filter; Retico et al. (2008) identified as the initial nodule candidates the local maxima in the dot-enhanced image and detected 97.3% internal nodules and 96.3% sub-pleural nodules with 170 false positives per scan; and Ye et al. (2009) achieved a sensitivity of 100% with 41 false positives per CT scan by using nodule-enhanced images. All these methods of using nodule-enhanced images achieved very high performance levels. Please note that Ye et al. (2009) employed both shape-index-based enhancement filter and dot-enhancement filter developed by Li et al. (2003b) to achieve a very high performance level.

In spite of the advantages of nodule enhancement, most CADe schemes to date did not employ nodule enhancement as a preprocessing step, and they attempted to identify initial nodule candidates directly from the original CT images by use of either a single (Bae et al. 2005; Marten et al. 2005; Pu et al. 2008) or a multiple thresholding technique (Brown et al. 2003; Zhao et al. 2003; Ozekes et al. 2008; Golosio et al. 2009; Messay et al. 2010). Some researchers further integrated the thresholding method with other techniques such as distance transform (Pu et al. 2008) for initial nodule identification. Because blood vessels have very high CT values in a CT scan, the thresholding techniques without the nodule enhancement would identify many blood vessels as *nodule* candidates and thus report a large number of false positives. Zhao et al. (2003) identified initial nodule candidates by thresholding the original CT images, and they reported a sensitivity of 94.4% with 906 false positives per CT scan; Bellotti et al. (2007) reported 88.5% of detected nodules with 2775 false positives per scan; Pu et al. (2008) identified 95.1% of nodules with 1200 false positives per scan; Golosio et al. (2009) detected 93% nodules with 522 false positives per scan; and Messay et al. (2010) reported a sensitivity of 97.5% with 450–600 false positives per scan. All these methods reported hundreds, or even thousands, of false positives per CT scan caused primarily by blood vessels.

Instead of thresholding, Ge et al. (2005) and Schilham et al. (2006) identified initial nodule candidates by use of a weighted k-means clustering segmentation with two output clusters, that is, a nodule cluster and a background cluster. They first calculated image features for each pixel from both the original image and a median-filtered image, and they used the image features to classify pixels into the nodule and background clusters. The criterion for classifying a pixel was the ratio of two distances, which measured how far the feature vector of the pixel was to the nodule cluster center and to the background cluster center. If the ratio was larger than a threshold, then the pixel was assigned to the nodule cluster; otherwise, it was assigned to the background cluster.

For initial nodule identification, investigators should address two important issues in their studies. The first is the definition of a criterion for determining whether a true nodule is correctly identified. Paik et al. (2004) considered a nodule candidate reported by their CADe as a detected true nodule if the distance between the center of the nodule candidate and the center of a *true* nodule (ground truth) was smaller than half of the diameter of the *true* nodule. Li et al. (2008) adopted a similar criterion based on the distance between the true nodule and the reported nodule candidate. Messay et al. (2010) considered a nodule candidate, a detected true nodule, if the segmented region of the nodule candidate included the center of the true nodule. Alternatively, if the center of a nodule candidate was located inside the reference outline delineated by radiologists, the nodule candidate can be regarded as a detected true nodule (Messay et al. 2010). No single criterion is universally reliable than the others. For example, using the distance criteria in Paik et al. (2004) and Li et al. (2008), a nodule candidate can be incorrectly judged as a detected true nodule even if there is no common pixels in the detected candidate region and the reference nodule region. On the other hand, with the criteria in Messay et al. (2010), any irrelevant but very large region that includes the center of the true nodule is considered as a detected true nodule. Therefore, in addition to the automated criteria for judging if a nodule is detected, visual confirmation by a radiologist or experienced physicist is highly recommended (Li et al. 2008).

The second issue is the explicit reporting of the performance level for initial nodule identification because it is an important step of the entire CADe system. Although some papers did not report the performance for initial nodule identification, more and more researchers in recent years have done this performance reporting (Zhao et al. 2003; Paik et al. 2004; Bellotti et al. 2007; Li et al. 2008; Pu et al. 2008; Retico et al. 2008; Golosio et al. 2009; Murphy et al. 2009; Ye et al. 2009; Messay et al. 2010).

9.2.4 Nodule Segmentation

Lung nodule segmentation is a crucial and challenging step in a CADe scheme because of the variability in nodule shape, pattern, and connection of the nodules to blood vessels and pleural surfaces. In many CADe schemes for lung nodule detection, the nodule segmentation is an implicit component included in initial nodule identification step; that is, the initial nodule identification and nodule segmentation are performed simultaneously. Therefore, as in the initial nodule identification, most CADe schemes segment nodule candidates by use of a single threshold technique (Bae et al. 2005; Marten et al. 2005; Pu et al. 2008), a multiple thresholding technique (Brown et al. 2003; Zhao et al. 2003; Ozekes et al. 2008; Golosio et al. 2009; Messay et al. 2010), or clustering technique (Ge et al. 2005; Schilham et al. 2006; Murphy et al. 2009).

However, an additional segmentation step is sometimes necessary for accurate nodule segmentation in some CADe schemes, particularly in those employing a nodule enhancement filter, because the segmented/identified nodule candidates in the nodule-enhanced image appear different from those in the original CT images. Li et al. (2008) developed a 3D constrained region-growing technique to segment each nodule candidate accurately in the original CT images. First, the 3D region of each initial nodule candidate segmented from the nodule-enhanced image was used as a seed region for the constrained region growing in the original CT images. They then calculated the mean and standard deviation of CT values for voxels inside the seed region. Next, they added some adjacent voxels to the seed region if the CT values of these adjacent voxels were within a range defined by the mean CT value of the seed region ±2 standard deviations. To prevent nodule regions from leaking into nearby structures such as blood vessels, the earlier region-growing process was constrained to five repetitions.

Pu et al. (2008) employed a progressive clustering operation to grow regions from seed points identified in the initial nodule identification. The progressive clustering is in principle similar to a region-growing algorithm as employed in Li et al. (2008), although it used a different *stop operation* rule. A unique feature of the progressive clustering operation is that it used not only the CT values in the original CT image, but also the distance transform information in the distance transformed image. Because of this unique feature, the progressive clustering operation generates a 3D volume in a manner that is similar to the skeletonization of an object. For example, the progressive clustering operation should generate a sphere-like shape for a nodule, a string-like shape for a blood vessel, and a plane-like shape for a fissure.

Ye et al. (2009) utilized a mixed statistical model for accurate segmentation of the initial nodule candidates. This method assumed that the ranges of image intensities could be modeled as Gaussian distributions and that the spatial constraints between adjacent voxels could be modeled by a Markov random field model. It then used an expectation–maximization algorithm to iteratively estimate the posterior probabilities that a given voxel belongs to the nodule class and the nonnodule class. For a voxel, if the posterior probability for the nodule class was greater than that for the nonnodule class, the voxel was considered as a nodule voxel; otherwise, it was considered as a nonnodule voxel.

Way et al. (2009) segmented the nodule candidate from its surrounding structured background in a local volume of interest (VOI) by use of a 3D active contour model. The 3D active contour model is based on the 2D one originally developed by Kass et al. (1987). The original active contour model includes two types of energies, that is, the internal energies and external energies. The internal energies impose constraints on the smoothness of contour itself, while the external energies push the contour toward salient image features such as strong edges. Way et al. (2009) added to the original energies three new energy components to take advantage of 3D information: (1) 3D gradient, which guides the active contour to seek the object surface; (2) 3D curvature, which imposes a smoothness constraint in the z direction; and (3) mask energy, which penalizes contours that grow beyond the pleura or thoracic wall. The search for the best energy weights in the 3D active contour model was guided by a simplex optimization method.

It is logical to segment nodules directly in 3D image space, as most nodule segmentation methods did. However, the nodule segmentation in 3D image space is typically complex and may be time consuming. Wang et al. (2007) developed a quasi-3D method to simplify nodule segmentation in 3D thin-section CT. First, a VOI was determined at the location of a nodule. The 3D VOI was transformed into a 2D image by use of a *spiral scanning* technique, in which a radial line originating from the center of the VOI spirally scanned the VOI from the *north pole* to the *south pole*. The voxels scanned by the radial line were arranged line by line to form a transformed 2D image. Because the surface of a nodule in the 3D image became a curve in the transformed 2D image, the spiral-scanning technique considerably simplified the segmentation method and enabled them to obtain reliable segmentation results. A dynamic programming technique was employed to delineate the *optimal* outline of a nodule in the 2D transformed image. The optimal outline in the 2D transformed image was then transformed back into 3D image space to provide the surface of the nodule. Figure 9.3 illustrates this nodule segmentation method for a nodule, in which (a) shows the slices of a VOI with the nodule at the center, (b) the transformed 2D image of the VOI, (c) the delineated optimal outline in the transformed 2D image, and (d) the reconstructed nodule volume in the 3D VOI.

The evaluation of nodule segmentation methods is a key issue in CADe scheme for nodule detection. There are at least two levels of evaluation for the nodule segmentations. The first (lower) level is the evaluation of the nodule segmentation method itself by looking at its accuracy measured with some metrics, such as the volume overlap ratio (also known as the Jaccard index), volume agreement, mean absolute distance, and maximum absolute distance between the automatically segmented nodules and the reference nodules (Wang et al. 2009). This level of evaluation is important for

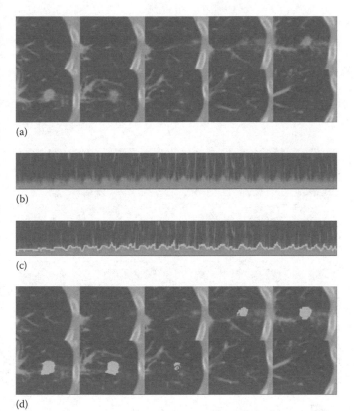

(a)

(b)

(c)

(d)

Figure 9.3 (See [c] and [d] in color insert.) Illustration of Wang's method for the segmentation of a nodule with an irregular shape in the LIDC data set: (a) the slices of a VOI with a nodule; (b) the transformed 2D image of the VOI; (c) the delineated optimal outline in the transformed 2D image; and (d) the reconstructed nodule volume in the 3D VOI.

assessing the volume and growth rate of the nodules. The second level of evaluation for the nodule segmentation is to assess how the accuracy of the nodule segmentation impacts the overall performance of the CADe scheme for nodule detection. This level of evaluation is particularly important for the CADe scheme development because a *more accurate* nodule segmentation method does not necessarily translate into a *better* nodule detection scheme. The second level of evaluation for the nodule segmentation in CT is extremely rare, if not none.

To date, some researchers have evaluated their nodule segmentation methods in the first level by use of the public Lung Image Database Consortium (LIDC) (Armato et al. 2004, 2007). Wang et al. (2007) employed 23 and 86 LIDC CT scans, respectively, to train and test their nodule segmentation method based on spiral scanning and dynamic programming. For the two data sets, six and four radiologists manually delineated the outlines of the nodules as reference standards for the evaluation of the nodule segmentation. The mean overlap ratios were 66% and 64% for the nodules in the training and test LIDC data

sets, respectively. Using the same LIDC, the reported mean overlap ratios were approximately 58% for the 3D active contour model (Way et al. 2009) and 63% for the multithresholding method developed by Messay et al. (2010).

9.2.5 Feature Extraction and Selection

As stated earlier, after initial nodule identification, there are generally hundreds or thousands of nodule candidates in each CT scan. Most of them are false positives and should be removed in the feature analysis and classification step. Features are some measurements made from the segmented regions to represent prominent and salient characteristics of the nodule candidates. For example, a nodule is generally spherical, and a blood vessel is a long linear structure; therefore, one can distinguish between the true nodules and blood vessels by use of a shape feature called sphericity. In addition, using features, instead of the large number of voxels inside the nodule region, enables one to markedly reduce the dimensionalities and thus the complexity of object classification task.

The most widely used features for a nodule candidate are probably the size feature (e.g., the effective diameter, volume, and the surface area), the shape features (the sphericity, irregularity, compactness, roundness, elongation, the maximum distance to the boundary, and the ratio of the volume of the object to the volume of a bounding box of the object), and the intensity features (the maximum, minimum, mean, standard deviation, skewness, kurtosis, and mass of CT values inside the nodule candidates) (Zhao et al. 2003; Schilham et al. 2006; Brown et al. 2007; Li et al. 2008; Golosio et al. 2009; Murphy et al. 2009; Ye et al. 2009; Messay et al. 2010). In addition to the original CT images, a variety of processed/enhanced images were employed for feature calculation, including shape-index image, curvedness image, nodule-enhanced image, blood vessel–enhanced image, distance transform image, edge-gradient image, and gradient field (Ge et al. 2005; Li et al. 2008; Murphy et al. 2009; Way et al. 2009; Ye et al. 2009; Messay et al. 2010).

Most researchers calculated features from the inside of the nodule candidate region, but features can also be determined from the outside band regions around the nodule candidate. The features calculated from the outside region can be very useful for distinction between benign and malignant nodules (Aoyama et al. 2002) and for distinction between nodules and nonnodules (Messay et al. 2010) because the outside region may include context information about nodules such as spiculation around malignant nodules.

Nearly all CADe schemes in thin-slice CT used global 3D features to represent the characteristics of an entire nodule. While this is reasonable, it is certainly not the only way or not even the best way, because it discards useful local 2D information for lung nodule detection. For instance, Guo and Li (2012) decomposed a 3D nodule into a set of reformatted 2D images

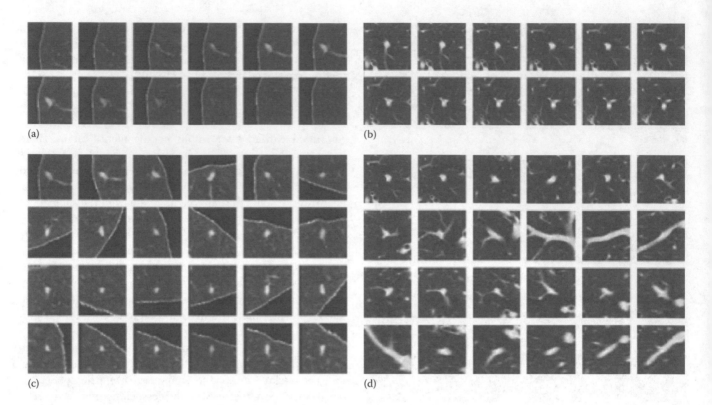

(a)

(b)

(c)

(d)

Figure 9.4 A nodule and a blood vessel in (a) and (b) the consecutive CT slices and (c) and (d) 2D reformatted images, respectively. The nodule appears circular in all consecutive CT slices and 2D reformatted images. Whereas the blood vessel appears as nodule-like circular objects in all consecutive CT slices, it shows clearly noncircular linear structures in some *effective* 2D reformatted images.

from multiple viewpoints and extracted local features from each of the 2D reformatted images. Figure 9.4 shows a nodule (left column) and a blood vessel (right column) in the consecutive CT slices ([a] and [b]) and the 2D reformatted images ([c] and [d]). As expected, the nodule appears circular in all the consecutive CT slices and 2D reformatted images. Although the blood vessel appears as nodule-like circular objects in all the consecutive CT slices, it appears clearly as noncircular linear structures in some *effective* 2D reformatted images. These *effective* 2D reformatted images are very useful to distinguish nodules from blood vessels. Guo and Li (2012) found that the local 2D information was more useful than the global 3D information in their nodule detection scheme, particularly, when it was integrated with 3D information.

Most CADe schemes calculated dozens of features to represent nodule candidates; some may calculate as few as three features (Zhao et al. 2003; Bellotti et al. 2007) and some as many as 245 features (Messay et al. 2010). Because of the curse of dimensionality, a few useful features have to be selected from the large number of features for better distinction between the nodules and nonnodules. A variety of feature selection methods have been employed in CADe schemes for lung nodules, including an iterative feature selection (Aoyama et al. 2002), a stepwise feature selection (Ge et al. 2005), and a sequential forward feature

selection method (Murphy et al. 2009; Messay et al. 2010). In principle, these feature selection methods are similar; a major difference is in the criteria to add/remove a feature to/from the current feature set. In the iterative feature selection method, Aoyama et al. (2002) utilized the Wilks' lambda and the F value to iteratively add/remove a feature to/from the current feature set. The Wilks' lambda is defined by the ratio of within-group variance to the total variance, whereas the F value is a cost function based on the Wilks' lambda, which measures the significance in the change of Wilks' lambda. A feature is added to the current feature combination if its addition results in a maximum decrease in the Wilks' lambda among all available features to be added and if the F value is larger than a threshold. A similar concept is applied to the deletion of a feature from the current feature set. After the selection step, the number of selected features is typically small (<20), although it can still be as large as 50 (Murphy et al. 2009) or 60 (Messay et al. 2010).

9.2.6 False-Positive Reduction

Whereas the initial nodule identification step locates suspicious nodule candidates in CT images and calculates features for each of the nodule candidates, the false-positive reduction step tries to classify the nodule candidates into nodule and false-positive (nonnodule) categories and, subsequently, remove false positives. One of the most frequently employed and simplest classifiers is the rule-based classifier. Many investigators have used a rule-based classifier to distinguish nodules from false positives (Zhao et al. 2003; Paik et al. 2004; Bae et al. 2005; Marten et al. 2005). Because the rule-based classifier generally has a clear semantic meaning, it can be readily comprehended or interpreted by human beings. However, rules were generally determined manually and empirically in the current CADe schemes, which leads to tediousness, long design time, and an overtraining effect. Li and Doi (2006a) devised an automated method to minimize the overtraining effect in the rule-based classifier, in particular, when a large number of rules were created. Often, the rule-based classifier was utilized as a first classifier followed by a second more sophisticated classifier such as a linear discriminant analysis or artificial neural network (ANN). In such a case, the rule-based classifier was employed in order to quickly remove obvious false positives (outliers) so that their influence on the training of the second classifier was eliminated. Instead of the rule-based classifier, Murphy et al. (2009) utilized a k-nearest-neighbor classifier as the first classifier to remove some *easy* false positives.

A variety of classifiers have been employed for reduction of false positives, including linear classifier (Ge et al. 2005; Li et al. 2008; Messay et al. 2010), quadratic classifier (Messay et al. 2010), k-nearest-neighbor classifier (Murphy et al. 2009), support vector machine (SVM) (Boroczky et al. 2006; Ye et al. 2009), and ANN (Bellotti et al. 2007; Golosio et al. 2009). The inputs to these classifiers are selected features of nodule candidates described in the previous section, and the output is generally an index value indicating the probability of being a true nodule. Although linear classifier appears to be less powerful than the other types of classifiers, it actually often outperforms more sophisticated ones such as quadratic classifier or ANN (Aoyama et al. 2002; Ge et al. 2005; Messay et al. 2010), probably because it is simpler and thus is more stable and robust to new unseen nodules.

The inputs to an ANN classifier can also be voxel values inside a nodule candidate rather than the features of a nodule candidate (Suzuki et al. 2003; Retico et al. 2008). Suzuki et al. (2003) developed a massive training artificial neural network (MTANN) for the reduction of false positives in computerized detection of lung nodules in low-dose CT. The MTANN is trained by use of a large number of subregions extracted from input images together with the teacher images containing the distribution for the *likelihood of being a nodule*. The input units to the MTANN are the pixel values in each subregion. The output image is obtained by scanning an input image with the MTANN. The distinction between a nodule and a nonnodule is made by use of a score that is defined from the output image of the MTANN. Retico et al. (2008) developed a voxel-based classification approach to classify each voxel, instead of each nodule

candidate, into a nodule voxel or a nonnodule voxel. Therefore, the output of the ANN indicates the probability of being a nodule voxel. For each voxel to be classified, the CT values of 147 voxels in its 3D neighborhood of $7 \times 7 \times 3$ voxels were employed as the input units of the ANN. Furthermore, six additional features representing the three eigenvalues of the gradient tensor matrix and the three eigenvalues of the Hessian matrix were computed for each voxel and employed as six additional input units to the ANN. Therefore, for each voxel of interest, the number of the input units to the ANN was 153.

Whereas linear classifier, ANN, and SVM are often employed in statistical pattern recognition tasks, the model-based semantic network used by Brown et al. (2003) is often employed in structural or semantic pattern recognition. Their model attempted to describe anatomic structures such as lungs and pulmonary vessels, and pathologic structures such as nodules. The model was represented by using a semantic network. In the structural model, each node contained a set of features, and each arc connecting two nodes represented structural relationships (part of, inside, etc.) between anatomic objects. To distinguish between blood vessels and nodules (the major opacities inside the lungs), candidates were matched to either nodule structures or vessel structures by use of fuzzy logic. A confidence score was calculated for each candidate based on the features of the candidates and a fuzzy membership function. Regions matched to the nodule structure in the model with a high confidence score were considered to be nodules, and those matched to the vessel structure with a high confidence score were considered to be blood vessels and were removed.

van Ginneken et al. (2010) and Camarlinghi et al. (2012) combined multiple CADe schemes to further improve the performance of computerized nodule detection in CT. van Ginneken et al. (2010) employed an ANODE09 database of 55 scans and a web-based framework for objective evaluation of multiple CADe schemes for nodule detection in CT. Six teams, including those in Bellotti et al. (2007), Retico et al. (2008), and Murphy et al. (2009), uploaded the detection results for the ANODE09 database to facilitate benchmarking. van Ginneken et al. (2010) first transformed each candidate output value from each individual system into a probability value and then calculated the sum of all probability values from the six systems as confidence score for the nodule candidate. Their results demonstrate that combining the output of multiple CADe systems leads to marked performance improvements. As of January 15, 2012, they have compared and integrated the performance of 12 CADe schemes on the ANODE09 website (http://anode09.isi.uu.nl/).

Camarlinghi et al. (2012) compared and integrated three CADe schemes to improve nodule detection performance by use of the LIDC with 138 CT scans. The three CADe schemes include one developed by Bellotti et al. (2007), one by Retico et al. (2008), and one called Channel Ant Model CADe.

They used the same combination method employed in van Ginneken et al. (2010), and their combined CADe scheme achieved higher performance than did the three individual CADe schemes.

9.2.7 Performance Evaluation for Nodule Detection

9.2.7.1 Performance Metrics for Evaluation of CADe Schemes

The output from a classifier for a nodule candidate indicates how likely the nodule candidate is a true nodule. Typically, a threshold selected for the output is employed to classify a nodule candidate into a nodule and a nonnodule category. For most CT scans, multiple candidates will be judged as *nodules*, which may include true nodules and false positives. For a fixed threshold, one can determine the nodule detection sensitivity (ratio of the number of detected nodules to the total number of nodules) and false-positive rate in terms of the number of false positives per CT scan. The pair of the sensitivity and false-positive rate constitutes an operating point for the CADe scheme and is the most important metric for measuring the performance of the CADe schemes for nodule detection. Changing the threshold to another value will provide another operating point. From multiple operating points, a free-response receiver operating characteristic (FROC) curve can be determined, in which the false-positive rate and the sensitivity are, respectively, the horizontal and vertical axes. An empirical FROC curve can be created by connecting the adjacent operating points; alternatively, a smooth FROC curve can be obtained from the multiple operating points by use of a maximum likelihood fitting (FROCFIT) program (Chakraborty 1989) for evaluating the overall performance of CADe schemes.

9.2.7.2 Evaluation Methods for CADe Schemes

In order to evaluate the performance level of a CADe scheme, the image database is often partitioned into at least two (generally disjoint) subsets, that is, a training set and a test set. The former is used for training a CADe scheme, and the latter is employed for testing the trained CADe scheme for providing an estimated performance level. Common methods for evaluating the performance of CADe schemes include the following:

1. *The resubstitution method*: The entire database is used for both training and testing of a CADe scheme.
2. *The k-fold cross-validation (CV) method*: The entire image database is first randomly partitioned into k disjoint subsets of nearly equal size, and then each of the k subsets is used, one by one, as a test set for the evaluation of a CADe scheme trained on the other (k – 1) subsets. The most frequently used method is the twofold CV method.

3. *The leave-one-out (LOO) method*: A special case of the k-fold CV method when the size of the subset is equal to 1.
4. *The holdout method*: The entire image database is first randomly partitioned into two disjoint subsets of nearly equal size, and then one subset is used for training and the other for testing the CADe scheme. Please note that this method is similar to, but different from, the twofold CV method.

9.2.7.3 Bias and Variance in the Estimated Performance

By use of one of the evaluation methods, the *estimated* performance of a CADe scheme is a random variable about its *true* performance, which is a fixed, but unknown, quantity. Therefore, the estimated performance may be biased from the true performance and has a variance. If the estimated performance is, on average, better (poorer) than the true performance, then the estimated performance is optimistically (pessimistically) biased. If there is large difference in the performance levels estimated from multiple evaluations of a CADe scheme (i.e., the estimated performance levels are quite inconsistent), then the variance in the estimated performance is large.

It is well known that the resubstitution evaluation method is optimistically biased and therefore is discouraged for the evaluation of CADe schemes. Both the LOO and CV methods provide more reliable evaluation results than does the resubstitution method and have been employed frequently for the evaluation of CADe schemes in recent years. Although the holdout evaluation method is similar to the twofold CV method, it is not as precise as the twofold CV method in which the average performance level estimated on two subsets of the entire database is reported.

Even with a good evaluation method such as LOO or CV, inappropriate use of the evaluation method may introduce significant bias or variance (Li and Doi 2006b). For example, it is important to train all steps of a CADe scheme on a training data set only, including image enhancement, nodule segmentation, feature selection, and classification. A common mistake is to train some of the steps such as feature selection using both training and testing data sets. Li and Doi (2006b) identified a number of inappropriate ways in the use of the evaluation methods, and they made recommendations to correct the potential mistakes in different situations.

9.2.8 Comparison of CAD Schemes for Nodule Detection in CT

Table 9.1 shows the databases, technical methods, and performance levels for the 14 nodule detection schemes developed by researchers in *academic* institutions. Two papers

TABLE 9.1 CADe SYSTEMS FOR LUNG NODULE DETECTION IN CT

Author	Year	Database	Lung Segmentation	Nodule Enhancement	Initial Nodule Identification	Number of Features	Classifier	Performance
Brown	2003	15 Patients 77 Micronodules (>1 mm) Partial CT scans	Anatomic model-based thresholding and region growing	None	Anatomic model-based thresholding and region growing	4 No feature selection	Fuzzy logic rules	Nodules < 3 mm: Sensitivity = 70% 15 FPs/scan Nodules ≥ 3 mm: Sensitivity = 100% 15 FPs/scan
Zhao	2003	8 Patients 266 Simulated nodules	Adaptive thresholding	None	Local density maximum detection	3 No feature selection	Rules	Sensitivity = 84.2% 5 FPs/scan
Paik	2004	8 Patients 46 Nodules (>6 mm)	Fixed thresholding	Surface normal overlap	Local maxima detection	None	Rule based on surface normal overlap	Sensitivity = 90% 5.6 FPs/scan
Bae	2005	20 Patients 164 Nodules (>3 mm)	Adaptive thresholding	Morphologic matching for juxtavascular nodules only	Region growing	Unknown	Rules	Sensitivity = 95.1% 6.9 FPs/scan
Ge	2005	56 Patients 82 Scans 116 Nodules Partial lungs	Thresholding and k-means clustering	None	Weighted k-means clustering	44 Feature selection	LDA	Sensitivity = 80% 0.34 FPs/section[a]
Bellotti	2007	15 Patients 26 Nodules (>5 mm)	Region growing	None	Region growing	3 No feature selection	ANN	Sensitivity = 88.5% 6.6 FPs/scan
Li	2008	117 Patients 153 Nodules (≥4 mm)	Fixed thresholding	Dot-enhancement filter	Fixed thresholding	18 Feature selection	LDA-based composite rules	Sensitivity = 86% 6.6 FPs/scan
Pu	2008	52 Scans 184 Nodules (≥3 mm)	Fixed thresholding	None	Fixed thresholding and distance transform	None	Shape matching with a sphere	Sensitivity = 81.5% 6.5 FPs/scan
Retico	2008	39 Patients 102 Nodules (≥4 mm)	Fixed thresholding	Dot-enhancement filter	Local maxima detection	None	Voxel-based ANN	Sensitivity = 80%–85% 10–13 FPs/scan
Ozekes	2008	16 Patients 16 Nodules (>5 mm) Partial CT scans	Genetic cellular neural network	None	Thresholding and directional searching	None	Voxel-based template matching	Sensitivity = 100% 13.4 FPs/scan

(Continued)

TABLE 9.1 (Continued)   CADe SYSTEMS FOR LUNG NODULE DETECTION IN CT

Author	Year	Database	Lung Segmentation	Nodule Enhancement	Initial Nodule Identification	Number of Features	Classifier	Performance
Ye	2009	108 Patients 220 Nodules	Fuzzy thresholding	Shape-index and dot-enhancement filter	Thresholding	15 Feature selection	SVM	Sensitivity = 90.2% 8.2 FPs/scan
Murphy	2009	Three databases with 813, 541, 541 scans and 1525, 1688, 768 nodules	Registration to a template lung	Shape index and curvedness	Fixed thresholding	135 Feature selection	KNN	For 3 databases: Sensitivity = 80% 4.2 FPs/scan Sensitivity = 72.4% 4.0 FPs/scan Sensitivity = 77.7% 4.2 FPs/scan
Golosio	2009	Two databases with 23 and 84 scans and 45 and 77 nodules (≥3 mm)	Fixed thresholding	None	Multiple thresholding	43 No feature selection	ANN	For 2 databases: Sensitivity = 84% 10 FPs/scan Sensitivity = 71% 4 FPs/scan
Messay	2010	84 Patients 143 Nodules	Fixed thresholding	None	Multiple thresholding	245 Feature selection	FLD QDA	Sensitivity = 90.2% 8.2 FPs/scan

ANN, artificial neural network; FLD, Fisher linear discriminant; KNN, k-nearest neighbors; LDA, linear discriminant analysis; QDA, quadratic discriminant analysis; SVM, supporting vector machine

[a] The number of false positives per section instead of per scan

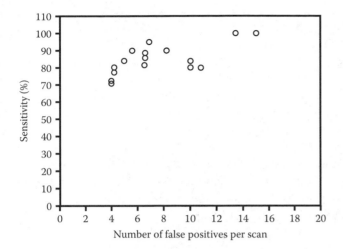

Figure 9.5 The sensitivities and false-positive rates for the CADe schemes listed in Table 9.1. The typical performance of current CADe schemes includes sensitivities of 80%–90% with four to eight reported false positives per scan.

presenting the integration of multiple CADe systems were not included (van Ginneken et al. 2010; Camarlinghi et al. 2012). The schemes were represented by the last names of the first authors and were listed in the order of publication year. The technical methods listed include the lung segmentation, nodule enhancement, initial nodule identification, number of features, and classification. For the database, information listed include the number of patients, number of nodules, the minimal size of nodules, and the extent of the CT scan (entire or partial lungs) whenever they were provided. Large nodules are generally easier to detect than small nodules. CADe schemes using CT scans of the entire lungs would report more false positives than those of partial lungs. Figure 9.5 shows the sensitivities and false-positive rates for the CADe schemes listed in Table 9.1. Typical performance of current CADe schemes includes sensitivities of 80%–90% and false-positive rates of four to eight per scan.

Direct comparison of the performance levels in Table 9.1 is discouraged because of the difference in a number of aspects, in particular, in the size of the database, the nature and characteristics of nodules, and the evaluation methods. Appropriate comparison should be made by use of the same CT databases, such as the LIDC and the ANODE09 database; readers can find more information on the public databases of lung nodules in Chapter 12. Excellent examples are the comparison of six CADe schemes by use of ANODE09 database (van Ginneken et al. 2010) and the comparison of three CADe schemes by use of the LIDC (Camarlinghi et al. 2012). van Ginneken et al. (2010) reported eight sensitivities at eight false-positive rates (from one-eighth to eight false positives per scan) for the detection of six types of nodules

(small, large, isolated, juxtavascular, juxtapleural, and perifissural nodules) with six CADe schemes. From this chapter, readers can understand how well each CADe scheme performs for each type of nodule at different operating points. They found that *a substantial performance difference exists between different CADe schemes*; for example, at a false-positive rate of two per scan, two schemes (A and E) reported sensitivities of 24.6% and 71.2%, respectively. Please note that, even in the case of evaluating CADe schemes using the same databases, a CADe scheme with a low performance does not necessarily mean that the CADe itself is poor; the database used for training the CADe may have a marked impact on the performance of the CADe scheme.

Table 9.2 shows the databases and performance levels for the commercial CADe systems developed by GE Healthcare (Milwaukee, WI), Philips Medical Systems (Cleveland, OH), R2 Technology (now Hologic, Sunnyvale, CA), Siemens Medical Solutions (Erlangen, Germany), and Toshiba Medical Systems (Tochigi, Japan) (Lee et al. 2005; Marten et al. 2005; Wiemker et al. 2005; Yuan et al. 2006; Beyer et al. 2007; White et al. 2008; Helm et al. 2009; Yanagawa et al. 2009; Roos et al. 2010; Song et al. 2011; Matsumoto et al. 2012). Because technical details typically were not presented in these papers, technical methods are not included in Table 9.2.

9.3 COMPUTERIZED DIAGNOSIS OF LUNG NODULE IN CT

When a nodule is detected, the next task is to characterize/diagnose the nodule, that is, to classify it as benign or malignant. A CADx scheme can be developed to perform this task by providing a score indicating the likelihood of malignancy for a nodule. The input to a CADx scheme is generally the location of a nodule, which can be provided by a human operator or a CADe scheme. The major steps in a CADx scheme include nodule segmentation, feature calculation, feature selection, as well as nodule classification. Technically, a majority of important techniques in a CADx scheme can be adopted from a CADe scheme. In some CADx schemes, major steps such as the nodule segmentation and feature determination are implemented manually or semi-automatically (Matsuki et al. 2002; Choi et al. 2008; Iwano et al. 2008; Okada et al. 2009). In this section, the unique characteristics of each automated CADx scheme are briefly presented.

9.3.1 Lung Nodule Diagnosis

Aoyama et al. developed a CAD scheme for nodule characterization in thick-section CT (Aoyama et al. 2003) and

TABLE 9.2   COMMERCIAL CADe SYSTEMS FOR LUNG NODULE DETECTION IN CT

Author	Year	Database	CADe System	Performance
Marten	2005	20 Scans 135 Nodules	Siemens ICAD	Sensitivity: 76.3% FP rate: 0.55/scan
Lee	2005	70 Scans 78 Nodules	R2 ImageChecker	Sensitivity: 60% FP rate: 1.6/scan
Wiemker	2005	12 Scans 330 Nodules (≥2 mm)	Philips CAD	Sensitivity: 95% FP rate: 4.4/scan
Yuan	2006	150 CT 628 Nodules	R2 ImageChecker	Sensitivity: 73% FP rate: 3.2/scan
Das	2006	25 Scans 116 Nodules (≥3 mm)	R2 ImageChecker Siemens NEV	R2 CADe: Sensitivity: 73% FP rate: 6/scan Siemens CADe: Sensitivity: 75% FP rate: 8/scan
Beyer	2007	50 Scans 340 Nodules (>1.1 mm)	Siemens LungCAD	Sensitivity: 43% FP rate: 1.3/scan
White	2008	109 Scans 91 Nodules	Philips CADe	Sensitivity: 66.7% FP rate: N/A
Yanagawa	2009	48 Scans 229 Nodules (≥4 mm)	GE VCAR	Sensitivity: 40.2% FP rate: 5.7/scan
Helm	2009	24 Scans of children 173 Nodules	R2 ImageChecker	Sensitivity: 34% (sensitivity: 80% for nodules ≥ 4 mm) FP rate: 0.9/scan
Song	2011	166 Scans 60 Nodules (≥4 mm)	Philips CADe	Sensitivity: 53% FP rate: 1.9/scan
Matsumoto	2012	60 Scans 122 Nodules (≥4 mm)	Toshiba CADe	Sensitivity: 70.5% FP rate: 3.2/scan

then transplanted the CAD scheme to thin-section CT by use of 3D image-processing techniques (Li et al. 2004). Their scheme first segmented a nodule automatically by use of a dynamic programming technique. Based on the extracted outline of the nodule, an inside region and an outside region were determined, which accounted for, respectively, the information inside the nodule region and the context information around the nodule. Forty-one and fifteen image features based, respectively, on 2D sectional data and 3D volumetric data were determined from quantitative analysis of the nodule outline and of pixel values. Eight features were automatically selected by use of a stepwise feature selection method, and they were input to a linear discriminant analysis classifier for distinction between benign and malignant nodules.

Shah et al. (2005b) employed a procedure to segment nodule regions, which were then reviewed, edited, and approved by one of three thoracic radiologists in their team. Each segmented nodule region was then further partitioned into two regions containing a solid portion and a nonsolid portion. For each of the two regions,

31 features were calculated, and important features were selected using a stepwise selection search based on the Akaike information criterion. It seemed that features extracted from the nonsolid portion were not very effective for distinguishing between benign and malignant nodules, regardless of whether they were used alone or combined with features extracted from the solid portion. Three classifiers, including linear and quadratic discriminant analysis as well as logistic regression, were employed to distinguish between benign and malignant nodules.

Mori et al. (2005) utilized a deformable surface model to extract nodule regions based on an initial surface placed within a nodule. They then extracted three features, that is, the attenuation, shape index, and curvedness value from the segmented nodule regions. A Fisher linear classifier was trained to provide a score for distinction between benign and malignant nodules. Each patient was scanned three times at three time points: before the injection of a contrast agent and 2 and 4 min after the start of contrast enhancement.

Chen et al. (2010) tried to classify nodules into three types (probably benign, uncertain, and probably malignant) rather than two types (benign and malignant). They segmented the nodules by using Canny's edge detection technique and, similar to Aoyama et al. (2003) scheme, determined 21 image features from the image analysis of the regions inside and outside of the segmented nodule outlines. They selected 15 image features that show statistical difference among the three types of the nodules by using the nonparametric Kruskal–Wallis test. From three types of ANNs (the back propagation algorithm-based feed-forward neural network, radial basis probabilistic neural network, and learning vector quantization algorithm-based neural network), a neural network ensemble classifier was constructed to classify nodules.

da Silva et al. (2008) segmented nodules with a region-growing method and calculated 504 texture features by use of the Ripley's K function analysis. The Ripley's K function is a tool for analyzing spatial patterns consisting of many *small* objects in 2D and 3D image space. It summarizes a point pattern, tests hypotheses about the pattern, estimates parameters, and fits models to the pattern. Therefore, the Ripley's K function can be used as features to assess spatial texture. da Silva et al. (2008) finally selected six features from the 504 Ripley features with a stepwise feature selection method and used an LDA classifier for distinguishing benign from malignant nodules.

Way et al. (2009) developed a CADx system to differentiate malignant and benign lung nodules on CT scans. They first designed a 3D active contour method to segment the nodule from its surrounding background in a local VOI and extracted image features from the segmented nodule for classification. The active contour was initialized with the boundary of a binary object that was generated by k-means clustering within the VOI and smoothed by morphological opening. They employed morphological, texture, and nodule surface features to characterize the lung nodule. A stepwise feature selection was trained using simplex optimization to select the most effective features. A linear discriminant analysis classifier and a supporting vector machine classifier were trained with a LOO resampling scheme to reduce the optimistic bias in estimating the test performance of the CAD system.

Lee et al. (2010) utilized 194 features (including the 2D, 2.5D, and 3D features) and three classifiers to characterize benign and malignant nodules. The 2.5D features were computed as a weighted average of 2D features calculated on all the native slices, where the weights were defined by the cross-sectional area of the nodule on each slice. The three classifiers included the ensemble classifier using the random subspace method (RSM), the ensemble classifier using the genetic algorithm (GA), and a two-step classifier that sequentially used a GA ensemble for the selection of the features and a subsequent RSM ensemble for nodule classification.

In addition to nodule features extracted from CT, Nie et al. (2006) further utilized features extracted from positron emission tomography (PET) for distinction between benign and malignant pulmonary nodules. They developed and evaluated 3 ANN-based CADx schemes by use of 16 features extracted from CT alone, 4 from 18F-FDG PEt alone, and 20 from both CT and 18F-FDG PET. The CADx scheme based on both PET and CT was better able to differentiate benign from malignant pulmonary nodules than were the CADx schemes based on PEt alone and CT alone.

9.3.2 Comparison of CAD Schemes for Nodule Diagnosis in CT

Table 9.3 shows the databases, technical methods, and performance levels for the CADx schemes reviewed. All CADx schemes were developed by researchers in academic institutions. Medical imaging companies do not put significant effort in developing CADx systems probably because it is difficult for them to have such CADx systems approved by the U.S. Food and Drug Agency.

9.3.3 Nodule Diagnosis Using Similar Images

In addition to the CADx schemes that provide the likelihood of malignancy for a nodule, radiologists may improve their diagnosis accuracy by using visual aid from a set of images of malignant and benign nodules that are similar to an unknown nodule to be diagnosed. Similar images may help radiologists diagnose nodules because radiologists learn diagnostic skills by observing many clinical cases during their training and clinical practice, and their knowledge obtained from visual impression of images with different type of nodules constitutes the foundation for their diagnosis. Li et al. (2003a) conducted two experiments to determine (1) a psychophysical similarity measure for selecting relevant similar images and (2) the usefulness of similar images to assist radiologists in the diagnosis of lung nodules in CT images.

Li et al. (2003a) developed and evaluated four similarity metrics to select the similar nodules, including the distance in the feature space between two nodules, the pixel-value difference, the image cross-correlation, and a psychophysical similarity measure by use of an ANN. The psychophysical similarity measure utilized radiologists' subjective similarity rating (i.e., the radiologists' knowledge in selecting similar images) as teacher to train an ANN and provided highly relevant similar nodules that correlated well with the radiologists' choice of similar nodules. The psychophysical similarity measure has also been studied and applied for the selection of

TABLE 9.3   CADx SYSTEMS FOR LUNG NODULE CHARACTERIZATION IN CT

Author	Year	Database	Segmentation	Number of Features	Classifier	Performance
Li	2004	244 Nodules 183 Benign 61 Malignant	Edge-based dynamic programming	58 Feature selection	LDA	AUC = 0.83
Shah	2005	35 Nodules 16 Benign 19 Malignant	Threshold-based region growing	31 or 62 Feature selection	LDA QDA Logistic regression	LDA: AUC = 0.91 QDA: AUC = 0.89 Logistic: AUC = 0.92
Mori	2005	62 Nodules 27 Benign 35 Malignant	Deformable surface model	3	Fisher linear classifier	AUC = 1.0
Nie	2006	92 Nodules 42 Benign 50 Malignant	N/A	16 CT features 4 PET features No feature selection	Artificial neural network	CT: AUC = 0.83 PET: AUC = 0.91 CT + PET: AUC = 0.95
da Silva	2008	39 Nodules 29 Benign 10 Malignant	Region growing	504 Feature selection	LDA	Sensitivity = 70% Specificity = 100%
Iwano	2008	107 Nodules 55 Benign 52 Malignant	Thresholding	2	LDA	Sensitivity = 77% Specificity = 80%
Way	2009	256 Nodules 132 Benign 124 Malignant	Active contour	16 New + old features Feature selection	LDA SVM	LDA: AUC = 0.857 SVM: Vary
Chen	2009	32 Nodules 13 Benign 19 Malignant	Canny's edge detection	21 Feature selection	Ensemble of three neural networks	AUC = 0.79
Lee	2010	125 Nodules 63 Benign 62 Malignant	Distance transform-based region growing	216 Feature selection	GA RSM GA + RSM	GA: AUC = 0.851 RSM: AUC = 0.866 GA + RSM: AUC = 0.889

AUC, area under ROC curve; GA, genetic algorithm; LDA, linear discriminant analysis; QDA, quadratic discriminant analysis; RSM, random subspace method; SVM, supporting vector machine

similar breast masses (Muramatsu et al. 2005) and similar clustered microcalcifications (Muramatsu et al. 2008) in mammography.

In order to verify the usefulness of similar images, Li et al. (2003a) conducted an observer study in which five radiologists made diagnostic decision for the unknown nodule without and with the aid of similar nodules. For each of the unknown nodules, a participating radiologist made diagnosis based on the observation of the unknown nodule only. Then, the 3 most similar malignant nodules and the 3 most similar benign nodules were automatically selected from an existing database of 76 confirmed malignant and 413 benign nodules, and these similar images were presented adjacent to the unknown nodule and were shown to the radiologist, as indicated in Figure 9.6 (benign: left-hand side; malignant: right-hand side). The radiologist was asked to re-rate the likelihood of malignancy for the unknown nodule after having observed the similar nodules. If the unknown nodule more closely resembles the similar malignant (benign) nodules, it is likely that the radiologist would increase (decrease) the likelihood of malignancy for the unknown nodule. They found that all radiologists improved their performance with the aid of similar nodules.

Lam et al. (2007) created an open-source content-based image retrieval framework for similar nodule searching based on the LIDC lung image database. Their system first extracted three kinds of features to represent a nodule, based on the Haralick co-occurrence, Gabor filters, and Markov random field models. For the Haralick co-occurrence features, they utilized three distances (Euclidean distance, Manhattan distance, and Chebyshev distance) to measure the similarity of two nodules. For the other two kinds of features, they utilized two metrics (the Chi-squared statistic

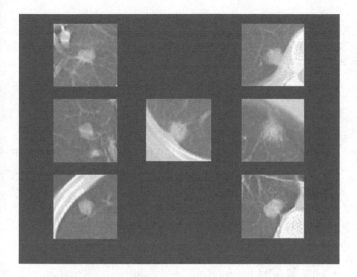

Figure 9.6 Illustration for the diagnosis of an unknown nodule with the aid of similar images for three benign nodules (left-hand side) and three malignant nodules (right-hand side).

and the Jeffrey divergence for comparison of feature histogram) to determine the similarity between the two nodules. They found that the Gabor and Markov features performed better at retrieving similar nodules than did the Haralick co-occurrence features.

9.4 OBSERVER STUDIES FOR LUNG NODULE IN CT

9.4.1 Observer Studies for Nodule Detection Schemes

The potential clinical usefulness of CADe systems for nodule detection in CT can be assessed by conducting an observer performance study in which the radiologists' performance without and with the aid of CADe systems is compared. Table 9.4 shows the observer studies using CADe detection systems, including commercial ones developed by GE, Philips Medical Systems, R2 Technology, Siemens Medical Solutions, and Toshiba Medical Systems (Brown et al. 2005; Lee et al. 2005; Das et al. 2006; Beyer et al. 2007; White et al. 2008; Park et al. 2009; Sahiner et al. 2009; Yanagawa et al. 2009; Roos et al. 2010). Provided in Table 9.4 are the first author's last name, the year the paper published, the databases used, the number of radiologists who participated in the study, the name of CADe system, the performance of CADe systems, and the radiologists' performance without and with the aid of CADe systems.

It is apparent from Table 9.4 that the CADe systems typically achieved a relatively low performance compared with the performance of radiologists. However, by use of these *low-performance* CADe systems, radiologists can still well

improve their detection sensitivity, with a slight increase in their false-positive rates. Technological improvements to the CADe systems would increase the sensitivity and specificity, and thus would further help radiologists reduce these false-positive detections. In four studies (Lee et al. 2005; White et al. 2008; Sahiner et al. 2009; Yanagawa et al. 2009), instead of using the sensitivity and false-positive rate, the authors also compared the performance of radiologists' with the area under the ROC curve (AUC) and the figure of merit (FOM) of the jackknife FROC (Chakraborty and Berbaum 2004). In all four studies, radiologists improved their nodule detection performance by use of the CADe systems.

Das et al. (2006) compared the effect of two commercial CADe systems on radiologists' detection of lung nodules in CT. The two CADe systems achieved similar performance levels for nodule detection, and their effect on radiologists' detection were also similar. Beyer et al. (2007) studied how to effectively utilize a CADe system in clinical practice; they found that a CADe system could improve radiologists' detection performance when used as a second reader in clinical practice, but could not when used as a concurrent reader.

9.4.2 Observer Studies for Nodule Diagnosis Schemes

Whereas the observer performance studies in Table 9.4 were conducted for the detection of lung nodules in thin-section CT, Table 9.5 shows the observer studies for nodule diagnosis using CADx systems developed by researchers in academic institutions (Matsuki et al. 2002; Li et al. 2004; Shah et al. 2005a; Awai et al. 2006; Way et al. 2010); none of the major medical imaging companies provides commercial CADx systems to clinicians. Provided in Table 9.5 are the first author's last name, the year the paper published, the databases used, the number of radiologists who participated in the study, the performance of CADx systems, and the radiologists' performance without and with the aid of CADx systems. In all five observer studies, the radiologists' performance levels with the CADx scheme were higher than those of the radiologists without CADx scheme, and the improvements were statistically significant. These studies indicated that the CADx scheme has the potential to improve radiologists' diagnostic accuracy in distinguishing benign nodules from malignant ones in thin-section CT.

9.5 DISCUSSIONS

A major concern in current CADe schemes is the high false-positive rate. When the nodule detection sensitivity is set at a reasonable level, the current CADe schemes typically report multiple false positives per scan. In contrast, radiologists

TABLE 9.4   OBSERVER STUDIES ON LUNG NODULE DETECTION IN CT BY USE OF CADe SYSTEMS

Author	Year	Database	Number of Readers	CADe System	Performance		
					CADe	Reader	Reader + CADe
Brown	2005	8 (Partial) scans 22 Nodules	13	UCLA CADe	Sensitivity: 86.4% FP rate: 2.6/scan	Sensitivity: 64.0% FP rate: 0.14/scan	Sensitivity: 81.9% FP rate: 0.17/scan
Lee	2005	70 Scans 78 Nodules	4	R2 ImageChecker	Sensitivity: 60.0% FP rate: 1.6/scan	Sensitivity: 83.0% FP rate: 0.13/scan AUC: 0.866	Sensitivity: 85.6% FP rate: 0.22/scan AUC: 0.878
Das	2006	25 Scans 116 Nodules (≥3 mm)	3	R2 ImageChecker Siemens NEV	R2 CADe: Sensitivity: 73% FP rate: 6/scan Siemens CADe: Sensitivity: 75% FP rate: 8/scan	Sensitivity: 76% FP rate: N/A	With R2 CADe: Sensitivity: 84% FP rate: N/A Siemens CADe: Sensitivity: 85% FP rate: N/A
Beyer	2007	50 Scans 340 Nodules (≥1.1 mm)	4	Siemens LungCAD	Sensitivity: 43% FP rate: 1.3/scan	Sensitivity: 62%–78% FP rate: N/A	Concurrent reading: Sensitivity: 62%–75% FP rate: N/A Second reader: Sensitivity: 69%–84% FP rate: N/A
White	2008	109 Scans divided into 436 quadrants 91 Nodules	10	Philips CADe	Sensitivity: 66.7% FP rate: N/A	AUC: 86.7%	AUC: 88.7%
Yanagawa	2009	48 Scans 229 Nodules (≥4 mm)	3	GE VCAR	Sensitivity: 40.2% FP rate: 5.7/scan	Sensitivity: 66% FP rate: 1.1/scan FOM: 0.659	Sensitivity: 77% FP rate: 1.4/scan FOM: 0.703
Sahiner	2009	85 Scans 241 Nodules (≥3 mm)	6	University of Michigan CADe	Sensitivity: 54% FP rate: 5.6/scan	Sensitivity: 56% FP rate: 0.67/scan FOM: 0.661	Sensitivity: 67% FP rate: 0.78/scan FOM: 0.705
Park	2009	49 Scans 121 Nodules	4	Seoul National University CADe	Sensitivity: 73% FP rate: 3.4/scan	Sensitivity: 88% FP rate: 1.1/scan	Sensitivity: 95% FP rate: 1.4/scan
Roos	2010	20 Scans 190 Nodules (≥3 mm)	3	Stanford University CADe	Sensitivity: 74% FP rate: N/A	Sensitivity: 53% FP rate: 1.15/scan	Sensitivity: 69% FP rate: 1.45/scan
Matsumoto	2012	60 Scans 122 Nodules (≥4 mm)	2	Toshiba CADe	Sensitivity: 70.5% FP rate: 3.2/scan	Two readers: FOM: 0.724 FOM: 0.682	Two readers: FOM: 0.768 FOM: 0.748

AUC, area under ROC curve; FOM, figure of merit of the jackknife free-response receiver operating characteristics

TABLE 9.5   OBSERVER STUDIES ON LUNG NODULE DIAGNOSIS IN CT BY USE OF CADx SYSTEMS

Author	Year	Database	Number of Readers	Performance		
				CADx	Reader	Reader + CADx
Matsuki	2002	155 Nodules 99 Malignant 56 Benign	12 Radiologists 4 Attending 4 Fellows 4 Residents	AUC = 0.951	AUC = 0.831	AUC = 0.959
Li	2004	56 Nodules 28 Malignant 28 Benign	16 Radiologists 7 Chest 9 Nonchest	AUC = 0.831	AUC = 0.785	AUC = 0.853
Shah	2005	28 Nodules 15 Malignant 13 Benign	8 Radiologists 2 Chest 2 Nonchest 1 Fellow 3 Residents	Unknown	AUC = 0.68	AUC = 0.81
Awai	2006	33 Nodules 18 Malignant 15 Benign	19 Radiologists 10 Attending 9 Residents	AUC = 0.795	AUC = 0.843	AUC = 0.924
Way	2010	256 Nodules 124 Malignant 132 Benign	6 Radiologists 6 Fellows	AUC = 0.857	AUC = 0.833	AUC = 0.853

report much fewer false positives than the CADe systems, generally below one false positive per CT scan. This weakness of CADe systems directly impacts radiologists' detection accuracy when they are aided by a CADe system (Rubin et al. 2005; Beyer et al. 2007; White et al. 2008; Roos et al. 2010). Roos et al. (2010) reported that when a CADe system output has few false positives at a reasonably high sensitivity, radiologists' detection sensitivity increased rapidly with CADe aid, with little increase in false-positive results; when the CADe system output has more false positives, radiologists had fewer opportunities to increase sensitivity and more opportunities to report false positives. Lee et al. (2005) reported that the most false positives were caused by blood vessels (62.4%) and scars (15.6%), whereas Yanagawa et al. (2009) reported that the false positives were typically induced by pleural changes (46%), blood vessels (38%), and scars (10%). Therefore, techniques for removing false positives caused by blood vessels and pleural changes should be able to markedly improve the performance of current CADe schemes.

Another issue in current CADe schemes is the low detection sensitivity for nonsolid nodules (also known as ground glass opacity [GGO]). Most current CADe schemes use only solid nodules in performance evaluation; some employ metastatic nodules or simulated nodules. All these nodules are easier to detect than nonsolid nodules because they are more circular and of higher contrast than nonsolid nodules.

Many factors can affect the performance levels of CADe schemes for nodule detection in thin-section CT. Among them, the dose level, section thickness, reconstruction interval, and reconstruction algorithm may have significant effects on computerized nodule detection. Kim et al. (2005) specifically studied the effect of section thickness and reconstruction interval on the performance level of their CADe scheme. They utilized three combinations of the section thickness and reconstruction interval to reconstruct CT data for 10 patients with lung nodules: thin group, 1 and 1 mm; overlap group, 5 and 1 mm; and thick group, 5 and 5 mm. The sensitivity and number of false positives per scan in their CADe scheme were thin group, 95.2% and 5.4; overlap group, 94.2% and 9.7; and thick group, 88.6% and 23.6. Their findings indicated that the performance of nodule detection was improved significantly with a smaller section thickness and a smaller reconstruction interval.

Another technical aspect to consider is the effect of radiation exposure on automated lung nodule detection using ultra-low-dose CT. In a study by Lee et al. (2008), 25 volunteers underwent CT scans using four different tube currents of 32, 16, 8, and 4 mAs. The sensitivities for detecting nodule decreased with reduced tube currents. Although the overall nodule detection performance was best at 32 mAs, no significant difference in nodule detectability was observed between scans at 16 or 8 mAs versus 32 mAs. However, scans performed at 4 mAs were significantly inferior to those performed at 32 mAs ($p < 0.001$).

9.6 CONCLUSIONS

The development and evaluation of CADe schemes for nodule detection in CT has been a hot topic in the past decade and will continue to be a hot one in the near future. Many CADe schemes have been developed by researchers from academic institutions in the United States, Europe, and Japan. In addition, major medical imaging companies have developed CADe systems in CT, and it is expected that these companies will distribute their CADe systems to more hospitals. Evidences have consistently shown that the CADe systems can help radiologists improve their nodule detection performance by using the CADe systems. The major issues in current CADe systems are the large number of false positives and low detection sensitivity for nonsolid nodules, and they represent major barriers for clinical application of the CADe systems. Further improvements to the current CADe schemes are needed to address major issues provided earlier.

Compared to CADe schemes, the development and evaluation of CADx schemes is slower. In particular, none of the major medical imaging companies have developed CADx system. Although the performance levels of current CADx schemes are quite high, radiologists are cautious and conservative in using the results of CADx schemes when it comes to the differential diagnosis of lung nodules. Continuous improvement of the current CADx schemes and the integration of confirmed similar nodules should be able to raise radiologists' confidence in using the CADx schemes in clinical practice.

ACKNOWLEDGMENTS

This work was supported by USPHS grants CA113820. Q.L. was a consultant to Riverain Medical Group, Miamisburg, OH. CAD technologies developed by Q.L. and his colleagues have been licensed to companies including R2 Technologies, Riverain Medical Group, Median Technology, Mitsubishi Space Software Co., General Electric Corporation, and Toshiba Corporation. It is the policy of Duke University that investigators disclose publicly actual or potential significant financial interests that may appear to be affected by research activities.

REFERENCES

Aberle, D. R., A. M. Adams et al. (2011). Reduced lung-cancer mortality with low-dose computed tomographic screening. *N Engl J Med* **365**(5): 395–409.

Aoyama, M., Q. Li et al. (2002). Automated computerized scheme for distinction between benign and malignant solitary pulmonary nodules on chest images. *Med Phys* **29**(5): 701–708.

Aoyama, M., Q. Li et al. (2003). Computerized scheme for determination of the likelihood measure of malignancy for pulmonary nodules on low-dose CT images. *Med Phys* **30**(3): 387–394.

Armato, S. G., 3rd, M. L. Giger et al. (1999). Computerized detection of pulmonary nodules on CT scans. *Radiographics* **19**(5): 1303–1311.

Armato, S. G., 3rd, M. L. Giger et al. (2001). Automated detection of lung nodules in CT scans: Preliminary results. *Med Phys* **28**(8): 1552–1561.

Armato, S. G., 3rd, F. Li et al. (2002). Lung cancer: Performance of automated lung nodule detection applied to cancers missed in a CT screening program. *Radiology* **225**(3): 685–692.

Armato, S. G., 3rd, G. McLennan et al. (2004a). Lung image database consortium: Developing a resource for the medical imaging research community. *Radiology* **232**(3): 739–748.

Armato, S. G., 3rd, M. F. McNitt-Gray et al. (2007). The Lung Image Database Consortium (LIDC): An evaluation of radiologist variability in the identification of lung nodules on CT scans. *Acad Radiol* **14**(11): 1409–1421.

Armato, S. G., 3rd, W. F. Sensakovic (2004b). Automated lung segmentation for thoracic CT impact on computer-aided diagnosis. *Acad Radiol* **11**(9): 1011–1021.

Awai, K., K. Murao et al. (2006). Pulmonary nodules: Estimation of malignancy at thin-section helical CT—Effect of computer-aided diagnosis on performance of radiologists. *Radiology* **239**(1): 276–284.

Bae, K. T., J. S. Kim et al. (2005). Pulmonary nodules: Automated detection on CT images with morphologic matching algorithm—Preliminary results. *Radiology* **236**(1): 286–293.

Bellotti, R., F. De Carlo et al. (2007). A CAD system for nodule detection in low-dose lung CTs based on region growing and a new active contour model. *Med Phys* **34**(12): 4901–4910.

Beyer, F., L. Zierott et al. (2007). Comparison of sensitivity and reading time for the use of computer-aided detection (CAD) of pulmonary nodules at MDCT as concurrent or second reader. *Eur Radiol* **17**(11): 2941–2947.

Boroczky, L., L. Zhao et al. (2006). Feature subset selection for improving the performance of false positive reduction in lung nodule CAD. *IEEE Trans Inform Technol Biomed* **10**(3): 504–511.

Brown, M. S., J. G. Goldin et al. (2003). Lung micronodules: Automated method for detection at thin-section CT—Initial experience. *Radiology* **226**(1): 256–262.

Brown, M. S., J. G. Goldin et al. (2005). Computer-aided lung nodule detection in CT: Results of large-scale observer test. *Acad Radiol* **12**(6): 681–686.

Brown, M. S., M. F. McNitt-Gray et al. (2001). Patient-specific models for lung nodule detection and surveillance in CT images. *IEEE Trans Med Imaging* **20**(12): 1242–1250.

Brown, M. S., R. Pais et al. (2007). An architecture for computer-aided detection and radiologic measurement of lung nodules in clinical trials. *Cancer Inform* **4**: 25–31.

Camarlinghi, N., I. Gori et al. (2012). Combination of computer-aided detection algorithms for automatic lung nodule identification. *Int J Comput Assist Radiol Surg* **7**(3): 455–464.

Chakraborty, D. P. (1989). Maximum likelihood analysis of free-response receiver operating characteristic (FROC) data. *Med Phys* **16**(4): 561–568.

Chakraborty, D. P., K. S. Berbaum (2004). Observer studies involving detection and localization: Modeling, analysis, and validation. *Med Phys* **31**(8): 2313–2330.

Chen, H., Y. Xu et al. (2010). Neural network ensemble-based computer-aided diagnosis for differentiation of lung nodules on CT images: Clinical evaluation. *Acad Radiol* **17**(5): 595–602.

Choi, E. J., G. Y. Jin et al. (2008). Solitary pulmonary nodule on helical dynamic CT scans: Analysis of the enhancement patterns using a computer-aided diagnosis (CAD) system. *Korean J Radiol* **9**(5): 401–408.

daSilva, E. C., A. C. Silva et al. (2008). Diagnosis of solitary lung nodules using the local form of Ripley's K function applied to three-dimensional CT data. *Comput Methods Prog Biomed* **90**(3): 230–239.

Das, M., G. Muhlenbruch et al. (2006). Small pulmonary nodules: Effect of two computer-aided detection systems on radiologist performance. *Radiology* **241**(2): 564–571.

Flehinger, B. J., M. Kimmel et al. (1992). The effect of surgical treatment on survival from early lung cancer. Implications for screening. *Chest* **101**(4): 1013–1018.

Flehinger, B. J., M. R. Melamed et al. (1984). Early lung cancer detection: Results of the initial (prevalence) radiologic and cytologic screening in the Memorial Sloan-Kettering study. *Am Rev Respir Dis* **130**(4): 555–560.

Fontana, R. S., D. R. Sanderson et al. (1984). Early lung cancer detection: Results of the initial (prevalence) radiologic and cytologic screening in the Mayo Clinic study. *Am Rev Respir Dis* **130**(4): 561–565.

Frost, J. K., W. C. Ball, Jr. et al. (1984). Early lung cancer detection: Results of the initial (prevalence) radiologic and cytologic screening in the Johns Hopkins study. *Am Rev Respir Dis* **130**(4): 549–554.

Ge, Z., B. Sahiner et al. (2005). Computer-aided detection of lung nodules: False positive reduction using a 3D gradient field method and 3D ellipsoid fitting. *Med Phys* **32**(8): 2443–2454.

Giger, M. L., K. T. Bae et al. (1994). Computerized detection of pulmonary nodules in computed tomography images. *Invest Radiol* **29**(4): 459–465.

Golosio, B., G. L. Masala et al. (2009). A novel multithreshold method for nodule detection in lung CT. *Med Phys* **36**(8): 3607–3618.

Guo, W., Q. Li (2012). High performance lung nodule detection schemes in CT using local and global information. *Med Phys* **39**(8): 5157–5168.

Helm, E. J., C. T. Silva et al. (2009). Computer-aided detection for the identification of pulmonary nodules in pediatric oncology patients: Initial experience. *Pediatr Radiol* **39**(7): 685–693.

Henschke, C. I., D. I. McCauley et al. (1999). Early Lung Cancer Action Project: Overall design and findings from baseline screening. *Lancet* **354**(9173): 99–105.

Henschke, C. I., D. F. Yankelevitz et al. (2006). Survival of patients with stage I lung cancer detected on CT screening. *N Engl J Med* **355**(17): 1763–1771.

Hu, S., E. A. Hoffman et al. (2001). Automatic lung segmentation for accurate quantitation of volumetric X-ray CT images. *IEEE Trans Med Imaging* **20**(6): 490–498.

Iwano, S., T. Nakamura et al. (2008). Computer-aided differentiation of malignant from benign solitary pulmonary nodules imaged by high-resolution CT. *Comput Med Imaging Graph* **32**(5): 416–422.

Jemal, A., R. Siegel et al. (2010). Cancer statistics, 2010. *CA Cancer J Clin* **60**(5): 277–300.

Kakeda, S., J. Moriya et al. (2004). Improved detection of lung nodules on chest radiographs using a commercial computer-aided diagnosis system. *Am J Roentgenol* **182**(2): 505–510.

Kass, M., A. Witkin et al. (1987). Snakes: Active contour models. *Int J Comput Vision* **1**: 11.

Kim, J. S., J. H. Kim et al. (2005). Automated detection of pulmonary nodules on CT images: Effect of section thickness and reconstruction interval—Initial results. *Radiology* **236**(1): 295–299.

Ko, J. P., M. Betke (2001). Chest CT: Automated nodule detection and assessment of change over time—Preliminary experience. *Radiology* **218**(1): 267–273.

Korfiatis, P. D., A. N. Karahaliou et al. (2010). Texture-based identification and characterization of interstitial pneumonia patterns in lung multidetector CT. *IEEE Trans Inform Technol Biomed* **14**(3): 675–680.

Kubik, A., J. Polak (1986). Lung cancer detection: Results of a randomized prospective study in Czechoslovakia. *Cancer* **57**(12): 2427–2437.

Lam, M. O., T. Disney et al. (2007). BRISC—An open source pulmonary nodule image retrieval framework. *J Digit Imaging* **20**(Suppl. 1): 63–71.

Leader, J. K., B. Zheng et al. (2003). Automated lung segmentation in X-ray computed tomography: Development and evaluation of a heuristic threshold-based scheme. *Acad Radiol* **10**(11): 1224–1236.

Lee, I. J., G. Gamsu et al. (2005). Lung nodule detection on chest CT: Evaluation of a computer-aided detection (CAD) system. *Korean J Radiol* **6**(2): 89–93.

Lee, J. Y., M. J. Chung et al. (2008). Ultra-low-dose MDCT of the chest: Influence on automated lung nodule detection. *Korean J Radiol* **9**(2): 95–101.

Lee, M. C., L. Boroczky et al. (2010). Computer-aided diagnosis of pulmonary nodules using a two-step approach for feature selection and classifier ensemble construction. *Artif Intell Med* **50**(1): 43–53.

Lee, Y., T. Hara et al. (2001). Automated detection of pulmonary nodules in helical CT images based on an improved template-matching technique. *IEEE Trans Med Imaging* **20**(7): 595–604.

Li, F., M. Aoyama et al. (2004). Radiologists' performance for differentiating benign from malignant lung nodules on high-resolution CT using computer-estimated likelihood of malignancy. *Am J Roentgenol* **183**(5): 1209–1215.

Li, F., S. Sone et al. (2002). Lung cancers missed at low-dose helical CT screening in a general population: Comparison of clinical, histopathologic, and imaging findings. *Radiology* **225**(3): 673–683.

Li, Q. (2007). Recent progress in computer-aided diagnosis of lung nodules on thin-section CT. *Comput Med Imaging Graph* **31**(4–5): 248–257.

Li, Q., K. Doi (2006a). Analysis and minimization of overtraining effect in rule-based classifiers for computer-aided diagnosis. *Med Phys* **33**(2): 320–328.

Li, Q., K. Doi (2006b). Reduction of bias and variance for evaluation of computer-aided diagnostic schemes. *Med Phys* **33**(4): 868–875.

Li, Q., S. Katsuragawa et al. (2001). Computer-aided diagnostic scheme for lung nodule detection in digital chest radiographs by use of a multiple-template matching technique. *Med Phys* **28**(10): 2070–2076.

Li, Q., F. Li et al. (2003a). Investigation of new psychophysical measures for evaluation of similar images on thoracic computed tomography for distinction between benign and malignant nodules. *Med Phys* **30**(10): 2584–2593.

Li, Q., F. Li et al. (2005). Computer-aided diagnosis in thoracic CT. *Semin Ultrasound CT MRI* **26**(5): 357–363.

Li, Q., F. Li et al. (2008). Computerized detection of lung nodules in thin-section CT images by use of selective enhancement filters and an automated rule-based classifier. *Acad Radiol* **15**(2): 165–175.

Li, Q., S. Sone et al. (2003b). Selective enhancement filters for nodules, vessels, and airway walls in two- and three-dimensional CT scans. *Med Phys* **30**(8): 2040–2051.

Lo, S. B., S. A. Lou et al. (1995). Artificial convolution neural network techniques and applications for lung nodule detection. *IEEE Trans Med Imaging* **14**(4): 711–718.

Marten, K., C. Engelke (2007). Computer-aided detection and automated CT volumetry of pulmonary nodules. *Eur Radiol* **17**(4): 888–901.

Marten, K., C. Engelke et al. (2005). Computer-aided detection of pulmonary nodules: Influence of nodule characteristics on detection performance. *Clin Radiol* **60**(2): 196–206.

Matsuki, Y., K. Nakamura et al. (2002). Usefulness of an artificial neural network for differentiating benign from malignant pulmonary nodules on high-resolution CT: Evaluation with receiver operating characteristic analysis. *Am J Roentgenol* **178**(3): 657–663.

Matsumoto, S., Y. Ohno et al. (2012). Potential contribution of multiplanar reconstruction (MPR) to computer-aided detection of lung nodules on MDCT. *Eur J Radiol* **81**(2): 366–370.

Messay, T., R. C. Hardie et al. (2010). A new computationally efficient CAD system for pulmonary nodule detection in CT imagery. *Med Image Anal* **14**(3): 390–406.

Mori, K., N. Niki et al. (2005). Development of a novel computer-aided diagnosis system for automatic discrimination of malignant from benign solitary pulmonary nodules on thin-section dynamic computed tomography. *J Comput Assist Tomogr* **29**(2): 215–222.

Muramatsu, C., Q. Li et al. (2005). Investigation of psychophysical measure for evaluation of similar images for mammographic masses: Preliminary results. *Med Phys* **32**(7): 2295–2304.

Muramatsu, C., Q. Li et al. (2008). Investigation of psychophysical similarity measures for selection of similar images in the diagnosis of clustered microcalcifications on mammograms. *Med Phys* **35**(12): 5695–5702.

Murphy, K., B. van Ginneken et al. (2009). A large-scale evaluation of automatic pulmonary nodule detection in chest CT using local image features and k-nearest-neighbour classification. *Med Image Anal* **13**(5): 757–770.

Nie, Y., Q. Li et al. (2006). Integrating PET and CT information to improve diagnostic accuracy for lung nodules: A semiautomatic computer-aided method. *J Nucl Med* **47**(7): 1075–1080.

Okada, T., S. Iwano et al. (2009). Computer-aided diagnosis of lung cancer: Definition and detection of ground-glass opacity type of nodules by high-resolution computed tomography. *Jpn J Radiol* **27**(2): 91–99.

Ozekes, S., O. Osman et al. (2008). Nodule detection in a lung region that's segmented with using genetic cellular neural networks and 3D template matching with fuzzy rule based thresholding. *Korean J Radiol* **9**(1): 1–9.

Paik, D. S., C. F. Beaulieu et al. (2004). Surface normal overlap: A computer-aided detection algorithm with application to colonic polyps and lung nodules in helical CT. *IEEE Trans Med Imaging* **23**(6): 661–675.

Park, E. A., J. M. Goo et al. (2009). Efficacy of computer-aided detection system and thin-slab maximum intensity projection technique in the detection of pulmonary nodules in patients with resected metastases. *Invest Radiol* **44**(2): 105–113.

Pu, J., B. Zheng et al. (2008). An automated CT based lung nodule detection scheme using geometric analysis of signed distance field. *Med Phys* **35**(8): 3453–3461.

Reeves, A. P., W. J. Kostis (2000). Computer-aided diagnosis of small pulmonary nodules. *Semin Ultrasound CT MRI* **21**(2): 116–128.

Retico, A., P. Delogu et al. (2008). Lung nodule detection in low-dose and thin-slice computed tomography. *Comput Biol Med* **38**(4): 525–534.

Roos, J. E., D. Paik et al. (2010). Computer-aided detection (CAD) of lung nodules in CT scans: Radiologist performance and reading time with incremental CAD assistance. *Eur Radiol* **20**(3): 549–557.

Rubin, G. D., J. K. Lyo et al. (2005). Pulmonary nodules on multi-detector row CT scans: Performance comparison of radiologists and computer-aided detection. *Radiology* **234**(1): 274–283.

Sahiner, B., H. P. Chan et al. (2009). Effect of CAD on radiologists' detection of lung nodules on thoracic CT scans: Analysis of an observer performance study by nodule size. *Acad Radiol* **16**(12): 1518–1530.

Schilham, A. M., B. van Ginneken et al. (2006). A computer-aided diagnosis system for detection of lung nodules in chest radiographs with an evaluation on a public database. *Med Image Anal* **10**(2): 247–258.

Shah, S. K., M. F. McNitt-Gray et al. (2005a). Solitary pulmonary nodule diagnosis on CT: Results of an observer study. *Acad Radiol* **12**(4): 496–501.

Shah, S. K., M. F. McNitt-Gray et al. (2005b). Computer aided characterization of the solitary pulmonary nodule using volumetric and contrast enhancement features. *Acad Radiol* **12**(10): 1310–1319.

Shiraishi, J., Q. Li et al. (2006). Computer-aided diagnostic scheme for the detection of lung nodules on chest radiographs: Localized search method based on anatomical classification. *Med Phys* **33**(7): 2642–2653.

Sluimer, I., M. Prokop et al. (2005). Toward automated segmentation of the pathological lung in CT. *IEEE Trans Med Imaging* **24**(8): 1025–1038.

Sluimer, I., A. Schilham et al. (2006). Computer analysis of computed tomography scans of the lung: A survey. *IEEE Trans Med Imaging* **25**(4): 385–405.

Sone, S., S. Takashima et al. (1998). Mass screening for lung cancer with mobile spiral computed tomography scanner. *Lancet* **351**(9111): 1242–1245.

Song, K. D., M. J. Chung et al. (2011). Usefulness of the CAD system for detecting pulmonary nodule in real clinical practice. *Korean J Radiol* **12**(2): 163–168.

Suzuki, K., S. G. Armato, 3rd et al. (2003). Massive training artificial neural network (MTANN) for reduction of false positives in computerized detection of lung nodules in low-dose computed tomography. *Med Phys* **30**(7): 1602–1617.

van Ginneken, B., S. G. Armato, 3rd et al. (2010). Comparing and combining algorithms for computer-aided detection of pulmonary nodules in computed tomography scans: The ANODE09 study. *Med Image Anal* **14**(6): 707–722.

Wang, J., R. Engelmann et al. (2007). Segmentation of pulmonary nodules in three-dimensional CT images by use of a spiral-scanning technique. *Med Phys* **34**(12): 4678–4689.

Wang, J., F. Li et al. (2009). Automated segmentation of lungs with severe interstitial lung disease in CT. *Med Phys* **36**(10): 4592–4599.

Way, T., H. P. Chan et al. (2010). Computer-aided diagnosis of lung nodules on CT scans: ROC study of its effect on radiologists' performance. *Acad Radiol* **17**(3): 323–332.

Way, T. W., B. Sahiner et al. (2009). Computer-aided diagnosis of pulmonary nodules on CT scans: Improvement of classification performance with nodule surface features. *Med Phys* **36**(7): 3086–3098.

White, C. S., R. Pugatch et al. (2008). Lung nodule CAD software as a second reader: A multicenter study. *Acad Radiol* **15**(3): 326–333.

Wiemker, R., P. Rogalla et al. (2005). Aspects of computer-aided detection (CAD) and volumetry of pulmonary nodules using multislice CT. *Br J Radiol* **78**(Spec. No. 1): S46–S56.

Xu, X. W., K. Doi et al. (1997). Development of an improved CAD scheme for automated detection of lung nodules in digital chest images. *Med Phys* **24**(9): 1395–1403.

Yanagawa, M., O. Honda et al. (2009). Commercially available computer-aided detection system for pulmonary nodules on thin-section images using 64 detectors-row CT: Preliminary study of 48 cases. *Acad Radiol* **16**(8): 924–933.

Ye, X., X. Lin et al. (2009). Shape-based computer-aided detection of lung nodules in thoracic CT images. *IEEE Trans Biomed Eng* **56**(7): 1810–1820.

Yuan, R., P. M. Vos et al. (2006). Computer-aided detection in screening CT for pulmonary nodules. *Am J Roentgenol* **186**(5): 1280–1287.

Zhao, B., G. Gamsu et al. (2003). Automatic detection of small lung nodules on CT utilizing a local density maximum algorithm. *J Appl Clin Med Phys* **4**(3): 248–260.

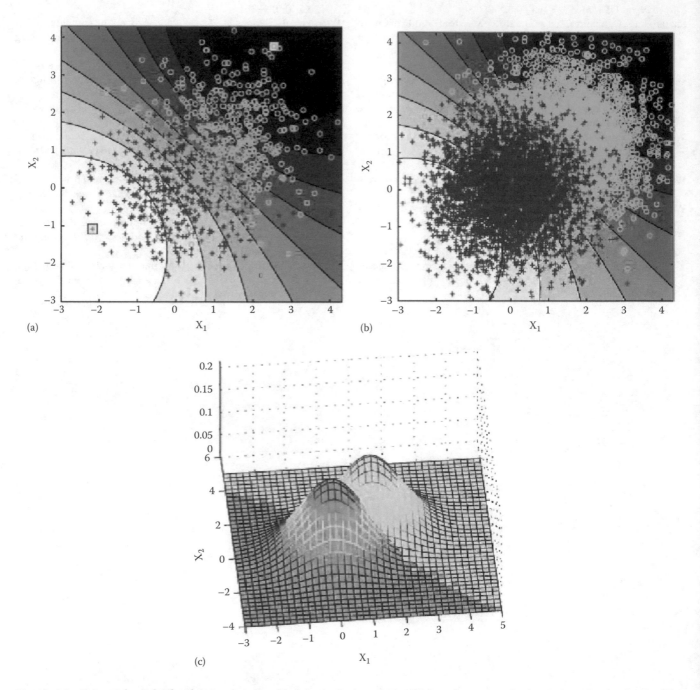

(a)

(b)

(c)

Figure 6.2 Data and results for the simulated problem in Argument 3. The ROC performance of a k-NN classifier for this problem was $A_z = 0.895$ while the optimal performance for this problem is $A_z = 0.90$. (a) Cases from development set (red crosses—positive, green circles—negative, yellow squares—selected by RMHC) and values of the k-NN classifier function based on two cases (contour plot in the background). (b) Cases from test set (red crosses—positive, green circles—negative, yellow squares—selected by RMHC) and values of the k-NN classifier function based on two cases (contour plot in the background). (c) Probability density function for positive (red) and negative (red) classes.

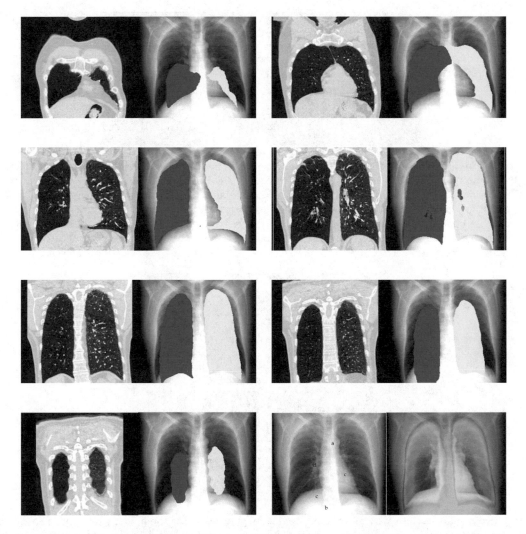

Figure 8.2 Where are the lungs? Seven equally spaced coronal slices are shown with the lungs superimposed on the radiograph simulated from the CT data. It is evident that the unobscured lung fields do not account for all of the lung volume. In the bottom-right image, a color-coding is shown indicating how much lung is behind each pixel in the projection image. In the bottom right figure, the areas indicated with labels a, b, c, d correspond approximately to the depth of 3 cm, 5 cm, 10 cm, and 20 cm, respectively.

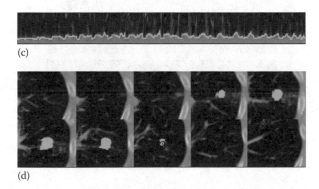

Figure 9.3 Illustration of Wang's method for the segmentation of a nodule with an irregular shape in the LIDC data set: (c) the delineated optimal outline in the transformed 2D image; and (d) the reconstructed nodule volume in the 3D VOI.

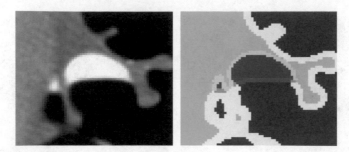

Figure 13.2 Picture on the left shows a portion of a CT slice image where the borders or interfaces between different materials are blurred due to PV effect. By our mixture image segmentation, we are able to detect those interfaces where the percentages of different materials in each image voxel are estimated. The red color shows the pure air material and blue indicates the pure tagged materials (colonic fluid and liquefied stool). The interface space of air and tagged materials are shown by pink/gray colors. The yellow color indicates the interface space of air and colon tissues. The light blue color shows the interface space of tagged materials and colon tissues. The PV layers are accurately identified where the polyps stay. By removing the percentages of non-colon wall materials in those voxels inside the PV layers, we obtain a layer that reflects the colon mucosa structure. An accurate mucosa structure is the key for accurate detection of polyps, especially small ones.

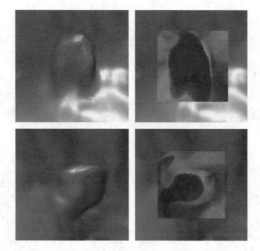

Figure 13.3 An illustration of texture features of small stool balls retained inside the lumen space after routine bowel cleansing. On the left are the endoscopic views, reflecting the geometrical features of the stool balls. On the right are the projections through the stool ball volumes, showing the texture features.

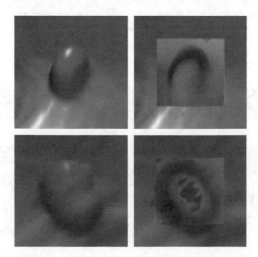

Figure 13.4 An illustration of texture features of small polyps. On the left are the endoscopic views, reflecting the geometrical features of the polyps. On the right are the projections through the polyp volumes. The top row shows a hyperplastic polyp and the bottom row shows an adenoma polyp.

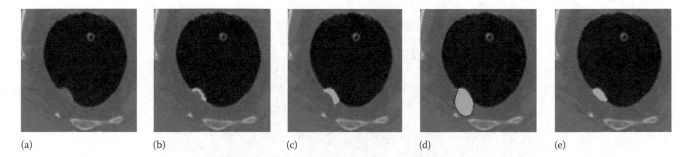

(a)   (b)   (c)   (d)   (e)

Figure 13.5   An experimental study of different VOI determination strategies. (a) A 12 mm sessile polyp in an axial slice, where the voxels in red color indicate the detected suspicious patch. (b) An initial VOI in the slice (including the red and green areas) generated by dilating the detected suspicious patch for a few steps. (c) The result from the previous method in Näppi et al. (2003). (d) The result from the previous method in Wang et al. (2005), where the blue curve represents the inner border found by the Harr transformation–based edge finder. (e) The result from the convex dilation process strategy. (From Zhu, H. et al., *Phys. Biol. Med.*, 55, 2087, 2010.)

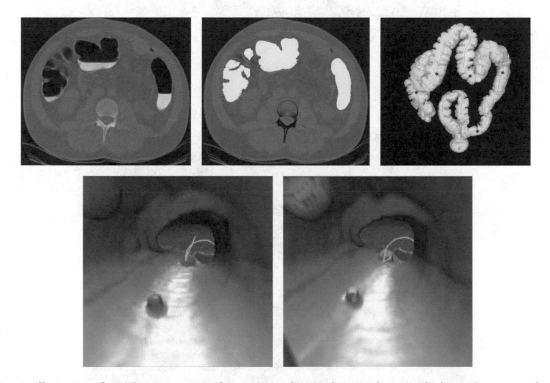

Figure 13.11   An illustration of a CADe system using the commercial V3D colon visualization platform. The top row shows the information processing from data acquisition (left) and image segmentation/ECC (middle) to colon model construction. On the bottom left is an endoscopic view inside the constructed colon model for polyp detection by human observer or radiologist. A CADe system or computer observer detects polyp candidates at their associated locations on the inner border of the colon model. The CADe output can be visualized by coloring the detected polyp candidates at their associated locations (bottom right).

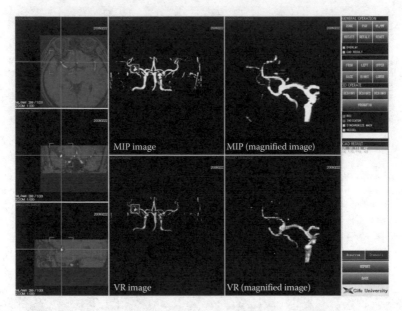

Figure 15.5   Illustration of a prototype CAD scheme for the detection of unruptured aneurysms.

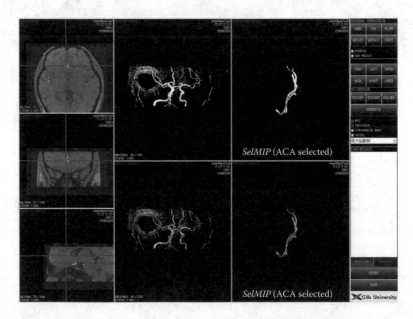

Figure 15.8   Illustration of *SelMIP* images.

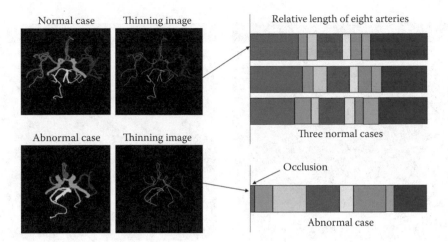

Figure 15.9 Relative lengths of the eight arteries obtained from three normal cases and one abnormal case with arterial occlusion. (From Yamauchi, M. et al., *SPIE Proc.*, 6514, 65142C-1, 2007.)

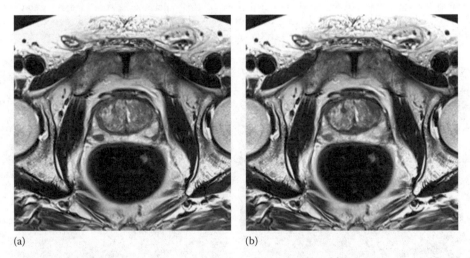

Figure 18.5 Demonstration of using blobness as a feature to detect prostate cancer. (a) Response of a multiscale blobness filter on the peripheral zone in a T2 MR image. (b) The image represents the same filter, but the response is restricted to the transition zone. A cancer is present in the left side of the images within the peripheral zone. These images show that such a feature is able to distinguish cancer from normal tissue.

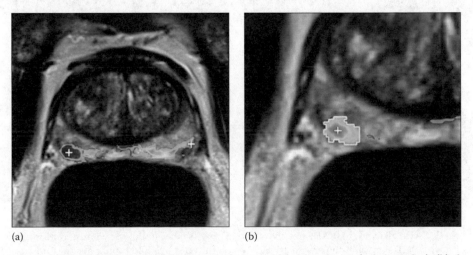

Figure 18.6 (a) The output (+) of a local maxima detection on the initial likelihood map (color overlay), (b) the results (yellow solid outline) of a bounded region-growing segmentation using the local maximum as a seed point.

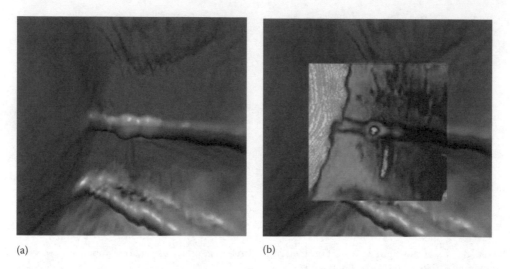

Figure 25.4 CADe reader FP caused by a small focus of tagged stool. (a) CADe detected a small raised area caused by stool on a fold. In the translucency view (b), a color map of the HU distribution shows central white consistent with tagged stool. This should have been recognized by the reader. Stool may be correctly identified by internal gas, tagging, or movement when comparing supine and prone views.

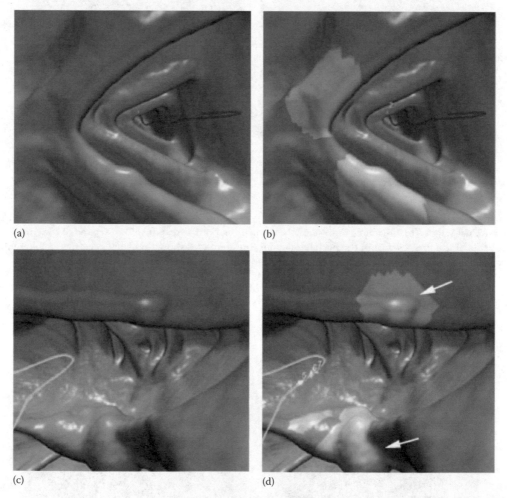

Figure 25.5 Top panel (a) (CADe off) and (b) (CADe on) show two FP marks on a shallow or <5 mm diminutive foci. The bottom panel ((c) with CADe off and (d) with CADe on) show a true-positive polyp on the apex of a fold (upper arrow) and fatty ileocecal valve (lower arrow).

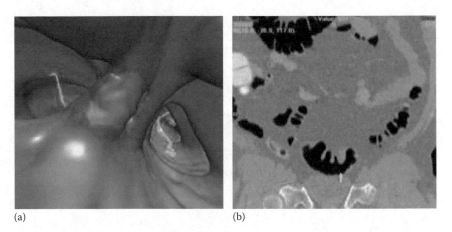

(a)   (b)

Figure 25.6 CADe FP caused by *flexural pseudotumor*. (a) Endoluminal view and (b) coronal 2D view show (arrow) a prominent fold mimicking a polyp at the inside of a sharp turn in the sigmoid colon. Note how all the adjacent folds appear thinner and normal.

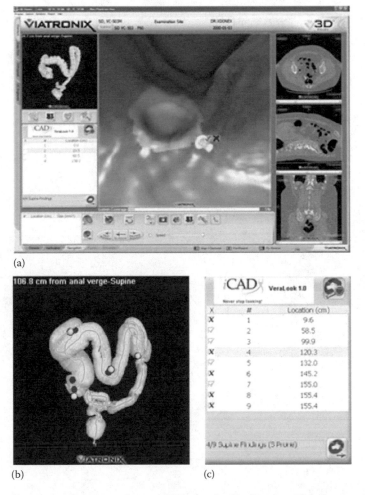

(a)

(b)   (c)

Figure 25.7 (a) CADe integrated into visualization software. CADe marks displayed as *Blue Caps* on the virtual colon wall in the 3D view. The green checkmark and red "X" marks displayed near each CADe mark in the 3D view enable users to accept or reject CADe marks as polyps. CADe marks are displayed as yellow circles on image slices in the 2D views. (b) CADe marks are displayed as yellow circles on the *full colon* view. (c) CADe findings are numbered and displayed in a list that indicates the distance from the anal verge and whether or not each CADe mark has been accepted or rejected as a polyp. The icon to the right of the logo enables users to toggle CADe marks on/off (defaulted off), as does the "C" key on the keyboard.

Chapter 10

Detection and Diagnosis of Interstitial Lung Disease

Shigehiko Katsuragawa, Takayuki Ishida, Kazuto Ashizawa, and Yoshikazu Uchiyama

CONTENTS

10.1 INTRODUCTION

Interstitial lung disease is a common clinical entity. Approximately 22% of lung abnormalities seen in chest radiographs at the University of Chicago Medical Center are due to interstitial abnormalities. Interstitial disease is defined as an abnormality of the interstitial compartments of the lung, which may be due to infiltration by inflammatory or neoplastic cells or may be a consequence of the accumulation of fluid or proteinaceous material (Genereux 1985). Despite of a common clinical entity, evaluation of interstitial lung diseases on chest radiographs and computed tomography (CT) images is considered a difficult task for radiologists. This is partly because interstitial diseases create numerous radiographic patterns to which we refer as lung textures that are generally ill-defined and that include complex variations. Therefore, if reliable quantitative measures of the lung textures related to interstitial diseases could be obtained from chest radiographs and CT images, it is likely that the accuracy and reproducibility in the evaluation of interstitial diseases could be improved.

Though CT technologies have advanced at a remarkable pace in recent years, chest radiography has played an important role for the evaluation of interstitial diseases because of low radiation exposure, low cost, and capacity to examine a wide image area at once. Therefore, we present computerized methods for the detection of interstitial diseases in chest radiographs by using a lung texture analysis and a geometric-pattern feature analysis as the first topic of this chapter. The texture analysis employed measures based on the power spectrum of the underlying lung textures that are related to interstitial diseases. In the geometric-pattern feature analysis, quantitative features related to the shape of interstitial infiltrates were extracted from chest radiographs.

The second topic of this chapter is an application of artificial neural networks (ANNs) for the differential diagnosis of interstitial lung diseases in chest radiographs. The ANNs were designed to distinguish between 11 interstitial lung diseases on the basis of 10 clinical parameters and 16 radiologic findings extracted by chest radiologists. As the final topic of this chapter, a quantitative analysis of diffuse lung diseases on high-resolution computed tomography (HRCT) images is presented by using physical measures on HRCT images in order to detect and characterize diffuse lung diseases.

10.2   COMPUTERIZED DETECTION OF INTERSTITIAL LUNG DISEASE IN CHEST RADIOGRAPHS

10.2.1   Lung Texture Analysis

The lung textures of interstitial diseases indicate particular patterns such as coarse and/or large variation of optical density on chest radiographs. Therefore, many investigators have attempted to develop computerized methods based on a lung texture analysis for the detection of interstitial lung diseases in chest radiographs. In the 1970s, investigators have been searching for an automated means of detecting and quantifying the severity of coal workers' pneumoconiosis as well as other forms of pulmonary infiltrates by using a computerized analysis of chest radiographs. Sutton and colleagues devised measures based on the statistical properties of the density distribution on a chest radiograph in order to differentiate a normal lung from a lung with pulmonary fibrosis (Sutton and Hall 1972). Kruger and colleagues attempted to classify coal workers' pneumoconiosis on radiographs by using two methods: one was a statistical approach in which they used 60 texture measures based on point-to-point variations in gray levels, and the other was based on an analysis of the optical Fourier spectrum (Kruger et al. 1974). Tully et al. (1978) used the

same statistical method to classify normal lungs, alveolar infiltrates, and interstitial infiltrates. Revesz and colleagues (1973) obtained the power spectrum of the lung texture by using the optical Fourier transform in order to distinguish between normal lungs and lungs with interstitial disease. Jagoe (1979) employed a method of coding the texture patterns in terms of the directions of the gray-level gradient vector, which was determined by sampling of the chest radiograph at 1.2 mm intervals, to investigate the severity of pneumoconiosis. These previous attempts to use computer analysis of lung texture for the diagnosis of interstitial disease have not been widely accepted, because digital imaging systems were not installed in many hospitals in the 1970s.

In the 1980s, new studies aimed at a computer-aided diagnosis (CAD) for the detection of interstitial diseases in digital chest radiographs were started with the widespread use of digital imaging systems in many hospitals. Katsuragawa and colleagues (1988, 1989) developed a computerized method for the detection and characterization of interstitial diseases in chest radiographs by using texture measures. Kido and colleagues (1995) obtained fractal dimensions of linear opacities extracted by using a Laplacian–Gaussian filter in order to differentiate between normal and abnormal lungs with interstitial diseases in chest radiographs. van Ginneken and colleagues (2002) attempted to find abnormal signs of a diffuse textural nature on chest radiographs by using texture features determined from the moments of responses to a multiscale filter bank.

In this section, we describe a computerized method that employs physical texture measures determined from the power spectrum of the lung texture in order to detect and characterize interstitial diseases in chest radiographs (Katsuragawa et al. 1988, 1989, 1990a,b).

10.2.1.1   Overall Scheme of Texture Analysis
The overall scheme of our approach to the texture analysis is described briefly here (Katsuragawa et al. 1988, 1990b). First, a large number (300–500) of square regions of interest (ROIs) with a 32×32 matrix size (5.6 mm × 5.6 mm area) were automatically selected in the peripheral lung regions, as shown in Figure 10.1 (Chen et al. 1993). The nonuniform background trend in each ROI was corrected by means of a 2D surface fitting technique in order to determine the fluctuating patterns of the underlying lung texture for subsequent computer analysis. The power spectrum of the lung texture was obtained from the 2D Fourier transform and was filtered by the visual system response of the human observer. Finally, the root-mean-square (rms) variation, R, and the first moment of the power spectrum, M,

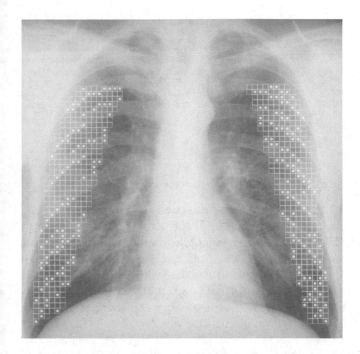

Figure 10.1 Selection of ROIs with a 5.6 mm × 5.6 mm matrix size for the lung texture analysis. ROIs are selected automatically in the peripheral regions by the elimination of some ROIs containing sharp rib edges that are marked by white dots.

were determined as quantitative texture measures for the magnitude and coarseness (or fineness), respectively, of the lung texture. These texture measures are defined as follows:

$$R = \sqrt{\iint_{-\infty}^{\infty} V^2(u,v)T^2(u,v)\,dudv} \,, \qquad (10.1)$$

$$M = \frac{\iint_{-\infty}^{\infty} \sqrt{u^2+v^2}\,V^2(u,v)T^2(u,v)\,dudv}{\iint_{-\infty}^{\infty} V^2(u,v)T^2(u,v)\,dudv}, \qquad (10.2)$$

where $V(u, v)$ and $T(u, v)$ correspond to the visual system response and the Fourier transform of the lung texture, respectively.

10.2.1.2 Image Database

An image database of chest radiographs used in this study included 100 normal cases and 100 abnormal cases with various interstitial diseases. These cases were selected by an experienced chest radiologist, over a period of time, from the clinical caseload. Each normal case was chosen on the basis of an unequivocally normal radiograph in a patient without clinically suspected cardiopulmonary disease.

Abnormal cases with interstitial infiltrates, which ranged from mild to severe, and included various etiologies, were selected based on the radiographic findings, together with clinical or biopsy data, and radiographic follow-up. All chest radiographs in the image database were exposed at 125 kV with a 12:1 grid, using Ortho-C films and Lanex medium screens (Eastman Kodak, Rochester, NY). Films were digitized using a laser scanner (KFDR-S; Konica, Tokyo, Japan) with a pixel size of 0.175 mm (2000 × 2430 matrix size) and a 10-bit gray scale (1024 gray levels).

10.2.1.3 Nonuniform Background Trend

The variation in optical density observed in the lung field includes two types: that due to the gross anatomy of the lung and chest wall (background trend) and that due to the fine underlying texture that is related to interstitial disease. Thus, it is important to isolate underlying density fluctuations from the actual overall lung texture. This preprocessing of chest radiographs is essential to derive sensitive measures of physical texture for the detection and characterization of interstitial lung disease. We estimated the background trend in a selected ROI by using a 2D surface fitting technique based on the least-squares method with a second-order polynomial. The effect of the background trend correction is demonstrated in Figure 10.2. The original image shown in Figure 10.2a is selected from a lower left portion of an abnormal lung, and it includes a large amount of background trend that is superimposed on a fluctuating pattern that represents the lung texture. Without the trend correction, the rms variation in this image is 26.6 pixel values. The trend corrected image in Figure 10.2b was obtained by subtraction of the background trend from the original image. After the trend correction, the overall background appears to be quite uniform. With this correction, the rms variation is reduced to 14.4 pixel values. This result clearly indicates that the background trend strongly affects the rms variation and that the rms variation of the underlying fluctuating pattern due to the lung texture can differ significantly from that of the fluctuating pattern seen in the original uncorrected chest image.

10.2.1.4 Filtering of Power Spectrum

The power spectra of lungs in a chest radiograph contain large low-frequency components, probably due to some residual uncorrected background trend. In addition, the power spectra include some components of very high frequencies due to radiographic mottle in the original chest radiograph. In order to suppress these unwanted components and to enhance the midfrequency components related to inherent lung texture, we chose to employ the visual system response of human observers, which filters

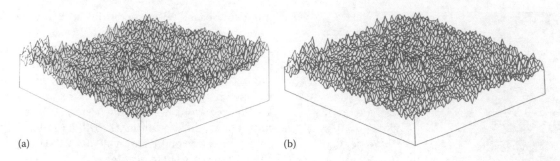

Figure 10.2 Demonstration of nonuniform background trend: (a) original image and (b) trend-corrected image.

the power spectrum (Chan et al. 1985). An equation of the visual system response is given by the following equation:

$$V(u,v) = \exp\left(-\frac{\left\{\ln\sqrt{u^2+v^2} - \ln\left(25\sqrt{u_0^2+v_0^2}\Big/D\right)\right\}^2}{2(0.973)^2}\right),$$

(10.3)

where u_0 and v_0 are the spatial frequencies with a maximum value of $V(u, v)$ at a viewing distance, D, of 25 cm. The filtered power spectra of the normal and abnormal lungs when the visual system response is used are shown in Figure 10.3.

10.2.1.5 Texture Measures for Typical Interstitial Infiltrates

The texture analysis was applied for four typical cases of one normal and three abnormal lungs with nodular, reticular, and honeycomb patterns as shown in Figure 10.4. The distribution of the texture measures obtained from ROIs selected in the four lungs is shown in Figure 10.5. The ellipse indicates the expected range (±1 standard deviation [SD]) of texture measures for the average normal lung, determined from 100 normal chest radiographs in the image database. The nodular pattern tends to have a low-frequency content, and its rms variation is slightly larger than that of the normal lung; the reticular pattern tends to have a large rms variation, and its frequency content is similar to that of the normal lung; and the honeycomb pattern tends to have a large rms variation and a low-frequency content. These results indicate that

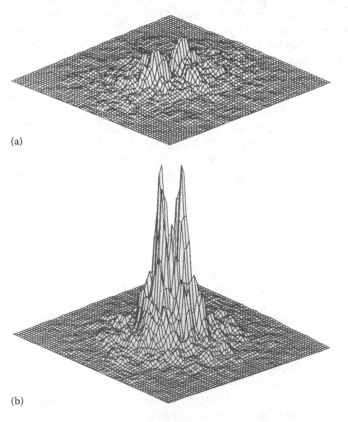

Figure 10.3 Power spectra filtered by the visual system response of human observers: (a) normal lung and (b) abnormal lung.

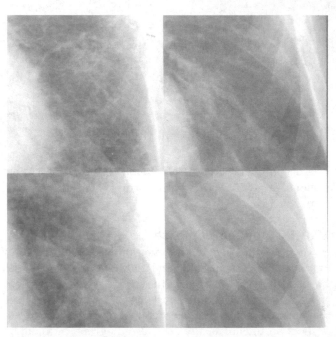

Figure 10.4 Chest radiographs of a normal lung (lower right) and abnormal lung with nodular (lower left), reticular (upper right), and honeycomb (upper left) patterns.

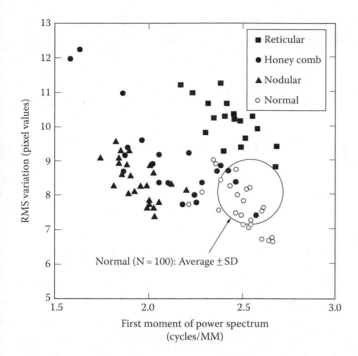

Figure 10.5 The distribution of texture measures obtained from ROIs selected in the four lungs illustrated in Figure 10.4.

the two texture measures can distinguish relatively obvious texture patterns in these abnormal lungs.

10.2.1.6 Computerized Classification of Normal and Abnormal Lungs

For subsequent computerized classification for the distinction between normal and abnormal lungs, the two texture measures R and M, which are obtained from a given chest image, are normalized by means of the average and the SD of texture measures determined from normal lungs that are included in the database:

$$R_N = \frac{R - \bar{R}}{\sigma_R}, \qquad (10.4)$$

$$M_N = \frac{M - \bar{M}}{\sigma_M}, \qquad (10.5)$$

where

R_N and M_N are the normalized rms variation and the normalized first moment of the power spectrum, respectively

$\bar{R}$ and $\bar{M}$ are the average values

σ_R and σ_M are the SDs obtained from normal lungs included in the image database

Based on the distribution features of texture measures for abnormal lungs with nodular, reticular, and honeycomb

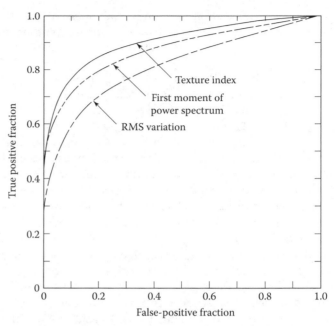

Figure 10.6 ROC curves for distinction between normal and abnormal lungs by the computerized method based on the rms variation, the first moment of the power spectrum, and the single texture index.

patterns as mentioned earlier, we formulated a single texture index, T, in order to facilitate the computerized classification as follows:

$$T = R_N \quad \text{for } M_N > 0 \text{ and } R_N > 0, \qquad (10.6)$$

$$T = \sqrt{M_N^2 + R_N^2} \quad \text{for } M_N < 0 \text{ and } R_N > 0, \qquad (10.7)$$

$$T = -M_N \quad \text{for } M_N < 0 \text{ and } R_N < 0, \qquad (10.8)$$

$$T = -\left[\text{Min}\left(M_N, |R_N| \right) \right] \quad \text{for } M_N > 0 \text{ and } R_N < 0. \quad (10.9)$$

The usefulness of the single texture index is demonstrated in Figure 10.6 by using receiver operating characteristic (ROC) curves that can represent the performance of the classification for the distinction between normal and abnormal lungs (Katsuragawa et al. 1989). The result indicates clearly that the single texture index is superior to either the normalized rms variation or the normalized first moment of the power spectrum in the automated classification of lung textures.

10.2.2 Geometric-Pattern Feature Analysis

In order to further improve the detection accuracy of interstitial infiltrates on chest radiographs, we have developed a geometric-pattern feature analysis method (Katsuragawa et al. 1996, Ishida et al. 1997). The geometric-pattern feature analysis can detect and evaluate the shape and size of interstitial infiltrates by extracting *area components* and *line components*, which are major components of interstitial infiltrates.

10.2.2.1 Initial Removal of Rib Edges and Background Trend Correction

First, approximately 34 ROIs were selected automatically with a 128×128 matrix size (22.4×22.4 mm^2), covering most of the peripheral lung regions. The Sobel operation (Rosenfeld and Kak 1982) was performed on the selected ROIs. The rib edges on the Sobel output image were detected by using a thresholding technique. Detected edges with small areas of less than 100 pixels (3.06 mm^2) were not considered to be rib edges. Detected rib edges were dilated by a morphological filter.

The nonuniform background trend was corrected by use of a 2D surface fitting technique with sixth-order polynomials (Katsuragawa et al. 1988). If an ROI included high-contrast edges, the 2D surface fitting function obtained with the least-squares method could oscillate near the edges. Therefore, the trend correction was made after initial rib edges had been removed.

10.2.2.2 Detection of Area and Line Components

To detect area components, a gray-level thresholding technique was applied to trend-corrected ROIs. The borders of all detected components were smoothed by morphological open and close filtering (Yoshimura et al. 1992). We determined the relative SD of the edge orientation histogram of all detected components for distinguishing between rib edges and other area components. After elimination of false positives by feature analysis, the ratio of the total area of area components to the area of the ROIs was determined as one of the geometric-pattern measures.

Line components were extracted by applying a line enhancement filter to the trend-corrected ROIs. The line enhancement filter has eight sets of three templates in eight different directions, as shown in Figure 10.7. Each set consists of three parallel templates with an interval between adjacent templates. The output value of the line enhancement filter is defined as follows:

$$E_i = 2B_i - A_i - C_i \quad \text{when } B_i > A_i \text{ and } B_i > C_i, \quad (10.10)$$

$$E_i = 0 \quad \text{otherwise,} \quad (10.11)$$

$$E = \max\{E_i\}, \quad i = 1,2,3,4,5,6,7,8, \quad (10.12)$$

where

A_i, B_i, and C_i are the summation of all pixel values in each template of a set

E_i is the output from one of the eight sets in different directions

The maximum value, E, from the outputs of the sets is the final output value of the line enhancement filter. A candidate of the line component is then identified when the output value of the line enhancement filter is larger than a predetermined threshold level. The detected line components overlapping the initially detected rib edges or the removed area components due to rib edges were eliminated. Finally, the ratio of the total length (number of pixels) of line components to the total number of pixels in an ROI was determined as another geometric-pattern measure.

10.2.2.3 Elimination of False Positives by Feature Analysis

To eliminate false area components, we evaluated the SD of the edge gradient–weighted edge orientation histogram and the area of all detected area components. The relative

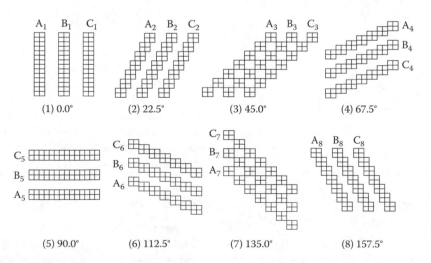

Figure 10.7 Line enhancement filter.

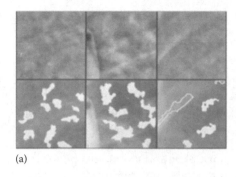
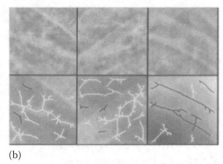

(a)   (b)

Figure 10.8   Detected (a) area components and (b) line components.

SD of the gradient-weighted edge orientation histogram is equal to the SD of accumulated edge gradients within the area of an area component relative to the average edge gradient, where the histogram represents accumulated edge gradients as a function of the orientation of edge gradient (Chen et al. 1993). The relative SD of the edge gradient–weighted edge orientation histogram can signify the magnitude of the variation in the histogram. Figure 10.8a shows detected area components and eliminated rib edges in three abnormal ROIs. ROIs on the top are trend-corrected images. In ROIs on the bottom, the detected area components and eliminated area components (as false positives) are indicated by white solid patterns and white contours, respectively.

False line components due to rib edges tend to be detected as long lines that produce sharp peaks in their edge orientation histogram. We used two features to remove false line components, namely, the relative SD of the edge orientation histogram obtained over the detected line component and the degree of linearity, which is defined by the ratio of the longest Euclidean distance to the total number of pixels over the detected line component. Figure 10.8b shows detected line components. The white lines and black lines indicate detected line components and eliminated components as false positives, respectively. Thus, the total area of area components and the total length of line components of each ROI are determined.

10.2.2.4 Classification by Geometric-Pattern Feature Analysis

For the evaluation of the classification performance, we randomly divided our image database into two sets. One set (50 normal cases and 50 abnormal cases) was used for training and another for testing. We partitioned the database into training and testing sets for 10 times. An ROC curve was obtained by averaging of 10 ROC curves derived from 10 different partitions of datasets.

The rule-based method alone, an ANN method alone, and a rule-based plus ANN method were employed for distinguishing between normal lungs and abnormal lungs with interstitial infiltrates. With the rule-based method, we determined the ratio of the number of abnormal ROIs to the total number of ROIs for distinction between normal lungs and abnormal lungs with interstitial disease. When the fraction of abnormal ROIs is greater than a threshold level, the chest image will be identified as abnormal lung. With the ANN method, an ANN was trained by entering the histogram of geometric-pattern features as input data. The output from the ANN represents the classification result (0: normal and 1: abnormal). For the rule-based plus ANN method, first, the rule-based method is applied for determination of *obviously normal* and *obviously abnormal* lungs. Then, the ANN is applied for the classification of the remaining *uncertain difficult cases*.

ROC curves obtained with several classification schemes (Monnier-Cholley et al. 1995, Katsuragawa et al. 1997) are shown in Figure 10.9. The ROC curve obtained with geometric-pattern feature analysis was better than that obtained with texture analysis. The combined rule-based approach

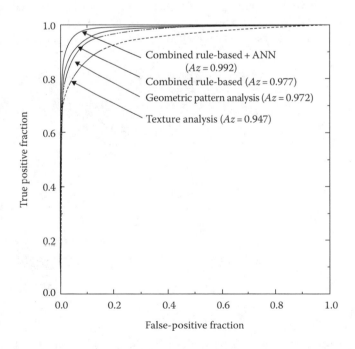

Figure 10.9   ROC curves obtained with various classification schemes.

was slightly better than that by geometric-pattern analysis. However, when we employed a rule-based method and the ANN, the overall performance was improved considerably, as indicated by a high Az value (0.992). The three-layer feedforward ANN, which trained by the histogram of texture index and/or geometric-pattern index for each image, was used for classification.

10.2.3 Effect of Computerized Analysis on Radiologists' Performance

We carried out an observer performance test to assess the effect of the computerized scheme for the detection of pulmonary interstitial infiltrates on radiologists' interpretations of chest radiographs by using ROC analysis (Monnier-Cholley et al. 1998). Twenty chest radiographs with normal findings and twenty chest radiographs with interstitial opacities were used in the test. The 20 normal radiographs were randomly selected from the image database of 100 cases with normal findings. The patients ranged in age from 16 to 82 years (mean ± SD, 37 ± 16 years). Normality was determined by two radiologists on the basis of unequivocally normal radiographs, clinical data (no suspected cardiopulmonary disease), and follow-up chest radiographs when available. The 20 abnormal radiographs were also selected from the image database of 100 cases with interstitial infiltrates on the basis of radiologic findings, clinical data, and follow-up chest radiographs. The patients ranged in age from 18 to 89 years (mean ± SD, 56 ± 19 years). In the absence of a CT scan, the presence of an interstitial opacity on a radiograph was confirmed by consensus of a panel of four

independent chest radiologists. The 20 abnormal radiographs included 15 subtle cases and five cases of more obvious disease. The interstitial diseases included miliary tuberculosis ($n = 3$), sarcoidosis ($n = 5$), silicosis ($n = 1$), interstitial pulmonary edema ($n = 2$), systemic sclerosis ($n = 1$), and indeterminate causes ($n = 8$). Each radiograph was divided into four quadrants (upper right, lower right, upper left, and lower left). When complete consensus was not reached by the panel as to whether a quadrant was normal or abnormal, this quadrant was designated indeterminate and removed from the database. Thirty-one quadrants in the abnormal cases were excluded because they were considered by one or more panel members to be equivocal. One hundred and twenty-nine quadrants (80 normal and 49 abnormal) were used for the observer performance testing.

The computer results obtained from the texture analysis were indicated on a chest image by superimposing various markers illustrating the normal and abnormal ROIs as shown in Figure 10.10. A plus symbol indicates a normal texture pattern. A square represents a predominantly reticular pattern (corresponding to large rms variation). A circle indicates a predominantly nodular pattern (corresponding to low first moment of the power spectrum). A triangle indicates a mixed pattern (corresponding to large rms variation and low first moment). The symbols have three possible sizes, with larger sizes indicating greater degrees of abnormality. The size was determined by the relative value of the texture index compared with the threshold level.

Sixteen observers, including ten residents and six attending radiologists, took part in the test. The observers were

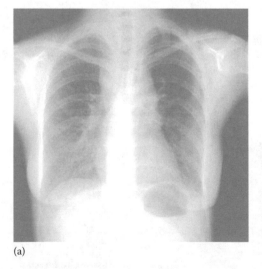

(a)

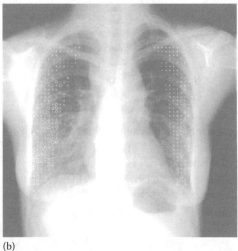

(b)

Figure 10.10   Computer results of the lung texture analysis: (a) chest image with diffuse interstitial infiltrates and (b) markers representing the types of patterns of interstitial infiltrates. A square, a circle, and a triangle correspond to reticular, nodular, and mixed patterns, respectively. The size of each marker indicates the degree of abnormality.

asked to rate each quadrant separately with regard to the presence or absence of an interstitial infiltrate. They used a continuous (0–100) rating scale on which zero indicated complete confidence that the lung was normal and 100 indicated complete confidence that at least 50% of the area of the quadrant in question showed an interstitial infiltrate. Neither scoring of severity was included in the rating scale, nor was any time limit for image interpretation imposed.

The test was designed to minimize potential bias due to reading order and learning effects. The observers were shown original films with patient identifiers masked. Every radiograph was interpreted twice by each observer during two separate sessions: once alone and once together with the result of the computerized analysis. The computer result showed the superimposed markers illustrating the normal and abnormal ROIs but did not specify the final computer classification (normal or abnormal). The two sessions were separated by at least 2 weeks so that recall bias was minimized. The ROC curves were obtained by using Metz's LABROC4 algorithm. The statistical significance of the difference between the Az value of the area under the ROC curve with and without the computer results was evaluated by a Student's two-tailed t-test for paired data.

The average ROC curves for the detection of interstitial infiltrates are shown in Figure 10.11. The Az value of all observers improved significantly when the computer results were available (0.948 versus 0.970, $P = 0.0002$). The detection performance of this computerized scheme was slightly below that of the radiologists, as evidenced by the somewhat smaller Az value (0.943 versus 0.948). However, most radiologists improved their diagnostic performance with the help of the computer result probably because false-positive and false-negative results tend to differ for the observers and the computer. Therefore, the result of the observer performance test indicates that the computerized scheme with the texture analysis can assist radiologists for the detection of interstitial diseases on chest radiographs.

10.3 COMPUTERIZED DIAGNOSIS OF INTERSTITIAL LUNG DISEASE IN CHEST RADIOGRAPHS

10.3.1 Application of Neural Network for Differential Diagnosis

The differential diagnosis of interstitial lung diseases in chest radiography is a difficult task for radiologists because of the similarity of radiologic patterns and the complexity of clinical parameters. The aim of CAD for the differential diagnosis of interstitial lung diseases is to provide the likelihood measure for each disease for the identification of interstitial lung disease among many possible diseases.

We applied a three-layer, feed-forward ANN with a back-propagation algorithm to determine the likelihood measure of each of 11 diseases (Asada et al. 1990, Ashizawa et al. 1999a, Abe et al. 2002). These 11 diseases, sarcoidosis, miliary tuberculosis, lymphangitis carcinomatosa, interstitial lung edema, silicosis, *Pneumocystis carinii* (*jiroveci*) pneumonia, scleroderma, eosinophilic granuloma, idiopathic pulmonary fibrosis, viral pneumonia, and pulmonary drug toxicity, were selected because they include most of the common interstitial lung diseases. Ten clinical parameters and sixteen subjective ratings of radiologic findings for each case were selected as input units by three chest radiologists independently, as shown in Figure 10.12. The ANN had 11 output units, which corresponded to 11 interstitial lung diseases to be identified. The output values of the ANN ranged from 0 to 1.0, which corresponds to the likelihood of each of the 11 possible diseases.

We used a round-robin method to determine ANN performance for each of the three databases including 110 hypothetical cases, 110 published cases, and 150 actual clinical cases. With this method, all but one case in each database was used for training, and the one case left out was used to test the trained ANN. The Az values with

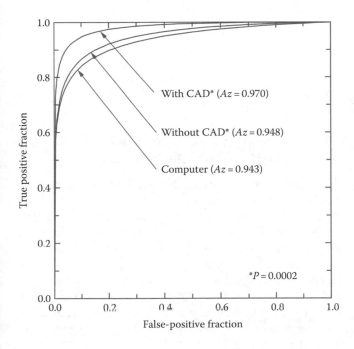

Figure 10.11 ROC curves for the detection of interstitial infiltrates by radiologists with and without CAD. ROC curves showed a significant improvement in the radiologists' detection accuracy with CAD output images. Note that the detection performance of the computerized scheme was slightly below that of the radiologists alone.

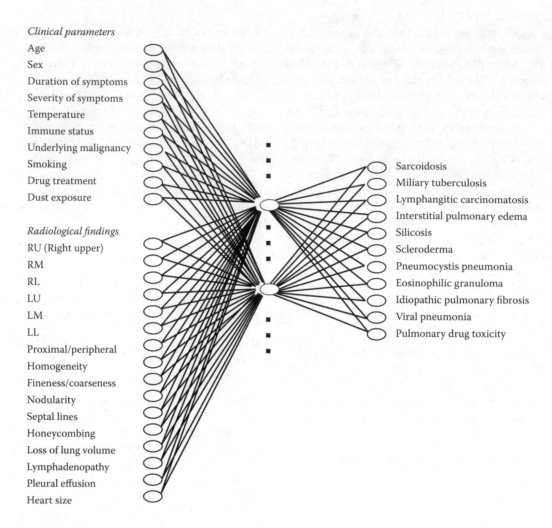

Figure 10.12   Structure of ANN for differential diagnosis of interstitial lung diseases.

hypothetical cases, published cases, and actual clinical cases by using ROC analysis were 0.938, 0.955, and 0.933, respectively. These results seem to indicate that ANN can consistently learn certain unique patterns associated with each disease in each of the three databases. To evaluate the overall performance of the ANN in distinguishing the actual clinical cases, we used a modified round-robin method. In this method, although a round-robin method was applied to all databases for training, only actual clinical cases were used for testing. The Az values for each disease ranged from 0.88 to 1.00, and the average Az value for the 11 diseases was 0.947. This Az value was higher than that obtained with the round-robin method in actual clinical cases alone ($Az = 0.933$). This result may indicate that hypothetical cases and published cases provided useful training data to improve the ANN performance in actual clinical cases. The ANN in this study can be trained to differentiate among 11 interstitial lung diseases.

10.3.2 Effect of Neural Network on Radiologists' Performance

An observer performance study with ROC analysis was carried out for investigation of the effect of the ANN outputs such as those shown in Figure 10.13b, on the radiologists' performance for the differential diagnosis of interstitial lung diseases (Ashizawa et al. 1999b). Thirty-three actual clinical cases (three cases per disease) were employed in this observer study. ROC analysis of the output values for the ANN found an Az value of 0.977 for the 33 cases (Figure 10.14). Eight radiologists who attended this observer study evaluated interstitial lung diseases on chest radiographs first without and then with the ANN output. The ROC curves indicate that the radiologists' performance in the differential diagnosis of interstitial lung diseases was improved ($P < 0.0001$) from an Az of 0.826–0.911 by use of the ANN output, as shown in Figure 10.14. This result suggests that the ANN can assist radiologists in the differential diagnosis of

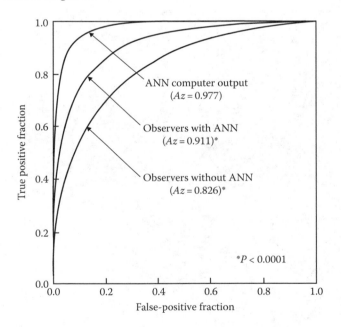

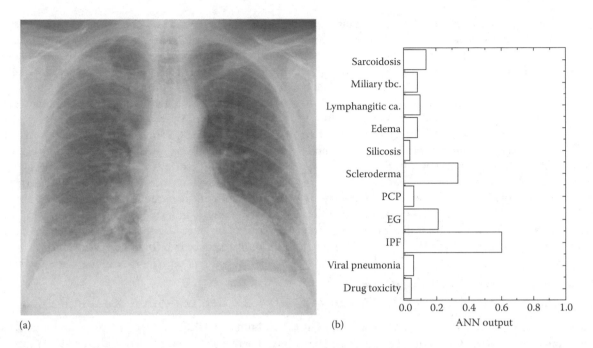

(a)

(b)

ANN output

Figure 10.13 Chest radiograph and computer outputs for the differential diagnosis of interstitial lung diseases: (a) chest radiograph with idiopathic pulmonary fibrosis and (b) corresponding ANN outputs. The largest output value among 11 diseases corresponds to the correct diagnosis.

ANN outputs. Therefore, when radiologists become familiar with the ANN outputs, their performance in the differential diagnosis of interstitial lung diseases might be increased further in the future.

10.4 COMPUTERIZED DETECTION OF INTERSTITIAL LUNG DISEASE IN CT

The differential diagnosis of diffuse lung diseases is a major subject in HRCT. However, it is considered a difficult task for radiologists, partly because of the complexity and variation in diffuse disease patterns on HRCT images and also because of the subjective terms used for describing diffuse lung diseases. Therefore, the goal of CAD scheme for diffuse lung diseases is to assist radiologists' image interpretation as a *second opinion*. A number of investigators (Uchiyama et al. 2003, Xu et al. 2006, Fetita et al. 2007, Park et al. 2009, 2011, Wang et al. 2009a) have attempted to develop CAD schemes for computerized detection and characterization of diffuse lung diseases using various methods and techniques. For example, Xu et al. (2006) developed a classification method of normal and three abnormal patterns using a support vector machine with 24 volumetric features, including statistical features, histogram, and fractal features. Wang et al. (2009a) employed statistical texture features such as run-length and co-occurrence matrix features to distinguish abnormal from normal lung. In order to explore a basis for selecting similar images to assist

Figure 10.14 ROC curves for the differential diagnosis of interstitial lung diseases on chest radiographs for ANN output alone and for all observers without and with ANN output.

interstitial lung diseases on chest radiographs. However, it should be noted that the Az for all radiologists with the ANN output (Az = 0.911) was considerably lower than that obtained with the ANN output alone (Az = 0.977). This result seems to reflect a lack of radiologists' experience with the radiologists' interpretation, Li et al. (2009) investigated the subjective similarity for pairs of images with various abnormal patterns of diffuse interstitial lung disease on CT images.

In this section, quantitative analysis of diffuse lung diseases on HRCT image is presented using a CAD scheme developed at the University of Chicago (Uchiyama et al. 2003). In this initial study, physical measures on HRCT images were determined in order to detect and characterize diffuse lung diseases, which will be the basis for application to the differential diagnosis of diffuse lung diseases in the future. The physical measures of normal slices were compared with those of abnormal slices, which included six typical patterns of diffuse lung diseases. The classification performance was also investigated for distinction between normal and abnormal slices.

10.4.1 *Gold Standard* for Normal and Abnormal Patterns on HRCT Images

It is important to establish reliable cases with typical normal and abnormal patterns, which will be used as *gold standard*, because the subjective terms and judgments by radiologists have generally been used to describe diffuse lung diseases.

The observer study was carried out to select areas with abnormal patterns as the *gold standard*. The database consisted of 315 HRCT images selected from 105 patients, which included normal and abnormal slices related to six different patterns, that is, ground-glass opacities, reticular and linear opacities, nodular opacities, honeycombing, emphysematous change, and consolidation. The areas that included specific diffuse patterns in the 315 HRCT images were marked by three radiologists independently on the CRT monitor in the same manner as they commonly describe them in their radiological reports. The areas with a specific pattern, which three radiologists marked independently and consistently as the same patterns, were used as *gold standard* for specific abnormal opacities. Figure 10.15 shows portion of enlarged HRCT images of one normal slice and six abnormal slices. The white lines indicate the abnormal area of the *gold standard* for each of the specific opacities.

10.4.2 Segmentation of Lung Region

The lungs in HRCT images were segmented from background in each slice by using a gray-level morphological opening and a thresholding technique. The gray-level morphological opening (Serra 1982) was applied for the removal

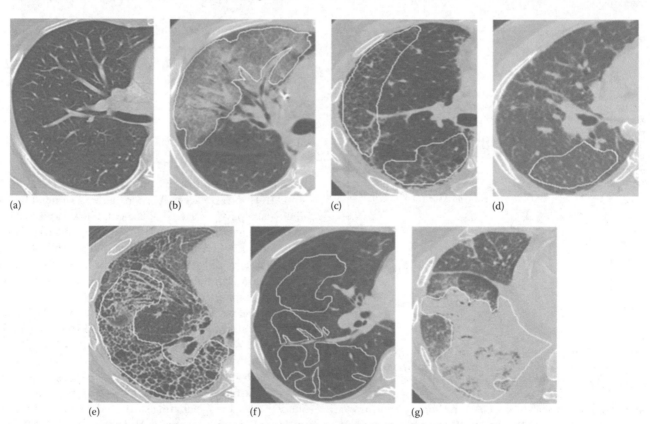

Figure 10.15   Illustration of *gold standard* for one normal and six abnormal patterns of diffuse lung diseases on HRCT images that were determined by the areas marked independently by three radiologists. (a) Normal, (b) ground-glass opacities, (c) reticular and linear opacities, (d) nodular opacities, (e) honeycombing, (f) emphysematous change, and (g) consolidation.

of small light structures such as vessels, while maintaining the overall gray levels and larger light structures. A gray-level histogram indicating the distribution of pixel values was constructed from pixels within the smoothed thorax, and the gray level that maximize the separation between the two main peaks of the histogram was used as a threshold to segment the lungs. The majority of the lungs in HRCT images were segmented by the use of this automated method. However, because 11 lungs with consolidation were not segmented correctly, a manual method was employed for the segmentation of the lung regions in these cases.

Accurate segmentation of lung with severe diffuse lung on CT images is an important and difficult task in the development of CAD scheme. Wang et al. (2009b) developed an automated segmentation method of lungs based on texture analysis. In their method, a CT value thresholding technique was first employed to obtain an initial lung estimate, and then texture-image was used to further identify abnormal regions. Finally, they combined the identified abnormal lung regions with the initial lungs to generate the final lung segmentation result. The segmentation result achieved a mean overlap rate of 96.7% using a database of 76 CT scans, including 31 normal cases and 45 abnormal cases. Korfiatis et al. developed a lung segmentation method using support vector machine with gray level and wavelet coefficient statistics features. Using a database of 22 HRCT cases, a mean overlap rate of 95.4% was obtained (Korfiatis et al. 2008).

10.4.3   Determination of Six Physical Measures

The segmented lungs were divided into many contiguous ROIs with a 32 × 32 (and/or 96 × 96) matrix. Six physical measures were determined in each ROI. These included three measures related to the gray-level distribution and three measures for geometric patterns. The gray-level distribution measures were the mean and the SD of CT values in an ROI and also the fraction of the area with air density components in an ROI. The air density component was defined by the area having CT values between −910 and −1000 HU. The air density component was quantified for the detection of some opacities, including air in the lung. The mean of CT values was a useful measure for distinguishing some opacities that included very light areas and very dark areas in HRCT images such as ground-glass opacities, consolidation, and emphysematous change. The SD of CT values was employed to characterize some opacities, which included a large variation in CT values due to the mixture of light and dark areas such as honeycombing. The distributions of the mean and the SD of CT values are shown in Figure 10.16, where some of the six different patterns listed earlier can be clearly distinguished even with the use of only two physical measures.

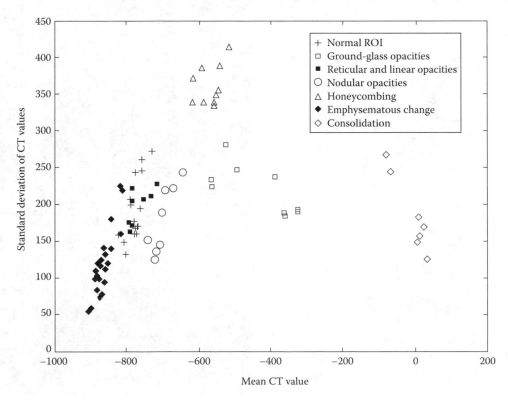

Figure 10.16   Illustration of the distribution of mean CT values and the standard deviation of CT values for six abnormal patterns and normal on high-resolution CT.

For example, the mean CT value for consolidation is larger than any other opacities, whereas the mean CT value for emphysematous change is smaller than any other opacities. The SD of CT value for honeycombing is much larger than that for all of the other categories. The ground-glass pattern has relatively large CT value comparable to those of honeycombing, but its SD is less than that of honeycombing. Although the measures obtained from the gray-level distribution are useful for the characterization of some diffuse lung diseases, it is difficult to detect nodular and reticular opacities because the gray-level distribution does not include shape information of opacities.

The geometric measures were employed for the characterization of some aspects of the nodular components, line components, and multilocular components. The morphological *white* top-hat transform (Serra 1982) was employed for detecting nodular components and line components, which is defined by the subtraction of the opening of an original image from the original image. This operation corresponds to extracting *white* patterns smaller than the structure element used. A gray-level thresholding

technique was applied to the morphological white top-hat transformed image for the determination of the initial candidates for nodular components and line components. The degree of circularity, which was defined by the fraction of the overlap area of the candidate with the circle having the same area as the candidate, was calculated for all of the detected candidate regions. All detected components with a degree of circularity greater than 0.7 were considered to be nodular components. On the other hand, all detected components with a degree of circularity smaller than or equal to 0.7 were considered to be line components. The nodular component and line component were useful for the detection of nodular opacities and reticular and linear opacities respectively, as illustrated in Figure 10.17. A measure for multilocular component was derived from the morphological *black* top-hat transform. The morphological black top-hat transform is given by subtraction of the original image from the opening of the original image. This operation corresponds to extracting *black* patterns that can fit into the area of the structure element used,

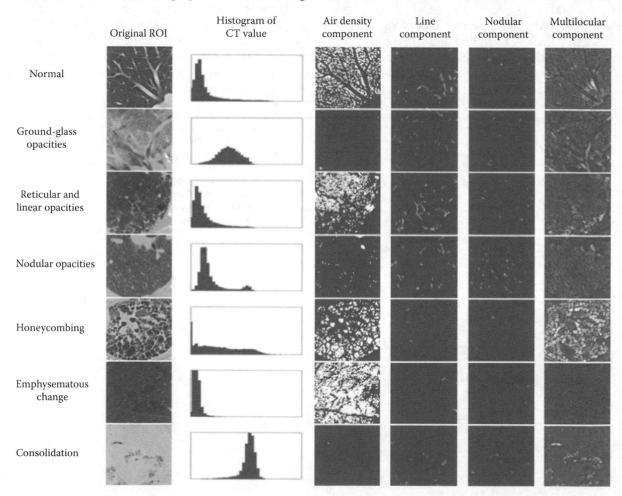

Figure 10.17   Illustration of images (96 × 96) selected from the seven slices in Figure 10.4.1, histogram of region-of-interest (ROI) images, and output images for air density components, line components, nodular components, and multilocular components.

as illustrated in Figure 10.17. Although the SD of the CT value was useful for detecting honeycombing, it was difficult to distinguish between honeycombing and very large vessels. Therefore, the measure for multilocular patterns was adapted as another feature.

10.4.4 Classification of Normal and Six Abnormal Patterns

A couple of classifiers, such as support vector machine (Xu et al. 2006, Park et al. 2009), quadratic classifier (Wang et al. 2009a), and Bayesian classifier (Xu et al. 2006), were employed for the classification of normal and different types of abnormal patterns. Uchiyama et al. (2003) employed a three-layered ANN with a back-propagation algorithm for distinguishing between seven different patterns, which included normal and the six patterns associated with diffuse lung diseases. The numbers of input, hidden, and output were 12, 10, and 7, respectively. The input data for the ANN consisted of six features obtained from a small ROI with a 32 × 32 matrix and another six features from a large ROI with a 96 × 96 matrix. A large (96 × 96) ROI was placed centered over the small (32 × 32) ROI, that is, one large ROI included nine contiguous small ROIs, and thus two adjacent large ROIs overlapped considerably. The six features for the large ROI were employed to take into account the information adjacent to the small ROIs. The output values for each of seven output units obtained with the ANN indicated likelihood of each of the normal pattern and six abnormal patterns. The output unit yielding the largest value was considered to be the result of classification. The sensitivity of this computerized method for the detection of the six abnormal patterns in each ROI was 99.2% (122/123) for GGOs, 100% (15/15) for reticular and linear opacities, 88.0% (132/150) for nodular opacities, 100% (98/98) for honeycombing, 95.8% (369/385) for emphysematous change, and 100% (43/43) for consolidation. The specificity in detecting a normal ROI was 88.1% (940/1067).

The classification performance for normal slices, abnormal slices, and suspicious normal/abnormal slices was also investigated. The normal slices were determined when there was no area identified by any of the three radiologists as abnormal. The abnormal slices were determined when there was an area identified by the three radiologists as abnormal even if they considered them as different abnormal patterns. The slices that did not belong to normal slices and abnormal slices were determined as *suspicious normal/abnormal slice*, that is, they were determined when there was an area identified by one or two of the radiologists as abnormal. The sensitivity and specificity for the detection of abnormal slices were 90.1% (192/213) and 83.7% (41/49), respectively. However, 52.8% (28/53) of the suspicious normal/abnormal slices

were classified as normal slices, whereas 47.2% (25/53) of the suspicious normal/abnormal slices were classified as abnormal slices. The results indicated the usefulness of the six physical measures for the distinction between normal and six different types of diffuse lung diseases. Therefore, this computerized method may be useful in assisting radiologists in their assessment of diffuse lung diseases on HRCT images.

10.5 CONCLUSION

CAD schemes for the detection and diagnosis of interstitial lung diseases on digital chest radiographs and CT images have been developed for assisting radiologists' image interpretation. Many observer performance studies indicate clearly that the radiologists' diagnostic accuracy was improved significantly by use of the computer output as a second opinion. Therefore, these CAD schemes will become increasingly important for radiologists' interpretation of diffuse lung diseases as long as the chest radiography and CT imaging in the PACS environment are playing a substantial role in hospitals and medical centers.

REFERENCES

Abe, H., K. Ashizawa, S. Katsuragawa, H. MacMahon, and K. Doi. 2002. Use of an artificial neural network to determine the diagnostic value of specific clinical and radiologic parameters in the diagnosis of interstitial lung disease on chest radiographs. *Acad. Radiol.* 9:13–17.

Asada, N., K. Doi, H. MacMahon et al. 1990. Potential usefulness of artificial neural network for differential diagnosis of interstitial lung diseases: A pilot study. *Radiology* 177:857–860.

Ashizawa, K., T. Ishida, H. MacMahon et al. 1999a. Artificial neural networks in chest radiographs: Application to differential diagnosis of interstitial lung disease. *Acad. Radiol.* 6:2–9.

Ashizawa, K., H. MacMahon, T. Ishida T et al. 1999b. Effect of an artificial neural network on radiologists' performance of differential diagnoses of interstitial lung disease using chest radiographs. *AJR* 172:1311–1315.

Chan, H. P., C. E. Metz, and K. Doi. 1985. Digital image processing: Optimal spatial filter for maximization of the perceived SNR based on a statistical decision theory model for the human observer. *Proc. SPIE* 535:2–11.

Chen, X., K. Doi, S. Katsuragawa, and H. MacMahon. 1993. Automated selection of regions of interest for quantitative analysis of lung textures in digital chest radiographs. *Med. Phys.* 20:975–982.

Fetita, C., K. C. Chang-Chien, P. Y. Brillet, F. Preteux, and P. Grenier. 2007. Diffuse parenchymal lung diseases: 3D automated detection in MDCT. *Med. Image Comput. Comput. Assist. Interv.* 10:825–833.

Genereux, G. P. 1985. Pattern recognition in diffuse lung disease. A review of theory and practice. *Med. Radiogr. Photogr.* 61:2–31.

Ishida, T., S. Katsuragawa, T. Kobayashi, H. MacMahon, and K. Doi. 1997. Computerized analysis of interstitial disease in chest radiographs: Improvement of geometric-pattern feature analysis. *Med. Phys.* 24:915–924.

Jagoe, J. R. 1979. Gradient pattern coding—An application to the measurement of pneumoconiosis in chest x rays. *Comput. Biomed. Res.* 12:1–15.

Katsuragawa, S., K. Doi, and H. MacMahon. 1988. Image feature analysis and computer-aided diagnosis in digital radiography: Detection and characterization of interstitial lung disease in digital chest radiographs. *Med. Phys.* 15:311–319.

Katsuragawa, S., K. Doi, and H. MacMahon. 1989. Image feature analysis and computer-aided diagnosis in digital radiography: Classification of normal and abnormal lungs with interstitial disease in chest images. *Med. Phys.* 16:38–44.

Katsuragawa, S., K. Doi, H. MacMahon et al. 1990a. Quantitative analysis of lung texture in the ILO pneumoconiosis standard radiographs. *RadioGraphics* 10:257–269.

Katsuragawa, S., K. Doi, H. MacMahon, L. Monnier, T. Ishida, and T. Kobayashi. 1997. Classification of normal and abnormal lungs with interstitial diseases by rule-based method and artificial neural networks. *J. Digital Imaging* 10:108–114.

Katsuragawa, S., K. Doi, H. MacMahon, L. Monnier-Cholley, J. Morishita, and T. Ishida. 1996. Quantitative analysis of geometric-pattern features of interstitial infiltrates in digital chest radiographs: Preliminary results. *J. Digital Imaging* 9:137–144.

Katsuragawa, S., K. Doi, N. Nakamori, and H. MacMahon. 1990b. Image feature analysis and computer-aided diagnosis in digital radiography: Effect of digital parameters on the accuracy of computerized analysis of interstitial disease in digital chest radiographs. *Med. Phys.* 17:72–78.

Kido, S., J. Ikezoe, H. Naito, S. Tamura, and S. Machi. 1995. Fractal analysis of interstitial abnormalities in chest radiography. *RadioGraphics* 15:1457–1464.

Korfiatis, P., C. Kalogeropoulou, A. Karahaliou, A. Kazantzi, S. Skiadopoulos, and L. Costaridou. 2008. Texture classification-based segmentation of lung affected by interstitial pneumonia in high-resolution CT. *Med. Phys.* 35:5290–5302.

Kruger, R. P., W. B. Thompson, and A. F. Turner. 1974. Computer diagnosis of pneumoconiosis. *IEEE Trans. Syst. Man Cybern.* SMC-4:40.

Li, F., S. Kumazawa, J. Shiraishi et al. 2009. Subjective similarity of patterns of diffuse interstitial lung diseases on thin-section CT: An observer performance study. *Acad. Radiol.* 16:477–485.

Monnier-Cholley, L., H. MacMahon, S. Katsuragawa, J. Morishita, and K. Doi. 1995. Computerized analysis of interstitial infiltrates on chest radiographs: A new scheme based on geometric-pattern features and Fourier analysis. *Acad. Radiol.* 2:455–462.

Monnier-Cholley, L., H. MacMahon, S. Katsuragawa, J. Morishita, T. Ishida, and K. Doi. 1998. Computer-aided diagnosis for detection of interstitial opacities on chest radiographs. *AJR* 171:1651–1656.

Park, S. C., J. Tan, X. Wang et al. 2011. Computer-aided detection of early interstitial lung diseases using low-dose CT images. *Phys. Med. Biol.* 56:1139–1153.

Park, S. O., J. B. Seo, N. Kim et al. 2009. Feasibility of automated quantification of regional diseases patterns depicted on high-resolution computed tomography in patients with various diffuse lung diseases. *Korean J. Radiol.* 10:455–463.

Revesz, G. and H. L. Kundel. 1973. Feasibility of classifying disseminated pulmonary diseases based on their Fourier spectra. *Invest. Radiol.* 8:345–349.

Rosenfeld, A. and A. C. Kak. 1982. *Digital Picture Processing*, 2nd edn., Vol. 2. Academic Press, New York, pp. 84–112.

Serra, J. 1982. *Image Analysis and Mathematical Morphology*. Academic Press, London, U.K.

Sutton, R. N. and E. L. Hall. 1972. Texture measures for automatic classification of pulmonary disease. *IEEE Trans. Comput.* COMM-21:667–676.

Tully, R. J., R. W. Conners, C. A. Harlow, and G. S. Lodwick. 1978. Toward computer analysis of pulmonary infiltration. *Invest. Radiol.* 13:298–305.

Uchiyama, Y., S. Katsuragawa, H. Abe et al. 2003. Quantitative computerized analysis of diffuse lung disease in high-resolution computed tomography. *Med. Phys.* 30:2440–2454.

van Ginneken, B., S. Katsuragawa, B. M. ter Haar Romeny, K. Doi, and M. A. Viergever. 2002. Automatic detection of abnormalities in chest radiographs using local texture analysis. *IEEE Trans. Med. Imaging* 21:139–149.

Wang, J., F. Li, K. Doi, and Q. Li. 2009a. Computerized detection of diffuse lung diseases in MDCT: The usefulness of statistical texture features. *Phys. Med. Biol.* 54:6881–6899.

Wang, J., F. Li, and Q. Li. 2009b. Automated segmentation of lung with severe interstitial lung disease in CT. *Med. Phys.* 36:4592–4599.

Xu, Y., E. J. van Beek, Y. Hwanjo, J. Guo, G. McLennan, and E. A. Hoffman. 2006. Computer-aided classification of interstitial lung diseases via MDCT: 3D adaptive multiple feature method (3D AMFM). *Acad. Radiol.* 13:969–978.

Yoshimura, H., M. L. Giger, K. Doi, H. MacMahon, and S. M. Montner. 1992. Computerized scheme for the detection of pulmonary nodules: Nonlinear filtering technique. *Invest. Radiol.* 27:124–129.

Chapter 11

Measurement of Change in Size of Lung Nodules

Anthony Reeves

CONTENTS

11.1 INTRODUCTION

The change of size of lesions is an important image bio-marker of patient health. Change-in-size measurement requires the availability of at least two time-separated images of the lesion. There are two main health applications for change-in-size measurement of pulmonary nodules: cancer diagnosis and response to therapy. In the diagnostic setting, the task is to assess the malignancy status of a (small) pulmonary nodule. The change-in-size assessment is made by estimating the growth rate from two time-separated images. A volumetric doubling time T_D of less than 400 days or a monthly volumetric growth rate G_I of more than 5.3% is typically considered to indicate malignancy. For response to therapy, the main objective has been to determine if there has been an increase in nodule size indicative of disease progression, a reduction in nodule size indicative of response to therapy, or no change in nodule size. An estimate of the amount of change would also be useful in this context if it could be reliably determined.

The uncertainty in a change-in-size measurement is the primary limitation in the clinical utility of change-in-size measurements. In the last 15 years, there has been considerable interest in developing computer methods for change assessment in the belief that they will have less uncertainty than conventional manual measurements made by physicians. The current challenge is to quantify both the uncertainty of the measurement method and the diagnostic significance of change measurements so that they may be used for the most effective diagnosis.

11.1.1 Change-in-Size Measurement Units

The units used for change-in-size measurement need to be considered. Conceptually, a size change is unitless; however, while the usual consideration of size is the volume of the lesion, traditional 2D imaging and history have provided a tradition of size change by radiologists using a uni-dimensional *diameter* measure providing an opportunity for confusion on the concept and the standard for the relative change-in-size measurement.

In medical contexts, size change is calculated for a second scan relative to a baseline initial measurement.

The definition for volumetric relative size change C_V is given by

$$C_V = \frac{V_2 - V_1}{V_1} \tag{11.1}$$

Therefore, for example, if a lesion increases in volume from $V_1 = 100$ mm^3 to $V_2 = 150$ mm^3, then the relative size change is 0.5 or 50%. Further, if $V_2 = 50$ mm^3, then the relative size change is −0.5 or −50%. Given a measured lesion diameter D_1 and a later diameter measure D_2, the relative change in diameter C_D may be defined as

$$C_D = \frac{D_2 - D_1}{D_1} \tag{11.2}$$

It is important to note that some of the literature reports on sizes and change-in-size based on unidimensional measures and that the fractional size change by diameter measurements are different than the fractional size change by volumetric measurements. These different measurements may be related to each if we assume that change is isotropic in all three spatial dimensions (i.e., the change amount is the same proportion in all directions) by the following:

$$C_D \approx \sqrt[3]{C_V + 1} - 1, \quad C_V \approx \left(C_D + 1\right)^3 - 1 \tag{11.3}$$

11.1.2 Change Measurement

Change measurement is a key diagnostic and disease evaluation tool in common use in medical practice; however, the quantitative treatment of change measurements is not well understood and harbors some misconceptions by the medical community. In making an estimate of change, we are interested in both the value of the measured change and the uncertainty in that measurement; without knowing the latter, the measurement itself has very limited clinical value. For example, consider that there is a measured change of 7% increase in the size of a lesion; this would normally reflect a significant biological change of progression; however, if the uncertainty in the measurement is 10%, then there may

actually be a reduction in the lesion size. Unfortunately, in the context of measuring change in the size of lesions in images, measurement errors much larger than 10% are common.

The issue of change measurement uncertainty is not well understood or reported in the literature. One current method for dealing with change uncertainty is the Response Evaluation Criteria for Solid Tumors (RECIST) criterion (Therasse et al. 2000, Eisenhauer et al. 2009), which is for manual single-dimension lesion measurements. The RECIST protocol, which has not been scientifically validated, specifies that at least a 20% increase in a single-diameter measurement ($C_D = 0.2$) is required for a biological progression of disease to be claimed and that at least a 30% decrease in a diameter measure is required for a response to therapy. This criterion has been used in clinical practice to conservatively accommodate the unknown uncertainty for change measurements. For volumetric measurements, the corresponding change requirements, assuming a spherical isotropic model, are $C_V = +0.73, -0.65$. That is, the uncertainty in the change in volumetric measurement is very conservatively set at more than 65%.

The uncertainty in a change measurement depends upon a number of different factors all of which must be considered in a given case to achieve an optimal clinical decision outcome. Usually, when quantitative measurements are made in medical practice, such as measuring blood pleasure or temperature, the measuring device is calibrated against a well-established reference *standard*. However, for change-in-size measurements for pulmonary nodules or lesions viewed in any imaging modality, there is no direct method to measure the lesion size precisely for such a reference. Even in cases where pathology analysis would permit the evaluation of size at a single time instance, this does not allow us a second evaluation and, therefore, a method to calibrate a change-in-size measurement. This lack of a comparison reference standard makes the evaluation of change-in-size measurement methods uniquely challenging.

Pulmonary nodules in CT images have been an early target for computer change-in-size measurement due to (a) the significance of size change for the diagnosis of lung cancer and (b) the high difference in image intensity between the nodule and the surrounding lung parenchyma, which simplifies the computer selection of the nodule region compared to most other lesion types. While traditionally physicians have typically estimated the size of a lesion in images by one or two caliper measures across the central image slice of the lesion, Yankelevitz et al. (1999) appreciated that the boundary of a nodule seen in a single image slice could also be robustly estimated by a computer method. The advantage of this approach is that the whole boundary is considered, and the estimation of the direction of the largest diameter, needed for the caliper method, is not required. The next innovation was to appreciate that the whole volume of the nodule could be assessed by considering all the image slices through the nodule as a single 3D image (Yankelevitz et al. 1999, 2000, Kostis et al. 2003, Reeves et al. 2006). A primary advantage of this approach is that all images in which the nodule is present are considered (i.e., all available data are considered), and the 2D method requirement of estimating which image slice has the largest presentation of the nodule is no longer required.

Since then, volumetric change-in-size methods have been explored in the context of lung cancer screening studies such as ELCAP in 2003 (Kostis et al. 2003) and NELSON in 2006 (Gietema et al. 2006, 2007) and have been made available by many commercial vendors. There has been considerable research to validate the clinical significance of growth rate (determined from change-in-size measurement) for diagnosing lung cancer and to determine and minimize the uncertainty in change-in-size measurements. Recently, the RSNA with funding from the NIH has created the Quantitative Imaging Biomarkers Alliance (QIBA) with the mission to improve the value and practicality of quantitative imaging biomarkers by establishing standardized protocols and by reducing variability across devices, patients, and time. The CT committee of QIBA has studied how to qualify change-in-size measurements on pulmonary nodules for the use as a surrogate endpoint in clinical trials (Buckler et al. 2010).

11.2 CHALLENGES TO PRECISE CHANGE-IN-SIZE MEASUREMENT

Pulmonary nodules present in a wide variety of sizes and forms; several different main morphological presentations are shown in Figure 11.1. The uncertainty in a change-in-size-measurement method depends upon a number of factors including the presentation of the nodule, the scanner parameters, the health of the patient, patient motion, and the evaluation method itself.

11.2.1 CT Scanner Parameters

As with any use of ionizing radiation, careful consideration must be made to the x-ray dose given to the patient; in general, the higher the dose, the better the quality of the image and therefore the better is the precision of the change-in-lesion-size measurement. However, due to the high contrast between soft tissue and the lung parenchyma, very good measurements for pulmonary nodules can be made from very low-dose scans, and other factors may have more impact on the change-in-size measurement precision.

There are a number of CT scanner acquisition parameters that impact the precision of lesion measurement: these include x-ray energy (kVp and mAs), and pitch. In addition, the image reconstruction parameters, also part of the scanner settings, affect measurement precision; these include the slice thickness and the pixel resolution. In general, for modern multidetector row CT scanners, the x-ray dose is set to the minimum required for clinical review. While increasing the

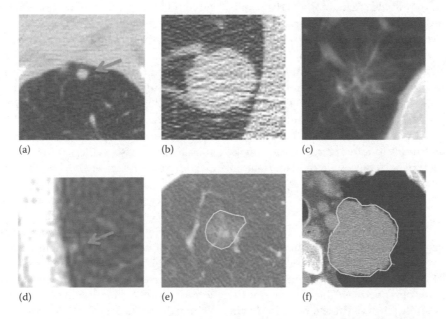

(a)   (b)   (c)

(d)   (e)   (f)

Figure 11.1 Several CT image presentations of pulmonary nodules: (a) a small isolated nodule, (b) a large isolated nodule, (c) a nodule with a complex structure, (d) a very small nodule that is visible but not measurable, (e) a nonsolid nodule, and (f) a large nodule that abuts the chest wall.

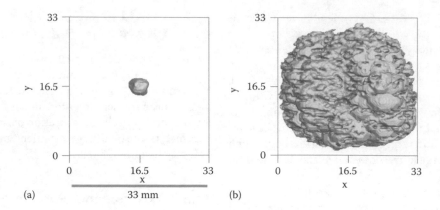

Figure 11.2 Light-shaded visualizations of the nodules shown in Figure 11.1a and b shown to the same scale.

dose would be expected to reduce noise and therefore provide more precise lesion measurements, a significant clinical benefit has not yet been shown in studies. For small nodules (less than 10 mm diameter), the pitch should be no greater than 1:1 recommendation), and the thinnest slice reconstruction should generally be set. For volumetric measurements, the nodule should be visible in four or more image slices.

Perhaps the most important issue is that the scanner parameters used for two time-separated scans should have comparable values and should ideally be made on the same model scanner. Further, one of the most critical parameters is the slice thickness, and any change in this parameter will likely bias the outcome of volumetric measurement methods. Both of these constraints present a challenge to current clinical practice; for the former, it is not usual for the prescription for a CT scan to provide such details as the acquisition parameters. For the latter, there is a preference among many physicians to read thick slice (2–3 mm) scans rather than the thinnest slice (0.5 mm) scans since the thicker slice provides a smaller number of images with less noise. However, for computer methods that work simultaneously in three dimensions, the near-isotropic thin slice images will provide superior size measurement outcomes. This issue should be resolvable in the future with newer PACS systems and the advent of multidetector row CT scanners that can satisfy the needs of both physicians and automated methods without any additional x-ray dose for the patient.

11.2.2 Nodule Presentation

Pulmonary nodules present in a number of different forms and in a very wide range of sizes. The size range deserves special consideration for quantitative evaluation from both the human and computer perspectives. The size range minimum is the limit of visibility in CT (in the order of 1 mm diameter) as shown in Figure 11.1d. Nodules are usually considered to have a maximum diameter of 30 mm; however, lesions much larger than this are possible in cases of advanced cancer. For size comparison, examples of a small and a large nodule are shown in Figure 11.2 at the same size scale. The equivalent volumetric size range is from a 0.52 to 14,137 mm^3 or about 1 to 30,000, which is an incredibly large measurement range to manage and characterize. Consider that for many clinical measurements (e.g., temperature, weight, and pressure), the range of values is often less than 1–10. The single measuring quanta of one voxel for a high-resolution chest scan with a 0.5 mm slice thickness will typically be in the order of 0.1 mm^3.

For small nodules, accurate nodule marking by a physician or by computer is challenging because of the partial voxel effect as the nodule spans only a small number of image slices. While for large nodules, the challenge is the very large number of slices (perhaps 50 or more) and the large boundary that the nodule spans on each image slice (typically several hundred pixels). For all nodule sizes, the attachments to other solid structures may present additional challenges; some nodules have a very complex appearance that makes the separation from attached structures very difficult. Finally, nodules may have a solid or nonsolid appearance; for solid nodules, the issue is separation from other solid structures, while for nonsolid nodules, the issue is confusion with other parenchymal health issues that may also give rise to increased image density and also with partial voxel effects between soft tissue and healthy lung parenchyma. Therefore, not all nodules may be measured with equal uncertainty; there also exists simple nodules of a moderate size with well-defined boundaries for which a very precise volume measurement should be possible. The Prevent Cancer Foundation public image database (Reeves et al. 2009b) provides a number of examples of pulmonary nodules and provides documentation on a number of different presentation issues. The database was developed primarily to assist computer algorithm developers; however, it also provides a useful online resource for physicians and others. The Lung Image Database Consortium (Reeves et al. 2007) has publicly made available over 1000 cases of documented CT chest scans with nodules annotated to aid algorithm developers, and this is discussed in the next chapter.

11.2.3   Subject Effects

Typically, lung scans with modern multirow detector CT scanners can be obtained in a single breath hold of a few seconds. In some cases, there is breathing artifact or similar patient motion during the scan that can severely compromise the scan for measurements in the region of a nodule. In general, the scanner technician may detect this during the scan in which case a second scan of the nodule region can be made. If the nodule is close to the pericardial region, then there is likely to be some heart motion that degrades the nodule image. Other typical artifacts include high noise in the lung apical regions due to local bony structures and the presence of major vessels in the nodule vicinity that complicates the identification of the nodule boundary.

11.2.4   Image Measurement Method

The image measuring method itself has an intrinsic uncertainty associated with it. There are a variety of different approaches to size change measurement ranging from single-dimension manual marking to totally automated volumetric marking to density change measurement. The uncertainty for a measurement method needs to be evaluated across the spectrum of conditions outlined earlier.

11.3   CLINICAL SIGNIFICANCE OF SIZE CHANGE

Change-in-size measurements for pulmonary nodules have two primary applications: the diagnosis of lung cancer though nodule growth rate and the response to therapy evaluated by the direction (larger/smaller) change in nodule size.

11.3.1   Screening for Lung Cancer

In lung cancer screening, the diagnostic challenge is to differentiate between benign and malignant pulmonary nodules. This is especially important for very small nodules not only where the malignant nodules are most treatable but also where the benign nodules are more numerous. In general, malignant pulmonary nodules grow more rapidly than benign nodules; further, it is generally assumed that the malignant cells have a constant (short) mitosis cycle and are therefore doubling in number after a fixed interval of time known as the doubling time T_D. The doubling time model implies an exponential increase in the number of malignant cells (and corresponding nodule volume) with time.

If we measure the volume of a lesion at two time points, obtaining the volume V_1 at time T_1 and V_2 at time T_2, then the volumetric doubling time T_D is given by

$$T_D = \frac{\Delta t \ln(2.0)}{\ln(V_2 / V_1)} \qquad (11.4)$$

where Δt is the time interval $(T_2 - T_1)$.

While the doubling time is informative to the biologist and is currently the most often used measure quoted in the literature, it is the growth rate of the nodule that provides a direct indication of malignancy and is more relevant as a quantitative clinical evaluation. The growth rate is inversely related to doubling time. For example, a nodule that is not growing has a growth rate of zero, and larger positive rates imply increased concern for malignancy, whereas the doubling time for no growth is infinity, and very large doubling time values (and also very large negative values) indicate low suspicion of malignancy. A direct measure of the growth rate, called the growth index (G_I), is defined as the percent volume increase in a nodule during the period of a month (Reeves 2005) and is defined by

$$G_I = 100 \left[\left(\frac{V_2}{V_1} \right)^{30.4375/\Delta t} - 1 \right] \qquad (11.5)$$

The (monthly) growth index and the (day) doubling time are related by the following equation:

$$G_I = 100 \left[2^{30.4375/T_D} - 1 \right] \qquad (11.6)$$

In the diagnosis of lung cancer, a growth rate of $G_I = 5.3\%$ per month or an annual doubling time of $D_T = 400$ days or less is considered an indication of lung cancer; in general, benign nodules do not exhibit that rapid a growth rate. Many lung cancers are adenocarcinomas that typically have a growth rate of around $G_I = 24$, $D_T = 100$, and some small cell cancers may have growth rates measured as fast as $G_I = 90$, $D_T = 33$. As the time between the scans increases, then so does the expected magnitude of the change, which reduces the uncertainty in the measurement. For effective lung cancer screening, a protocol must be established that optimizes the time interval between scans given the nodule size, the nodule characteristics, and the measurement uncertainty, see Henschke (2011) for a current screening protocol.

In screening for lung cancer using low-dose CT images, nodule size change is a primary consideration for additional follow-up decisions for the periodic (typically annual) screening cycles. This change-in-size evaluation is made by comparing the current CT scan to the previous screening CT scan. The baseline, or first initiation to the screening program, is a different situation and is similar to an incidental

TABLE 11.1 ZERO-CHANGE MEASUREMENT STUDIES

Study	# Nodules	Slice (mm)	Size Range (mm)	% Vol. Change Confidence Interval	Software
Gietema et al. (2007)	218	0.75	3.2–9.7	−21.2 to 23.8	Siemens LungCare
Goodman et al. (2006)	43	1.25	4–19	−25.6 to 25.6	GE Adv. Lung.
Wormanns et al. (2004)	151	1.25	2.2–20.5	−20.4 to 21.9	Siemens LungCare

CT chest exam since there is no previous scan with which to compare. For effective lung cancer screening, it is critical that a precise protocol is followed to ensure the earliest possible diagnosis with the minimum number of false positives. This protocol should be based on the most recent research information available since both CT technology and research knowledge concerning lung cancer screening continue to rapidly evolve; the International Early Lung Cancer Action Program (I-ELCAP) protocol (Henschke 2011) is one such protocol that we will consider here. The I-ELCAP protocol specifies that on a repeat screening scan, the result of the initial low-dose CT test is positive if at least one noncalcified solid or part-solid nodule 3 mm or larger or a solid endobronchial nodule 5.0 mm or larger in diameter with interim growth is identified, whether newly seen or seen in retrospect but not previously identified.

On the baseline-screening scan or for an incidental chest CT scan (given no previous scan with which to rule out stable benign nodules), there is a higher prevalence of small nodules that are stable and benign, and a less aggressive follow-up protocol is indicated. On evaluating a nodule in a CT scan, the decision on the best follow-up and the length of time to wait for a second CT scan for volumetric growth analysis should be based on recommendations derived from recent scientific evidence as is provided by ongoing studies such as the I-ELCAP.

11.3.2 Response to Therapy

For response to therapy, the challenge is to select an appropriate time between scans that is minimized to allow for therapeutic decisions to be made as timely as possible; however, the time interval must be long enough for the actual change to be reliably determined, that is, the magnitude of the change measure must exceed the change measurement uncertainty.

Several studies have been conducted to estimate the change measurement uncertainty by using zero-change image datasets. That is, the two scans are made just a few minutes apart (the subject may change position during this interval); therefore, the actual physical change in the nodule is known to be zero, and therefore, any measured change should be representative of the intrinsic variation in the measuring system. Several studies of this type have been conducted for commercial measuring systems, and their results are summarized in Table 11.1.

From these studies, we see that a variation of the order of 20%–25% is possible with the methods studied. As mentioned in Section 11.1.1, the RECIST criterion is the established protocol for response to therapy, and it provides overly conservative error bounds (which translate to a volumetric equivalent of over 65%). Refining the significance criterion for volumetric size assessment would have a dramatic effect on both clinical studies that use nodule change as a criterion and also in the assessment of response to therapy for clinical practice. QIBA is actively addressing the challenge of establishing a replacement for RECIST for volumetric measurements of pulmonary nodules that may be qualified for use in FDA-reviewed clinical trials.

11.4 TYPES OF PULMONARY NODULES

There are three main types of nodules by radiological appearance: solid nodules, nonsolid nodules, and part-solid nodules. These different types are illustrated in Figure 11.3. Solid nodules have the same density as soft tissue (typically in the order of water density, 0 HU) and are the most common type of nodules. Nonsolid nodules are formed by layers of cells on the epithelium of the airways and alveoli. This provides a more dense presentation of the lung parenchyma than healthy parenchyma, but there is still some space for air in the affected airways and alveoli. The resulting image is an increased density of the lung parenchyma. There also exists benign calcified nodules that are easily distinguished from other nodule types by their high density and will be not be considered further in this chapter.

Solid nodules have received the most attention in studies since cancers seen on 2D chest x-rays are of this type. Malignant solid nodules consist of rapidly growing invasive masses driven by a given cancer cell type. There are also many benign nodules especially for the small sizes less than 10 mm in diameter. Also some infections may have the appearance of a pulmonary nodule.

Nonsolid nodules have received much less attention than solid nodules and are clearly visible only in CT images. They appear as a single layer of cells that grow along the epithelium of the airways, and in general, nonsolid nodules have

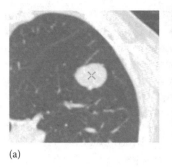 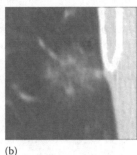 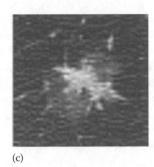

(a)   (b)   (c)

Figure 11.3 The three main presentations for small pulmonary nodules: (a) a solid nodule, (b) a nonsolid nodule, and (c) a part-solid nodule.

a much slower growth rate than solid nodules; there have been few studies to characterize their growth rates.

The part-solid nodules have both a nonsolid component and an inner solid component. It is hypothesized that the inner component may be where the cancer becomes invasive and a solid tumor starts to grow. For part-solid nodules, a prudent strategy is to measure the growth rate of both components with special significance given to the rate for the solid component (which may be considered as a nodule of the solid type). Early results indicate that nonsolid nodules are more likely to be malignant than solid nodules and that part-solid nodules are more likely to be malignant than pure nonsolid nodules (Henschke et al. 2002).

11.5 CHANGE-IN-SIZE MEASUREMENT METHODS

The earliest approach to size change measurement was to use the segmentations of two separate images to define the two volumetric estimates V_1 and V_2 from which the relative size change C_V is defined by Equation 11.1.

A basic problem with this approach is that difficult decisions with respect to the precise location of the nodule boundary in the image need to be made. Other methods have been proposed and developed that avoid making such decisions: chief among these are density change and registration-based techniques. The outcome of the measurement process must be visually inspected, and in some cases, the user may modify the decisions made by the automated computer algorithms.

11.5.1 Volumetric Change Measurement Methods

Key to the volumetric approach is determining exactly which pixels of voxels in the image belong to just the nodule. Usually, region measurement commences with the identification of a single seed point or location within the nodule; many methods also permit the specification of two

seed points that provide the system with both the location and approximate size of the nodule. The seed points may be manually specified by a user or may be automatically computed by a nodule detection algorithm (e.g., Enquobahrie et al. 2007). There are many commercial pulmonary nodule detection systems available.

One common segmentation approach is to filter the image to minimize the impact of noise, threshold the outcome to identify the pixels with a density of soft tissue (excluding pixels of the normal lung parenchyma that has a density much closer to that of air), and finally use shape information to separate the nodule identified by the seed point from attached soft tissue density structures such as the chest wall, vessels, or airways.

A critical aspect of this process is to partition the image between the nodule and any attached vessels. Since there is frequently no significant intensity difference between these structures, decisions are made on the geometry (or shape) of the high-intensity image regions. Many different technical approaches to this problem have been explored, but it is still necessary, currently, for the user to review the outcome to be sure that no gross errors have been made. All systems allow the user to view the segmentation outcome, and many systems permit the user to manually modify or correct these outcomes.

In difficult segmentation situations, the computer algorithm may make different decisions between the two scans on the exact location of the nodule boundary with respect to an attached structure. One method to address this is to register the two 3D images and to use a rule-based decision scheme to ensure that exactly the same partition strategy is used on both images (Reeves et al. 2006).

11.5.2 Density Change Measurement Methods

The density-based approach considers a regular geometrically shaped region of space (typically a sphere or a cube) that surrounds the nodule and computes the average density of that region. The change in density between two scans will then reflect the size change of the nodule if exactly the same special region of space is selected for each time instance and if the only change is due to the nodule (Jirapatnakul et al. 2009). The main advantage of this approach is that it can reliably measure the size change of very complex nodules such as the nodule shown in Figure 11.1c for which explicit segmentation is both very difficult and unreliable. The computer method to realize this approach must identify the nodule region and carefully register the same location for the nodule in both images, so exactly the same region of space is selected. The second requirement is that the correlation relationship between density change and size change needs to be established; one approach to doing this would be to use phantom studies.

Review of the computer algorithm outcome is also important for the density method. In this case, there should be a careful visual image review by the user that the two regions selected for comparison represent the same regions of space in the subject.

11.6 ROLE OF IMAGE PHANTOMS

The major challenge in the development of size change methods is that we do not know the correct value for a size change in a real pulmonary nodule. One approach is to use a synthetic object to represent a pulmonary nodule for which we have precise information on its size through other measurement methods (such as displacement or weight if the density of the material is known). To simulate the human imaging environment, the phantom can be scanned in an anthropomorphic phantom of the chest.

The phantom approach has some shortcomings. First, the nodule has an idealized shape and density and does not closely resemble true nodules. Second, a real pulmonary nodule appears to be shaped by its environment, and when it *grows* into vessels, its shape is modified by the presence of the vessel; in contrast, a spherical phantom that abuts a cylinder (vessel phantom) does not exhibit the same kind of involvement that occurs when a growing nodule meets a vessel. Second, phantoms do not grow; therefore, we are restricted to zero-change experiments.

The FDA has been active in establishing anthropomorphic phantoms for pulmonary nodules and chest CT (Gavrielides et al. 2010). Nodule phantoms include spheres and a number of different geometric shapes at different sizes and densities. These phantoms have been scanned on a number of different scanners, and the results have been made available for public access as a resource for algorithm developers.

A second use of phantoms is to assist in the calibration of the density and geometry properties of the scanner.

This may directly provide for more precise change-in-size evaluation. In this context, the phantoms generally contain a number of spheres of constant density. The concept is that they provide a characterization of the CT scanner at the time when the subject is scanned. Therefore, characteristics such as any scanner drift since its last calibration and the modulation transfer function of the specific scanner settings can be accurately determined. Calibration phantoms are small and compact and may be scanned by placing on the patient or built into the scanner table as for bone mineral density phantoms or scanned separately without the patient. Early studies on pulmonary nodules used spherical phantoms to determine basic measurement properties (Yankelevitz et al. 2000). NIST has been active in developing various calibration phantoms for CT imaging of the chest (Levine et al. 2008), and Kitware has developed a calibration device suitable for commercial use.

11.7 MEASUREMENT PERFORMANCE

There are two aspects in change-in-size measurement methods: the first is the technical performance, that is, what is the uncertainty in the measurement made in a change-in-size measurement method, and the second is the clinical performance, that is, what is the uncertainty in determining the state of health of the subject given a change-in-size measurement by some method. We would like to characterize each of these separately so that we can directly evaluate the relative performance of different technical methods and further so we can optimize the usage protocol given an improved measurement method. Unfortunately, for pulmonary nodules, we have no direct method for characterizing the technical performance of a method, and consequently indirect methods have been employed. For technical performance, studies have been conducted with phantom datasets and zero-change datasets. For overall clinical performance, volumetric methods are compared to other diagnostic methods in a clinical study environment.

11.7.1 Measurement Performance Studies

The technical performance of a measurement method is related to the uncertainty associated with making a measurement. Ideally, to characterize measurement uncertainty, we would compare a set of change-in-size measurements with a known reference standard and analyze the results using a method such as that proposed by Bland and Altman (1986). The problem with automated measurement methods for pulmonary nodules is that we have no reliable reference *standard* method with which to compare the computer method.

11.7.2 Challenges in Establishing Ground Truth

In introducing new diagnostic methods such as change analysis to pulmonary nodules, the usual practice is to compare such methods against the reference *standard* for clinical practice. The current standard practice for pulmonary nodule measurement is manual marking by an experienced physician. Unfortunately, this method has been shown to have a very high measurement uncertainty (see, e.g., Reeves et al. 2007). The goal of computer methods is to obtain an improved performance of the current *gold standard*; therefore, a direct comparison to this standard is not sufficient to validate these methods. One indirect approach to this problem is the zero-change studies such as those outlined in Table 11.1. Unfortunately, these studies characterize only a single point on the change continuum, namely, the case when the change is zero. One novel approach is the VOLCANO'09 study (Reeves et al. 2009a) that compares the performance of a number of different computer algorithms on a set of cases (including some zero-change cases). The main goal of this study is to create a set of benchmark cases that can be used to characterize new computer methods that is not dependent on human judgment.

In addition to the studies in Table 11.1 that showed an order of 25% variation for zero-change measurements, the VOCANO'09 results compared the performance of 17 different semiautomated computer change measurement methods applied to 50 nodule image pairs. Although there was a large variation in the computer methods over the 50 image pairs (and also in the amount of user editing that these methods incorporated), there was no statistical difference detected between the methods. There was a significant bias in the methods for the subset of zero-change data where there was a change in slice thickness between the scans.

11.8 CLINICAL PRACTICE WITH CAD TOOLS

Current commercial tools are available with CT scanners and also from third-party vendors in enhanced image viewing workstations. These tools at the least provide for the volumetric measurement of pulmonary nodules at two time intervals and the calculation of the resulting growth rate; further, when automated algorithms are involved, these tools provide annotated visualizations of CT image data indicating where the location of the nodule boundary has been determined. For effective use of these tools, the operator should carefully inspect these visualizations to assert that boundaries have the correct locations for all parts of the nodule surface. At this time, the computer algorithms have a precise evaluation of image intensities

and are highly repeatable given the same data; however, in general, they have a very limited knowledge of human anatomy. In contrast, physicians have extensive knowledge of human anatomy but are not as good as computers at precisely evaluating image intensities and making repeatable 3D measurements. Most systems have a facility that permits the physician to modify the computed nodule boundary to correct for the *computer's* obvious errors (the most common of such errors are confusing a part of an attached structure such as a vessel as part of the nodule).

Missing from current systems are two important components: first is an evaluation of measurement uncertainty and a corresponding specification of measurement accuracy and precision. Second is a precise protocol for measurement use that mandates strict quality conditions required for making measurements. These components are necessary for a quality clinical evaluation of the measurement outcome. One approach that is possible in lung cancer screening and in some cases of response to therapy is to take additional CT scans beyond the required two (Reeves 2005). In this case, consistency over multiple scans can be analyzed both for value and for measurement variation; thus, we can obtain an estimate of measurement uncertainty that is directly related to the given subject and scanning environment. This may be used both to provide high confidence when the measured change is small and also to highlight conditions where the measurement variation and therefore uncertainty are unusually high.

11.9 CONCLUSION

The evaluation of change-in-size of pulmonary nodules offers the potential for a very effective diagnosis for cancer and evaluation of therapy; however, improved characterization of the uncertainty in such measurements is necessary before the full benefit of this approach can be realized. A major challenge to establish and validate these methods is the lack of a reference standard alternative measurement approach with which a comparison can be made; that is, how to validate a measurement method when we do not know what the correct answer is.

Commercial products are available that provide change-in-size estimates for sequential CT scans of pulmonary nodules. Studies indicate that when these methods are used correctly, for the context of response to therapy, they should provide a significant improvement over the current convention of RECIST measurements. Current efforts, especially by QIBA, are directed to provide compelling evidence for this claim.

For the diagnosis of lung cancer by growth rate, research studies have shown that computer volumetric measurements can be highly effective and that timely evaluations can be made on pulmonary nodules that are too small for evaluation by other conventional methods. The studies to date are reported on research programs in screening where the technical quality of the images is carefully reviewed for each case. Attention to image quality is key for the success of quantitative measurement-based methods when used in clinical practice.

When used with due care, computer volumetric growth measurement is a very effective diagnostic tool with a sensitivity and specificity far higher than alternative methods. Misconceptions about the understanding of uncertainty on change measurements and a focus on one-size-fits-all currently diminish the effectiveness of this approach in clinical practice. For the future, improved protocols that include case-specific measurement uncertainty estimation and multiple scans to increase diagnostic accuracy may offer a superior diagnostic tool compared to alternative methods such as biopsy and PET.

Key to the optimal performance of change-in-size measurements is quality control and standardized high-resolution imaging protocols that are currently not part of accepted clinical practice. Future CT scanners may be expected to include improvements for making high-quality multiple scans including automated protocol scanner settings and image calibration phantoms. Further research is indicated to improve the protocol and evaluation of uncertainty for these methods. Current system development is limited by the availability of example cases for system training; future technical advances may be anticipated in computer methods once larger training databases of documented nodules and benchmark nodule datasets are available to system developers.

REFERENCES

Bland, J. M. and D. G. Altman. 1986. Statistical methods for assessing agreement between two methods of clinical measurement, *Lancet*, 1(8476):307–310.

Buckler, A. J., L. H. Schwartz, N. Petrick et al. 2010. Data sets for the qualification of volumetric CT as a quantitative imaging biomarker in lung cancer, *Optics Express*, 18(14):15267–15282.

Eisenhauer, E. A., P. Therasse, J. Bogaerts et al. 2009. New response evaluation criteria in solid tumours: Revised RECIST guideline (version 1.1), *European Journal of Cancer*, 45(2):228–247.

Enquobahrie, A., A. P. Reeves, D. F. Yankelevitz, and C. I. Henschke. 2007. Automated detection of small solid pulmonary nodules in whole lung ct scans from a lung cancer screening study, *Academic Radiology*, 14(5):579–593.

Gavrielides, M. A., L. M. Kinnard, K. J. Myers et al. 2010. A resource for the assessment of lung nodule size estimation methods: Database of thoracic CT scans of an anthropomorphic phantom, *Optics Express*, 18(14):15244–15255.

Gietema, H. A., C. M. Schaefer-Prokop, W. P. T. M. Mali, G. Groenewegen, and M. Prokop. 2007. Pulmonary nodules: Interscan variability of semiautomated volume measurements with multisection CT—Influence of inspiration level, nodule size, and segmentation performance, *Radiology*, 245(3):888–894.

Gietema, H. A., Y. Wang, D. Xu et al. 2006. Pulmonary nodules detected at lung cancer screening: Interobserver variability of semiautomated volume measurements, *Radiology*, 241(1):251–257.

Goodman, L. R., M. Gulsun, L. Washington, P. G. Nagy, and K. L. Piacsek. 2006. Inherent variability of CT lung nodule measurements in vivo using semiautomated volumetric measurements, *American Journal of Roentgenology*, 186:989–994.

Henschke, C. I. 2011. International early lung cancer action program: Enrollment and screening protocol. http://www.ielcap.org/professionals/docs/ielcap.pdf. (Accessed November 11, 2011).

Henschke, C. I., D. F. Yankelevitz, R. Mirtcheva et al. 2002. CT screening for lung cancer: Frequency and significance of part-solid and nonsolid nodules, *American Journal of Roentgenology* 178(5):1053–1057.

Jirapatnakul, A. C., A. P. Reeves, A. M. Biancardi, D. F. Yankelevitz, and C. I. Henschke. 2009. Semi-automated measurement of pulmonary nodule growth without explicit segmentation. *Biomedical Imaging: From Nano to Macro, 2009.* ISBI 2009. *IEEE International Symposium.* pp. 855–858. IEEE, Boston.

Kostis, W. J., A. P. Reeves, D. F. Yankelevitz, and C. I. Henschke. 2003. Three-dimensional segmentation and growth-rate estimation of small pulmonary nodules in helical CT images, *IEEE Transactions on Medical Imaging*, 22:1259–1274.

Levine, Z. H., S. Grantham, D. S. Sawyer IV, A. P. Reeves, and D. F. Yankelevitz, 2008. A low-cost fiducial reference phantom for computed tomography, *Journal of Research of the National Institute of Standards and Technology*, 113(6):335–340.

Reeves, A. P. 2005. Computer-aided measurement and analysis of CT images of the lungs. In S. G. Armato III and M. S. Brown, editors, *2005 Syllabus, Multidimensional Image Processing, Analysis, and Display: RSNA Categorical Course in Diagnostic Radiology Physics*. pp. 153–164. RSNA Education, Chicago, IL.

Reeves, A. P., A. M. Biancardi, T. V. Apanasovich et al. 2007. The lung image database consortium (LIDC): A comparison of different size metrics for pulmonary nodule measurements, *Academic Radiology*, 14(12):1475–1485.

Reeves, A. P., A. M. Biancardi, D. Yankelevitz et al. 2009b. A public image database to support research in computer aided diagnosis. *31st Annual International Conference of the IEEE Engineering in Medicine and Biology Society*, Minneapolis, MN, September 3, 2009–September 6, 2009. pp. 3715–3718.

Reeves A. P., A. B. Chan, D. F. Yankelevitz, C. I. Henschke, B. Kressler, and W. J. Kostis. 2006. On measuring the change in size of pulmonary nodules, *IEEE Transactions on Medical Imaging*, 25:435–450.

Reeves, A. P., A. C. Jirapatnakul, A. M. Biancardi et al. 2009a. The VOLCANO'09 challenge: Preliminary results, In M. Brown, M. de Bruijne, B. van Ginneken, A. Kiraly, J-M. Kuhnigk, C. Lorenz, J. McClelland, K. Mori, A. Reeves, and J. Reinhardt, editors, *The Second International Workshop on Pulmonary Image Analysis*, London, U.K., September 20, 2009. pp. 353–364.

Therasse, P., S.G. Arbuck, E. A. Eisenhauer et al. 2000. New guidelines to evaluate the response to treatment in solid tumors, *Journal of the National Cancer Institute*, 92(3):205–216.

Wormanns, D., G. Kohl, E. Klotz et al. 2004. Volumetric measurements of pulmonary nodules at multi-row detector CT: In vivo reproducibility, *European Radiology*, 14:86–89.

Yankelevitz, D. F., A. P. Reeves, W. J. Kostis, B. Zhao, and C. I. Henschke. 2000. CT small pulmonary nodules: Volumetrically determined growth rates based on CT evaluation, *Radiology*, 217(1):251–256.

Yankelevitz, D. F., R. Gupta, B. Zhao, and C. I. Henschke. 1999. Small pulmonary nodules: Evaluation with repeat CT-preliminary experience, *Radiology*, 212(2):561–566.

Chapter 12

Public Lung Image Databases*

Samuel G. Armato III

CONTENTS

12.1 INTRODUCTION

Essential to the conduct of research in the field of computer-aided diagnosis (CAD) is a collection of clinical images that capture the range of the disease state under investigation. Such an image collection, known as a *database*, preferably requires metadata, supplied by a domain expert radiologist, on the nature, extent, and/or location of the abnormality. Herein lies a major impediment to investigators wishing to contribute to CAD research: the collection of image databases is a laborious and expensive task. Limited capabilities of the hospital information system or radiology information system may complicate the initial search for relevant clinical images. Limited institutional informatics infrastructure and restricted access to the clinical picture archiving and communications system that stores clinical images may physically hinder access to required images. Issues of patient confidentiality, codified in the Health Insurance Portability and Accountability Act (Department of Health and Human Services 2002), mandate strict anonymization schemes. The time required for radiologists to review, assess, and annotate images as required by the research may be quite onerous and infringes on their clinical responsibilities. Finally, some institutions not affiliated with a medical center may not even have access to

clinical data of any kind. Consequently, for those investigators able to collect an image database from their own institutional resources, the number of accumulated cases is often smaller than desired, and the rigor of the associated "truth" is often less than preferred.

A complication with image databases, once collected, is their limited utility. Research groups that expend the time and money to create a database will likely use it for a single project and typically are reluctant to share their database with other groups. Consequently, each research group struggles to gather a passable number of cases in their own image database for their own research, and many grant applications state, as the first specific aim, "We will collect a database of images...." A further consequence of this isolation of databases is the inability to compare directly the performance of CAD methods reported in the literature, and since database composition is a known source of variability in CAD performance (Nishikawa et al. 1994, Nishikawa and Yarusso 1998), such disparate databases could be expected to slow down the US Food and Drug Administration's (FDA) approval process for the commercialization of successful CAD technologies.

One solution that is emerging in an attempt to overcome these difficulties, especially for lung-image-based

---

* Disclosure statement: SGA receives royalties and licensing fees through the University of Chicago related to computer-aided diagnosis.

CAD research, is the creation and dissemination of public databases. Various models exist for both the collection and the distribution of publicly available image databases; the task is not as simple as depositing a local collection of images on an accessible website. While an organized collection of anonymized clinical images alone would provide a valuable resource to investigators (Kallergi et al. 1997), some level of information provided by a domain expert would greatly enhance the practical utility of the database. The acquisition of this "truth" information could occur on a variety of levels for a variety of tasks and is itself a complex endeavor. This chapter will explore various lung image databases, the source of the images, the level of acquired "truth," and practical implementations for thoracic CAD research.

12.2 CHEST RADIOGRAPHY

Public databases of medical images were first introduced in mammography. The most notable of these databases is the Digital Database for Screening Mammography (DDSM) (Bowyer et al. 1996, Heath et al. 1998, 2000), which contains digitized mammograms acquired from a breast cancer screening program during the 1990s. An expert radiologist annotated lesions with a keyword description, Breast Imaging-Reporting and Data System rating, subtlety score, and a manual outline, and each case includes metadata such as patient age, breast density rating, and digitizer technical parameters. The DDSM has made a substantial contribution to the medical imaging community.

The detection of lung nodules is a key diagnostic task in chest radiography and was one of the first challenges of thoracic imaging CAD research (Giger et al. 2008). In 1998, the Japanese Society of Radiological Technology (JSRT), in conjunction with the Japanese Radiological Society, created a public database of chest radiographs for education, training, and research. The JSRT database contains 247 digitized posteroanterior chest radiographs with either a solitary pulmonary nodule (n = 154) or no nodule (n = 93), as confirmed by CT and reviewed by three experienced thoracic radiologists (Shiraishi et al. 2000). The database may be accessed at http://www.jsrt.or.jp/jsrt-db/eng.php. Each case includes metadata such as patient age, patient gender, nodule size, malignancy status, subtlety, anatomic location, and nodule centroid position.

The success of any image database designed to facilitate research is ultimately demonstrated by the published studies that incorporate the database. The JSRT lung nodule chest radiograph database has been used by researchers internationally. For example, Schilham et al. (2006) developed an automated lung nodule detection method based on multiscale blob detection and segmentation followed by classification of nodule candidates as either nodules or nonnodules. Oda et al. (2009) used the JSRT database to compare the abilities of radiologists to identify lung nodules on chest radiographs without and with novel rib-suppression processing (Figure 12.1); similarly, Li et al. (2011) used the database to conduct an observer study to compare radiologists' abilities to identify lung nodules in bone suppression images created by commercial software relative to standard chest radiographs.

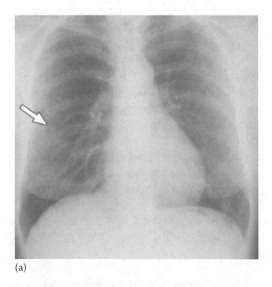 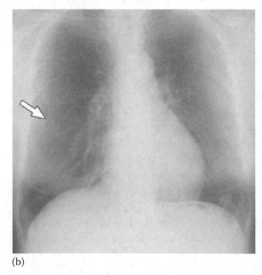

(a)   (b)

Figure 12.1 Lung nodule (arrow) in (a) an example chest radiograph from the JSRT database and (b) the software-generated rib-suppressed version of the radiograph. (Reprinted with permission from Oda et al., *Am. J. Roentgenol.*, 193, W397, 2009.)

Hardie et al. (2008) used the JSRT database as a test set for the evaluation of their multiscale-convergence-index-based nodule detection technique. In an investigation of low-contrast signal visual perception, Andia et al. (2009) used the database to show statistically significant improvements in nodule detection by use of a dynamic cues algorithm, and Usami et al. (2006) investigated liquid crystal display monitors.

A rewarding aspect of public databases is the use of the database in a manner or for a purpose that was not anticipated by the database architects. The potential utility of public databases, therefore, is limited only by the creativity of those who use them. Loog and van Ginneken (2006), for example, developed an automated technique to segment the posterior ribs within the lung fields of chest radiographs. These investigators used the images from the JSRT database but had their own radiologists supplement the "truth" data of the JSRT database (which was developed specifically for lung nodules) with manual outlines of the rib boundaries for their evaluation. The JSRT database was similarly adapted by van Ginneken et al. (2006), who had their own radiologists manually segment the lung fields, heart, and clavicles in the chest radiographs to evaluate the performance of their supervised methods to segment these anatomic structures (Figure 12.2).

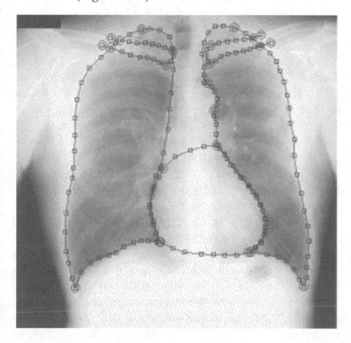

Figure 12.2 Manual delineations of the lungs, heart, and clavicles independently constructed by researchers on a chest radiograph from the JSRT database in preparation for the development of an automated method to segment anatomic structures. (Reprinted with permission from van Ginneken, B. et al., *Med. Image Anal.*, 10, 19, 2006.)

12.3 LUNG CANCER SCREENING PROGRAMS

Public databases could be created from the images acquired during lung cancer screening trials if the organizers of these trials choose to make the scans publicly available and spend the not-insignificant amount of time required to organize, curate, and post the image data and any associated metadata. The Early Lung Cancer Action Program (ELCAP) (Henschke et al. 1999) made available the ELCAP Public Lung Image Database in 2003 as a prototype web-based image archive. The database, which may be found at http://www.via.cornell.edu/databases/lungdb.html, consists of 50 low-dose CT scans along with the locations of nodules identified by ELCAP radiologists. The database is intended to serve as a common dataset for the performance evaluation of computer-aided detection systems. The website also includes interactive image-viewing tools for the CT images and the radiologists' annotations.

Cornell University, in conjunction with the National Cancer Institute (NCI) and funding from the Prevent Cancer Foundation, has created a growing database of serial CT scans as a public resource (http://www.via.cornell.edu/databases/crpf.html). Included with the images are lung nodule outlines provided by radiologists (Reeves et al. 2009). The Public Lung Database to Address Drug Response is meant to facilitate the development of computerized methods for the assessment of tumor response to therapy, so lesion measurements and growth analyses are included with the database. The NCI-funded Reference Image Database to Evaluate Response to therapy in lung cancer (RIDER) project extends the scope of public databases that allow for the quantitative analysis of serial CT scans, an activity that merges radiologic and oncologic research (Armato et al. 2008, Meyer et al. 2009). This database, which will be available through the Cancer Imaging Archive (TCIA) of the NCI (http://cancerimagingarchive.net), contains serial CT scans of lung cancer patients on different treatment regimens and with different durations of time between scans. Some of these scans have annotations that capture Response Evaluation Criteria in Solid Tumors (RECIST) (Therasse et al. 2000) measurements made by radiologists. The RIDER database was intended to provide a common dataset for the development, optimization, validation, and benchmarking of tumor change analysis software tools prior to their use in clinical therapy trials.

The two-arm Lung Screening Study (LSS) of the National Lung Screening Trial (NLST) randomized 17,309 subjects at high risk for lung cancer to annual low-dose screening chest CT scans, with an equal number of subjects receiving annual screening chest radiographs instead. From among the 48,723 CT scans acquired at the 12 participating screening centers under a common image-acquisition protocol, 48,547 scans were archived in the centralized CT Image

Library (CTIL) (Clark et al. 2007, 2009, Cody et al. 2010) with appropriate local institutional review board (IRB) approval. A strict quality assurance (QA) protocol was applied to each scan received at the central site to ensure that the image-acquisition requirements had been met and that the image headers contained no protected health information (PHI). The QA protocol also included the visual inspection of images to verify appropriate image quality without significant artifacts, to confirm that PHI was not contained within the actual images, and to ensure that no image annotations were present. Although the images were not annotated with lesion locations or attributes, correlation with demographic and clinical data was maintained. The CTIL was established as a resource for NLST investigators, clinical researchers in pulmonary disease, and developers of CAD algorithms. The CTIL has distributed subsets of CT images and associated data to groups of internal NLST investigators; these projects have included a reader variability study, the development of CAD methods, and a comparison of emphysema in two groups of participants. The CTIL is expected to become publicly available once NLST follow-up data have been collected.

The NELSON (Nederlands Leuvens Longkanker Screeningsonderzoek) trial is the *Dutch-Belgian lung cancer screening trial* and has accrued 15,822 participants across four institutions since 2003 (van Iersel et al. 2007, Xu et al. 2006). Annual screening CT scans are uploaded to a central site for a secondary review after an initial review at the local institution. CT scans from the NELSON study have been used by investigators associated with the project to investigate, for example, interobserver variability of semiautomated lung nodule volume measurements (Gietema et al. 2006), the discrimination between benign and malignant nodules (Xu et al. 2008, 2009), automated lung nodule detection (Murphy et al. 2009, van Ginneken et al. 2010), and automated lung segmentation (van Rikxoort et al. 2009).

The ITALUNG trial is a randomized controlled trial in Italy that assigned 3206 current or former smokers to four annual lung cancer screening examinations with low-dose CT or to a no-screen control arm (Lopes Pegna et al. 2009, Picozzi et al. 2005). Of those randomized to screening, 1406 participants completed the four CT examinations (Mascalchi et al. 2011). Although the public availability of the ITALUNG data is not clear. CT scans acquired during this trial have been used by local investigators in studies designed to improve the automated segmentation of small juxtavascular lung nodules using local shape analysis (Diciotti et al. 2011), to develop a semiautomated lung nodule segmentation technique (Diciotti et al. 2008), to develop an automated method for nodule size computation based on a scale-space representation (Diciotti et al. 2010), to develop a 3D method for the segmentation of lungs from thoracic CT scans as a preprocessing step for automated lung nodule

detection techniques (De Nunzio et al. 2011), and to develop lung nodule CAD methodologies (Bellotti et al. 2007, Golosio et al. 2009).

12.4 THORACIC CT SCANS

In April 2000, the NCI announced a request for applications (RFA) entitled "Lung Image Database Resource for Imaging Research." The purpose of this RFA was to create a consortium of institutions that would establish a set of consensus-based guidelines for the design and formation of a lung nodule reference database of CT scans (Clarke et al. 2001). The resulting Lung Image Database Consortium (LIDC), comprised of Weill Cornell Medical College, University of California, Los Angeles, University of Chicago, University of Iowa, and University of Michigan, developed a web-accessible resource for the development, training, and evaluation of CAD methods for lung nodules that includes a repository of screening and diagnostic thoracic CT scans, associated metadata such as image acquisition parameters, patient diagnostic information, and nodule "truth" information (Dodd et al. 2004) based on the subjective assessments of multiple experienced radiologists with regard to nodule location, nodule boundary, and subjective ratings of nodule characteristics (Armato et al. 2004).

The Foundation for the National Institutes of Health, under the premise that "public-private partnerships are essential to accelerating scientific discovery for human health" (Carrillo et al. 2009), created the Image Database Resource Initiative (IDRI) in 2004 to complement the LIDC. The IDRI added two cancer centers (MD Anderson Cancer Center and Memorial Sloan-Kettering Cancer Center) and eight medical imaging companies (AGFA Healthcare, Carestream Health, Inc., Fuji Photo Film Co., GE Healthcare, iCAD, Inc., Philips Healthcare, Riverain Medical, and Siemens Medical Solutions) to the five LIDC institutions. The combined LIDC/IDRI was designed to facilitate the development of CAD methods for lung nodule detection, classification, and quantitative assessment and required a substantial commitment of time and resources to create the standards and infrastructure necessary to accommodate the data collection process. The consensus-based creation of the LIDC/IDRI Database required careful planning and consideration of practical issues such as CT scan inclusion criteria, a definition of target lesions and associated "truth" requirements, and a process model to guide population of the Database (Armato et al. 2004, McNitt-Gray et al. 2007). The LIDC/IDRI Research Group has stressed that a solid understanding of the process through which the Database was created, along with important caveats on its use, is required to ensure that investigators conduct studies that are compatible with valid uses of the Database while at the same time allowing investigators to take full advantage of the available information (Armato et al. 2011).

The LIDC/IDRI Database contains 1018 thoracic CT scans from 1010 distinct patients retrospectively collected from the clinical archives of the participating institutions; in addition, nearly 300 digital chest radiographic images associated with a subset of these CT scans were collected. For 268 of the patients with CT scans in the Database, pathologic information was collected retrospectively and is available along with the Database. All images were collected under protocols approved by each local IRB and were anonymized. The Database intentionally includes a range of scanner models and technical parameters to represent the spectrum of clinical imaging protocols at the participating sites: 17 different scanner models from four manufacturers; tube current from 40 to 627 mA (to include both standard-dose diagnostic CT scans and lower-dose CT scans from lung cancer screening examinations); slice thickness from 0.6 to 5.0 mm (mode: 1.25 mm); reconstruction interval from 0.45 to 5.0 mm (mean: 1.74 mm); and three broad categories of convolution kernel for image reconstruction. Scans were limited to approximately six lung nodules with longest dimension between 3 and 30 mm (Austin et al. 1996), although this guideline was not strictly enforced. Scans with other pathology, high levels of noise, and artifacts were allowed unless nodule visualization was hindered.

The LIDC/IDRI Database may be accessed at the NCI's publicly available TCIA (http://cancerimagingarchive.net/). The purpose of TCIA is to organize and catalog, for public download, clinical and research images from cancer clinical trials and other cancer-related studies, including the LIDC/IDRI Database. Although registration is required to access the TCIA, the DICOM images and associated metadata (XML files in the case of the LIDC/IDRI Database) are downloadable without charge to registered users. Documentation for the LIDC/IDRI Database is available on the NIH wiki page at https://wiki.nci.nih.gov/display/CIP/LIDC, which includes information on the XML file format, radiologist instructions during the image annotation process (see Section 12.5), nodule sizes according to a standard metric (Reeves et al. 2007), and the pathology spreadsheet.

12.5   FROM DATABASE TO REFERENCE STANDARD

Along with the images, the LIDC/IDRI Database includes annotations of lesions observed in the CT scans by experienced thoracic radiologists, thus making it a reference standard for CAD researchers. Three lesion categories were of interest: (1) *nodule ≥ 3 mm* (any lesion considered to be a nodule with greatest in-plane dimension between 3 and 30 mm regardless of presumed histology), (2) *nodule < 3 mm* (any lesion considered to be a nodule with greatest in-plane dimension less than 3 mm that is not clearly benign), and (3) *nonnodule ≥ 3 mm* (any other pulmonary lesion with greatest in-plane dimension greater than or equal to 3 mm) (McNitt-Gray et al. 2007) (Figure 12.3). A two-phase interpretation/annotation process, involving an initial "blinded read" followed by an "unblinded read," was developed that required a thoracic radiologist at each of four different LIDC/IDRI institutions; the purpose of this process was to identify as completely as possible all lung nodules in a scan without requiring forced consensus (McNitt-Gray et al. 2007). This process was completely independent of the clinical interpretation that had been rendered previously for each scan.

The initial blinded read required each of the four radiologists to independently review a scan and identify lesions in each of the three lesion categories. For each *nodule ≥ 3 mm* (the main lesion of interest in the LIDC/IDRI Database) identified by a radiologist, that radiologist used a computer interface to construct outlines around the nodule in every CT section in which it appeared; for each lesion in one of the other two lesion categories identified by a radiologist, that radiologist used the computer interface to mark the approximate 3D center-of-mass location. The subsequent unblinded read required the same four radiologists to again independently review the scan, but this second review

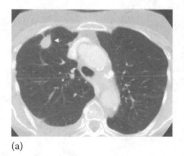
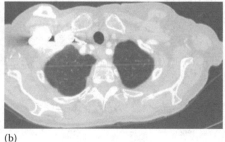
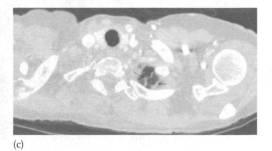

(a)   (b)   (c)

Figure 12.3   Examples of lesions considered to satisfy the LIDC/IDRI definition of (a) a *nodule ≥ 3 mm*, (b) a *nodule < 3 mm*, and (c) a *nonnodule ≥ 3 mm*. (Reprinted with permission from McNitt-Gray et al., *Acad. Radiol.*, 14, 1464, 2007.)

included annotations from the blinded read (with radiologist identity withheld); each radiologist could then modify their marks as they felt appropriate in light of the newly provided information from their colleagues.

For each lesion that a radiologist identified as a *nodule ≥ 3 mm* after the unblinded read, that radiologist independently assessed several nodule characteristics (e.g., subtlety, internal structure, spiculation, and margin) (McNitt-Gray et al. 2007). The post-unblinded-read lesion category designations, associated annotations, and nodule characteristic ratings from each radiologist were stored in a single XML file for each scan. The efficient execution of this complete process required the development of a common data format with a standardized structure so that data could be shared among institutions and eventually recorded in the final set of XML files. Each XML file contains the spatial coordinates of lesion annotations from each of the four radiologists grouped by radiologist (whose identities have been anonymized); however, the associations of lesions across radiologists are not explicitly provided.

The final XML file created for each scan was subjected to a manual QA protocol (Armato et al. 2007b). All *nodule ≥ 3 mm* and *nodule < 3 mm* marks recorded in the XML file for a particular scan were superimposed on the corresponding images at the appropriate spatial locations and visually reviewed (along with any spatially associated *nonnodule ≥ 3 mm* marks) on a computer interface; isolated *nonnodule ≥ 3 mm* marks were not reviewed, since the nonnodule marks were meant to supplement the two nodule categories and provide a guide for users of the Database rather than a complete record of all other abnormalities in the scan. The interface displayed marks of each radiologist as color-coded symbols to distinguish among the marks of different radiologists and among the different lesion categories (for a *nodule ≥ 3 mm*, the complete nodule outline

was displayed). Several QA categories were defined, including errant marks outside the lungs, marks from more than one lesion category assigned to the same lesion by the same radiologist, and discontinuous or aberrant *nodule ≥ 3 mm* outlines. Potential errors identified through the visual QA review were referred to the appropriate radiologist for correction or confirmation that the mark was intentional. The importance of a QA protocol for any database effort is demonstrated by the fact that QA issues were identified in 449 of the 1018 LIDC/IDRI cases (Armato et al. 2011).

The LIDC/IDRI Database contains 7371 lesions annotated with *nodule ≥ 3 mm* or *nodule < 3 mm* marks from at least one of the four radiologists, of which 2669 lesions are annotated specifically with at least one *nodule ≥ 3 mm* mark (Armato et al. 2011). Only 19 cases contain no *nodule ≥ 3 mm* or *nodule < 3 mm* marks from any radiologist. A key feature of the LIDC/IDRI Database is that it captures differences of opinion among the four radiologists; many lesions were annotated differently (or not at all) by the different radiologists (Figure 12.4). Only 1940 (26.3%) of the 7371 lesions considered to be a nodule by at least one radiologist demonstrated complete agreement with all four radiologists assigning either a *nodule ≥ 3 mm* mark or all four radiologists assigning a *nodule < 3 mm* mark (although 2562 nodules [34.8%] received one of the two nodule marks from all four radiologists). Of these 7371 nodules, 1481 (20.1%) received only a single *nodule ≥ 3 mm* mark or a single *nodule < 3 mm* mark. The main focus of the LIDC/IDRI effort was the identification of lesions considered to be a *nodule ≥ 3 mm*. Of the 2669 lesions marked by at least one radiologist as a *nodule ≥ 3 mm*, 777 (29.1%) were assigned *nodule ≥ 3 mm* marks by only a single radiologist, while 928 (34.8%) received *nodule ≥ 3 mm* marks from all four radiologists.

The LIDC/IDRI Database was made publicly available in several installments. The first sizable release

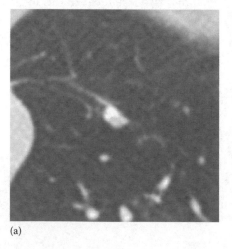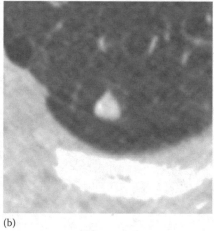

(a)   (b)

Figure 12.4   Examples of lesions marked as a *nodule ≥ 3 mm* (a) by only a single radiologist (the other three radiologists identified this lesion as a *nonnodule ≥ 3 mm*) and (b) by all four radiologists. (Reprinted with permission from Armato et al., *Med. Phys.*, 38, 915, 2011.)

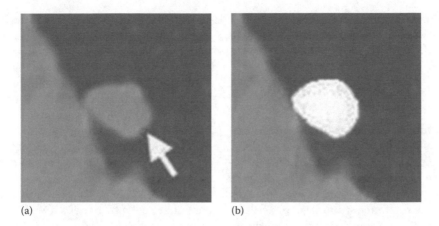

(a)   (b)

Figure 12.5   (a) A *nodule ≥ 3 mm* from the LIDC/IDRI Database (arrow) and (b) the results of an automated nodule segmentation method applied to this nodule. (Reprinted with permission from Wang et al., *Med. Phys.*, 34, 4678, 2007.)

occurred in 2009 (400 CT scans and associated XML files). The full database of 1018 cases became available in 2011. A PubMed search on the keywords "LIDC," "Lung Image Database Consortium," or "Lung Imaging Database Consortium" (an incorrect variant of the LIDC acronym) performed at the time of this writing yielded 75 relevant articles. Nine of these articles were authored by the LIDC/IDRI research group and address conceptual database issues, database design, or database process models (Armato et al. 2004, 2007b, 2011, Clarke et al. 2001, McNitt-Gray et al. 2007), nodule segmentation variability or variability in nodule size metrics (Meyer et al. 2006, Reeves et al. 2007a), nodule "truth" considerations (Dodd et al. 2004), and radiologist variability in the identification of lung nodules (Armato et al. 2007a).

Other investigators around the world have used the LIDC/IDRI database for a wide variety of studies, including segmentation of lungs and pulmonary anatomy (De Nunzio et al. 2011, Korfiatis et al. 2007, Ochs et al. 2007), nodule segmentation (Chen et al. 2011, Diciotti et al. 2008, 2010, 2011, Kubota et al. 2011, Sensakovic et al. 2008, Wang et al. 2007, 2009) (Figure 12.5), lung nodule detection (Camarlinghi et al. 2011, Golosio et al. 2009, Messay et al. 2010, Ozekes and Osman 2010, Ozekes et al. 2008, Riccardi et al. 2011, Tan et al. 2011), lung nodule classification (Way et al. 2006), radiologist nodule detection performance (Sahiner et al. 2009) (Figure 12.6), CAD performance assessment (Choudhury et al. 2010), image data visualization and mining (Lin et al. 2011, Tan et al. 2010), content-based nodule image retrieval (Lam et al.

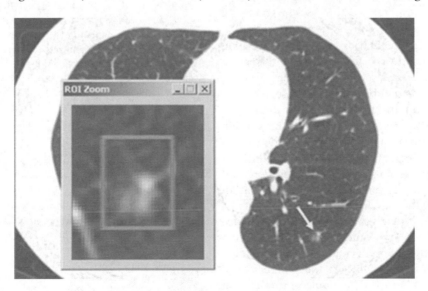

Figure 12.6   A lung nodule (arrow and inset) from the LIDC/IDRI Database that was detected by one and four study radiologists without and with, respectively, the benefit of an automated nodule detection method. (Reprinted with permission from Sahiner et al., *Acad. Radiol.*, 16, 1518, 2009.)

2007), radiologist semantic assessment (Opulencia et al. 2011), and "truth" assessment (Biancardi et al. 2010, Ross et al. 2007, Turner et al. 2006).

12.6 CONCLUSION

Publicly available databases of thoracic CT and radiographic images, especially those that include associated clinical, demographic, and radiologist annotation information, are a valuable resource for the medical imaging research community. Moreover, such databases have the potential to become true reference standards to facilitate the direct comparison of CAD methods and, eventually, to streamline the FDA approval process for new technologies developed for well-defined radiologic tasks. The presence of variability, error, and noise confounds any task, but robust CAD systems will need to accommodate these effects; public databases that incorporate real-world variability provide an added benefit to researchers.

Researchers who use a public database should document the specific cases included in their study when reporting results. The training/testing approach should be described along with the distribution of cases between the training and test sets. Researchers should describe the approach used to establish their task-specific "truth" from the information provided with the database along with the manner in which agreement between the output of the method and the reference "truth" was determined. For example, in the context of the development of automated lung nodule detection algorithms using the LIDC/IDRI Database, researchers should explicitly define the detection targets, which could range from only those nodules marked by all four radiologists to all nodules marked by at least one radiologist. The performance evaluation method also should be described for the given task, dataset, training/testing paradigm, "truth" metric, and scoring approach.

Isolated public image databases are themselves powerful research resources; the impact of such databases, however, may be greatly enhanced by their incorporation in more widespread research initiatives and informatics infrastructure developments, including NCI-funded caBIG Imaging Workspace projects (e.g., the Annotation and Image Markup [AIM] project and the Algorithm Validation Tool [Rubin et al. 2009]) and the Radiological Society of North America's Quantitative Imaging Biomarker Alliance effort (Buckler et al. 2010). For example, the caBIG Imaging Workspace has facilitated the conversion of data contained in the LIDC/IDRI Database XML files to the AIM format to make these data accessible to AIM-enabled visualization and analysis tools.

The creation of a public database of clinical images requires an image review paradigm, an image annotation scheme, a QA protocol, and the specification of a database format. The LIDC/IDRI Database, for example, required consideration of important technical and clinical issues such as guidelines for scan inclusion, well-defined lesion categories, a rationale for the information collected from lesions in each category, detailed instructions to the LIDC/IDRI radiologists, a unique image interpretation paradigm, an electronic workflow to transmit images and associated annotations across multiple institutions, a thorough QA protocol, detailed documentation, and an infrastructure for maintaining and distributing the data (Armato et al. 2011). These details are essential for a database that seeks to benefit a wide array of studies. Users of public databases will certainly adapt the database to applications beyond those considered by the database developers; the process through which each database was created must be understood so that appropriate studies may be designed.

ACKNOWLEDGMENTS

The author would like to recognize all investigators who participated in the formulation, development, and collection of the LIDC/IDRI Database.

REFERENCES

Andia, M. E., J. Plett, C. Tejos, M. W. Guarini, M. E. Navarro, D. Razmilic, L. Meneses et al. 2009. Enhancement of visual perception with use of dynamic cues. *Radiology* 250:551–557.

Armato, S. G. III, G. McLennan, L. Bidaut, M. F. McNitt-Gray, C. R. Meyer, A. P. Reeves, B. Zhao et al. 2011. The Lung Image Database Consortium (LIDC) and Image Database Resource Initiative (IDRI): A completed reference database of lung nodules on CT scans. *Medical Physics* 38:915–931.

Armato, S. G. III, G. McLennan, M. F. McNitt-Gray, C. R. Meyer, D. Yankelevitz, D. R. Aberle, C. I. Henschke et al. 2004. Lung Image Database Consortium: Developing a resource for the medical imaging research community. *Radiology* 232:739–748.

Armato, S. G. III, G. McLennan, C. R. Meyer, A. P. Reeves, M. F. McNitt-Gray, B. Y. Croft, and L. P. Clarke. 2008. The Reference Image Database to Evaluate Response to therapy in lung cancer (RIDER) project: A resource for the development of change analysis software. *Clinical Pharmacology and Therapeutics* 84:448–456.

Armato, S. G. III, M. F. McNitt-Gray, A. P. Reeves, C. R. Meyer, G. McLennan, D. R. Aberle, E. A. Kazerooni et al. 2007a. The Lung Image Database Consortium (LIDC): An evaluation of radiologist variability in the identification of lung nodules on CT scans. *Academic Radiology* 14:1409–1421.

Armato, S. G. III, R. Y. Roberts, M. F. McNitt-Gray, C. R. Meyer, A. P. Reeves, G. McLennan, R. M. Engelmann et al. 2007b. The Lung Image Database Consortium (LIDC): Ensuring the integrity of expert-defined "truth". *Academic Radiology* 14:1455–1463.

Austin, J. H. M., N. L. Mueller, P. J. Friedman, D. M. Hansell, D. P. Naidich, M. Remy-Jardin, W. R. Webb et al. 1996. Glossary of terms for CT of the lungs: Recommendations of the nomenclature committee of the Fleischner Society. *Radiology* 200:327–331.

Bellotti, R., F. De Carlo, G. Gargano, S. Tangaro, D. Cascio, E. Catanzariti, P. Cerello et al. 2007. A CAD system for nodule detection in low-dose lung CTs based on region growing and a new active contour model. *Medical Physics* 34:4901–4910.

Biancardi, A. M., A. C. Jirapatnakul, and A. P. Reeves. 2010. A comparison of ground truth estimation methods. *International Journal of Computer Assisted Radiology and Surgery* 5:295–305.

Bowyer, K., D. Kopans, W. P. Kegelmeyer, R. Moore, M. Sallam, K. Chang, and K. Woods. 1996. The digital database for screening mammography. In: K. Doi, M. L. Giger, R. M. Nishikawa, and R. A. Schmidt eds. *Digital Mammography '96: Proceedings of the 3rd International Workshop on Digital Mammography*. Amsterdam: Elsevier, 431–434.

Buckler, A. J., P. D. Mozley, L. Schwartz, N. Petrick, M. McNitt-Gray, C. Fenimore, K. O'Donnell et al. 2010. Volumetric CT in lung cancer: An example for the qualification of imaging as a biomarker. *Academic Radiology* 17:107–115.

Camarlinghi, N., I. Gori, A. Retico, R. Bellotti, P. Bosco, P. Cerello, G. Gargano et al. 2011. Combination of computer-aided detection algorithms for automatic lung nodule identification. *International Journal of Computer Assisted Radiology and Surgery*.

Carrillo, M. C., C. A. Sanders, and R. G. Katz. 2009. Maximizing the alzheimer's disease neuroimaging initiative II. *Alzheimer's and Dementia* 5:271–275.

Chen, B., T. Kitasaka, H. Honma, H. Takabatakc, M. Mori, H. Natori, and K. Mori. 2011. Automatic segmentation of pulmonary blood vessels and nodules based on local intensity structure analysis and surface propagation in 3D chest CT images. *International Journal of Computer Assisted Radiology and Surgery*.

Choudhury, K. R., D. S. Paik, C. A. Yi, S. Napel, J. Roos, and G. D. Rubin. 2010. Assessing operating characteristics of CAD algorithms in the absence of a gold standard. *Medical Physics* 37:1788–1795.

Clark, K. W., D. S. Gierada, G. Marquez, S. M. Moore, D. R. Maffitt, J. D. Moulton, M. A. Wolfsberger et al. 2009. Collecting 48,000 CT exams for the Lung Screening Study of the National Lung Screening Trial. *Journal of Digital Imaging* 22:667–680.

Clark, K. W., D. S. Gierada, S. M. Moore, D. R. Maffitt, P. Koppel, S. R. Phillips, and F. W. Prior. 2007. Creation of a CT image library for the Lung Screening Study of the National Lung Screening Trial. *Journal of Digital Imaging* 20:23–31.

Clarke, L. P., B. Y. Croft, E. Staab, H. Baker, and D. C. Sullivan. 2001. National cancer institute initiative: Lung image database resource for imaging research. *Academic Radiology* 8:447–450.

Cody, D. D., H. J. Kim, C. H. Cagnon, F. J. Larke, M. F. McNitt-Gray, R. L. Kruger, M. J. Flynn et al. 2010. Normalized CT dose index of the CT scanners used in the National Lung Screening Trial. *American Journal of Roentgenology* 194:1539–1546.

De Nunzio, G., E. Tommasi, A. Agrusti, R. Cataldo, I. De Mitri, M. Favetta, S. Maglio et al. 2011. Automatic lung segmentation in CT images with accurate handling of the hilar region. *Journal of Digital Imaging* 24:11–27.

Department of Health and Human Services. 2002. Standards for privacy of individually identifiable health information: Final rules. *Federal Register* 67:53182–53272.

Diciotti, S., S. Lombardo, G. Coppini, L. Grassi, M. Falchini, and M. Mascalchi. 2010. The LoG characteristic scale: A consistent measurement of lung nodule size in CT imaging. *IEEE Transactions on Medical Imaging* 29:397–409.

Diciotti, S., S. Lombardo, M. Falchini, G. Picozzi, and M. Mascalchi. 2011. Automated segmentation refinement of small lung nodules in CT scans by local shape analysis. *IEEE Transactions on Bio-Medical Engineering* 58:3418–3428.

Diciotti, S., G. Picozzi, M. Falchini, M. Mascalchi, N. Villari, and G. Valli. 2008. 3-D segmentation algorithm of small lung nodules in spiral CT images. *IEEE Transactions on Information Technology in Biomedicine* 12:7–19.

Dodd, L. E., R. F. Wagner, S. G. Armato III, M. F. McNitt-Gray, S. Beiden, H.-P. Chan, D. Gur et al. 2004. Assessment methodologies and statistical issues for computer-aided diagnosis of lung nodules in computed tomography: Contemporary research topics relevant to the Lung Image Database Consortium. *Academic Radiology* 11:462–475.

Gietema, H. A., Y. Wang, D. Xu, R. J. van Klaveren, H. de Koning, E. Scholten, J. Verschakelen et al. 2006. Pulmonary nodules detected at lung cancer screening: Interobserver variability of semiautomated volume measurements. *Radiology* 241:251–257.

Giger, M. L., H.-P. Chan, and J. Boone. 2008. Anniversary paper: History and status of CAD and quantitative image analysis: The role of *Medical Physics* and AAPM. *Medical Physics* 35:5799–5820.

Golosio, B., G. L. Masala, A. Piccioli, P. Oliva, M. Carpinelli, R. Cataldo, P. Cerello et al. 2009. A novel multithreshold method for nodule detection in lung CT. *Medical Physics* 36:3607–3618.

Hardie, R. C., S. K. Rogers, T. Wilson, and A. Rogers. 2008. Performance analysis of a new computer aided detection system for identifying lung nodules on chest radiographs. *Medical Image Analysis* 12:240–258.

Heath, M., K. Bowyer, D. Kopans, W. P. Kegelmeyer, R. Moore, K. Chang, and S. Munishkumaran. 1998. Current status of the digital database for screening mammography. In: N. Karssemeijer, M. Thijssen, J. Hendriks, and L. van Erning, eds. *Digital Mammography '98: Proceedings of the 4th International Workshop on Digital Mammography*. Dordrecht: Kluwer, 457–460.

Heath, M., K. Bowyer, D. Kopans, R. Moore, and W. P. Kegelmeyer. 2000. The digital database for screening mammography. In: M. J. Yaffe, ed. *Digital Mammography 2000: Proceedings of the 5th International Workshop on Digital Mammography*. Madison: Medical Physics Publishing, 212–218.

Henschke, C. I., D. I. McCauley, D. F. Yankelevitz, D. P. Naidich, G. McGuinness, O. S. Miettinen, D. M. Libby et al. 1999. Early lung cancer action project: Overall design and findings from baseline screening. *The Lancet* 354:99–105.

Kallergi, M., R. A. Clark, and L. P. Clarke. 1997. Medical image databases for CAD applications in digital mammography: Design issues. *Studies in Health Technology & Informatics* 43 Pt B:601–605.

Korfiatis, P., S. Skiadopoulos, P. Sakellaropoulos, C. Kalogeropoulou, and L. Costaridou. 2007. Combining 2D wavelet edge highlighting and 3D thresholding for lung segmentation in thin-slice CT. *The British Journal of Radiology* 80:996–1004.

Kubota, T., A. K. Jerebko, M. Dewan, M. Salganicoff, and A. Krishnan. 2011. Segmentation of pulmonary nodules of various densities with morphological approaches and convexity models. *Medical Image Analysis* 15:133–154.

Lam, M. O., T. Disney, D. S. Raicu, J. Furst, and D. S. Channin. 2007. BRISC-an open source pulmonary nodule image retrieval framework. *Journal of Digital Imaging* 20 (Suppl. 1):63–71.

Li, F., T. Hara, J. Shiraishi, R. Engelmann, H. MacMahon, and K. Doi. 2011. Improved detection of subtle lung nodules by use of chest radiographs with bone suppression imaging: Receiver operating characteristic analysis with and without localization. *American Journal of Roentgenology* 196:W535–W541.

Lin, H., Z. Chen, and W. Wang. 2011. A pulmonary nodule view system for the Lung Image Database Consortium (LIDC). *Academic Radiology* 18:1181–1185.

Loog, M. and B. van Ginneken. 2006. Segmentation of the posterior ribs in chest radiographs using iterated contextual pixel classification. *IEEE Transactions on Medical Imaging* 25:602–611.

Lopes Pegna, A., G. Picozzi, M. Mascalchi, F. Maria Carozzi, L. Carrozzi, C. Comin, C. Spinelli et al. 2009. Design, recruitment and baseline results of the ITALUNG trial for lung cancer screening with low-dose CT. *Lung Cancer* 64:34–40.

Mascalchi, M., L. N. Mazzoni, M. Falchini, G. Belli, G. Picozzi, V. Merlini, A. Vella et al. 2011. Dose exposure in the ITALUNG trial of lung cancer screening with low-dose CT. *The British Journal of Radiology*.

McNitt-Gray, M. F., S. G. Armato III, C. R. Meyer, A. P. Reeves, G. McLennan, R. Pais, J. Freymann et al. 2007. The Lung Image Database Consortium (LIDC) data collection process for nodule detection and annotation. *Academic Radiology* 14:1464–1474.

Messay, T., R. C. Hardie, and S. K. Rogers. 2010. A new computationally efficient CAD system for pulmonary nodule detection in CT imagery. *Medical Image Analysis* 14:390–406.

Meyer, C. R., S. G. Armato III, C. P. Fenimore, G. McLennan, L. M. Bidaut, D. P. Barboriak, M. A. Gavrielides et al. 2009. Quantitative imaging to assess tumor response to therapy: Common themes of measurement, truth data and error sources. *Translational Oncology* 2:198–210.

Meyer, C. R., T. D. Johnson, G. McLennan, D. R. Aberle, E. A. Kazerooni, H. MacMahon, B. F. Mullan et al. 2006. Evaluation of lung MDCT nodule annotation across radiologists and methods. *Academic Radiology* 13:1254–1265.

Murphy, K., B. van Ginneken, A. M. Schilham, B. J. de Hoop, H. A. Gietema, and M. Prokop. 2009. A large-scale evaluation of automatic pulmonary nodule detection in chest CT using local image features and k-nearest-neighbour classification. *Medical Image Analysis* 13:757–770.

Nishikawa, R. M., M. L. Giger, K. Doi, C. E. Metz, F.-F. Yin, C. J. Vyborny, and R. A. Schmidt. 1994. Effect of case selection on the performance of computer-aided detection schemes. *Medical Physics* 21:265–269.

Nishikawa, R. M. and L. M. Yarusso. 1998. Variations in measured performance of CAD schemes due to database composition and scoring protocol. *SPIE Proceedings* 3338:840–844.

Ochs, R. A., J. G. Goldin, F. Abtin, H. J. Kim, K. Brown, P. Batra, D. Roback et al. 2007. Automated classification of lung bronchovascular anatomy in CT using AdaBoost. *Medical Image Analysis* 11:315–324.

Oda, S., K. Awai, K. Suzuki, Y. Yanaga, Y. Funama, H. MacMahon, and Y. Yamashita. 2009. Performance of radiologists in detection of small pulmonary nodules on chest radiographs: Effect of rib suppression with a massive-training artificial neural network. *American Journal of Roentgenology* 193:W397–W402.

Opulencia, P., D. S. Channin, D. S. Raicu, and J. D. Furst. 2011. Mapping LIDC, RadLex, and lung nodule image features. *Journal of Digital Imaging* 24:256–270.

Ozekes, S. and O. Osman. 2010. Computerized lung nodule detection using 3D feature extraction and learning based algorithms. *Journal of Medical Systems* 34:185–194.

Ozekes, S., O. Osman, and O. N. Ucan. 2008. Nodule detection in a lung region that's segmented with using genetic cellular neural networks and 3D template matching with fuzzy rule based thresholding. *Korean Journal of Radiology* 9:1–9.

Picozzi, G., E. Paci, A. Lopez Pegna, M. Bartolucci, G. Roselli, A. De Francisci, S. Gabrielli et al. 2005. Screening of lung cancer with low dose spiral CT: results of a three year pilot study and design of the randomised controlled trial "Italung-CT". *La Radiologia Medica* 109:17–26.

Reeves, A. P., A. M. Biancardi, T. V. Apanasovich, C. R. Meyer, H. MacMahon, E. J. R. van Beek, E. A. Kazerooni et al. 2007. The Lung Image Database Consortium (LIDC): A comparison of different size metrics for pulmonary nodule measurements. *Academic Radiology* 14:1475–1485.

Reeves, A. P., A. M. Biancardi, D. Yankelevitz, S. Fotin, B. M. Keller, A. Jirapatnakul, and J. Lee. 2009. A public image database to support research in computer aided diagnosis. In: *31st Annual International Conference of the IEEE Engineering in Medicine and Biology Society*, 3715–3718.

Riccardi, A., T. S. Petkov, G. Ferri, M. Masotti, and R. Campanini. 2011. Computer-aided detection of lung nodules via 3D fast radial transform, scale space representation, and Zernike MIP classification. *Medical Physics* 38:1962–1971.

Ross, J. C., J. V. Miller, W. D. Turner, and T. P. Kelliher. 2007. An analysis of early studies released by the Lung Imaging Database Consortium (LIDC). *Academic Radiology* 14:1382–1388.

Rubin, D. L., P. Mongkolwat, and D. S. Channin. 2009. A semantic image annotation model to enable integrative translational research. *AMIA Summit on Translational Bioinformatics*.

Sahiner, B., H. P. Chan, L. M. Hadjiiski, P. N. Cascade, E. A. Kazerooni, A. R. Chughtai, C. Poopat et al. 2009. Effect of CAD on radiologists' detection of lung nodules on thoracic CT scans: Analysis of an observer performance study by nodule size. *Academic Radiology* 16:1518–1530.

Schilham, A. M., B. van Ginneken, and M. Loog. 2006. A computer-aided diagnosis system for detection of lung nodules in chest radiographs with an evaluation on a public database. *Medical Image Analysis* 10:247–258.

Sensakovic, W. F., A. Starkey, R. Y. Roberts, and S. G. Armato III. 2008. Discrete-space versus continuous-space lesion boundary and area definition. *Medical Physics* 35:4070–4078.

Shiraishi, J., S. Katsuragawa, J. Ikezoe, T. Matsumoto, T. Kobayashi, K. Komatsu, M. Matsui et al. 2000. Development of a digital image database for chest radiographs with and without a lung nodule: Receiver operating characteristic analysis of radiologists' detection of pulmonary nodules. *American Journal of Roentgenology* 174:71–74.

Tan, J., J. Pu, B. Zheng, X. Wang, and J. K. Leader. 2010. Computerized comprehensive data analysis of Lung Imaging Database Consortium (LIDC). *Medical Physics* 37:3802–3808.

Tan, M., R. Deklerck, B. Jansen, M. Bister, and J. Cornelis. 2011. A novel computer-aided lung nodule detection system for CT images. *Medical Physics* 38:5630–5645.

Therasse, P., S. G. Arbuck, E. A. Eisenhauer, J. Wanders, R. S. Kaplan, L. Rubinstein, J. Verweij et al. 2000. New guidelines to evaluate the response to treatment in solid tumors. *Journal of the National Cancer Institute* 92:205–216.

Turner, W. D., T. P. Kelliher, J. C. Ross, and J. V. Miller. 2006. An analysis of early studies released by the Lung Imaging Database Consortium (LIDC). *Medical Image Computing and Computer-Assisted Intervention 2006* 9:487–494.

Usami, H., M. Ikeda, T. Ishigaki, H. Fukushima, and K. Shimamoto. 2006. The influence of liquid crystal display (LCD) monitors on observer performance for the detection of nodular lesions on chest radiographs. *European Radiology* 16:726–732.

van Ginneken, B., S. G. Armato III, B. de Hoop, S. van Amelsvoort-van de Vorst, T. Duindam, M. Niemeijer, K. Murphy et al. 2010. Comparing and combining algorithms for computer-aided detection of pulmonary nodules in computed tomography scans: The ANODE09 study. *Medical Image Analysis* 14:707–722.

van Ginneken, B., M. B. Stegmann, and M. Loog. 2006. Segmentation of anatomical structures in chest radiographs using supervised methods: A comparative study on a public database. *Medical Image Analysis* 10:19–40.

van Iersel, C. A., H. J. de Koning, G. Draisma, W. P. T. M. Mali, E. T. Scholten, K. Nackaerts, M. Prokop et al. 2007. Risk-based selection from the general population in a screening trial: Selection criteria, recruitment and power for the Dutch-Belgian randomised lung cancer multi-slice CT screening trial (NELSON). *International Journal of Cancer* 120:868–874.

van Rikxoort, E. M., B. de Hoop, M. A. Viergever, M. Prokop, and B. van Ginneken. 2009. Automatic lung segmentation from thoracic computed tomography scans using a hybrid approach with error detection. *Medical Physics* 36:2934–2947.

Wang, J., R. Engelmann, and Q. Li. 2007. Segmentation of pulmonary nodules in three-dimensional CT images by use of a spiral-scanning technique. *Medical Physics* 34:4678–4689.

Wang, Q., E. Song, R. Jin, P. Han, X. Wang, Y. Zhou, and J. Zeng. 2009. Segmentation of lung nodules in computed tomography images using dynamic programming and multidirection fusion techniques. *Academic Radiology* 16:678–688.

Way, T. W., L. M. Hadjiiski, B. Sahiner, H. P. Chan, P. N. Cascade, E. A. Kazerooni, N. Bogot et al. 2006. Computer-aided diagnosis of pulmonary nodules on CT scans: Segmentation and classification using 3D active contours. *Medical Physics* 33:2323–2337.

Xu, D. M., H. Gietema, H. de Koning, R. Vernhout, K. Nackaerts, M. Prokop, C. Weenink et al. 2006. Nodule management protocol of the NELSON randomised lung cancer screening trial. *Lung Cancer* 54:177–184.

Xu, D. M., R. J. van Klaveren, G. H. de Bock, A. Leusveld, Y. Zhao, Y. Wang, R. Vliegenthart et al. 2008. Limited value of shape, margin and CT density in the discrimination between benign and malignant screen detected solid pulmonary nodules of the NELSON trial. *European Journal of Radiology* 68:347–352.

Xu, D. M., R. J. van Klaveren, G. H. de Bock, A. L. M. Leusveld, M. D. Dorrius, Y. Zhao, Y. Wang et al. 2009. Role of baseline nodule density and changes in density and nodule features in the discrimination between benign and malignant solid indeterminate pulmonary nodules. *European Journal of Radiology* 70:492–498.

Chapter 13

Detection and Diagnosis of Colonic Polyp in CT Colonography

Jerome Zhengrong Liang

CONTENTS

13.1 INTRODUCTION

According to the most recent statistics from American Cancer Society (http://www.cancer.org/docroot/home/index.asp), colorectal carcinoma ranks as the fourth most commonly diagnosed cancer and the second leading cause of death from cancers in the United States (Jemal et al. 2010). It was estimated that more than 142,000 new cases will be diagnosed with more than 50,000 dying from the disease in 2010 (Jemal et al. 2010). Similar to other cancers, colon cancer is often diagnosed at an advanced stage, after the patient has developed symptoms. Different from other cancers, most colon cancers can be avoided because they arise from adenomatous polyps, a precursor that takes a long time period over several years of malignant transformation and can be detected during the transformation period. For example, it takes more than 2 years for an adenomatous polyp to grow to 5 mm size with far less than 1% cancer risk, an additional 3 or more years to 10 mm size with

cancer risk approaching to 1%, and another 5 or more years to 20 mm size and 10% cancer risk (Grandqvist 1981, Stryker et al. 1987, Potter and Slattery 1993, Jass 2007, Yoo et al. 2007). Therefore, screening of an asymptomatic patient at an adequate time interval and removal of detected adenomatous polyps of less than 10 mm can effectively cure the patient (Morimoto et al. 2002, Winawer and Zauber 2002). There are several options currently available for the screening purpose, such as (1) fecal occult blood testing (Mandel et al. 2000), (2) fecal immunochemical or immunoassay testing (Allison et al. 2007), (3) stool DNA testing (Ahlquist et al 2008), (4) double-contrast or air-contrast barium enema (Brady et al. 1994), (5) flexible sigmoidoscopy (Levin et al. 2005), and (6) optical colonoscopy (OC) (Hafner 2007). Each has advantages and drawbacks (Liang and Richards 2010), where OC is the gold standard for the evaluation of the entire colon wall mucosal (or inner) surface with therapeutic capability of resection of found abnormalities.

Prior to the OC procedure, the patient must undergo full oral bowel preparation of (1) taking liquid diet in one or more days and (2) ingesting laxative solutions for colon cleansing the evening before the examination. The procedure starts by inserting a flexible scope into the colon from the rectum up to the cecum. When withdrawing the scope, a camera at the tip of the scope captures the images of the inner surface of the colon. If a polyp is found, a resection can be performed through a channel inside the scope. Sedation is commonly used to relieve the discomfort during the procedure, and, therefore, an escort is needed to accompany the patient to home. In current practice, OC removes all findings, regardless if adenomatous or hyperplastic polyps, where the latter kind of polyp is benign (Morimoto et al. 2002).

While it is accurate and can biopsy detected polyps, OC has several drawbacks: (1) It is an uncomfortable invasive procedure, and sedation may be needed. (2) The bowel preparation prior to the procedure is stressful, requiring full oral laxative colon cleansing, and may cause abdominal discomfort, cramps, faintness, etc. (Cai et al. 2009). (3) It is time consuming (especially for elders), ranging from 30 min up to an hour. (4) It carries a small risk of perforation and death (colonic perforation in 1 in 500–1000 cases and death in 1 in 2000–5000 cases) (Orsoni et al. 1997). (5) It fails to demonstrate the entire colon in 10%–15% of cases (i.e., the scope cannot reach the cecum) and thus misses 10%–20% of lesions (Pickhardt et al. 2004, Heresbach et al. 2008). For the purpose of screening, the asymptomatic patient population aged over 50, since the polyps ranging from 6 to 9 mm would be 8%–9% and polyps of 10 mm and larger would be 5%–7% (Heresbach et al. 2008, Lieberman et al. 2008), that is, a total of less than 20%, therefore OC could generate more than 80% negative cases (no finding) as a screening tool. The risk and cost on these negative cases would be unnecessary. Furthermore, since the small advanced adenomas of 6–9 mm would be 0.17%–0.46% and all adenomas would be 3%–4% (Lieberman et al. 2008), so among the 16% detected polyps (9% for the size of 6–9 mm and 7% for the size of 10 mm and larger) in the best performance, less than one-third is adenomatous (others are hyperplastic). The resection of the other two-thirds, that is, the hyperplastic polyps, by current OC practice may not be necessary. Overall, the miss rate of OC for large adenomas and cancer has been shown to be about 12% and 5%, respectively (Heresbach et al. 2008).

Because of the high prevalence, lack of screening resource (including both manpower and devices), and low compliance rate, these explain the current high mortality rate of colorectal incidence. A convenient, effective screening method for the evaluation of the entire colon and detection and diagnosis of polyps as small as 5 mm is desired.

Since 1994, several pilot studies (Vining et al. 1994, Hong et al. 1995) of evaluating the feasibility of an alternative means for screening the entire colon have motivated a great amount of research interests ranging from image formation and processing to visualization (Hong et al. 1997, Reed and Johnson 1997, Wan et al. 1999), although there was an early report in 1983 (Coin et al. 1983). This alternative means is called computed tomography (CT)-based virtual colonoscopy (VC) or CT colonography (CTC). It utilizes medical imaging and computer techniques to visualize the inner surface of the colon wall in the CT images, looking for polyps. More specifically, it can mimic the OC procedure by first constructing a three-dimensional (3D) patient-specific colon model using the patient's abdominal CT images and then building a virtual-reality environment inside the model. A radiologist can use the computer mouse to control a talking navigation inside the model as if he/she is walking inside the colon and looking for abnormalities. In practice, CTC procedure starts by inflating a cleansed colon by room air or CO_2 gas introduced through rectal insert. Then, abdominal CT slice images are taken in seconds (during a single breath-holding) with sub mm resolution in both axial and transverse directions and excellent contrast between the colon wall and the lumen (filled by air/CO_2). The slice images are stacked together as a volume image, from which the patient-specific colon model is constructed. Image segmentation is necessary for the construction of an accurate colon model (Liang et al. 1999). Computer graphics are heavily involved to navigate or fly through inside the 3D virtual colon model.

The potential of CTC to be a screening option has been demonstrated by two large clinical trials (Pickhardt et al. 2003, Johnson et al. 2008), indicating that by the same full oral bowel cleansing, both CTC and OC have a similar performance for detecting polyps of 8 mm and larger.

However, there are several obstacles preventing CTC from becoming a screening modality, as evidenced by the recent refusal of CTC to be included in Medicare coverage: http://www.cms.hhs.gov/mcd/viewpubliccomments.asp?nca_id=220, such as the risk from x-ray radiation, the challenge in detecting small polyps (less than 10 mm in size), the reluctance of going through the full oral bowel cleansing as OC does, the readers' variation and efficiency, etc. Researches to overcome these obstacles have been in progress. This chapter reviews mainly one of the research topics, that is, computer-aided detection and diagnosis of polyps (CADpolyp, including both computer-aided detection [CADe] and computer-aided diagnosis [CADx]) for the possibility of maximizing the reader's efficiency, minimizing the readers' variation, improving the detection of small polyps, alleviating the stress of bowel preparation, etc.

13.2 COMPUTERIZED DETECTION OF COLONIC POLYP IN CT COLONOGRAPHY

The detection of polyps is expected to be performed on the colon wall in the acquired CT abdominal volumetric image. While constructing a virtual colon model from a cleansed CT volume image for the inspection of the entire colon inner surface could be achieved currently by a commercial system, for example, the V3D Colon Module (Viatronix, Inc., Stony Brook, NY), searching for abnormalities and identifying polyps along the long colon *pipe* would be a challenging task because of the involved intensive user interaction during the fly-through navigation. In addition, the variation among readers with different experience has been widely noticed. Conceptually, CADe can reduce the readers' interaction effort and minimize the variation among readers' assessments. However, a series of investigations turned out that developing an effective CADe system is very challenging (Vining et al. 1997, Summers et al. 2001, Yoshida and Nappi 2001, Wang et al. 2005, Taylor et al. 2006, Bielen and Kiss 2007), because of various causes of false positives (FPs), such as imperfect bowel cleansing, complicated colon fold structures, image noise, and motion artifacts. This chapter reviews some of the major challenges and their related research progresses from the view point of image information processing (a description of image content from image formation and processing to visualization [Liang et al. 2007]).

13.2.1 Acquisition of Abdominal Volumetric Images

Image acquisition for CTC is currently achieved by helical or spiral scanning using a multi-detector band CT system. Within a single breath-holding of less than 20 s, the spiral scanning can cover the entire abdomen, generating a set of more than 400 slice images of 512 × 512 array size. The image resolution can be less than 1 mm isotropically. If each image element or voxel has an intensity value of 16 bits (or two bytes) in computer space, the image volume of 512 × 512 × 400 array size will take 200 MB space in a computer. Manipulating such high image volume quantity of 200 MB is computationally intensive even by a currently available powerful computer.

By current CTC practice, the patient will be frequently scanned at two (supine and prone) positions. Sometimes, a third (lateral) position will be scanned, resulting in three sets of slice images each set taking 200 MB of computer space. By current data acquisition protocol and image reconstruction techniques, each of the two or three scans carries approximately 3.0 mSv radiation dose. As the most efficient algorithm, an analytical filtered back-projection (FBP)-type reconstruction technique, for example (Kachelrieβ

et al. 2001), can produce more than two slice images per second in a modern CT system.

The CT-associated radiation risk is a concern for the screening purpose (Brenner and Hall 2007). Research for reducing the radiation is under progress, mostly by delivering less x-ray energy (e.g., lowering mAs or kVp parameters in data acquisition protocol) to the patient and developing adaptive statistical algorithms to model the data properties of the low-dose acquisition protocols and to reconstruct the images from the modeled low-dose data (Lu et al. 2003, Wang et al. 2008a). The statistical reconstruction requires more computing time than the analytical FBP-type algorithm. The increase can be significant if iterative calculation is necessary (Wang et al. 2006b).

The desired information in each acquired CTC volumetric image is the colon wall. Extracting the wall volume from the large image quantity of over 200 MB size is the major task of the following image processing tasks.

13.2.2 Processing of Volumetric Image Data for Colon Wall Model

Given a set of the acquired slice images, the main goal of image data processing is to construct a patient-specific virtual colon model as stated earlier. By stacking all the slice images together, we have a volumetric image data, representing the patient's abdomen. If the colon lumen is fully filled with air or CO_2 gas, which has a very small image intensity value close to −1000 in Hounsfield Unit (HU) as compared to that of the colon wall with an image intensity value around zero in HU, then by the use of a threshold, the lumen space can be extracted. All the image elements or voxels on the border of the lumen volume make up the inner surface of the colon wall, reflecting the virtual colon model.

In reality, the model construction is much more complicated because of imperfect colon cleansing and insufficient colon insufflations of the complex colon structure as well as other causes. For example, the colonic residues (stool and fluid), which were retained inside the lumen space after bowel cleansing, have similar image intensities as that of the colon wall and are indistinguishable from the wall.

To obtain good image contrasts between the colon wall and the colonic residues for the colon model construction, oral contrast solutions may be needed to tag the residues (Liang et al. 1997). Because of the variation in tagging, sophisticated image segmentation is necessary. The combination of tagging the colonic materials and segmenting the images is termed electronic colon cleansing (ECC) (Liang et al. 1997, Wang et al. 2006a). More detailed review on this topic can be found in Chapter 15 of this book and Liang (2008).

An ideal tagging contrast would be to decrease the densities of the colonic fluid and stool for less x-ray attenuation similar to that of the air/CO_2, so that the colon lumen becomes *dark* in the CT images. In the absence of such ideal contrast solution, a suboptimal choice is to increase the densities for enhanced image intensities on the colonic materials (Liang et al. 1997). Because of the enhanced image intensities, there are several drawbacks associated with the suboptimal choice, for example, the presence of partial volume (PV) effect at the interface between the colon wall and the colonic materials with nonuniformly enhanced image intensities, and, therefore, sophisticated image segmentation and pre- and postsegmentation processing algorithms are needed to address the PV effect and the nonuniformly enhanced image intensity distribution (e.g., Näppi et al. 2007, Wang et al. 2008b, Zhang et al. 2011a).

A major drawback of the suboptimal choice of positive tagging is the cause of burying of small polyps inside the tagged materials in the acquired image volume, as shown in the left column of Figure 13.1. Without considering the burying effect via a restoration operation, a segmentation algorithm would generate the results of the middle column, representing shrunken objects. By a restoration operation, for example, an adaptive scaling operation (Zhang et al. 2011a), the size of the submerged objects can be noticeably

recovered. While the burying effect can be reduced by a restoration operation, the PV effect remains.

For the purpose of detecting small polyps, the PV effect occurring at the inner border of the colon wall shall be considered and the image intensities around the border shall be preserved when constructing the virtual colon model and performing the task of CADpolyp. Toward that end, segmenting tissue mixtures inside each image voxel has shown the potential to minimize the PV effect while preserving the image information for the detection of small polyps (Wang et al. 2008b). Figure 13.2 shows an example of our mixture-based image segmentation. The theoretical details of the mixture-based image segmentation are given in Liang and Wang (2009). Other segmentation methods for the colon wall model can be seen in Chen et al. (2000), Serlie et al. (2003), and Cai et al. (2006).

By the mixture segmentation, we obtain a shell volume enclosing the inner border of the colon wall, where each voxel contains the percentages of all different tissues inside. The shell volume can be shrunk to a surface for CADpolyp as seen in most CADe reports in the past. By our opinion, CADpolyp shall be performed on the shell volume because of the preserved image information about the colon mucosal layer where the clinical significance resides.

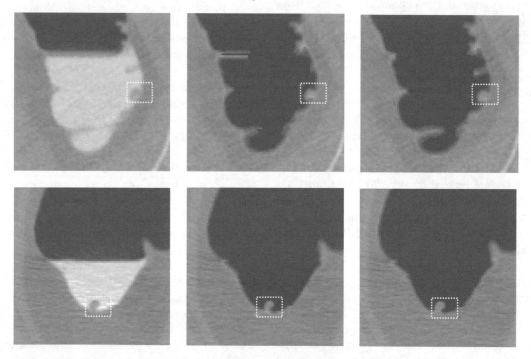

Figure 13.1   An illustration of the cause of burying small polyps in the positive tagging regime. The left column shows the original CT images, where the submerged colonic structures and polyps become smaller in visual inspection. The middle column shows the segmentation results without restoration on the burying effect. (From Wang et al., *Med. Phys.*, 35, 5787, 2008a.) On the right column are the segmentation results after restoration on the burying effect. (From Zhang, G., Lu, H., and Liang, Z., A feasibility study on the differentiation of polyps types for CADx. *Lab Technical Report*, Department of Radiology, Stony Brook University, 2011b.)

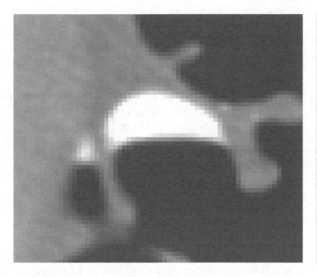
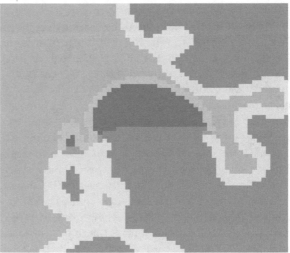

Figure 13.2   (See color insert.) Picture on the left shows a portion of a CT slice image where the borders or interfaces between different materials are blurred due to PV effect. By our mixture image segmentation, we are able to detect those interfaces where the percentages of different materials in each image voxel are estimated. The red color shows the pure air material and blue indicates the pure tagged materials (colonic fluid and liquefied stool). The interface space of air and tagged materials are shown by pink/gray colors. The yellow color indicates the interface space of air and colon tissues. The light blue color shows the interface space of tagged materials and colon tissues. The PV layers are accurately identified where the polyps stay. By removing the percentages of non-colon wall materials in those voxels inside the PV layers, we obtain a layer that reflects the colon mucosa structure. An accurate mucosa structure is the key for accurate detection of polyps, especially small ones.

If the ECC is successful, only one scan of the patient would be sufficient for CTC at either the supine, prone, or lateral position, resulting in the reduction of the x-ray radiation by a half or more. Furthermore, the routine laxative colon cleansing may no longer be necessary (Liang et al. 2005), achieving cathartic-free (or minimal or free laxative bowel preparation) CTC and therefore relieving the patient stress on bowel preparation.

Prior to a successful ECC being developed, two to three scans of the patient remain the choice of the CTC practice. From each scan, we will construct a virtual colon model. Registration of the colon models from the multiple scans remains a research topic despite noticeable progress in the past decade (Wang et al. 2009).

From the registered colon models, a true detection shall occur at the same location in all the models. Because of registration error, such true detection may not be achievable. In reality, such true detection might not be achievable. However, all the scans may provide information supplemental to each other. The registered colon models can facilitate the image interpretation when the radiologists look at the models for clinical assessment. It remains an interesting research topic if the registration will improve CADe performance.

In the following, the presentation assumes a single colon model from one scan at either the supine, prone, or lateral position.

13.2.3 Localization of Initial Polyp Candidates from Colon Wall Model

From the mixture segmentation, a shell volume is extracted, which encloses the inner border or mucosal layer of the colon wall and represents the colon model. Then, sensitive shape geometry measures, such as curvature (or related metrics, e.g., shape index, sphericity ratio), surface normal (or related metrics), and more (Summers et al. 2001, Yoshida and Nappi 2001, Kiss et al. 2002, Konlukoglu et al. 2007, van Wijk et al. 2010), can be applied to the colon model volume to localize suspicious patches as initial polyp candidates (IPCs) (Wang et al. 2008c, Zhu et al. 2010). The goal of this step is to localize all suspects without missing any true polyp or true positives (TPs) in an efficient way so that we will thereafter focus our interest to the patches of small areas and ignore the other normal large areas on the colon model. Of course, there are many FPs. It still remains a challenging task to detect small candidates with reasonable number of FPs in an efficient manner (Zhu et al. 2010, 2011).

Removing FPs from the IPCs has been a major focus in CADe research in the past decade. One approach is to find more geometry-based features and/or improved classifiers. Examples of this approach are described in Göktürk et al. (2001), Acar et al. (2002), Kiss et al. (2002), Jeroebko et al. (2003), Chowdhury et al. (2006), van Wijk et al. (2010), and

Zhu et al. (2011). Another approach is to extract texture-related features from the volume of each suspicious patch. Examples of this latter approach are described in Liang et al. (2002), Näppi and Yoshida (2002, 2003), Yoshida et al. (2002), Wang et al. (2005), Liang et al. (2008), Lu et al. (2008), and Zhu et al. (2009, 2010a).

In the former approach, most features are related to the curvature and generated by convolving specific operators with the image intensities of the segmented 3D colon wall (Monga et al. 1992, Monga and Benayoun 1992, Sundaram et al. 2008). Unfortunately, the colons are densely structured, and different topological structures may be located in one neighborhood area. The adjacent unrelated structures are possibly involved in the convolution. Therefore, the feature calculation remains a research topic. Improved feature calculation can render a noticeable gain in the localization of IPCs (Zhu et al. 2011). Also improved convolution among topological structures by an adequate means, for example, level set method, and the associated distance transform function have shown better distinguishing of different colon structures for feature extraction, leading to improved CADe performance (Zhu et al. 2009). In addition to the research interest in exploring more geometry-related features and improved feature calculations, the development of high-performance classifiers has been remaining a major focus in the CADe research field (Yao et al. 2005, Suzuki et al. 2008, Song et al. 2011).

Regarding the latter approach, the usefulness of texture-related features for CADpolyp can be seen from the following experiments. A projection was performed through the 3D object of either stool ball or polyp to form a 2D planar image or view (Wan et al. 2001). The intensity value of each pixel in the 2D projected image is a weighted integral value along each projection ray through the object. Figure 13.3 shows an example of the projection view through two stool balls, respectively. Figure 13.4 shows an example of the projection view through hyperplastic and adenoma polyps, respectively. While there is some small variation in the geometry characteristics among stool ball, hypoplastic polyp and adenoma polyp, as seen in the left columns of these two figures, the texture-related features are noticeably different, as seen in the right columns of the figures. This observation indicates that CADe is highly likely to differentiate polyps from stool because of the very different textures between polyps and stool. Furthermore, the texture difference between the hypoplastic and adenoma polyps may indicate the possibility of differentiating the hypoplastic polyps and adenoma ones or the feasibility of CADx of polyp types. More detailed description on the latter approach of how to extract texture-related features is given by the following sections.

13.2.4 Determination of Volumes of Interest for Initial Polyp Candidates

For each localized patch, its volume contains the essential information while its surrounding would provide more or less supplementary information for the description of its characteristics. Determining the volume of interest (VOI) remains a research topic. Up to now, two strategies have been reported, both of which use the detected portion of the patch protruded into the lumen space as the base. One strategy explores the image contrast between the lesion and its surrounding normal tissue. Since the image contrast between the lesion and its surrounding normal tissue inside the colon wall volume is usually very small, this strategy could fail in some cases. The other strategy utilizes dilation techniques to grow the detected portion into the colon wall space. Since the detected patch varies significantly in shape and the dilation depends on the patch shape, this latter strategy could provide variable results depending on the patch and stopping criterion on the dilation process.

The first strategy, Wang et al. (2005), selected several rays, which start on the detected border of the patch and go into the wall along the normal directions. A wavelet-based edge detector was developed to find the edge of the suspect patch inside the wall. From the found edge points inside the wall and those points on the detected patch border protruding into the lumen, the surface of a VOI was fitted by surface fitting. Other researchers, for example, Yao et al. (2004) and van Wijk et al. (2010), have used different deformable models to segment the VOIs of IPCs.

In the second strategy, conditional dilation was employed to dilate the detected portion of the patch (i.e., the portion that protrudes into the lumen) into the wall (Nappi 2003). Later, the conditional dilation was further improved with a convex dilation process, which stops when a concave shape is reached (Zhu et al. 2010). Figure 13.5 shows an example from the convex dilation process strategy with comparison to the results of other methods.

Because of lack of image contrast between the detected patch and its surrounding, the challenge of extracting the VOI of each IPC remains. The latest report of utilizing the convex dilation seems robust to patch shape variation and always gives a reasonable VOI (Zhu et al. 2010a). However, without the ground truth, evaluation of the accuracy of the convex dilation method seems unrealistic. In the following, we assume that the extracted VOI is sufficiently accurate for the generation of texture-related features. Our focus will then turn to what features can be generated from the VOI.

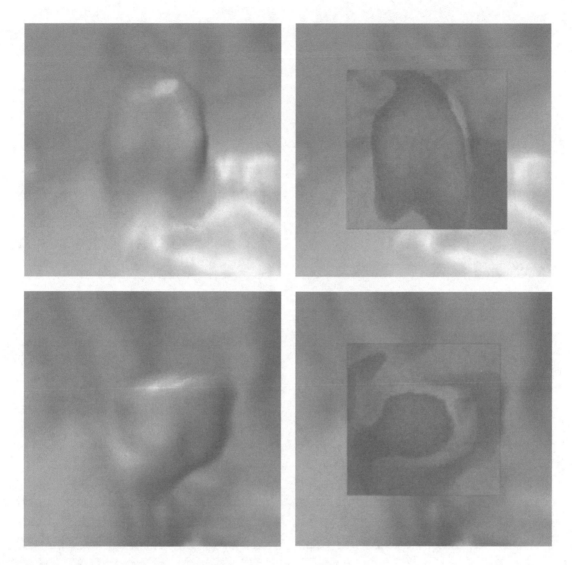

Figure 13.3   (See color insert.) An illustration of texture features of small stool balls retained inside the lumen space after routine bowel cleansing. On the left are the endoscopic views, reflecting the geometrical features of the stool balls. On the right are the projections through the stool ball volumes, showing the texture features.

13.2.5   Extraction and Selection of Features from Volumes of Interest

Given a VOI, various geometry- and texture-related features can be extracted by the use of the VOI border geometry and the intensity distribution inside VOI (Nappi 2003, Zhu et al. 2009). The top two rows of Table 13.1 show some examples of the geometry- and texture-related features.

In addition to the two feature types referred earlier, other feature types have been recently explored from the VOI. For example, Wang et al. (2005) investigated some morphology-related features from an ellipsoid VOI; see the third row in Table 13.1. Lu et al. (2008) studied a few co-occurrence matrix texture features from any shape VOI; see the fourth row in Table 13.1. Zhu et al. (2010a) took advantage of the projection views through a 3D object and explored the texture features in the projected planar images; see the bottom row in Table 13.1. It is expected that more features will be extracted from the VOI in the future. At the present time, a total of more than 30 features can be extracted from each VOI of the IPCs.

Classifying a large number of features for polyp detection is an undesirable task because of the dimension problem, named curse of dimensionality (Powell 2007, Wang et al. 2010). Some features may not be important, and inclusion of these features can degrade the classification

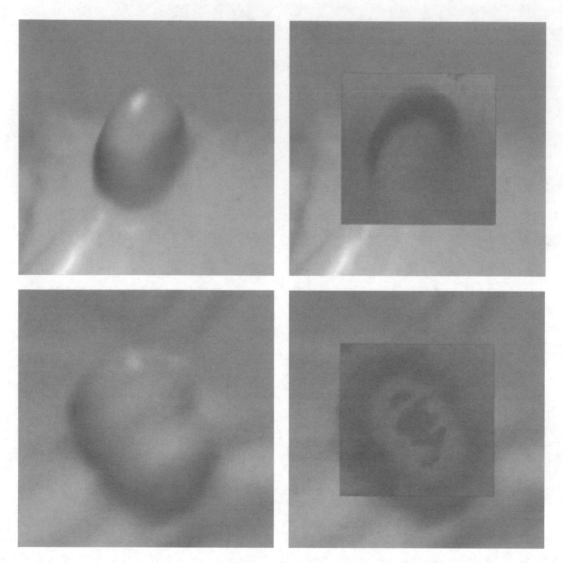

Figure 13.4   **(See color insert.)** An illustration of texture features of small polyps. On the left are the endoscopic views, reflecting the geometrical features of the polyps. On the right are the projections through the polyp volumes. The top row shows a hyperplastic polyp and the bottom row shows an adenoma polyp.

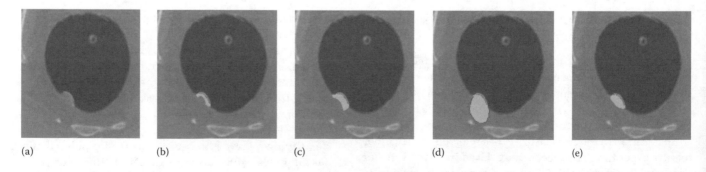

(a)   (b)   (c)   (d)   (e)

Figure 13.5   **(See color insert.)** An experimental study of different VOI determination strategies. (a) A 12 mm sessile polyp in an axial slice, where the voxels in red color indicate the detected suspicious patch. (b) An initial VOI in the slice (including the red and green areas) generated by dilating the detected suspicious patch for a few steps. (c) The result from the previous method in Näppi et al. (2003). (d) The result from the previous method in Wang et al. (2005), where the blue curve represents the inner border found by the Harr transformation–based edge finder. (e) The result from the convex dilation process strategy. (From Zhu, H. et al., *Phys. Biol. Med.*, 55, 2087, 2010.)

TABLE 13.1   LIST OF EXAMPLE FEATURES USED IN CTC

	Features	Description
Geometry-related features	Mean(SI), var(SI), skew(SI), etc.	Statistics of shape index, like mean, variance, and skewness
	Mean(CV), var(CV), skew(CV), etc.	Statistics of curvedness, like mean, variances, and skewness
	AR	The axis ratio
Texture-related features	Mean(CT), var(CT), skew(CT), kurtosis(CT), entropy(CT), etc.	Statistics of CT density distribution, like mean, variance, and skewness
Morphology-related features	CR, RR	Coverage ratio on the VOI border, radiation ratio on the VOI border distribution
Co-occurrence matrix texture features	GLCM, GLGCM	Gray-level co-occurrence matrix, gray-level-gradient co-occurrence matrix
Projection texture features	HR, DL	The highlighting ratio and disk-likeness from the axial gray image
	LRC, LRS	The lightness ratios of the coronal and sagittal gray images
	$POS_x^C(L), POS_y^C(L), POS_x^C(B), POS_y^C(B)$ $POS_x^S(L), POS_y^S(L), POS_x^S(B), POS_y^S(B)$	The normalized positions of the light and bright patches in the coronal and sagittal images
	$f_{hue}, f_{saturation}, f_{intensity}$	The three components of the dominant color of the core area in the axial color image

performance. Selection of important features for classification purpose remains a challenging task. In general, feature selection or intrinsic dimensionality is a relatively rich field and has been widely studied in signal processing, model selection, etc. It is expected that more research effort will be devoted in the future to explore its application in CTC.

One example of recent effort to explore feature selection for CTC is reported in Wang et al. (2010), which adapts a constrained energy minimization strategy from signal band selection to application in CTC. Another example is described in Zhu et al. (2010b), where principal component analysis (PCA)-based strategy is used to reduce the feature correlation. The eigenvalue is believed to be part of the corresponding feature and should be combined with the associated principal component to yield a new feature. Therefore, each principal component is adaptively weighted with its corresponding eigenvalue, and thus the feature selection is partially implemented by the different weights. The gain by the use of PCA for feature selection for CADe in CTC can be seen from an experimental study, as shown in Figure 13.6.

Based on these two examples, we further explored other feature selection strategies for CTC application. By the use of the area under the receiver operating characteristic (ROC) curve, that is, AUC, as the merit, we examined

the conventional PCA, Laplacian eigenmap, neighborhood preserving embedding, partial least squares, and minimum redundancy maximum relevance strategies with comparison to our most recent method (i.e., graph embedding method in a semi-supervised style—SemiGE [Fan et al. 2012a]). The comparison results are shown in Figure 13.7, where the well-known support vector machine (SVM) classifier was used. The feature selection method of SemiGE showed most robust performance in terms of AUC measure.

13.2.6 Reduction of False Positives in Initial Polyp Candidates

Given a set of selected features from a VOI of IPC, our next task is to classify these features to determine if the IPC is a TP. Several classifiers have been widely used, such as SVM (Burges 1998, Chang and Lin 2001) and artificial neural network (ANN) (Egmont-Petersen et al. 2002). Adapting these two well-known classifiers with various implementation strategies for CADe in CTC can be seen in Jeroebko et al. (2003), Yao et al. (2005), Suzuki et al. (2008), and Zhu et al. (2009).

A review of alternative polyp classification strategies, which are specific to the application for CADe in CTC, can be a long list (Bielen and Kiss 2007). Typical

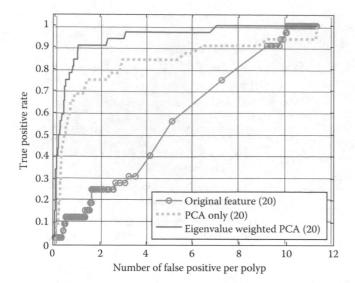

Figure 13.6 An experimental study on the use of PCA for feature selection. A total of 20 features were extracted from each VOI of IPCs. The artificial neural network (ANN) classifier was used to generate the results, and the results were represented by the plot of free-response receiver operating characteristic (FROC). The curve with circles shows the result from the original 20 features. The curve with solid dots shows the result from the PCA-transformed features (or the principal components). It is observed that the decorrelation PCA operation among the 20 features improves the CADe performance noticeably. The curve of solid line represents the result from the eigenvalue-weighted principal components or the new features. The gain by the eigenvalue-weighted PCA strategy is obvious.

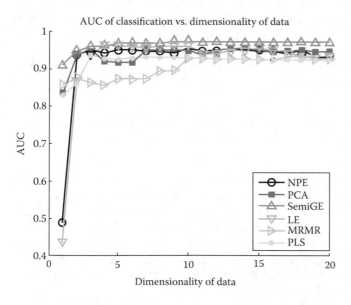

Figure 13.7 A 21D feature vector is extracted from each VOI. There are a total of 786 VOIs, in which 64 are true polyps. After selection of the first seven features, the SemiGE strategy generated the best result in terms of AUC.

examples of these alternative strategies are briefly outlined as follows.

Göktürk et al. (2001) explored a statistical pattern processing strategy on the inner border of the colon wall for polyp classification.

Kiss et al. (2002) reported a polyp classification strategy, which utilizes surface normal and sphere fitting to the inner border of the colon wall.

Acar et al. (2002) presented a polyp classification strategy by the use of edge displacement field over the inner border of the colon wall.

Yao et al. (2004) utilized deformable modeling and fuzzy clustering means to detect polyps and measure their sizes.

Wang et al. (2005) proposed a polyp classifier that includes a transform function on the selected features and a two-level classification operation of training and linear discrimination.

Chowdhury et al. (2006) applied a 3D surface fitting on the inner border of the colon wall for polyp classification.

Konlukoglu et al. (2007) adapted a level set evolution processing to enhance the variation on the inner surface of the colon wall for polyp classification.

van Wijk et al. (2010) explored a flow model of second principal curvatures on an isosurface describing the inner border of the colon wall for polyp classification.

By our conjecture, some of the descriptions of the colon wall in the earlier alternative polyp classification strategies can be formatted as features. If so, the feature dimension will increase, and, therefore, more powerful feature selection (as shown earlier) and classification (to be discussed later) are desired.

In addition to the two well-known classifiers of SVM and ANN, other widely used classifiers in different applications include linear discriminant analysis (LDA) (Mika et al. 1999), random forest (RF) (Breiman 2001), adaboost (Freund and Shapire 1995), and more.

Our preliminary studies indicate that the SVM, LDA, and RF classifiers perform similarly and can outperform others (Song et al. 2011, 2012). With an adaptive kernel, the SVM classifier can have a noticeable gain (Fan et al. 2012b), as shown by Figure 13.8, which shows a preliminary study of comparing the performance of our modified SVM with adaptive kernel (AK-SVM) and the conventional SVM with the well-known RBF kernel (SVM). Further investigation on combining some of these classifiers for improved CADe performance is under progress.

Since feature selection and classification are two essential components for CADe in CTC, it is expected that more research effort will be seen in the future in advancing the knowledge about these two topics. By our conjecture, an

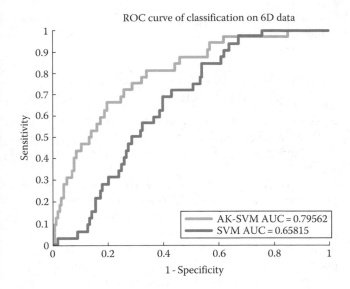

ROC curve of classification on 6D data

AK-SVM AUC = 0.79562
SVM AUC = 0.65815

Figure 13.8 A 6D feature vector is extracted from each VOI. There are a total of 786 VOIs, in which 64 are true polyps.

interleaved approach of integrating feature selection in classification would be an example of the future endeavor for CADe in CTC.

13.2.7 Evaluation of Computerized Detection Performance

The pipeline from image processing and feature selection to feature classification is termed a CADe system. The pipeline is task specific, that is, it focuses on the desired information embedded in the acquired image volume and processes the information for the ultimate clinical goal of detecting colonic polyps. Figure 13.9 shows a flowchart of a typical CADe pipeline.

The first component or module is image processing, which aims to segment the colon wall from the large image volume and localize suspicious patches on the colon wall as IPCs. The performance of this module can be evaluated by the measures of colon segmentation accuracy and detection sensitivity. The accuracy measures the preservation of the information about the colon wall after it is segmented from the abdominal image. The sensitivity measures the quantity of how many TPs are detected.

We hope to detect polyps as small as possible with a reasonable number of FPs in the IPCs.

The second module is feature extraction, which aims to obtain as much information as possible from the localized suspicious patches or IPCs. The efficacy of the extracted features is measured by a classifier in the following third module in Figure 13.9.

The third module performs feature selection and classification and aims to reduce FPs as much as possible while remaining the TPs in the IPC pool.

The most important measures on the performance of a CADe system (or the pipeline of Figure 13.9) are the detection sensitivity and the discrimination specificity. The former indicates the proportion of TPs being detected, while the latter indicates the proportion of FPs remaining in the detection. To obtain these two measures, the ground truth must be known. At the present time, the report from OC is the gold standard of representing the ground truth.

The performance evaluation is also task specific. For example, the outputs of sensitivity and specificity measures will depend on the task of what sized polyps are concerned. The measures will get worse in detecting smaller polyps. Given the clinical task of detecting polyps of size 5 mm and larger, we wish to reach over 95% sensitivity and less than 10 FPs in each patient.

To compare the performance of different CADe systems, the curves plotting the sensitivity and specificity, that is, the ROC curve (Chakraborty 2000) and the free-response ROC (fROC) curve (Chakraborty and Berbaum 2004), are often used (Summers et al. 2001, Yoshida and Nappi 2001, Wang et al. 2005, Zhu et al. 2009, 2010a). Figure 13.6 shows the fROC representation.

To generate the ROC and/or fROC results, the leave-one-out or cross-validation strategy across various data acquired from different medical centers is also necessary to validate the robustness of different CADe systems (Zhu et al. 2009).

In summary, CADe in CTC remains an active research topic. The three steps in the CADe pipeline of Figure 13.9 still face challenges. Segmentation of the colon wall or virtual cleansing of the colonic materials from the abdominal image volume is an essential task. Based on the segmentation, another essential task is the analysis of the segmented

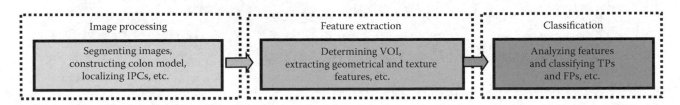

Image processing
Segmenting images, constructing colon model, localizing IPCs, etc.

Feature extraction
Determining VOI, extracting geometrical and texture features, etc.

Classification
Analyzing features and classifying TPs and FPs, etc.

Figure 13.9 Flowchart of a typical CADe pipeline.

colon wall characteristics for the detection of the TPs, where the detection of IPCs, feature selection, and classification are the main concerns.

13.3 COMPUTERIZED DIAGNOSIS OF COLONIC POLYP IN CT COLONOGRAPHY

At present, research interest is mainly at the stage of computerized detection of both adenomas and hyperplastic polyps of a given size range. Given the rich image intensity information inside the VOI of a suspicious patch, computerized diagnosis (i.e., CADx) of the detected polyps may be feasible. Some preliminary results are reported in the work (Pickhardt 2004). Some examples are given later in the chapter.

13.3.1 Differentiation of Adenomas from Hyperplastic Polyps

By the use of a projection through the determined VOI of a polyp, the projected image intensity distribution on a 2D plane reveals some specific patterns between adenomas and hyperplastic polyps. An example is given in Figure 13.4 in the differentiation between adenoma and hyperplastic polyps. Characterization of the texture patterns for the differentiation of adenoma from hyperplastic

polyps is an interesting topic and is under investigation (Zhang et al. 2011b).

13.3.2 Differentiation of Different Adenoma Polyps

By the same projection strategy, we can see the different texture patterns between different adenomas polyps as shown in Figure 13.10 with a comparison to the bottom of Figure 13.4.

The feasibility of CADx for differentiating different polyp types can be realized from the following experiment. Based on the pathological reports from the resected polyps of variable size larger than 5 mm, we grouped a total of 191 polyps into four categories or types: (1) hyperplastic (H), (2) tubular adenoma (Ta), (3) tubulovillous adenoma (Va), and (4) adenocarcinoma (A) polyps (see Table 13.2).

From each detected IPC of the 191 polyps, a VOI was segmented semiautomatically (Zhang et al. 2012). The co-occurrence matrix texture features (see Table 13.1) from both the polyp image density distribution and the polyp image density gradient distribution were extracted. A total of 38 features were considered for each VOI. By the use of the PCA, the first seven components were used for the purpose of matching the dimension of the polyp type A. The paired Hotelling T-square testing was applied to differentiate the texture feature vectors. The testing results are shown in Table 13.3.

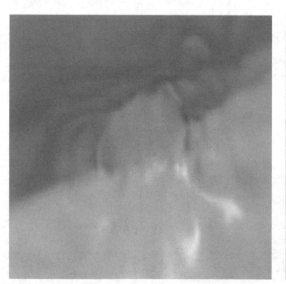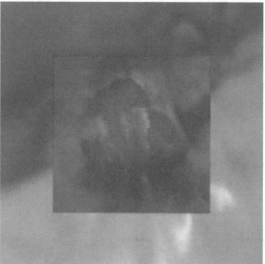

Figure 13.10   An illustration of different types of adenoma polyps—tubulovillous adenoma.

TABLE 13.2   DETAILS OF THE DATABASE FOR CADX FEASIBILITY STUDY

Pathology Type	Abbreviation	Cases	Risk Rate
Adenocarcinoma	A	7	
Tubulovillous adenoma	Va	34	
Tubular adenoma	Ta	94	
Hyperplastic	H	56	
Total	4	191	

TABLE 13.3   PAIRED HOTELLING T-SQUARE TESTS OF THE FOUR POLYP TYPES

N =	56	94	34	7
	H	Ta	Va	A
H		*	‡	‡
Ta			‡	‡
Va				†

* To be statistically significant, a larger feature dimension, that is, 20, is needed.
† Statistically significant ($P < 0.05$).
‡ Statistically significant ($P < 0.001$).

By the matched dimension of seven between the feature size and the data sample size, except for the H and Ta types, the differentiations among other polyp types were statistically significant. When the feature dimension was increased to 20, the differentiations among all polyp types were statistically significant.

In summary, computerized detection (or CADe) of polyps has been under development in the past two decades, and significant progress has been made. Very limited progress has been made for computerized diagnosis (or CADx) of polyps. The main challenge for CADx of polyps is related to the small variation of x-ray attenuation among the polyps and the colon wall tissue. By the use of the high order co-occurrence matrix texture features from the gradient and even curvature distributions (in addition to the texture features the image density distribution), mimicking the amplification in pathology, CADx of polyps seems feasible.

13.4 COMMERCIAL SYSTEMS FOR COMPUTERIZED POLYP DETECTION IN CT COLONOGRAPHY

By the use of the commercial V3D Colon Module of Viatronix Inc. as a visualization platform, all the commercial CADe systems can be described by Figure 13.11. The top row represents the computerized operations of image acquisition from a patient with fecal tagging (left), image segmentation (middle), and colon model construction (right). The bottom left is a computer-generated endoscopic view, by which the human observer or radiologists will perform the task of polyp detection. A CADe system or computer observer can detect the polyp candidates and color them in the endoscopic view (bottom right).

The first CADe software of receiving FDA 510(k) approval for commercial use in CTC is the iCAD system (Global Headquarters, iCAD, Inc.; 98 Spit Brook Road, Suite 100 Nashua, NH 03062 USA) (http://www.icadmed.com/index.cfm).

Another CADe software, which recently received FDA 510(k) approval for commercial use in CTC, is the ColonCAD system of Medicsight, Inc. (Medicsight PLC; Kensington Centre; 66 Hammersmith Road; London, W14 8UD; United Kingdom) (http://www.medicsight.com/medicsight/).

Another commercial CADe system for colon is from IM 3D (im3D S.P.A., Medical Imaging Lab; Via Lessolo, 3; 10153—Torino; Italy) (http://www.i-m3d.com/en/).

The performance of the earlier commercial CADe systems varies significantly similar to the research CADe pipelines described in Section 13.2.6 and other sections. This indicates that the CADe technologies for polyp detection via CTC are still under development.

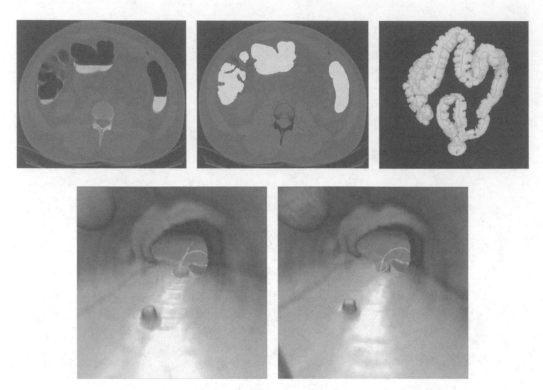

Figure 13.11   (See color insert.) An illustration of a CADe system using the commercial V3D colon visualization platform. The top row shows the information processing from data acquisition (left) and image segmentation/ECC (middle) to colon model construction. On the bottom left is an endoscopic view inside the constructed colon model for polyp detection by human observer or radiologist. A CADe system or computer observer detects polyp candidates at their associated locations on the inner border of the colon model. The CADe output can be visualized by coloring the detected polyp candidates at their associated locations (bottom right).

13.5   CONCLUSION

By current CT technologies and image processing and rendering methodologies, experienced radiologists can detect polyps of size 8 mm and greater using a sophisticated CTC system with comparable performance to the OC outcome of experienced GI physicians if the patient undergoes a routine bowel cleansing regime (Pickhardt et al. 2003, Johnson et al. 2008). Reducing the patient stress from the routine bowel cleansing regime and optimizing the virtual colon cleansing for CTC have been a research interest. With improved image processing algorithms and rendering technologies, experienced radiologists may be able to detect polyps smaller than 8 mm by CTC at a similar performance level as OC outcome of experienced GI physicians.

Current commercially available CADe systems can help less experienced radiologists to improve their clinical assessment but may help very little for experienced radiologists. Therefore, further research in the CADe field is desired. Further improvement in image processing would lead to a more accurate colon model and preserve more image information in the colon model for detection purposes. Improved feature selection and classification would lead to higher sensitivity with less FPs.

Regarding CADx, the research is at the very early stage. We have a great opportunity and also many severe challenges ahead for both CADe and CADx of colonic polyps (i.e., CADpolyp).

ACKNOWLEDGMENTS

This work was supported in part by the NIH/NCI under Grant #CA082402, #CA120917, and #CA143111. The author appreciates the contributions from the following researchers when they were in the author's research lab: Dr. Chaijie Duan, PhD; Prof. Lihong Li, PhD; Prof. Hongbing Lu, PhD; Dr. Su Wang, PhD; Dr. Zigang Wang, PhD; Dr. Hongbin Zhu, PhD; Mr. Lei Fan; Mr. Bowen Song; Mr. Guopeng Zhang; and Mr. Hao Zhang. In addition, the English editing effort from Ms. Donna Carroll shall be acknowledged.

REFERENCES

Acar, B., Beaulieu, C., Paik, D. et al., 2002. Edge displacement field-based classification for improved detection of polyps in CTC. *IEEE Transactions on Medical Imaging*, 21: 1461–1467.

Ahlquist, D., Sargent, D., Loprinzi, C. et al., 2008. Stool DNA and occult blood testing for screen detection of colorectal neoplasia. *Annals of Internal Medicine*, 149(7): 441–450.

Allison, J., Sskoda, I., Ransom, L. et al., 2007. Screening for colorectal neoplasms with new fecal occult blood tests: Update on performance characteristics. *Journal of the National Cancer Institute*, 99(11): 1462–1470.

Bielen, D. and Kiss, G., 2007. CADe for CTC: Update 2007. *Abdominal Imaging*, 32: 571–581.

Brady, A., Stevenson, G., and Stevenson, I., 1994. Colorectal cancer overlooked at barium enema examination and colonoscopy: A continuing perceptual problem. *Radiology*, 192(2): 373–378.

Breiman, L., 2001. Random forests. *MachineLearning*, 45(1): 5–32. doi:10.1023/A:1010933404324.

Brenner, D. and Hall, E., 2007. CT—An increasing source of radiation exposure. *The New England Journal of Medicine*, 357: 2277–2284.

Burges, C., 1998. A tutorial on support vector machines for pattern recognition. *Data Mining and Knowledge Discovery*, 2: 121–167.

Cai, S., Zhang, S., Zhu, H., and Zheng, S., 2009. Barriers to colorectal cancer screening: A case-control study. *World Journal of Gastroenterology*, 15(12): 2531–2536.

Cai, W., Zalis, M., Nappi, J. et al., 2006. Structure-based digital cleansing for CADe of polyps in CTC. *The Proceedings of the Annual Meeting of the Computer Assisted Radiology and Surgery Society*, Osaka, Japan, pp. 369–371.

Chakraborty, D., 2000. The FROC, AFROC and DFROC variants of the ROC analysis. *Handbook of Medical Imaging*, vol. 1, *Physic and Psychophysics*, pp. 771–796, SPIE Press, Bellingham, WA.

Chakraboty, D. and Berbaum, K., 2004. Observer studies involving detection and localization: Modeling, analysis, and validation. *Medical Physics*, 31: 2313–2330.

Chang, C. and Lin, C., 2001. LIBSVM: A library for support vector machines. Software description available on October 2014 at http://www.csie.ntu.edu.tw/~cjlin/libsvm.

Chowdhury, T., Whelan, P., and Ghita, O., 2006. The use of 3D surface fitting for robust polyp detection and classification in CTC. *Computerized Medical Imaging and Graphics*, 30(8): 427–436.

Chen, D., Liang, Z., Wax, M. et al., 2000. A novel approach to extract colon lumen from CT images for VC. *IEEE Transactions on Medical Imaging*, 19(12): 1220–1226.

Coin, C., Wollett, F., Coin, J. et al., 1983. Computerized radiology of the colon: A potential screening technique. *Computed Radiology*, 7(2): 215–221.

Egmont-Petersen, M., de Ridder, D., and Handels, H., 2002. Image processing with neural networks—A review. *Pattern Recognition*, 35(10): 2279–2301.

Fan, L., Song, B., Gu, X., and Liang, Z., 2012a. Feature selection for CADe of polyps using semi-supervised graph embedding. *Lab Technical Report*, Department of Radiology, Stony Brook University.

Fan, L., Song, B., Gu, X., and Liang, Z., 2012b. Improved CADe of polyps using a modified SVM classifier with adaptive kernel. *Lab Technical Report*, Department of Radiology, Stony Brook University.

Freund, Y. and Shapire, R., 1995. A decision-theoretic generalization of on-line learning and an application to boosting. *The Proceedings of the Second European Conference on Computational Learning Theory*, Barcelona, Spain, pp. 23–37.

Göktürk, S., Tomasi, C., Acar, B. et al., 2001. A statistical 3D pattern processing method for CADe of polyps in CTC. *IEEE Transactions on Medical Imaging*, 20: 1251–1260.

Grandqvist, S., 1981. Distribution of polyps of the large bowel in relation to age: A colonoscopic study. *Scandinavian Journal of Gastroenterology*, 16(11): 1025–1031.

Hafner, M., 2007. Conventional colonoscopy: Technique, indications, limits. *European Journal of Radiology*, 61(2): 409–414.

Heresbach, D., Barrioz, T., Lapalus, M. et al., 2008. Miss rate for colorectal neoplastic polyps: A prospective multi-center study of back-to-back video colonoscopies. *Endoscopy*, 40(4): 282–290.

Hong, L. Kaufman, A., Wei, Y., Viswambharan, A., Wax, M., and Liang, Z., 1995. 3D VC. *IEEE Biomedical Visualization Symposium*, IEEE CS Press, CA, pp. 26–32.

Hong, L., Liang, L., Viswambharan, A. et al., 1997. Reconstruction and visualization of 3D models of colonic surface. *IEEE Transactions on Nuclear Science*, 44(11): 1297–1302.

Jass J., 2007. Classification of colorectal cancer based on correlation of clinical, morphological and molecular features. *Histopathology*, 50(1): 113–130.

Jemal, A., Siegel, R., Xu, J., and Ward, E., 2010. Cancer statistics, 2010. *A Cancer Journal for Clinicians*, 60(5): 277–300.

Jeroebko, A., Malley, J., Franaszek, M., and Summers, R., 2003. Multiple neural network classification scheme for detection of colonic polyps in CTC datasets. *Academic Radiology*, 10: 154–160.

Johnson, C., Chen, M., Toledano, A. et al., 2008. Accuracy of CTC for detection of large adenomas and cancers. *The New England Journal of Medicine*, 359(12): 1207–1217.

Kachelrieβ, M., Watzke, O., and Kalender, W., 2011. Generalized multi-dimensional adaptive filtering for conventional and single-slice, multi-slice, and cone-beam CT. *Medical Physics*, 28: 475–490.

Kiss, G., van Cleynenbreugel, J., Thomeer, M. et al., 2002. Computer aided diagnosis in VC via combination of surface normal and sphere fitting methods. *European Journal of Radiology*, 12: 77–81.

Konlukoglu, E., Acar, B., Paik, D. et al., 2007. Polyp enhancement level set evolution of colon wall: Method and pilot study. *IEEE Transactions on Medical Imaging*, 26(12): 1649–1656.

Levin, T., Farraye, F., Schoen, R. et al., 2005. Quality in the technical performance of screening flexible sigmoidoscopy: Recommendations of an international multi-society task group. *Gut*, 54(6): 807–813.

Liang, Z., Yang, F., Wax, M. et al., 1997. Inclusion of *a priori* information in segmentation of colon lumen for 3D VC, *Conf Record of IEEE NSS-MIC*, in CD-ROM.

Liang, Z., Chen, D., Li, B. et al., 1999. On segmentation of colon lumen for VC. *Proceedings of SPIE Medical Imaging*, 3660: 270–278.

Liang, Z. Wang, Z., Li, L., and Harrington, D., 2002. Feature-based approach toward computer aided detection and diagnosis—An application to VC. *The Proceeding of the Annual Meeting of the Computer Assisted Radiology and Surgery Society*, Paris, France, pp. 755–760.

Liang, Z., Chen, D., Wax, M. et al., 2005. A feasibility study on laxative-free bowel preparation for VC. *Proceedings of SPIE Medical Imaging*, 5746: 415–423.

Liang, Z., Lu, H., Metaxas, D., and Reinhardt, J., 2007. Medical Imaging Informatics—An information processing from image formation to visualization. In: Editorial to the Special Issue of Medical Image Reconstruction, Processing and Visualization for *The International Journal of Image and Graphics*, 7(1), 1–15.

Liang, Z., 2008. Electronic colon cleansing techniques: Past, present, and future. *The 11ᵗʰ International Conference on Medical Image Computing and Computer Assisted Intervention (MICCAI) Workshop*—"New Era of VC", New York City, NY, September 6, pp. 26–32.

Liang, Z., Cohen, H., Posniak, E. et al., 2008. Texture-based CADx improves diagnosis for low-dose CTC. *Proceedings of SPIE Medical Imaging*, in CD-ROM.

Liang, Z. and Wang, S., 2009. An EM approach to MAP solution of segmenting tissue mixtures: A numerical analysis. *IEEE Transactions on Medical Imaging*, 28(2): 297–310.

Liang, Z. and Richards, R., 2010. VC vs OC. *Expert Opinion on Medical Diagnostics Journal*, 4: 149–158.

Lieberman, D., Moravec, M., Holub, J. et al., 2008. Polyp size and advanced histology in patients undergoing colonoscopy screening: Implications for CTC. *Gastroenterology*, 135(4): 1100–1105.

Lu, H., Li, X., Li, L., Chen, D., Xing, Y., Wax, M., Hsieh, J., and Liang, Z., 2003. Adaptive noise reduction toward low-dose CT. *Proceedings of SPIE Medical Imaging*, 5030: 759–766.

Lu, H., Zhang, G., Wang, T., Jiao, C., Wang, J., and Liang, Z., 2008. Computer-aided polyp detection based on 3D texture analysis for VC. *The 11th International Conference of MICCAI, Workshop on Computational and Visualization Challenges in the New Era of Virtual Colonoscopy*, pp. 52–57, September 6, New York.

Mandel, J., Church, T., Bond, J. et al., 2000. The effect of fecal occult blood screening on the incidence of colorectal cancer. *The New England Journal of Medicine*, 343(22): 1603–1607.

Mika, S., Ratsch, G., Weston, J. et al., 1999. Fisher discriminant analysis with Kernels. *The IEEE Conference on Neural Networks for Signal Processing IX*, Madison, WI, pp. 41–48.

Monga, O., Ayache, N., and Sander, P., 1992. From voxel to intrinsic surface features. *Image and Vision Computing*, 10(6): 403–417.

Monga, O. and Benayoun, S., 1992. Using partial derivatives of 3D images to extract typical surface features. In: *The Proceedings of the 3ʳᵈ Annual Conference, AI, Simulation and Planning in High Autonomy Systems, Integrating Perception, Planning and Action*, Perth, Australia, pp. 225–236.

Morimoto, L. Newcomb, P., Ulrich, C. et al., 2002. Risk factors for hyperplastic and adenomatous polyps: Evidence for malignant potential. *Cancer Epidemiology, Biomarkers and Prevention*, 11(10): 1012–1018.

Näppi, J. and Yoshida, H., 2002. Automated detection of polyps with CTC: Evaluation of volumetric features for reduction of false-positive findings. *Academic Radiology*, 9: 386–397.

Näppi, J. and Yoshida, H., 2003. Feature-guided analysis for reduction of false positives in CADe of polyps for CTC. *Medical Physics*, 30(7): 1592–1601.

Näppi, J., Yoshida, H., Zalis, M. et al., 2007. Pseudo-enhancement correction for CADe in fecal-tagging CTC. *Proceedings of SPIE Medical Imaging*, 6514: 65140A.

Orsoni, P., Berdah, S., Verrier, C. et al., 1997. Colonic perforation due to colonoscopy: A retrospective study of 48 cases. *Endoscopy*, 29(1): 160–164.

Pickhardt, P., Choi, R., Hwang, I. et al., 2003. Computed tomographic VC to screen for colorectal neoplasia in asymptomatic adults. *The New England Journal of Medicine*, 349: 2191–2200.

Pickhardt, P., Nugent, P., Mysliwiec, P. et al., 2004. Location of adenomas missed by optical colonoscopy. *Archives of Internal Medicine*, 141(2): 352–359.

Pickhardt, P., 2004. Translucency rendering in 3D endoluminal CTC: A useful tool for increasing polyp specificity and decreasing interpretation time. *American Journal of Roentgenology*, 183: 429–436.

Potter, J. and Slattery, M., 1993. Colon cancer: A review of the epidemiology. *Epidemiologic Reviews*, 15(3): 499–545.

Powell, W., 2007. *Approximate Dynamic Programming: Solving the Curses of Dimensionality*. Wiley, New York (ISBN: 0470171553).

Reed, J. and Johnson, C., 1997. Automatic segmentation, tissue characterization, and rapid diagnosis enhancements to the CTC analysis workstation. *Journal of Digital Imaging*, 10(1): 70–73.

Serlie, I., Truyen, R., Florie, J. et al., 2003. *Computed Cleansing for VC using a Three-material Transition Model. MICCAI*, Montreal, Canada, pp. 175–183.

Song, B., Zhu, H., Zhu, W., and Liang, Z., 2011. Evaluation of Classifiers for CADe in CTC. *The Conf Record of IEEE NSS-MIC*, in CD-ROM, IEEE Publisher, NJ.

Song, B., Zhang, G., Zhu, W., and Liang, Z., 2012. A study on random forests for CADe in CTC. *The Proceedings of the 26ᵗʰ International Congress and Exhibition of CARS*, Pisa, Italy, *Intl. J. CARS*, vol. 7, (Suppl): pp. S275.

Stryker, S., Wolff, B., Culp, C. et al., 1987. Natural history of untreated colonic polyps. *Gastroenterology*, 93(5): 1009–1013.

Summers, R., Johnson, C., Pusanik, L. et al., 2001. Automated polyp detection at CTC: Feasibility assessment in a human population. *Radiology*, 219(1): 51–59.

Sundaram, P., Zomorodian, A., Beauleu, C., and S. Napel, S., 2008. Colon polyp detection using smoothed shape operator: Preliminary results. *Medical Image Analysis*, 12: 99–119.

Suzuki, K., Yoshida, H., Nappi, J. et al., 2008. Mixture of expert 3D massive-training ANNs for reduction of multiple types of false positives in CADe for detection of polyps in CTC. *Medical Physics*, 35(2): 694–703.

Taylor, S., Halligan, S., Burling, D. et al., 2006. Computer-assisted reader software versus expert reviewers for polyp detection on CTC. *American Journal of Roentgenology*, 186: 696–702.

van Wijk, C., van Ravesteijn, V., Vos, F., and van Vliet L., 2010. Detection and segmentation of colonic polyps on implicit isosurfaces by second principal curvature flow. *IEEE Transactions on Medical Imaging*, 29(3): 688–698.

Vining, D., Gelfand, D., Bechtold, R. et al., 1994. Technical feasibility of colon imaging with helical CT and virtual reality. *Annual Meeting of American Roentgen Ray Society*, New Orleans, LA, pp. 104.

Vining, D., Hunt, G., Ahn, D., and Stelts, D., 1997. CADe of colon polyps and masses. *Radiology*, 205(P): 705.

Wan, M., Tang, Q., Kaufman, A., and Liang, Z., 1999. Volume rendering based interactive navigation within the human colon. *Proceedings of IEEE Computer Graphics and Applications*, pp. 397–400.

Wan, M., Dachille, F., Kreeger, K., Lakare, S., Sato, M., Kaufman, A., Wax, M., and Liang, Z., 2001. Interactive electronic biopsy for 3D VC. *Proceedings of SPIE Medical Imaging*, 4321: 483–488.

Wang, Z., Liang, Z., Li, L. et al., 2005. Reduction of false positives by internal features for polyp detection in CT-based VC. *Medical Physics*, 32(12): 3602–3616.

Wang, Z., Liang, Z., Li, X. et al., 2006a. An improved electronic colon cleansing method for detection of colonic polyps by VC. *IEEE Transactions on Biomedical Engineering*, 53(8): 1635–1646.

Wang, J., Li, T., Lu, H., and Liang, Z., 2006b. Penalized weighted least-squares approach to sinogram noise reduction and image reconstruction for low-dose x-ray CT. *IEEE Transactions on Medical Imaging*, 25(10), 1272–1283.

Wang, J., Wang, S., Li, L., Lu, H., and Liang, Z., 2008a. VC screening with ultra low-dose CT & less-stressful bowel preparation: A computer simulation study. *IEEE Transactions on Nuclear Science*, 55(5): 2566–2575.

Wang, S., Li, L., Cohen, H., Mankes, S., Chen, J., and Liang, Z., 2008b. An EM approach to MAP solution of segmenting tissue Mixture percentages with application to CT-based VC. *Medical Physics*, 35(12): 5787–5798.

Wang, S., Zhu, H., Lu, H., and Liang, Z., 2008c. Volume-based feature analysis of mucosa for automatic initial polyp detection in VC. *International Journal of Computer Assisted Radiology and Surgery*, 3(1–2): 131–142.

Wang, S., Yao, J., Liu, J. et al., 2009. Registration of prone and supine CTC scans using correlation optimized warping and canonical correlation analysis. *Medical Physics*, 36(12): 5595–5603.

Wang, S., Zhu, H., Fan, Y., Lu, H., and Liang, Z., 2010. Feature selection by adaptive weighting and reordering for computer-aided polyp detection in CTC. *Proceedings of SPIE Medical Imaging*, in CD-ROM.

Winawer, S. and Zauber, A., 2002. The advanced adenomas as the primary target of screening. *Gastrointestinal Endoscopy Clinics of North America*, 232(3): 784–790.

Yao, J., Miller, M., Franaszek, M., and R. Summers, R., 2004. Colonic polyp segmentation in CTC based on fuzzy clustering and deformable models. *IEEE Transactions on Medical Imaging*, 23(11): 1344–1352.

Yao, J., Summers, R., and Hara, A., 2005. Optimizing the support vector machine committee configuration in a colonic polyp CADe System. *Proceedings of SPIE Medical Imaging*, 5746: 384–392.

Yoo, T., Park, D., Kim, Y. et al., 2007. Clinical significance of small colorectal adenoma less than 10mm: The KASID study. *Hepatogastroenterology*, 54(74): 418–421.

Yoshida, H. and Nappi, J., 2001. 3D Computer-aided diagnosis scheme for detection of colonic polyps. *IEEE Transactions on Medical Imaging*, 20(8): 1261–1274.

Yoshida, H., Masutani, Y., Maceneaney, P. et al., 2002. Computerized detection of colonic polyps at CTC on the basis of volumetric features: Pilot study. *Radiology*, 222: 327–336.

Zhang, H., Li, L., Zhu, H., Lin, Q., Harrington, D., and Liang, Z., 2011a. An integrated electronic colon cleansing for CTC via MAP-EM segmentation and scale-based scatter correction. *Lab Technical Report*, Department of Radiology, Stony Brook University.

Zhang, G., Lu, H., and Liang, Z., 2011b. A feasibility study on the differentiation of polyps types for CADx. *Lab Technical Report*, Department of Radiology, Stony Brook University.

Zhang, G., Lu, H., and Liang, Z., 2012. CADx in CADx. *The 26th International Congress and Exhibition of CARS 2012*, Pisa, Italy, to appear.

Zhu, H., Duan, C., Pickhardt, P., Wang, S., and Liang, Z., 2009. CADe of colonic polyps with level set-based adaptive convolution in volumetric mucosa to advance CTC toward a screening modality. *Journal of Cancer Management and Research*, 1(1): 1–13.

Zhu, H., Fan, Y., Lu, H., and Liang, Z., 2010. Improving initial polyp candidate extraction for CTC. *Physics in Biology and Medicine*, 55(3): 2087–2102.

Zhu, H., Liang, Z., Barish, M. et al., 2010a. Increasing CADe specificity by projection features for CTC. *Medical Physics*, 37: 1468–1481.

Zhu, H., Wang, S., Fan, Y., Lu, H., and Liang, Z., 2010b. Eigenvalue-weighted feature selection for CADe of polyps in CTC. *Proceedings of SPIE*, 7624: 76241V-1.

Zhu, H., Fan, Y., Lu, H., and Liang, Z., 2011. Improved curvature estimation for CADe of colonic polyps in CTC. *Academic Radiology*, 18(8): 1024–1034.

Emerging Computer-Aided Detection and Diagnosis

Chapter 14

Detection and Characterization of Brain Tumor

Walter G. O'Dell, Robert Ambrosini, Anitha Priya Krishnan, Mathews Jacob, and Delphine Davis

CONTENTS

14.1 INTRODUCTION

This chapter addresses the application of computer-aided imaging processing for detection, segmentation, diagnosis, and treatment planning of brain cancer. There are additional potential applications of brain image processing that are not addressed here, including diagnosis and assessment of arteriovenous malformations, multiple sclerosis (MS), brain trauma, Alzheimer's disease, stroke, vasculature disease, and aging. Individuals interested in the application of computer-aided detection (CAD) for MS lesions are directed to an article by Yamamoto et al. (2010) and an excellent review by Mortazavi et al. (2012).

14.1.1 Clinical Utility of Computer-Aided Detection for Primary Brain Cancer

Each year in the United States, approximately 17,000 new cases of primary brain cancer are diagnosed (Ries et al. 2006). The common primary brain tumors are anaplastic astrocytomas, glioblastoma multiforme (GBM or simply glioblastoma), oligodendrogliomas, meningiomas, and medulloblastomas.

GBM is an aggressive primary brain tumor that spreads diffusely. The World Health Organization (WHO) has classified astrocytomas into four grades based on histological features: grade I (pilocytic astrocytoma), grade II (diffuse astrocytoma), grade III (anaplastic astrocytoma), and grade IV (GBM) (Louis et al. 2007). Of these grades, III and IV are considered malignant gliomas. Even with the current standard of care, which includes surgery, radiation therapy, and chemotherapy, for patients 45 years or older with GBM, the local control rate is only 9%, and the 5-year survival rate is less than 2%. Those with anaplastic astrocytoma experience a similarly discouraging 16% 5-year survival rate (ACS 2005). The median survival, from the time of initial diagnosis, for patients with glioblastoma was recently reported to be 16.9 months, the 1-, 2-, and 3-year survival rates were 72%, 23%, and 14%, respectively (Biswas et al. 2009).

Complete resection, whenever possible, is typically the initial therapy. Even if the tumor cannot be completely resected, partial resection helps to reduce pressure on the brain and to reduce the size of the tumor to be treated by radiation or chemotherapy. Complete surgical resection of tumors has been shown to result in increased survival duration of patients (Ammirati et al. 1987). Chemotherapy is used as a complement to surgical resection and radiotherapy/radiosurgery. Currently, the most frequently administered drugs are temozolomide (Temodar, Merck & Co., Inc., Whitehouse Station, NJ) (Quinn et al. 2003), bevacizumab (Avastin, Genentech, San Francisco, CA) (Norden et al. 2008), and bis-chloroethyl nitrosourea (Brandes et al. 2004).

Aided by the fact that a patient's head can be rigidly fixed to the radiosurgery table for precise localization of the internal target, external beam radiation in the form of stereotactic radiosurgery (SRS) and radiotherapy (SRT) offers the most intriguing and promising treatment option for brain cancer. SRS is a treatment modality that allows for single high-dose radiation applications to small lesion targets (up to 3–4 cm in diameter) with a sharp dose falloff outside the lesion (Bajaj et al. 2005; Jagannathan et al. 2007; van den Bent 2001). Consequently, SRS serves as a minimally invasive brain tumor therapy option that spares surrounding normal tissue while providing high local tumor control, even in the case of tumor histologies often regarded as radioresistant, such as melanoma and renal cell carcinoma (Barker 2005). One notable limitation of single-dose radiotherapy is that its ability to kill tumor cells depends heavily upon the hypoxic cell fraction; hypoxic cells are only one-third as sensitive to radiation damage as oxygenated cells (Hall 2000; Suit et al. 1977). In SRT, the treatment is fractionated (dividing the radiation dose over multiple sessions) to permit revascularization and reoxygenation of the core of hypoxic tumors during the time interval between applications.

Unfortunately, at present, the role of CAD for early detection of primary brain cancer through screening is limited because of the low incidence of disease in the general population and because a large, well-defined, high-risk group on whom to perform image-based screening does not exist. Instead, patients typically present initially with neurological deficits, such as seizure, headache, dizziness, altered perception, memory loss, change in personality, or paralysis, that lead to additional tests, including magnetic resonance imaging (MRI) and computed tomography (CT) (Weller 2011). Thus, when a brain tumor is diagnosed, the primary tumor mass is typically large and conspicuous to the unaided radiologist.

14.1.2　Clinical Utility of Computer-Aided Detection for Metastatic Cancer

Unlike primary brain cancer, brain metastases represent a facet of cancer where CAD is likely to play an increasingly prominent role. Brain metastasis is often a life-limiting diagnosis for many common primary cancers, including breast and prostate cancers, for which a well-defined, high-risk group can be readily identified, and modern screening

tools hold promise for early detection. Moreover, several clinical approaches are available to directly improve patient outcomes. Because systemically active antineoplastic drugs allow for coverage of not only detected metastases but also any undetected disease reservoirs, chemotherapy has long represented the backbone of treatment for metastatic disease. Advances in surgical tools and techniques have enabled metastasectomy, the surgical resection of metastases, to become a viable option for the treatment of accessible secondary tumors in the brain and other organs, offering symptomatic relief and a survival benefit (Khatri et al. 2005). Newly developed immunotherapy drugs promote the abilities of a patient's immune system to battle metastatic disease through the administration of cytokines, monoclonal antibodies, or vaccine therapy (Mc Dermott 2009). Hormone therapy drugs achieve their efficacy by acting upon the endocrine system and, as a result, can be used as an additional means of systemic therapy for metastatic disease originating in hormone-responsive tissues, such as the breast, prostate, ovaries, or endometrium. Whole-brain radiation therapy (WBRT), which has long served as the core option for brain metastasis treatment, has been shown to increase survival from 2 to 6 months from the time of diagnosis (Martin and Kondziolka 2005). However, in light of the adverse effects of radiation applied to the entire brain, including long-term memory loss, ataxia, and dementia, the superior local control rates of radiosurgery when compared with WBRT (Martin and Kondziolka 2005) suggest that SRS can provide prominent therapeutic effect for many patients with brain metastases. Often described as ideal targets for radiosurgery (Noel et al. 2004), brain metastases are normally smaller than 3 cm in diameter with well-defined borders when detected (Boyd and Mehta 1999; Gupta 2005).

14.1.3　Clinical Utility of Computer-Aided Segmentation of Brain Tumors

Once a primary brain tumor is identified, the active tumor must be segmented out from the surrounding healthy brain and regions of edema. Modern image-guided surgical interventions permit the excision of tissue with order-millimeter precision, motivating the careful and consistent definition of boundaries of the observable tumor in order to remove the maximum amount of cancer while preserving the maximum amount of healthy tissue.

14.1.4　Clinical Utility of Assessing the Extent of the Primary Tumor

Primary brain cancer often has an infiltrative component that leads to poorly defined tumor borders and the likelihood for distant migration of cancer cells that are too small to be visualized directly using conventional imaging methods.

As early as 1940, Scherer (1940) documented that migrating cancer cells pass through the brain parenchyma to aggregate around the surfaces of major vessels (perivascular satellitosis), near the brain's outer surfaces (subpial/subarachnoid spread), and around the ventricles (subependymal spread) and major fiber bundles (perineuronal satellitosis) in patterns of invasion referred to as the secondary structures of Scherer. For example, if fiber tracts are present adjacent to the primary tumor, more migrating cancer cells move large distances away from the tumor along the fibers than through the general brain parenchyma.

After surgical resection of the observable glioma mass, in more than 90% of the cases, the tumor recurs within 2–3 cm of the resection cavity (Burger et al. 1988). To account for the microscopic spread of tumor cells, radiation oncologists often include a 20–25 mm isotropic margin when planning for SRS/SRT. The treatment margin is usually either (1) the extent/size of the primary brain tumor/surgical cavity seen in postcontrast T1-weighted magnetic resonance images and an additional 2–2.5 cm margin or (2) the size of the primary tumor and edema visualized in the T2-weighted magnetic resonance images (with or without contrast) and an additional 2 cm margin. In certain cases, no margin may be used to spare a critical structure.

Improved assessment of the microscopic extent of primary brain cancer could have great clinical impact. The migration of tumor cells in the brain is not isotropic; hence, the isotropic treatment margin currently used can be improved with a higher dose and/or greater margin in the areas of high tumor cell concentration and a lower dose and/or smaller margin in areas lacking tumor cells.

14.2 APPEARANCE OF BRAIN TUMORS IN MEDICAL IMAGES

14.2.1 MRI Sequences (T1, T2, DWI)

The typical MRI exam is comprised of several imaging sequences during a 1 h session. Four to seven sequences provide various types of information about the brain tissue environment. Perhaps the most commonly utilized are a comparison of precontrast to postcontrast T1-weighted and T2-weighted images. Gadolinium-based contrast agents alter the MRI T1 relaxation rate of tissue. Postcontrast T1-weighted images show enhanced contrast in the region around the tumor. In this context, precontrast and postcontrast T2-weighted images show enhancement that is generally associated with edema; hence, the area of T2 enhancement is larger than the area of T1 enhancement. In grade IV gliomas, the regions of edema are assumed to carry an elevated risk for harboring infiltrative disease and are usually targeted for SRS.

Diffusion-weighted imaging (DWI) achieves contrast related to the relative motion of water molecules on a length of scale associated with water diffusion (Le Bihan et al. 1986; Taylor and Bushell 1985). DWI does not require the administration of a contrast agent but does necessitate the acquisition of four or more images (one being the baseline), each with a different set of applied directional bipolar magnetic field gradients. Water diffusion in tissue is often directionally dependent. With only three directional gradients, one can merely compute the average weighted diffusion of water (AWD). Regions of edema have a higher AWD than healthy gray or white matter; thus, changes in AWD can indicate edema surrounding a tumor. Densely packed cells or tissue matrix can restrict water diffusion leading to decreased AWD in these areas. If six or more directional gradients are used, the full three-dimensional (3D) diffusion tensor can be computed for each pixel (Basser et al. 2000). From the resulting diffusion tensor image, one can compute the direction of maximal diffusion as the principal eigenvector of the 3D diffusion tensor. In areas with a preferred directional component to water diffusion, the principal eigenvector aligns with the direction of the prominent underlying fiber network (Pierpaoli et al. 1996), such as muscle fibers or white matter tracts. The ratio of the coefficient of diffusion along the principal eigenvector to the coefficients of diffusion in the remaining two eigenvectors indicates the relative prominence of the underlying fiber bundle and is measured as the fractional anisotropy (FA) index. A decrease in FA in a white matter region can indicate the effect of infiltrative disease or the presence of edema in the neighborhood of a tumor mass. The effects of radiation, chemotherapy, and disease can cause edema or nerve fiber demyelination that can also result in a decrease in local FA.

14.2.2 Contrast and Determinants of Variable Enhancement

In the healthy brain, gadolinium-based contrast agents cannot normally penetrate the blood brain barrier; hence, there is no contrast enhancement save for the exchange of water molecules between the blood vessels and the extracellular tissue space (Mathews et al. 1997). Larger tumors are generally associated with angiogenesis, abnormal vascular architecture, and leaky vessels that permit contrast agents to enter the extravascular space. Changes in tissue MRI enhancement can be seen immediately after the contrast injection but can be confused by the enhanced pixel intensity of the intravascular space. Thus, one should wait long enough for contrast to wash out of the vascular space. Once contrast has infiltrated into the extravascular space, several hours may be needed for the agent to fully wash out, thereby creating a range of time in which the vessels are clear of contrast while the extravascular space retains contrast enhancement. A limitation of conventional contrast enhancement is that the contrast targets the tissue surrounding leaking vessels and not the cancer cells directly. Tumors that are either too small to promote angiogenesis or that are able to induce increased blood flood of the native vasculature (via increased vessel size and flow rates) without creating new vessels (Sakariassen et al. 2006) will be invisible to such contrast agents. Moreover, the core of larger (>1 cm) tumors typically is necrotic; therefore, there may be no vessels (leaky or not) that permeate to the tumor center. These features contribute to the contrast enhancement of primary brain tumors that are often nonuniform, blotchy, and unpredictable.

14.2.3 Magnetic Resonance Spectroscopic Imaging

Magnetic resonance spectroscopy imaging (MRSI) provides information about individual molecular species, such as the number of chemical bonds, neighboring nuclei, and overall molecular structure. The identification of individual molecular species and the ability to quantify the relative concentration provide information about the metabolic state of the underlying tissue (Glunde and Bhujwalla 2011). MRSI uses localization techniques to provide MRS spectra at individual voxels within the brain. However, the MRSI voxel size (in single-voxel mode) in the clinical setting is large compared to that of conventional MRI—approximately 1 cm^3 or roughly that of positron emission tomography (PET) imaging. Through its ability to noninvasively map brain metabolite concentrations, MRSI has been demonstrated to detect microscopic tumor spread (Gillard et al. 2004; Nelson et al. 2002) and differentiate therapy effects from recurrence (Dhermain et al. 2010; Srinivasan et al. 2006; Weybright et al. 2004). The brain metabolites that are routinely observed with MRSI are N-acetyl aspartate (NAA), creatine, and choline (choline-containing compounds). NAA is a neurotransmitter that is found only in functioning normal neurons and is a marker for viable neurons. Since most brain tumors are of non-neuronal origin, decreased NAA concentration is commonly observed in brain cancers (Black and Loeffler 2005; Gillard et al. 2004). The level of creatine indicates a tissue's energetic status and is typically utilized as a reference for estimating alterations in other metabolites (Srinivasan et al. 2006). Choline plays an important role in membrane turnover and is an accepted marker for malignancy that increases with tumor presence and aggressiveness (Ackerstaff et al. 2003; Gillard et al. 2004). In vivo choline levels have been shown to correlate with proliferative potential, as determined by immunohistochemical analysis of tumor biopsies of gliomas (Herminghaus et al. 2002; Shimizu et al. 2000). The choline-to-NAA index (CNI) is positively associated with areas of increased proliferation

and cell density within and surrounding the tumor (Laprie et al. 2008), and its use to identify microscopic lesions is now well accepted. This approach considerably improves the detection of regions with cancer infiltration (Nelson et al. 2002). CNI also can differentiate tumor recurrence from radiation therapy effects (pseudo-progression) (Weybright et al. 2004). NAA, creatine, and choline can be reliably measured on most clinical scanners using manufacturer-provided sequences and reconstruction algorithms.

There are additional theoretically measurable metabolites that may be more relevant to the diagnosis of microscopic glioma infiltration, including myo-inositol and glutamate. Using unconventional hardware and protocols, several human in vivo studies have reported the dramatic increase in glutamate concentrations in tumors (Hu et al. 2007). Significant increases in glutamate have been detected in normal-appearing white matter with microscopic infiltration using MRS (Kallenberg et al. 2009). Unfortunately, due to the overlap of its peaks with glutamine, glutamate is especially difficult to detect from MRSI. Myo-inositol has been characterized as a specific marker of astrocytes in the adult brain (Brand et al. 1993). Recent studies have shown that microscopic infiltration in newly diagnosed gliomas elicits a brain inflammatory response with extensive astrocytosis (Fitzgerald et al. 2008; Kallenberg et al. 2009; Takano et al. 2001). These cells secrete factors that increase the growth potential of glioma cells in vitro (Fitzgerald et al. 2008). Myo-inositol is increased in newly diagnosed gliomas because of astrocytic proliferation (Hattingen et al. 2008; Norfray et al. 1999). Consistent with astrocytosis, mean myo-inositol levels are significantly increased in contralateral normal-appearing white matter of patients with GBM (Kallenberg et al. 2009). Recent ex vivo MRS studies have indicated that myo-inositol/choline levels may also be valuable for separating low-grade gliomas from high-grade gliomas and for distinguishing gliosis from recurrent grade IV gliomas (Laprie et al. 2008). These metabolites do not directly measure the metabolic signatures of the glioma cancer cells; instead, they indicate changes in the brain as a response to tumor infiltration. The resulting amplification can, in theory, enable the imaging of infiltrative disease, even when the extensions are much smaller than the voxel dimensions.

However, the technical challenges associated with MRSI are the main factors that limit the widespread use of MRS in the clinic. The low signal-to-noise ratio of the MRSI metabolites restricts the number of samples that can be reliably acquired in a specified acquisition time, thus limiting resolution or spatial coverage. The resulting large voxels (volumes of ~1 cc) can cause the signal from the surrounding normal tissue to dilute the metabolic variations due to microscopic tumors within the voxels, thus making the detection of microscopic tumor spread challenging.

In addition, the MRSI data at a specified voxel will have contributions from the metabolic variations in a large neighboring region (due to large side-lobes in the reconstructed point-spread function). Inhomogeneity of the primary magnetic field (B0), due to tissue susceptibility differences, results in broadening of the peaks in the MRS spectrum; this result makes the unambiguous separation of the contribution from neighboring metabolite peaks difficult. Furthermore, the signal from extracranial lipids and unsuppressed water (due to B0 inhomogeneity) is approximately two orders of magnitude stronger than that of the metabolites. The leakage from these signals results in strong baseline fluctuations and additional masking of metabolite peaks. To avoid these problems, it is a general practice to restrict imaging to rectangular regions within the brain to minimize the fat leakage. However, this often severely limits the spatial coverage, thereby preventing the evaluation of cancer infiltration close to the head surface (Park et al. 2007). The quantitative parameters resulting from MRSI data are important for predicting the tumor grade, managing tissue sampling during biopsy or precise surgical resection, defining the spatial scope of the tumor for focal therapy planning, and assessing the therapeutic effect. Therefore, since these MRSI techniques provide information that is valuable for making decisions regarding patient care, further work is warranted to standardize data acquisition and computer-aided post-processing across institutions and scanners from various manufacturers (Laprie et al. 2008).

14.2.4 Positron Emission Tomography

PET imaging enables the assessment of molecular processes, such as glucose consumption and downstream effects of altered protein synthesis (Jacobs et al. 2002; Prieto et al. 2011; Ullrich et al. 2008). The most common application is the study of altered metabolism using the glucose analog 2-deoxy-2-(^{18}F)fluoro-D-glucose (FDG, also commonly referred to as fluorodeoxyglucose and fludeoxyglucose). The amount of metabolic activity is reflected in the amount of radioactive tracer uptake and is quantified using the standardized uptake value (SUV). Typically, the SUV of malignant tissue is ≥2.5 greater than that of normal tissue. PET with ^{18}F-FDG has become an essential imaging modality in oncology for diagnosing, staging, and predicting prognosis (Kato et al. 2008); however, the benefit of ^{18}F-FDG in neuro-oncology is limited by the high rate of physiologic glucose metabolism in normal brain tissue. Low-grade tumors present lower uptake than do normal gray matter (Chung et al. 2002). Therefore, tracers such as ^{11}C-methionine (Herholz et al. 1998), which present a high tumor-to-normal brain contrast, play an important role in improving diagnostic procedures. Spence et al. (2004) introduced dual-time-point ^{18}F-FDG PET in neuro-oncology, resulting in improved diagnostic sensitivity and specificity for brain cancer where delayed images were studied visually and quantitatively using volumes of interest. They examined the behavior of model-derived kinetic rate constants over time and concluded that ^{18}F-FDG is dephosphorylated faster from normal tissue than from tumors, thus improving image contrast. In 2011, Prieto et al. (2011) first demonstrated the ability to quantitatively analyze dual-time-point imaging voxelwise. Their results established a considerable improvement in sensitivity for brain tumor diagnosis using dual-time-point imaging, as compared with standard ^{18}F-FDG. Notwithstanding their findings, the methodology was limited for tumor volume delineation, with time interval and type of tumor being exposed as critical factors. While their analysis provides encouraging results, further study with a larger prospective succession of patients is required.

The minimal voxel dimension of a typical PET scan is 6–10 mm. The minimal lung-nodule size that can be detected by PET is 7 mm (Shields 2005); thus, PET is more often employed for cancer staging and confirmation of malignancy found on CT or MRI. For this reason, computer-aided segmentation of lesions is not commonly applied directly to PET image data; rather, PET is used to indicate an area of suspicion; CAD is then performed on the abnormal lesion found within that area on the coregistered CT or MRI.

14.3 COMPUTERIZED DETECTION OF BRAIN TUMORS IN MRI

The heterogeneous appearance of primary brain cancer makes it challenging for computer-automated detection. This fact, in addition to the lack of both an identifiable high-risk group and support for image-based screening, at least partially explains the absence of publications related specifically to initial detection of primary brain tumors; indeed, effort is currently concentrated on delineating the microscopic extent of disease and discerning active tumors from treatment effects. The application of computer-assisted approaches to these tasks is discussed in the next section.

Because brain metastases typically displace rather than infiltrate normal brain matter, they typically present with pronounced margins in contrast-enhancement imaging studies (Boyd and Mehta 1999; Gupta 2005). Moreover, brain metastases have been described as spherical or spheroid structures that are well circumscribed (Jagannathan et al. 2007; Ranasinghe and Sheehan 2007). In principle, CAD algorithms can be designed to take advantage of these features. We applied a 3D spherical template-matching approach, which was previously shown to successfully detect lung metastases on volumetric CT scans, to brain metastases MR datasets (Wang et al. 2007). In our approach, we created a library of 3D templates in which each template was generated by computing the appearance of a solid sphere in a given CT exam, taking into consideration the scan's voxel dimensions and the partial volume effects at the edges of the sphere. Three variants of each template were created for each sphere, representing different offsets of the image cut-planes intersecting the sphere. A halo of zero-valued pixels around the sphere ensured preferential selection of objects with limited extent in all three directions. Additional realism was imparted to each template image by imposing a Gaussian filter (to approximate the point-spread function of the image reconstruction) and gray-scale intensity fluctuations (noise) matched to the level of noise found in the given scan. A library of templates was generated from 12 spherical template image sets with radius values evenly distributed from 4 to 20 times the in-plane voxel size. The similarity between the pixel values in the 3D region around a point of interest in the image, $f(u,v,w)$, and the pixel values in a given spherical template image, $t(x,y,z)$, was quantified using the normalized cross-correlation coefficient (NCCC). NCCC depends upon the average pixel value in the region of interest, $\bar{f}$, and the template, $\bar{t}$, as follows:

$$\text{NCCC}(u,v,w)$$

$$= \frac{\sum_{x,y,z}\left[f(x,y,z)-\bar{f}_{u,v,w}\right]\cdot\left[t(x-u,y-u,z-w)-\bar{t}\right]}{\sqrt{\sum_{x,y,z}\left[f(x,y,z)-\bar{f}_{u,v,w}\right]^2\cdot\sum_{x,y,z}\left[t(x-u,y-u,z-w)-\bar{t}\right]^2}}.$$

$$(14.1)$$

Subtraction of the average pixel value from each region and normalization by the individual self-correlations (the terms in the denominator) create a matching coefficient that is independent of absolute voxel intensity, alleviating contributions from low-frequency background intensity variations that can occur in MRI due to different scan parameters, RF receiver coil placement, and differential contrast agent dispersal across the brain spatially and over time. Normal anatomical structures, such as blood vessels, are avoided in the final detection results due to poor matching of their 3D extent with the zero-padded halo region of the template images. The template-matching approach with the NCCC metric is similar to approaches for lung nodule detection that use multiple 2D and 3D classifiers because both select nodule candidates based primarily on 2D and 3D size, shape, edge features, and texture (Figure 14.1).

In our study, CAD was performed on 22 patient datasets consisting of 1320 coronal MRI slices containing 161 total nodules. Figure 14.2 demonstrates representative MR images of brain metastases and their NCCC maps. The average patient MRI dataset contained 60 slices, and the CAD processing time was approximately 30 min (using MATLAB 7.2 running on a Power Mac G5 with quad 2.5 GHz processors and 4 gigabytes of RAM). The resultant CAD

performance metrics were a sensitivity of 87.6% with a false positive rate of 0.58 per image slice (Ambrosini et al. 2010). Although these performance outcomes are lower than that typical of CAD applied to the lung, they are on par with that typically encountered for CAD of primary tumors of the breast using conventional clinical imaging modalities and protocols (Wang et al. 2007).

14.4   COMPUTER-AIDED SEGMENTATION OF BRAIN TUMORS

In the application of computer-aided image processing technology to brain cancer, much of the focus has been on the accurate delineation of the tumor from the surrounding healthy brain tissue and edema. In part, this effort is due to the need to combine spatial information from multiple MRI modalities, where precontrast and postcontrast T1- and T2-weighted images are most commonly employed. The quest for the optimal means of combing this information, while being robust to contrast variability (i.e., due to differential contrast uptake), has led to the development of a variety of competing approaches. The first class of techniques is based on a multispectral histogram analysis/clustering that seeks to segment the tumor from edema from normal tissue (including white matter, gray matter, and cerebrospinal fluid). These efforts have included fuzzy clustering (Clark et al. 1998; Fletcher-Heath et al. 2001; Karayiannis and Pai 1999; Phillips et al. 1995) and statistical classification schemes (Kaus et al. 2001; Prastawa et al. 2003). Although pure intensity-based schemes lack a spatial connectivity constraint, which can lead to the inclusion of spurious voxels, this problem can be solved with the addition of knowledge through an atlas (Prastawa et al. 2003), a separate connectivity step (Fletcher-Heath et al. 2001), or their iterative integration (Kaus et al. 2001). In addition, one can apply level sets and/or snakes to extract connected boundaries (Ho et al. 2002; Zhu and Yan 1997); however, for this to work for each tissue component (e.g., tumor, edema, CSF, and normal), each component must have an accurate classification and a separate level set or snake. Analysis of the limitations of these approaches has motivated more sophistication schemes to better integrate both spatial and intensity information, such as support vector machines (Lee et al. 2008) and Bayesian probability models based on training data (Corso et al. 2008). In the latter approach, Corso et al. began with 20 patient datasets consisting of precontrast T1- and T2-weighted images, a fluid-attenuated inversion recovery (FLAIR) image, and a postcontrast T1-weighted image. In this approach, an expert segments each patient dataset to delineate not only normal brain matter, the region outside the head, edema, and the tumor but also where the tumor is further subdivided into

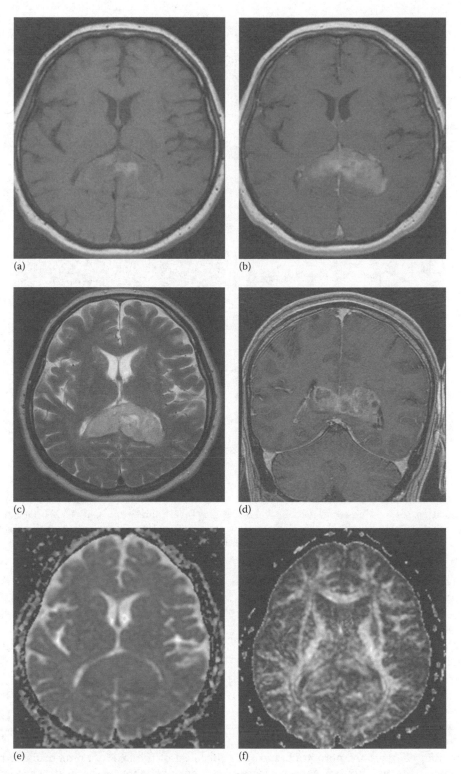

Figure 14.1 MR axial (a–c, e, f) and coronal (d) image slices of a patient's brain harboring a grade IV primary brain tumor (glioblastoma) in the splenium of the corpus callosum. The following are shown: (a) T1-weighted axial MR image acquired prior to the administration of gadolinium-based contrast; (b) T1-weighted axial image acquired postcontrast; (c) T2-weighted axial, postcontrast image; (d) T1-weighted postcontrast image in a coronal slice orientation; (e) average diffusion coefficient image in axial orientation; and (f) axial fractional anisotropy image. All of the axial slices were selected to be in nearly the same slice location, with the differences due to varying slice thickness and slice locations among the sequences and possible patient movement between scans.

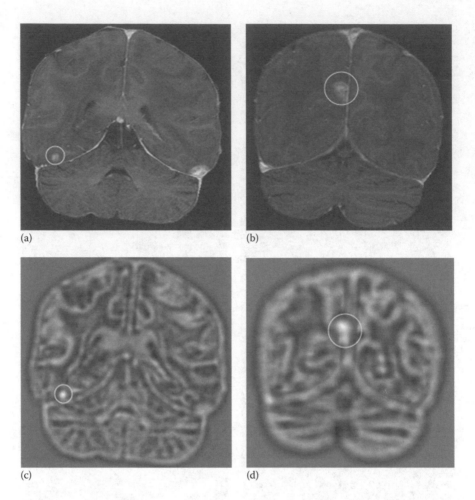

Figure 14.2 (a–b) MR coronal image slices of extracted patient's brain where locations of known metastases are indicated by circles. (c–d) Correlation maps at corresponding slice locations where the gray-level values represent the 3D normalized cross-correlation coefficient (NCCC) at each voxel between the 3D spherical template and the 3D patient image dataset. A template diameter of 6.88 mm in (c) and 7.74 mm in (d) was optimal. A uniform zero-padding width of 1.29 mm was used with both templates.

enhancing tumor, nonenhancing tumor, necrotic tissue, regions of possible tumor infiltration, and ambiguous tissue between necrotic and enhancing. The training datasets and expert ground truth are used to optimally classify each tissue type based on the four different MRI measurements. Thereafter, to segment a new dataset, voxels are linked (or not) to neighboring voxels as part of a connected cluster that identifies with a particular tissue type based on a probability derived from the training set classifiers and aggregate MRI outcomes of the cluster. The algorithm uses a multilevel clustering scheme wherein at the first level, a large number of possible clusters are permitted, and the segmentation is optimized for that number. At each successive level, the number of possible clusters is reduced by 50%, which forces the creation of larger groups from neighboring clusters on the previous level. Levels are added until only one or two clusters remain. Each voxel is then assigned the

tissue type corresponding to that of the strongest cluster to which it belonged across all levels. Thus, this approach has contributions from a priori knowledge of tissue-type features (gathered from the training set) and spatial connectivity from the multilevel clustering algorithm.

14.5 COMPUTERIZED DETECTION OF TUMOR EXTENT AND DIAGNOSIS OF BRAIN TUMORS IN MRI

Because of the lack of an identifiable high-risk group and the current state of the healthcare economy, there is no role at present for computer-aided early (presymptomatic) detection of primary brain cancer. The primary roles of computer-aided image analysis in brain cancer are to identify regions of tumor infiltration and to differentiate tumor recurrence from normal tissue response and damage following treatment. Therapy-induced changes in brain tissue include reactive astrocytosis and disruptions in vasculature; these can result from either surgery, radiation necrosis, or antiangiogenic therapies. Accurate and timely estimates of recurrence can greatly facilitate the reoptimization of therapy, minimize unwanted surgery or biopsy, and determine which patients should stay in clinical trials. Applying computer assistance in this task allows one to incorporate multimodality, multiparametric data in a fast and objective decision-making process. Currently, there are few examples of actual CAD applications in the literature. Jensen and Schmainda (2009) trained and tested four classifier systems for the task of differentiating invading tumor from edematous brain tissue. The input data consisted of MR-measured morphological, diffusion-weighted, and perfusion-weighted parameters, specifically the standardized FLAIR signal, the standardized precontrast and post-contrast T1-weighted signal, the average diffusion coefficient, the mean diffusivity, diffusion fractional isotropy (FA), the relative cerebral blood volume from a gradient-echo image ($rCBV_{GE}$), the relative cerebral blood volume from a spin-echo image ($rCBV_{SE}$), and the ratio of change in T2-star relaxivity to change in T2-relaxivity ($\Delta R_2^* / \Delta R_2$). The four classifier systems were a logistic linear regression model; a multilayer perception neural network consisting of two hidden layers containing 17 and 9 perceptions, respectively; a Sugeno-type fuzzy inference system using fuzzy subtractive clustering; and the same fuzzy clustering approach with an added neuroadaptive learning technique.

As described earlier, PET, MRSI, and MR-DWI have been applied in the clinic to achieve these goals, but they face the challenges of overcoming poor signal-to-noise performance, low image resolution (large voxel size), a limited ability to unambiguously identify or separate the molecular peaks of interest in MRSI, and difficulty in distinguishing tumor markers from the effects of edema and normal-tissue treatment response. Therefore, much effort has been made to apply multiparameter MR approaches for this task (Nelson 2011). Further utility may be found in combining information gathered from MRI with PET indices of tumor biology and activity (Ullrich et al. 2008). Although such approaches show promise, computer automation of such tasks has yet to be applied clinically.

14.6 CONCLUSIONS AND FUTURE OUTLOOK

At present, computer-aided image processing for brain cancer detection and diagnosis has not had a significant clinical impact. The primary challenges in the application of CAD for screening for primary brain cancer are the low incidence of disease, the lack of a readily identifiable high-risk group on whom to perform screening, and the heterogeneous and unpredictable appearance of lesions on contrast-enhanced images. Once detected, grade III and IV primary cancers (the most common diagnosis) have extremely poor prognosis. Targeted surgical and SRS therapies are fundamentally limited by the inability of current imaging schemes to identify microscopic tumor spread, and some in the field doubt whether improved delineation will lead to a meaningful improvement in patient outcomes due to the highly infiltrative nature of the disease. Moreover, the inability of imaging schemes to reliably discriminate tumor recurrence from pseudo-progression poses a challenge in the current clinical management of glioblastoma patients. The ability to apply MRSI techniques to better quantify and localize the measurement of common metabolites that illustrate microscopic tumor spread not seen by conventional MRI and new molecules of interest (e.g., glutamate and myo-inositol) holds great promise; however, at present, these metabolites cannot be reliably measured in the clinic with sufficient resolution and sensitivity in a reasonable amount of time. Since the imaging results are often inconclusive, choices to perform additional biopsy or continue with treatment can vary based on the experience and aggressiveness of the attending oncologists. Accurate and timely estimates of recurrence can greatly facilitate the reoptimization of therapy, minimize unwanted surgery or biopsy, and determine which patients should stay in clinical trials, so there remains a potential role for CAD in this arena. If the current technical challenges are overcome in the future, we will be able to utilize a clinically feasible multiparametric assay to detect microscopic infiltrations around the primary tumor and to detect tumor progression.

The future of CAD for the brain is probably most optimistic in the role of screening and surveillance for early detection of metastases to the brain from primary cancers from other organs. The advent of new treatment options (SRS/SRT) has created the exciting opportunity to apply brain tumor CAD with potentially life-changing benefit to patients with all cancers that have metastatic potential. Three-dimensional CAD techniques formerly applied to the lung can be successfully reformulated and reoptimized to the task of automated detection of brain metastases. We expect to see more effort put forth toward adapting other existing approaches to the brain and hope that the expected success of these efforts will rejuvenate interest in the detection of other brain anomalies, notably MS lesions. As CAD for brain metastases gains acceptance, it should accelerate the opening of clinical screening and surveillance trials for high-risk patient populations.

REFERENCES

Ackerstaff, E., K. Glunde, and Z. M. Bhujwalla. 2003. Choline phospholipid metabolism: A target in cancer cells? *J Cell Biochem* 90(3):525–533.

ACS. 2005. Treatment of specific types of brain and spinal cord tumors. Detailed guide: Brain/CNS tumors in adults. *Am Cancer Soc.* http://www.cancer.org/cancer/braincnstumorsinadults/detailedguide/.

Ambrosini, R. D., P. Wang, and W. G. O'Dell. 2010. Computer-aided detection of metastatic brain tumors using automated three-dimensional template matching. *J Magn Reson Imaging* 31(1):85–93.

Ammirati, M., N. Vick, Y. L. Liao, I. Ciric, and M. Mikhael. 1987. Effect of the extent of surgical resection on survival and quality of life in patients with supratentorial glioblastomas and anaplastic astrocytomas. *Neurosurgery* 21(2):201–206.

Bajaj, G. K., L. Kleinberg, and S. Terezakis. 2005. Current concepts and controversies in the treatment of parenchymal brain metastases: Improved outcomes with aggressive management. *Cancer Invest* 23(4):363–376.

Barker, F. G. 2nd. 2005. Surgical and radiosurgical management of brain metastases. *Surg Clin North Am* 85(2):329–345.

Basser, P. J., S. Pajevic, C. Pierpaoli, J. Duda, and A. Aldroubi. 2000. In vivo fiber tractography using DT-MRI data. *Magn Reson Med* 44(4):625–632.

Biswas, T., P. Okunieff, M. C. Schell, T. Smudzin, W. H. Pilcher, R. S. Bakos, G. E. Vates, K. A. Walter, A. Wensel, D. N. Korones, and M. T. Milano. 2009. Stereotactic radiosurgery for glioblastoma: Retrospective analysis. *Radiat Oncol* 4:11.

Black, P. M. and J. S. Loeffler. 2005. *Cancer of the Nervous System.* 2nd edn., Philadelphia: Lippincott Williams & Wilkins.

Boyd, T. S. and M. P. Mehta. 1999. Radiosurgery for brain metastases. *Neurosurg Clin N Am* 10(2):337–350.

Brand, A., C. Richter-Landsberg, and D. Leibfritz. 1993. Multinuclear NMR studies on the energy metabolism of glial and neuronal cells. *Dev Neurosci* 15(3–5):289–298.

Brandes, A. A., A. Tosoni, P. Amista, L. Nicolardi, D. Grosso, F. Berti, and M. Ermani. 2004. How effective is BCNU in recurrent glioblastoma in the modern era? A phase II trial. *Neurology* 63(7):1281–1284.

Burger, P. C., E. R. Heinz, T. Shibata, and P. Kleihues. 1988. Topographic anatomy and CT correlations in the untreated glioblastoma multiforme. *J Neurosurg* 68(5):698–704.

Chung, J. K., Y. K. Kim, S. K. Kim, Y. J. Lee, S. Paek, J. S. Yeo, J. M. Jeong, D. S. Lee, H. W. Jung, and M. C. Lee. 2002. Usefulness of 11C-methionine PET in the evaluation of brain lesions that are hypo- or isometabolic on 18F-FDG PET. *Eur J Nucl Med Mol Imaging* 29(2):176–182.

Clark, M. C., L. O. Hall, D. B. Goldgof, R. Velthuizen, F. R. Murtagh, and M. S. Silbiger. 1998. Automatic tumor segmentation using knowledge-based techniques. *IEEE Trans Med Imaging* 17(2):187–201.

Corso, J. J., E. Sharon, S. Dube, S. El-Saden, U. Sinha, and A. Yuille. 2008. Efficient multilevel brain tumor segmentation with integrated bayesian model classification. *IEEE Trans Med Imaging* 27(5):629–640.

Dhermain, F. G., P. Hau, H. Lanfermann, A. H. Jacobs, and M. J. van den Bent. 2010. Advanced MRI and PET imaging for assessment of treatment response in patients with gliomas. *Lancet Neurol* 9(9):906–920.

Fitzgerald, D. P., D. Palmieri, E. Hua, E. Hargrave, J. M. Herring, Y. Qian, E. Vega-Valle, R. J. Weil, A. M. Stark, A. O. Vortmeyer, and P. S. Steeg. 2008. Reactive glia are recruited by highly proliferative brain metastases of breast cancer and promote tumor cell colonization. *Clin Exp Metastasis* 25(7):799–810.

Fletcher-Heath, L. M., L. O. Hall, D. B. Goldgof, and F. R. Murtagh. 2001. Automatic segmentation of non-enhancing brain tumors in magnetic resonance images. *Artif Intell Med* 21(1–3):43–63.

Gillard, J. H., A. D. Waldman, and P. B. Barker. 2004. *Clinical MR Neuroimaging: Diffusion, Perfusion and Spectroscopy*, Vol. 1. Cambridge, U.K.: Cambridge University Press.

Glunde, K. and Z. M. Bhujwalla. 2011. Metabolic tumor imaging using magnetic resonance spectroscopy. *Semin Oncol* 38(1):26–41.

Gupta, T. 2005. Stereotactic radiosurgery for brain oligometastases: Good for some, better for all? *Ann Oncol* 16(11):1749–1754.

Hall, E. J. 2000. *Radiobiology for the Radiologist.* 5th ed. Philadelphia, PA: Lippincott Williams & Wilkins.

Hattingen, E., P. Raab, K. Franz, H. Lanfermann, M. Setzer, R. Gerlach, F. E. Zanella, and U. Pilatus. 2008. Prognostic value of choline and creatine in WHO grade II gliomas. *Neuroradiology* 50(9):759–767.

Herholz, K., T. Holzer, B. Bauer, R. Schroder, J. Voges, R. I. Ernestus, G. Mendoza, G. Weber-Luxenburger, J. Lottgen, A. Thiel, K. Wienhard, and W. D. Heiss. 1998. 11C-methionine PET for differential diagnosis of low-grade gliomas. *Neurology* 50(5):1316–1322.

Herminghaus, S., U. Pilatus, W. Moller-Hartmann, P. Raab, H. Lanfermann, W. Schlote, and F. E. Zanella. 2002. Increased choline levels coincide with enhanced proliferative activity of human neuroepithelial brain tumors. *NMR Biomed* 15(6):385–392.

Ho, S., E. Bullitt, and G. Gerig. 2002. Level-set evolution with region competition: Automatic 3-D segmentation of brain tumors. In *16th International Conference on Pattern Recognition, 2002, Proceedings 1,* pp. 532–535. Vol. 1. doi:10.1109/ICPR.2002.1044788.

Hu, J., S. Yang, Y. Xuan, Q. Jiang, Y. Yang, and E. M. Haacke. 2007. Simultaneous detection of resolved glutamate, glutamine, and gamma-aminobutyric acid at 4 T. *J Magn Reson* 185(2):204–213.

Jacobs, A. H., C. Dittmar, A. Winkeler, G. Garlip, and W. D. Heiss. 2002. Molecular imaging of gliomas. *Mol Imaging* 1(4):309–335.

Jagannathan, J., J. H. Sherman, G. U. Mehta, and L. S. Chin. 2007. Radiobiology of brain metastasis: Applications in stereotactic radiosurgery. *Neurosurg Focus* 22(3):E4.

Jensen, T. R. and K. M. Schmainda. 2009. Computer-aided detection of brain tumor invasion using multiparametric MRI. *J Magn Reson Imaging* 30(3):481–489.

Kallenberg, K., H. C. Bock, G. Helms, K. Jung, A. Wrede, J. H. Buhk, A. Giese, J. Frahm, H. Strik, P. Dechent, and M. Knauth. 2009. Untreated glioblastoma multiforme: Increased myo-inositol and glutamine levels in the contralateral cerebral hemisphere at proton MR spectroscopy. *Radiology* 253(3):805–812.

Karayiannis, N. B. and P. I. Pai. 1999. Segmentation of magnetic resonance images using fuzzy algorithms for learning vector quantization. *IEEE Trans Med Imaging* 18(2):172–180.

Kato, T., J. Shinoda, N. Nakayama, K. Miwa, A. Okumura, H. Yano, S. Yoshimura, T. Maruyama, Y. Muragaki, and T. Iwama. 2008. Metabolic assessment of gliomas using 11C-methionine, [18F] fluorodeoxyglucose, and 11C-choline positron-emission tomography. *Am J Neuroradiol* 29(6):1176–1182.

Kaus, M. R., S. K. Warfield, A. Nabavi, P. M. Black, F. A. Jolesz, and R. Kikinis. 2001. Automated segmentation of MR images of brain tumors. *Radiology* 218(2):586–591.

Khatri, V. P., N. J. Petrelli, and J. Belghiti. 2005. Extending the frontiers of surgical therapy for hepatic colorectal metastases: Is there a limit? *J Clin Oncol* 23(33):8490–8499.

Laprie, A., I. Catalaa, E. Cassol, T. R. McKnight, D. Berchery, D. Marre, J. M. Bachaud, I. Berry, and E. C. Moyal. 2008. Proton magnetic resonance spectroscopic imaging in newly diagnosed glioblastoma: Predictive value for the site of postradiotherapy relapse in a prospective longitudinal study. *Int J Radiat Oncol Biol Phys* 70(3):773–781.

Le Bihan, D., E. Breton, D. Lallemand, P. Grenier, E. Cabanis, and M. Laval-Jeantet. 1986. MR imaging of intravoxel incoherent motions: Application to diffusion and perfusion in neurologic disorders. *Radiology* 161(2):401–407.

Lee, C. H., S. Wang, A. Murtha, M. R. Brown, and R. Greiner. 2008. Segmenting brain tumors using pseudo-conditional random fields. *Med Image Comput Comput Assist Interv* 11(Pt 1):359–366.

Louis, D. N., H. Ohgaki, O. D. Wiestler, W. K. Cavenee, P. C. Burger, A. Jouvet, B. W. Scheithauer, and P. Kleihues. 2007. The 2007 WHO classification of tumours of the central nervous system. *Acta Neuropathol* 114(2):97–109.

Martin, J. J. and D. Kondziolka. 2005. Indications for resection and radiosurgery for brain metastases. *Curr Opin Oncol* 17(6):584–587.

Mathews, V. P., K. S. Caldemeyer, J. L. Ulmer, H. Nguyen, and W. T. Yuh. 1997. Effects of contrast dose, delayed imaging, and magnetization transfer saturation on gadolinium-enhanced MR imaging of brain lesions. *J Magn Reson Imaging* 7(1):14–22.

Mc Dermott, D. F. 2009. Immunotherapy of metastatic renal cell carcinoma. *Cancer* 115(10 Suppl):2298–2305.

Mortazavi, D., A. Z. Kouzani, and H. Soltanian-Zadeh. 2012. Segmentation of multiple sclerosis lesions in MR images: A review. *Neuroradiology* 54(4):299–320.

Nelson, S. J. 2011. Assessment of therapeutic response and treatment planning for brain tumors using metabolic and physiological MRI. *NMR Biomed* 24(6):734–749.

Nelson, S. J., E. Graves, A. Pirzkall, X. Li, A. Antiniw Chan, D. B. Vigneron, and T. R. McKnight. 2002. In vivo molecular imaging for planning radiation therapy of gliomas: An application of 1H MRSI. *J Magn Reson Imaging* 16(4):464–476.

Noel, G., G. Boisserie, L. Feuvret, and J. J. Mazeron. 2004. Radiosurgery of brain metastasis: Reflexions, controversies and unanswered questions in 2004. *Bull Cancer* 91(1):81–93.

Norden, A. D., G. S. Young, K. Setayesh, A. Muzikansky, R. Klufas, G. L. Ross, A. S. Ciampa et al. 2008. Bevacizumab for recurrent malignant gliomas: Efficacy, toxicity, and patterns of recurrence. *Neurology* 70(10):779–787.

Norfray, J. F., T. Tomita, S. E. Byrd, B. D. Ross, P. A. Berger, and R. S. Miller. 1999. Clinical impact of MR spectroscopy when MR imaging is indeterminate for pediatric brain tumors. *Am J Roentgenol* 173(1):119–125.

Park, I., G. Tamai, M. C. Lee, C. F. Chuang, S. M. Chang, M. S. Berger, S. J. Nelson, and A. Pirzkall. 2007. Patterns of recurrence analysis in newly diagnosed glioblastoma multiforme after three-dimensional conformal radiation therapy with respect to pre-radiation therapy magnetic resonance spectroscopic findings. *Int J Radiat Oncol Biol Phys* 69(2):381–389.

Phillips, W. E. 2nd, R. P. Velthuizen, S. Phuphanich, L. O. Hall, L. P. Clarke, and M. L. Silbiger. 1995. Application of fuzzy c-means segmentation technique for tissue differentiation in MR images of a hemorrhagic glioblastoma multiforme. *Magn Reson Imaging* 13(2):277–290.

Pierpaoli, C., P. Jezzard, P. J. Basser, A. Barnett, and G. Di Chiro. 1996. Diffusion tensor MR imaging of the human brain. *Radiology* 201(3):637–648.

Prastawa, M., E. Bullitt, N. Moon, K. Van Leemput, and G. Gerig. 2003. Automatic brain tumor segmentation by subject specific modification of atlas priors. *Acad Radiol* 10(12):1341–1348.

Prieto, E., J. M. Marti-Climent, I. Dominguez-Prado, P. Garrastachu, R. Diez-Valle, S. Tejada, J. J. Aristu, I. Penuelas, and J. Arbizu. 2011. Voxel-based analysis of dual-time-point 18F-FDG PET images for brain tumor identification and delineation. *J Nucl Med* 52(6):865–872.

Quinn, J. A., D. A. Reardon, A. H. Friedman, J. N. Rich, J. H. Sampson, J. M. Provenzale, R. E. McLendon et al. 2003. Phase II trial of temozolomide in patients with progressive low-grade glioma. *J Clin Oncol* 21(4):646–651.

Ranasinghe, M. G. and J. M. Sheehan. 2007. Surgical management of brain metastases. *Neurosurg Focus* 22(3):E2.

Ries, L. A. G., D. Harkins, M. Krapcho, A. Mariotto, B. A. Miller, E. J. Feuer, L. Clegg et al. 2006. *SEER Cancer Statistics Review, 1975–2003*. Bethesda, MD: National Cancer Institute.

Sakariassen, P. O., L. Prestegarden, J. Wang, K. O. Skaftnesmo, R. Mahesparan, C. Molthoff, P. Sminia et al. 2006. Angiogenesis-independent tumor growth mediated by stem-like cancer cells. *Proc Natl Acad Sci USA* 103(44):16466–16471.

Scherer, H. J. 1940. The forms of growth in gliomas and their practical significance. *Brain* 63(1):1–35.

Shields, T. W. 2005. *General Thoracic Surgery*, Vol. 2. Philadelphia, PA: Lippincott Williams & Wilkins.

Shimizu, H., T. Kumabe, R. Shirane, and T. Yoshimoto. 2000. Correlation between choline level measured by proton MR spectroscopy and Ki-67 labeling index in gliomas. *Am J Neuroradiol* 21(4):659–665.

Spence, A. M., M. Muzi, D. A. Mankoff, S. F. O'Sullivan, J. M. Link, T. K. Lewellen, B. Lewellen, P. Pham, S. Minoshima, K. Swanson, and K. A. Krohn. 2004. 18F-FDG PET of gliomas at delayed intervals: Improved distinction between tumor and normal gray matter. *J Nucl Med* 45(10):1653–1659.

Srinivasan, R., C. Cunningham, A. Chen, D. Vigneron, R. Hurd, S. Nelson, and D. Pelletier. 2006. TE-averaged two-dimensional proton spectroscopic imaging of glutamate at 3 T. *Neuroimage* 30(4):1171–1178.

Suit, H. D., A. E. Howes, and N. Hunter. 1977. Dependence of response of a C3H mammary carcinoma to fractionated irradiation on fractionation number and intertreatment interval. *Radiat Res* 72(3):440–454.

Takano, T., J. H. Lin, G. Arcuino, Q. Gao, J. Yang, and M. Nedergaard. 2001. Glutamate release promotes growth of malignant gliomas. *Nat Med* 7(9):1010–1015.

Taylor, D. G. and M. C. Bushell. 1985. The spatial mapping of translational diffusion coefficients by the NMR imaging technique. *Phys Med Biol* 30(4):345–349.

Ullrich, R. T., L. W. Kracht, and A. H. Jacobs. 2008. Neuroimaging in patients with gliomas. *Semin Neurol* 28(4):484–494.

van den Bent, M. J. 2001. New perspectives for the diagnosis and treatment of oligodendroglioma. *Expert Rev Anticancer Ther* 1(3):348–356.

Wang, P., A. DeNunzio, P. Okunieff, and W. G. O'Dell. 2007. Lung metastases detection in CT images using 3D template matching. *Med Phys* 34(3):915–922.

Weller, M. 2011. Novel diagnostic and therapeutic approaches to malignant glioma. *Swiss Med Wkly* 141:w13210.

Weybright, P., P. Maly, D. Gomez-Hassan, C. Blaesing, and P. C. Sundgren. 2004. MR spectroscopy in the evaluation of recurrent contrast-enhancing lesions in the posterior fossa after tumor treatment. *Neuroradiology* 46(7):541–549.

Yamamoto, D., H. Arimura, S. Kakeda, T. Magome, Y. Yamashita, F. Toyofuku, M. Ohki, Y. Higashida, and Y. Korogi. 2010. Computer-aided detection of multiple sclerosis lesions in brain magnetic resonance images: False positive reduction scheme consisted of rule-based, level set method, and support vector machine. *Comput Med Imaging Graph* 34(5):404–413.

Zhu, Y. and H. Yan. 1997. Computerized tumor boundary detection using a Hopfield neural network. *IEEE Trans Med Imaging* 16(1):55–67.

Chapter 15

Detection of Cerebrovascular Diseases

Yoshikazu Uchiyama and Hiroshi Fujita

CONTENTS

15.1 INTRODUCTION

Recently, the concept of CAD has been expanded to the cerebral region. A screening system called the *Brain Check-up* is widely employed in Japan. A number of CAD schemes are being developed in Japan to assist radiologists in the early detection of cerebrovascular diseases at screening centers and hospitals (Arimura et al. 2004, Hayashi et al. 2003, Kobayashi et al. 2006, Uchiyama et al. 2005, 2007a, Yokoyama et al. 2007). Figure 15.1 shows the trend in leading causes of death in Japan. The number of cerebrovascular diseases has gradually decreased every year. However, it should be noted that the numbers of cases of subarachnoid hemorrhage (SAH) and cerebral infarction are on the increase. Therefore, it is important to reduce the incidence of these conditions. In this chapter, CAD schemes developed at Gifu University (Fujita et al. 2008) and observer performance studies are presented, with reference to related works and with an emphasis on potential clinical applications in the future. Subjects for these CAD schemes included in the following sections are (1) detection of intracranial unruptured aneurysms in magnetic resonance angiography (MRA), (2) a new viewing technique for the detection of unruptured aneurysms, (3) detection of arterial occlusion in MRA, (4) detection of lacunar infarcts in T_1- and T_2-weighted images, and (5) classification of lacunar infarcts and enlarged Virchow–Robin spaces in T_1- and T_2-weighted images.

15.2 COMPUTERIZED DETECTION OF UNRUPTURED ANEURYSMS IN MR ANGIOGRAPHY

The detection of unruptured aneurysms in MRA studies is an important task because aneurysm rupture is the main cause of SAH, which is a serious disorder with high mortality and morbidity (Fogelholm et al. 1993). The rate of rupture of asymptomatic aneurysms has been estimated to be 1%–2% per year (Wardlaw and White 2000). However, it is often difficult and time consuming for radiologists to detect small aneurysms, and it may not be easy to detect even medium-sized aneurysms in the MRA studies because of the overlap between an aneurysm and adjacent vessels on maximum-intensity projection (MIP) images. Therefore, CAD schemes would be useful in assisting radiologists in detecting unruptured aneurysms (Arimura et al. 2004, Hayashi et al. 2003, Kobayashi et al. 2006, Uchiyama et al. 2005).

15.2.1 Vessel Segmentation

Figure 15.2 shows the overall scheme used for the detection of unruptured aneurysms in MRA images (Uchiyama et al. 2008a). The vessel region was segmented first to avoid false positives (FPs) located outside the vessel region. A linear gray-level transformation was applied to the three-dimensional (3D) MRA image so that the minimum voxel value became zero, and voxels with values greater than the 99% margin depicted in a cumulative histogram were assigned a maximum value of 1024. After the linear gray-level transformation, the vessel regions were segmented from the background by using the gray-level thresholding method with an empirically selected threshold level of 700. Using this method, large vessel regions were successfully segmented. However, it is difficult to segment small vessels using this method because the voxel values in the small vessel regions are low. Therefore, a region-growing technique was subsequently applied to segment the small vessel regions. The segmented large vessel regions were used as *seed* points, and the neighboring voxels with values greater than 500 were appended to the seed points.

Accurate segmentation of vessel regions on MRA images is an essential and often difficult task in the development of a CAD scheme. Gao et al. (2011) have developed a fast, fully automatic segmentation algorithm for extracting the 3D cerebral vessels in MRA images, based on statistical

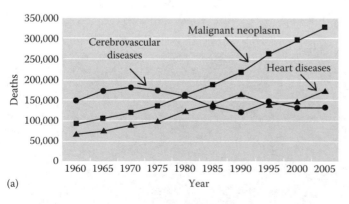

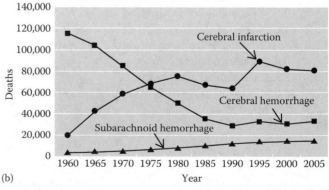

Figure 15.1 (a) Trend in leading causes of death in Japan. Cerebrovascular diseases are the third leading cause of death. (b) Trend in deaths from cerebrovascular diseases in Japan. The numbers of subarachnoid hemorrhages and cerebral infarctions are increasing.

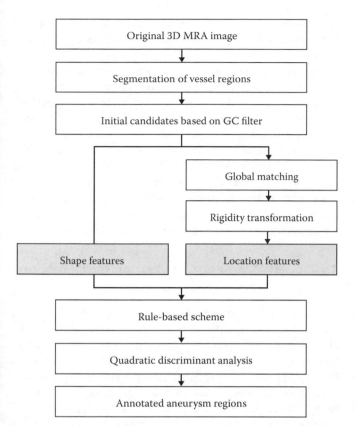

Figure 15.2 Overall scheme for the detection of unruptured aneurysms in magnetic resonance angiography. (From Uchiyama, Y. et al., *SPIE Proc.*, 6915, 69151Q-1, 2008a.)

model analysis and improved curve evolution. Quantitative comparisons with 10 sets of manual segmentation results showed that the average volume sensitivity, average branch sensitivity, and average mean absolute distance error were 93.6%, 95.98%, and 0.333 mm, respectively. By applying the algorithm to 200 clinical datasets from three hospitals, it has been demonstrated that the proposed algorithm can provide good-quality segmentation capable of extracting a vessel with a one-voxel diameter in less than 2 min.

15.2.2 Initial Identification of Unruptured Aneurysms

For the enhancement of aneurysms, a 3D gradient concentration (GC) filter was employed. This filter was designed to enhance the regions of a sphere by measuring the degree of convergence of the gradient vectors around a point of interest, which is defined by

$$GC(p) = \frac{1}{M} \sum_{R} \cos\theta_j. \qquad (15.1)$$

Figure 15.3 illustrates GC filter. The output value of the GC filter at the point of interest $p(x, y, z)$ was computed within

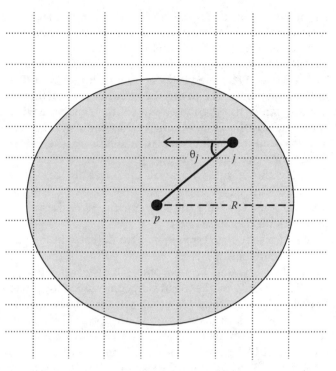

Figure 15.3 Illustration of gradient concentration filter.

the regions of a sphere with radius R at the center of $p(x, y, z)$. The angle θ_j is the angle between the direction vector from $p(x, y, z)$ to $j(x, y, z)$ and the gradient direction vector located at $j(x, y, z)$. M is the number of voxels when the gradient magnitude located at $j(x, y, z)$ was greater than zero. The gradient magnitude and gradient direction were determined by the first-order difference filter with a matrix size of $3 \times 3 \times 3$. The output value of GC filter ranges from 0.0 to 1.0. If the candidate region is in spherical form, the GC filter takes a value of 1.0. For the initial identification of aneurysm candidates, the gray-level thresholding technique with a threshold level of 0.5 was applied to the image obtained using the GC filter. After thresholding, regions lager than 10 voxels were determined as the initial candidates.

Other investigator (Arimura et al. 2004) employed a 3D selective enhancement filter (Li et al. 2003) for the enhancement of aneurysms. This filter can enhance objects of a specific shape (e.g., dot-like aneurysms) and suppress objects of other shapes (e.g., line-like vessels). For identifying initial candidates, multiple gray level thresholding technique was applied to the dot-enhanced image processed using a selective multiscale enhancement filter.

15.2.3 Feature Extraction

The initially selected candidates included many FPs. To eliminate these FPs, features of shape and anatomical location of each candidate region were determined. The shape features were size, degree of sphericity, and mean and maximum values of the GC image. The size was given as the number of voxels in the initial candidate region and was considered a useful feature for eliminating FPs because the sizes of some FPs were either smaller or larger than those of the aneurysms. The degree of sphericity was defined by the fraction of the overlap volume of the candidate with a sphere having the same volume as the candidate. The mean and maximum values of the GC image were given as the mean and maximum values in the candidate region processed by the GC filter. These features were also considered useful for distinguishing between vessels and aneurysms because some FPs were line-like or more irregular in comparison with the aneurysms.

Unruptured aneurysms were often detected in the anterior communicating artery, branch points of the middle cerebral artery, and branch points between the internal carotid artery and the posterior communicating artery. Therefore, the anatomical location is an important piece of information for the detection of unruptured aneurysms. In order to obtain anatomical location features, a reference (normal) MRA image was selected. The vessel regions in the reference image were then semi-manually segmented for image registration. The segmented vessel regions in the target image were shifted to align with the reference image by using a global matching procedure and rigid transformation, which is described in Section 15.4.3. After the rigid transformation, the locations x, y, and z in the target image were shifted into common coordinates on the reference image, thereby providing anatomical location information.

Other investigators have proposed a number of image features for the elimination of FPs. For example, Arimura et al. (2006) have developed a shape-based difference image (SBDI) technique for extracting small protrusions or small aneurysms. The SBDI technique is based on the shape difference between an original segmented vessel and a vessel with a suppressed local change in thickness. The SBDI technique is useful for obtaining local changes in vessel thickness, that is, shape-based difference (SBD) regions, which could be small aneurysms in the case of true positives, but thin or very small regions in the case of FPs. Yang et al. (2011) used other features to reduce FPs, such as distance to the trunk, radius of the vessel, planeness, cylinder surface, Gaussian and mean curvature, and shape index.

15.2.4 False-Positive Reduction

Four shape features and three anatomical location features were obtained from the initial candidate regions. The rules in rule-based schemes were then set using these values. First, the maximum and minimum values of each of these seven features were obtained from all the aneurysms. All 14 cutoff thresholds were determined on the basis of these values.

The rule-based schemes were then used for the first step in the elimination of FPs; that is, when a candidate was located outside the range determined by the cutoff thresholds in the feature space, the candidate was considered as an FP. For further eliminating FPs, a quadratic discriminant analysis (QDA) was employed using the four shape features and three anatomical location features. The QDA generates a decision boundary that optimally partitions the feature space into two classes, that is, an aneurysm class and FP class. The decision boundary for the QDA was a quadratic surface given by a discriminant function. The output value of the discriminant function indicates the likelihood of the occurrence of the aneurysm. By changing the threshold level, the performance of the CAD scheme can be determined.

15.2.5 Performance Evaluation for Detection of Unruptured Aneurysms

The database consisted of 100 MRA studies (72 normal and 28 abnormal) with 30 unruptured aneurysms (diameter: 2.3–3.5 mm; mean: 2.8 mm). These MRA studies were acquired by using a 1.5 T magnetic image scanner. In the first step toward identifying the initial aneurysm candidate regions, 93.3% (28/30) aneurysms were accurately detected, with 27.32 (2732/100) FPs per patient. This result indicates that the GC filter was useful in the detection of aneurysms because almost all the aneurysms were detected accurately. However, many FPs were also detected using this method. To eliminate FPs, the rule-based scheme and QDA with seven features were employed. The results revealed that CAD scheme achieved a sensitivity of 90.0% (27/30) with 1.52 (152/100) FPs per patient. Figure 15.4 shows the free-response receiver operating characteristic (FROC) curves for the overall performance of the detection of aneurysms with and without location features. The graphs show that the number of FPs decreased from 3.47 (without location features) to 1.52 (with location features) while maintaining a sensitivity of 90.0%. This result indicates that the three location features were useful for distinguishing between aneurysms and FPs. Figure 15.5 shows a prototype of the CAD scheme for the detection of unruptured aneurysms, where MIP images and volume rendering images can be displayed. In this case, the CAD scheme indicated two candidate regions containing an unruptured aneurysm.

15.3 OBSERVER STUDY FOR DETECTION OF UNRUPTURED ANEURYSMS

Other investigators (Hirai et al. 2006, Kakeda et al. 2008) have carried out observer performance studies to retrospectively evaluate the effect of CAD on radiologists'

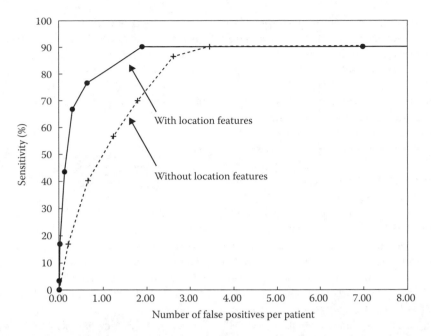

Figure 15.4   FROC curves for the overall performance of the CAD scheme in the detection of unruptured aneurysms with and without anatomical location features. (From Uchiyama, Y. et al., *SPIE Proc.*, 6915, 69151Q-1, 2008a.)

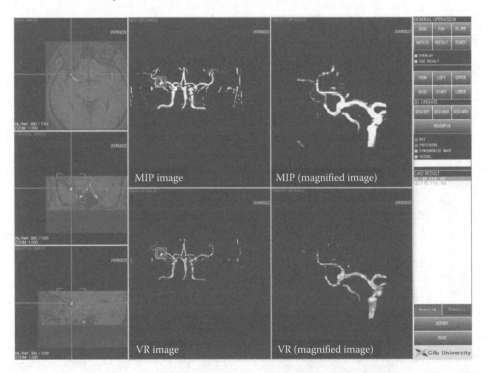

Figure 15.5   (See color insert.) Illustration of a prototype CAD scheme for the detection of unruptured aneurysms.

performance in the detection of intracranial aneurysms using MRA. Hirai et al. (2006) used 50 MIPs of MR angiograms in their study. The dataset included 50 patients, 22 (age range, 43–86 years) with intracranial aneurysms and 28 (age range, 32–80) without aneurysms. Fifteen radiologists, including eight neuroradiologists and seven general

radiologists, participated in the observer performance test, which was carried out using a sequential test method. Each observer read the MR angiograms displayed on a monitor first without computer output and rated his or her confidence level in determining the presence or absence of an aneurysm. Next, the computer output, marked by circles that indicated potential aneurysms, was superimposed on the MR angiograms. The observer then viewed the image with the computer output and rated it again. The observers were allowed to select the direction of the MR angiograms and the magnification of the image on the monitor. The following information was provided to the observers: (a) a description of the sequential test method used, (b) the presence of only one aneurysm in each patient, and (c) the type of aneurysm being either saccular or fusiform. The observers were blinded to the number of patients with aneurysms and the performance level of the CAD scheme. There was no limit on the reading time.

The observers' performance without and with the computer output was evaluated by receiver operating characteristic (ROC) analysis. For all 15 observers, average area under the receiver operating characteristic curve (AUC) value for detection of aneurysms was increased significantly from 0.931 to 0.983 ($p = 0.001$) with the computer output, as shown in Table 15.1. AUC values for general radiologists and neuroradiologists increased from 0.894 to 0.983 ($p = 0.022$) and from 0.963 to 0.984 ($p = 0.014$), respectively.

The improvement in the performance of general radiologists in terms of the AUC value was much greater than that of neuroradiologists. These results indicate that the use of the CAD scheme helped to improve the performance of both neuroradiologists and general radiologists for the detection of intracranial aneurysms in MR angiograms.

15.4 VIEWING TECHNIQUE FOR DETECTION OF UNRUPTURED ANEURYSMS

To facilitating the detection of small aneurysms by radiologists, Uchiyama et al. (2006) developed a new viewing technique termed a *SelMIP* image. This involved the generation of a new type of MIP image containing target vessel regions only, by manually selecting a desired cerebral artery from a list. By using a *SelMIP* image, the selected vessel region can be observed from various directions, and small aneurysms are easier to detect. For this technique, a new method was developed for the automated labeling of eight arteries in MRA studies.

15.4.1 Reference Image

For the automated labeling of eight arteries, a 3D reference image was used as a reference for the locations of the eight arteries to be segmented in all MRA studies. The eight cerebral arteries were prelabeled in the 3D reference image. These were the anterior cerebral artery (ACA), right middle cerebral artery (MCA), left MCA, right internal carotid artery (ICA), left ICA, right posterior cerebral artery (PCA), left PCA, and basilar artery (BA). Image registration was performed on the 3D reference image and an image to be classified, referred to as a target image, with the former kept unchanged. Figure 15.6 shows a representative target image and a reference image.

15.4.2 Global Matching

Global matching was used in initial image registration. As the locations of the corresponding vessel regions in the target image and the reference image are likely to be different due to variations in patient positioning, registration of corresponding vessel regions is necessary. Segmentation of the vessel regions in a target image was performed by using the thresholding and region-growing techniques, as described in Section 15.2.1. The segmented vessel regions in the target image were then shifted to align with the reference image. The translation vector was defined so as to maximize the overlapping of the vessel regions in the target image and the reference image. By using the global matching technique, the corresponding vessel regions in the two images were brought close to each other.

TABLE 15.1 AUC VALUES FOR RADIOLOGISTS IN THE DETECTION OF INTRACRANIAL ANEURYSMS

Observers	Without CAD	With CAD
Neuroradiologists		
1	0.939	0.964 ↑
2	0.986	0.994 ↑
3	0.989	0.998 ↑
4	0.969	0.970 ↑
5	0.969	0.984 ↑
6	0.952	0.993 ↑
7	0.942	1.000 ↑
8	0.958	0.967 ↑
Mean	0.963	0.984 ↑
General radiologists		
9	0.916	0.961 ↑
10	0.909	0.984 ↑
11	0.871	0.978 ↑
12	0.909	0.989 ↑
13	0.871	0.989 ↑
14	0.872	0.984 ↑
15	0.910	0.993 ↑
Mean	0.894	0.983 ↑
Overall	0.931	0.983 ↑

Source: Hirai, T. et al., *Radiology*, 237, 605, 2006.

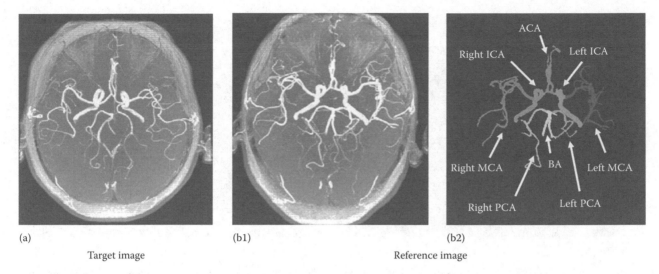

Figure 15.6   Target image and reference image. (a) MIP image of target image. The target image was changed to register the reference image. (b1) MIP image of the reference image. (b2) The eight prelabeled arteries shown on the reference image in (b1).

15.4.3   Rigid Transformation of the Target Image

After the global matching procedure, the rigid transformation was used to achieve a more accurate matching between the target and reference images. A number of control points were predetermined in the reference image, and the template matching method was used to determine the locations of the corresponding control points in the target image. In the template matching procedure, the normalized cross-correlation value $C(x, y, z)$ was used as a similarity measure. The normalized cross-correlation value $C(x, y, z)$ between the template $A(i, j, k)$ centered at a predetermined feature point (i, j, k) on the reference image and a region $B(x + i, y + j, z + k)$ located at $(x + i, y + j, z + k)$ on the target image that corresponds to the feature point (i, j, k) is given by

$$C(x,y,z) = \frac{1}{IJK}\sum_{k=1}^{K}\sum_{j=1}^{J}\sum_{i=1}^{I}$$

$$\frac{\left\{A(i,j,k)-\bar{a}\right\}\left\{B(x+i,y+j,z+k)-\bar{b}\right\}}{\sigma_A \sigma_B},$$

(15.2)

where $\bar{a}$ and $\bar{b}$ are mean voxel values of template $A(i, j, k)$ and region $B(x + i, y + j, z + k)$, respectively, and σ_A and σ_B are the corresponding standard deviations. The size of the template $I \times J \times K$ was set to be $21 \times 21 \times 21$. The normalized cross-correlation value indicates the resemblance between the candidate region and the template. If the images A and B are identical, C will take on the value 1.0. Twelve templates were located manually in the cerebral region of the reference image. Figure 15.7a shows the center points of the 12 templates in black dots. The size of search region

associated with each template in the target image was $41 \times 41 \times 41$. Figure 15.7b shows the 12 corresponding points found in the target image using the template matching method. A set of corresponding control points determined by the template matching method were used to determine the translation and rotation vectors, T and R, between the two images for the rigid transformation. If P and p represent the corresponding points in the reference and target images, respectively, assuming the coordinates of the corresponding points in the images after global matching are $\{p_i = (x_i, y_i, z_i), P_i = (X_i, Y_i, Z_i): i = 1,...,12\}$, the relation between the corresponding points in the images can be written as

$$P_i = R p_i + T.$$

(15.3)

The translation vector T and the rotation vector R can be determined by minimizing

$$E^2 = \sum_{i=1}^{12} P_i - \left(R p_i + T\right)^2.$$

(15.4)

15.4.4   Classification of Cerebral Arteries

After the rigid transformation, all voxels in the segmented vessel regions of the target image were classified into eight cerebral arteries. Classification was based on the Euclidean distance between a voxel $v(x, y, z)$ in the target image and a voxel $a^i(x^i, y^i, z^i)$, $\{i = 1,...,8\}$ in the eight labeled vessel regions in the reference image, that is,

$$d\left(v, a^i\right) = \sqrt{\left(v_x - a_x^i\right)^2 + \left(v_y - a_y^i\right)^2 + \left(v_z - a_z^i\right)^2}.$$

(15.5)

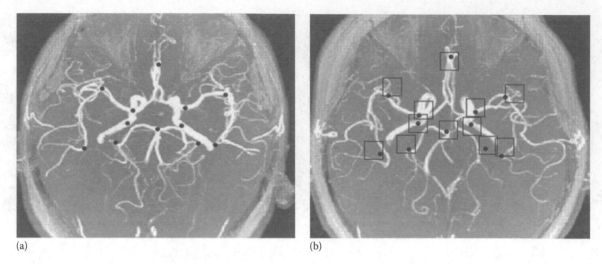

(a)   (b)

Figure 15.7   Corresponding control points for the rigid transformation. (a) The center points of the 12 templates (black dots) projected onto the MIP image of the reference MRA study. (b) Corresponding points (black dots) in the MIP image of the target MRA study were found using the template matching method. Square boxes indicate search areas for individual control points.

The classification result yielding the minimum Euclidean distance was considered to be the best initial result. A few small regions were not classified correctly at this stage because of slight deviations in vessel length and location in individual cases. To rectify any potential misclassification, the label of the largest component in each of the eight arteries was kept unchanged, and the rest of the regions were relabeled based on their distances from the earlier eight labeled components. Figure 15.8 shows the *SelMIP* image of the ACA. By selecting the ACA from the list of cerebral arteries, a *SelMIP* image containing interested vessel alone can easily be generated. By using our new viewing technique, the selected vessel region can be observed from various directions, and small aneurysms are easy to detect.

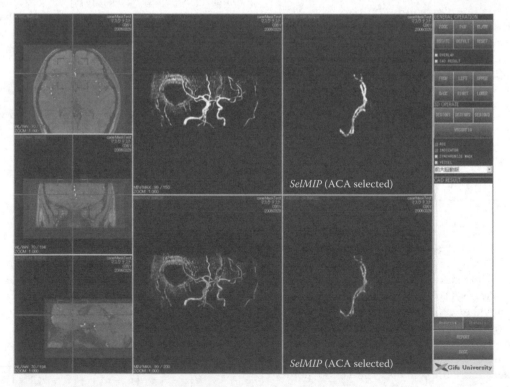

Figure 15.8   (See color insert.) Illustration of *SelMIP* images.

15.5   COMPUTERIZED DETECTION OF ARTERIAL OCCLUSION IN MRA

In the previous section, a new method for automated labeling of eight arteries in MRA studies was described. By using this method, the lengths of these eight arteries can be calculated. The lengths of vessels with arterial occlusion are shorter than those of normal vessels. Thus, the lengths of arteries can be used as a feature to distinguish between normal vessels and abnormal cases with arterial occlusion. This section describes a CAD scheme for the detection of arterial occlusion in MRA studies based on the relative lengths of these eight arteries (Yamauchi et al. 2007).

15.5.1   Detection of Arterial Occlusion Based on Relative Length of Arteries

In order to eliminate the effect of vessel thickness, 3D thinning transformation was applied to the labeled vessel regions, as shown in left-side images of Figure 15.9. The absolute lengths of the eight arteries, obtained by counting the total number of labeled voxels, were found to be different in different MRA studies. However, the relative lengths of the eight arteries were similar among normal cases. The relative length of an artery RL_i is defined as

$$RL_i = \frac{L_i}{TL} \quad i = 1,\dots,8, \tag{15.6}$$

where
  L_i is the length of the ith labeled artery
  TL is the total length of all eight labeled arteries

Right-side images of Figure 15.9 indicate the relative lengths of the eight arteries obtained from three normal cases and one abnormal case with arterial occlusion. As shown in the figure, the relative lengths of the eight arteries obtained from the normal cases are similar. However, the relative lengths of the eight arteries obtained from the abnormal case are quite different from those obtained from the normal cases because the artery containing the occlusion is shortened. In building the classification for detecting arterial occlusion, the relative lengths of the eight arteries were used as eight features. The features were then normalized using the average values and standard deviations of the eight features obtained from the normal cases. In the feature space, the distribution of the eight features was centered around the origin in normal cases, whereas this distribution was generally shifted from the origin in abnormal cases. The distance from the origin indicates the likelihood of abnormality. A classifier based on the distance of a case from the origin was employed for the detection of abnormal cases with arterial occlusion. In calculating the distance from the origin, three types of distance were investigated, that is, Euclidean distance, chessboard distance, and city block distance.

15.5.2   Performance Evaluation for Detection of Arterial Occlusions

The method was evaluated by applying it to 100 MRA studies, consisting of 85 normal cases and 15 abnormal cases with arterial occlusion. To evaluate the performance of the CAD scheme using the chessboard, Euclidean, or city block distances, ROC analysis was employed. The distances obtained from the normal cases and the abnormal cases were used as decision scores in the ROC analysis. Figure 15.10 shows the ROC curves obtained from CAD schemes using the chessboard, Euclidean, and city block distances, respectively; the AUC values for CAD schemes using each of these three methods of calculating distance were 0.765, 0.854,

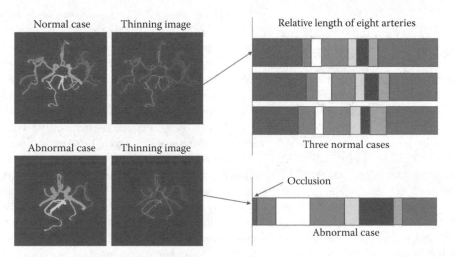

Figure 15.9   (See color insert.) Relative lengths of the eight arteries obtained from three normal cases and one abnormal case with arterial occlusion. (From Yamauchi, M. et al., *SPIE Proc.*, 6514, 65142C-1, 2007.)

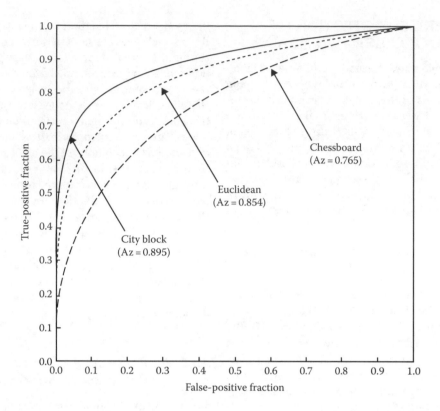

Figure 15.10   ROC curves showing the difference between normal cases and abnormal cases with arterial occlusion using the city block, Euclidean, and chessboard distances, respectively. (From Yamauchi, M. et al., *SPIE Proc.*, 6514, 65142C-1, 2007.)

and 0.895, respectively. The results indicate that the CAD scheme based on city block distance achieved the best performance. Using the CAD scheme based on city block distance, the sensitivity and specificity for the detection of abnormal cases with arterial obstruction were found to be 80.0% (12/15) and 95.3% (81/85), respectively.

15.6   COMPUTERIZED DETECTION OF LACUNAR INFARCTS IN MR IMAGES

The detection of asymptomatic lacunar infarcts in MR images is important because their presence indicates an increased risk of severe cerebral infarction (Kobayashi et al. 1997, Shintani et al. 1998, Vermeer et al. 2003). However, accurate identification of lacunar infarcts on MR images is difficult for radiologists because of the difficulty in distinguishing lacunar infarcts from enlarged Virchow–Robin spaces (Bokura et al. 1998). The Virchow–Robin space is a normal change caused by age-related atrophy of brain tissue. Figure 15.11 indicates a lacunar infarct and an enlarged Virchow–Robin space. Both have low signal intensity in T_1-weighted image and high signal intensity in T_2-weighted image. It is therefore difficult to make a clear-cut distinction between lacunar infarcts and enlarged

Virchow–Robin spaces. Therefore, a CAD scheme for the detection and/or characterization of lacunar infarct on MR images would be useful in assisting image interpretation by radiologists (Uchiyama et al. 2007a,b).

15.6.1   Extraction of Cerebral Region

Lacunar infarcts are generally detected in the basal ganglia region and in the white matter regions. Therefore, the cerebral parenchymal region was segmented first in order to avoid detecting false findings located outside the cerebral parenchymal region. A 3 × 3 median filter was applied to the T_1-weighted image for eliminating impulse noise, and a histogram of the T_1-weighted image was obtained. All pixels having the mode value of pixel values greater than 120 in the histogram were used as seed points. The region was then grown by appending a neighboring pixel to each seed point when the difference between a seed point and a neighboring pixel was less than 15. Small islands were eliminated using size-based feature analysis. Black islands such as the lateral ventricle were filled. The remaining largest white island was determined as the cerebral parenchymal region. Figure 15.12 illustrates the process adopted for segmentation of the cerebral parenchymal region.

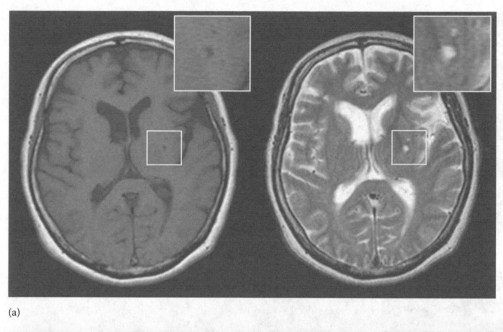

(a)

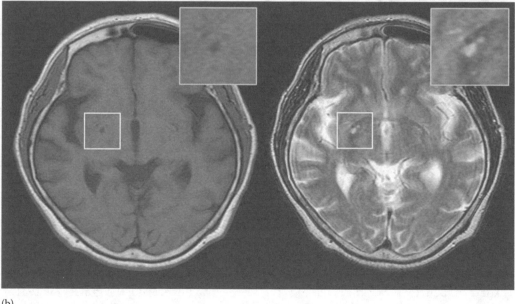

(b)

Figure 15.11   Illustration of (a) lacunar infarct and (b) enlarged Virchow–Robin space in T_1-weighted image (on left) and T_2-weighted image (on right).

15.6.2   Initial Identification of Lacunar Infarcts

The lacunar infarcts were classified into two types based on their location: isolated lacunar infarcts and lacunar infarcts adjacent to the lateral ventricle, as shown in Figure 15.13a and b. The former can easily be extracted using a simple thresholding technique. However, it is difficult to extract the latter because the adjacent lateral ventricle also has a high-intensity value with pixel values similar to that of the lacunar infarct. Therefore, to enhance the lacunar infarcts while suppressing normal structures, white top-hat transform was employed. Figure 15.13c and d shows images obtained by white top-hat transform. It is clearly illustrated that this operation enhances white patterns smaller than the structure element used. Thus, extraction of the lacunar infarct adjacent to the cerebral ventricle is rendered easy using a thresholding technique.

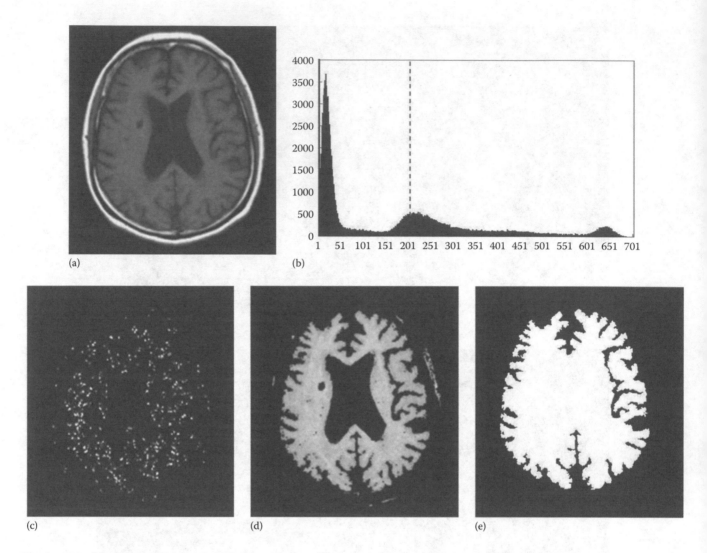

Figure 15.12 Extraction of cerebral parenchymal region. (a) T_1-weighted image. (b) Histogram of T_1-weighted image. (c) Seed points. (d) Resulting image of region growing. (e) Extracted cerebral parenchymal region.

By applying a thresholding technique to the image after white top-hat transform, initial candidates for lacunar infarcts were determined. However, the pixel values of lacunar infarcts on MR images change according to the phases (acute, subacute, or chronic). Therefore, it is difficult to detect lacunar infarcts using a fixed threshold value. To solve this problem, a multiple-phase binarization technique was employed. In this procedure, thresholding techniques with several threshold values were applied to the T_2-weighted images after white top-hat transformation. The thresholds for multiple-phase binarization were determined by increasing the pixel value from 55 to 205 at 15-pixel intervals. The total phase number of threshold values was 11. The size and degree of circularity were then calculated for each candidate region in the 11 binarized images. Regions were considered to be candidates for lacunar infarcts when the size was between 33 and

285 pixels and the degree of circularity was greater than 0.59. Initial candidate lacunar infarct regions were determined by integrating the gravity centers of all candidates detected by multiple-phase binarization. If the center of a candidate region appeared two or more times within a 3×3 square region around the gravity center of the candidate, it was considered as lacunar infarct candidate. However, if it appeared only once, it was regarded as FP and was eliminated.

15.6.3 Feature Extraction

Using the techniques described in the previous section, almost all lacunar infarcts were detected accurately. However, the initially selected candidates also included many FPs. To eliminate these, 12 features were determined for each initial candidate. These features included x and y coordinates,

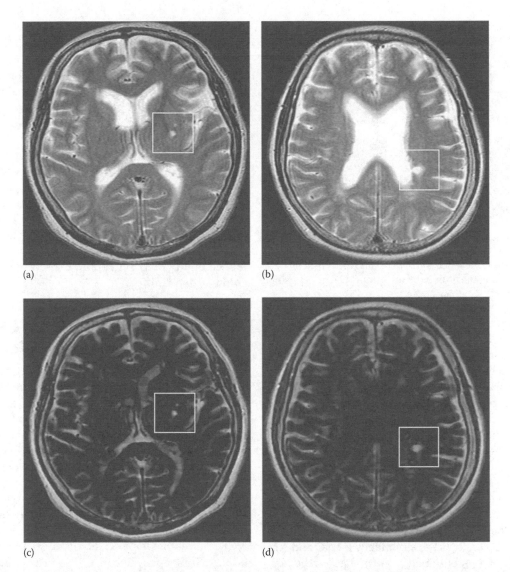

(a)

(b)

(c)

(d)

Figure 15.13 Efficacy of white top-hat transform in the enhancement of lacunar infarcts. (a) T_2-weighted image with an isolated lacunar infarct. (b) T_2-weighted image with a lacunar infarct adjacent to lateral ventricle. (c) The result of white top-hat transform of image (a). (d) The result of white top-hat transform image of (b). The white rectangular areas indicate lacunar infarct. (From Uchiyama, Y. et al., *Acad. Radiol.*, 14, 1554, 2007a.)

signal intensity differences in the T_1- and T_2-weighted images, nodular components (NCs) on a scale of 1–4, and nodular and linear components (NLCs) on a scale of 1–4.

15.6.3.1 Location

The x and y coordinates were defined based on the center of gravity of the candidate regions. Because lacunar infarcts occur within cerebral vessel regions, candidates on the periphery of the cerebral region have a strong possibility of being FPs.

15.6.3.2 Signal Intensity Difference

The signal intensity differences on T_1- and T_2-weighted images were determined by the difference between the average pixel value of the lacunar infarct region and the average pixel value of the peripheral region. The lacunar infarct region was defined as the region of maximum area when multiple-phase binarization was applied. The peripheral region was defined as the differential region between the binary image of the lacunar infarct and its surrounding regions. The surrounding region was determined by applying a dilation process to the binarized region of the lacunar infarct three times in succession.

15.6.3.3 NCs and NLCs

NCs and NLCs were calculated on a scale of 1–4 using a new filter bank technique (Nakayama et al. 2006). This filter bank consists of an analysis bank and a synthesis bank.

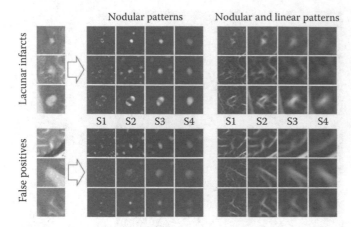

Figure 15.14 Nodular patterns and nodular and linear patterns on scale 1–4 (S1–S4). These patterns were obtained from lacunar infarcts and FPs using the filter bank technique. (From Uchiyama, Y. et al., *Acad. Radiol.*, 14, 1554, 2007a.)

The analysis bank yields second-derivative images in various sizes in the horizontal, vertical, and diagonal directions. The value of the second derivative for nodular structures tends to be in the negative in all directions. However, the value of the second derivative for linear structures tends to be zero in the direction of the axis of the linear structure, and negative in the direction perpendicular to the axis of the linear structure. The smallest and largest values of the second derivatives in all directions can be calculated by the smallest eigenvalue and the largest eigenvalue of the Hessian matrix. Thus, the NC image was defined based on the absolute value of the largest eigenvalue of the Hessian matrix. On the other hand, the NLC image was defined based on the absolute value of the smallest eigenvalue of the Hessian matrix. Figure 15.14 shows the subimages for NC and NLC both on a scale of 1–4, obtained from images of the lacunar infarcts and FPs. As shown in this figure, small lacunar infarcts are enhanced at the small scale, while large lacunar infarcts are enhanced at the large scale. For determining NCs and NLCs, an ROI with a matrix size of 100 × 100 was selected at the center of the candidate region. Using the ROI, we plotted cumulative histograms of the subimages for NCs and NLCs. NCs were identified by an average pixel value higher than 95% of the cumulative histogram of the subimage for nodular patterns at each point on a scale from 1 to 4. NLCs were determined in the same manner by using the subimage for nodular and linear patterns at each point on a scale from 1 to 4.

15.6.4   False-Positive Reduction

A support vector machine (SVM) with 12 features was employed for the elimination of FPs. For training and testing the SVM, twofold cross-validation was employed.

In this method, the database was randomly divided into two sets (A and B). The former was used for training and the latter for testing. This was then reversed, that is, set B was used for training and set A for testing. In this process, we finalized the following variables: the type of kernel function, its associated parameter, and the regularization parameter C in the structural risk function. To optimize these parameters, we employed the AUC that indicates the accuracy with which lacunar infarcts were distinguished from FPs. In this study, a polynomial kernel with kernel order 1 was used. The parameter C was set at 50. The numbers of input and output units for the SVM were set at 12 and 1, respectively. The output value of the SVM indicates the likelihood of lacunar infarcts. By changing the threshold level of the output, the performance of our CAD scheme in detecting lacunar infarcts could be determined.

15.6.5   Performance Evaluation for Detection of Lacunar Infarcts

In the first step toward identifying initial candidates for lacunar infarcts, 96.8% (90/93) of the lacunar infarcts were detected accurately with 6.88 (6771/1063) FPs per slice (51.3 FPs per patient). This indicates that a combination of white top-hat transformation and multiple-phase binarization was useful in the detection of lacunar infarcts, since most of the lacunar infarcts were detected accurately. To eliminate FPs, an SVM with 12 features was employed. Two FROC curves for the overall performance of our CAD scheme were obtained, because twofold cross-validation was used for training and testing the SVM. Averaging of the two FROC curves yielded a sensitivity of 96.8% (90/93) with 0.76 (813/1063) FPs per slice (6.2 FPs per patient). Figure 15.15 shows a prototype of the CAD scheme for the detection of lacunar infarcts in T_1- and T_2-weighted images.

15.7   OBSERVER STUDY FOR DETECTION OF LACUNAR INFARCTS

A retrospective observer study was carried out to evaluate the performance of radiologists in detecting lacunar infarcts on T_1- and T_2-weighted images without and with use of the CAD scheme. Thirty T_1-weighted and 30 T_2-weighted MR images obtained from 30 patients were used for evaluating observer performance. The group included 15 patients (age range: 48–83 years; mean: 67.2 years; 10 men and 5 women) with a lacunar infarct and 15 patients (age range: 39–76 years; mean: 64.0 years; 8 men and 7 women) without lacunar infarcts. Nine radiologists participated in the observer study. A sequential method was used in the observer performance study.

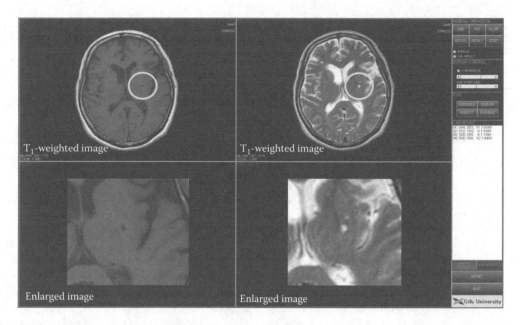

Figure 15.15 Illustration of a prototype CAD scheme for the detection of lacunar infarct.

T_1- and T_2-weighted images were displayed together at the same transverse location. The observers could manually control the speed or sequence of the slice image display, and they were allowed to change the window level and width on the monitor. Each observer reads all of the slice images for T_1- and T_2-weighted images displayed on the LCD monitor initially without computer output. The observer marked his or her confidence level regarding the likelihood of the presence of a lacunar infarct. After the observer marked the initial level of confidence, the computer outputs were superimposed on the T_1- and T_2-weighted images. The observer again marked his or her confidence level if he or she wished to change the initial result.

The observers were given the following information: (a) The purpose of the study was to evaluate the performance of radiologists in detecting lacunar infarcts without and with the CAD scheme on T1- and T2-weighted images; (b) the role of the CAD output as a *second opinion* would be evaluated; (c) the observer study consisted of 30 MRI studies that did not or did contain a lacunar infarct and/or nonlacunar lesions such as enlarged Virchow–Robin spaces; (d) the defined diameter of *lacunar infarcts* was 3–15 mm; (e) computer performance yielded a sensitivity of 96% and 0.76 FP per slice on average, and this result was not obtained from the 30 cases in this observer study; and (f) the observers were instructed to click on the screen using a mouse (1) to indicate on a bar their confidence level regarding the presence (or absence) of a lacunar infarct and (2) to locate the most likely position in each case. Each observer used a continuous rating scale displayed on the monitor. The observers were blinded to the number of patients with a

lacunar infarct. The selected cases for the observer performance study were presented in the same randomized order to the observers. There was no limit on reading time.

ROC analysis was used for comparison between the radiologists' performances without and with the computer output for the detection of lacunar infarcts on T_1- and T_2-weighted images. Figure 15.16 shows ROC curves obtained from all

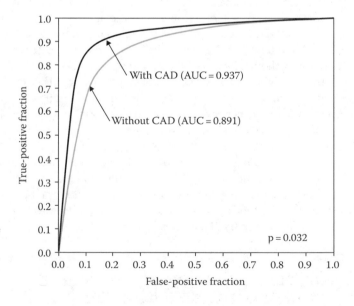

Figure 15.16 Average ROC curves obtained from nine radiologists for the detection of lacunar infarcts without and with computer output. The average AUC value was significantly improved from 0.886 to 0.930 when observers used the computer output (p = 0.032).

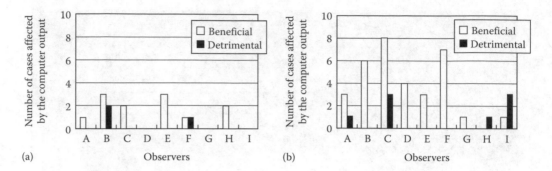

Figure 15.17   Graphs showing the number of cases (>15%) affected by CAD output in confidence level with regard to patients (a) with a lacunar infarct and (b) without a lacunar infarct.

the radiologists without and with the computer output. The average AUC values for all the radiologists improved from 0.891 (without the computer output) to 0.937 (with the computer output), and this difference was statistically significant (p = 0.032). Figure 15.17a shows clinically relevant changes in the confidence ratings of each observer with regard to patients with a lacunar infarct. The average number of cases affected beneficially was 1.33 (8.9%). However, the average number of cases affected detrimentally was 0.33 (2.2%). In two out of the three detrimentally affected cases, the CAD scheme could not accurately detect the lacunar infarct. In one of the three detrimentally affected cases, the observers changed his/her confidence level into a lower value even though the CAD scheme accurately detected the lacunar infarct. Figure 15.17b shows clinically relevant changes in the confidence ratings of each observer with regard to patients without a lacunar infarct. The average number of cases affected beneficially and detrimentally were 3.67 (24.4%) and 0.89 (5.9%), respectively. The average number of patients without a lacunar infarct that were affected beneficially was higher than that of patients with a lacunar infarct. These beneficial effects were caused by the fact that observers first marked lesions such as enlarged Virchow–Robin spaces with a relatively high confidence level indicating the presence of lacunar infarcts. However, the confidence level was changed to a lower value after taking into account the absence of lesions detected by CAD. Therefore, observers were able to make the correct diagnosis using the computer output. On the other hand, eight detrimentally affected cases were caused by FPs detected by the CAD scheme.

15.8   CLASSIFICATION OF LACUNAR INFARCTS AND ENLARGED VIRCHOW–ROBIN SPACES

In the observer study described earlier, we realized that the majority of FPs detected by the computer are different from those detected by radiologists, and radiologists

can therefore disregard these obvious FPs identified by the computer. However, it is of interest to note that some FPs due to enlarged Virchow–Robin spaces detected by the computer were difficult for radiologists to distinguish from lacunar infarcts. These FPs were the main sources to the detrimental effects of the CAD scheme. A strong influence on radiologists by these FPs might result in unnecessary medical treatment for the patient. Therefore, a CAD scheme for the classification of lacunar infarcts and enlarged Virchow–Robin spaces was developed to assist radiologists' image interpretation (Uchiyama et al. 2008b).

15.8.1   Feature Extraction

The database consisted of T_1- and T_2-weighted images obtained from 109 patients, which included 89 lacunar infarcts and 20 enlarged Virchow–Robin spaces. These images were acquired using a 1.5 T MR scanner. The radiologist selects regions of interest (ROIs) including a lesion. The morphological white top-hat transform was first employed for the enhancement of small focal hyperintensity lesions in ROIs of T_2-weighted images. The gray-level thresholding technique was then employed for the segmentation of the lesions. To measure the characteristics of lacunar infarcts and enlarged Virchow–Robin spaces, six features were determined from the segmented lesions. These features included the x and y coordinates, size, degree of irregularity, and signal intensity differences in T_1- and T_2-weighted images. The x and y coordinates were defined based on the centroid of the segmented region. Size was defined as the number of pixels in the segmented region. The degree of irregularity was given as 1-C/L, where C is the length of circumference of the circle having the same area as the segmented region, and L is the boundary length of the segmented region. The signal intensity differences in the T_1- and T_2-weighted images were defined as the difference between the average pixel value of the segmented region and the average pixel value of the peripheral region. Figure 15.18 shows the distribution of the six features obtained from 89 lacunar infarcts and

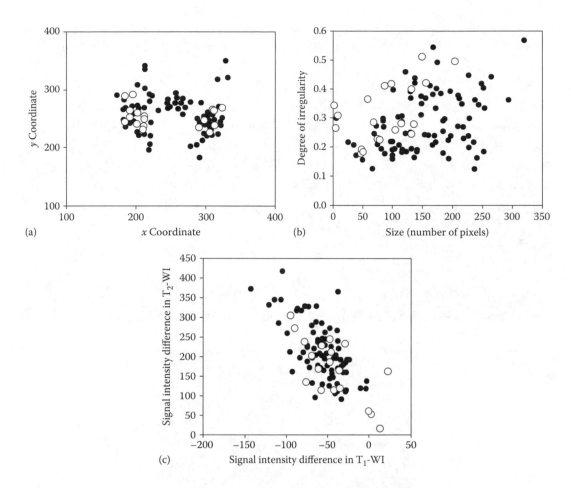

Figure 15.18 Distribution of six features obtained from lacunar infarcts and enlarged Virchow–Robin spaces. (a) Relation between x and y coordinates. (b) Relationship between size and degree of irregularity. (c) Relationship between signal intensity difference in T_1-weighted image (WI) and signal intensity difference in T_2-weighted image (WI). (From Uchiyama, Y. et al., *Conf. Proc. IEEE Eng. Med. Biol.*, 3908, 2008b.)

20 enlarged Virchow–Robin spaces. Black and white circles indicate lacunar infarcts and enlarged Virchow–Robin spaces, respectively. Enlarged Virchow–Robin spaces are located at the central region on the right and left sides, as shown in Figure 15.18a. The sizes of enlarged Virchow–Robin spaces are relatively small comparable to those of lacunar infarcts, as shown in Figure 15.18b. Signal intensity differences in T_2-weighted image appear to be smaller for enlarged Virchow–Robin spaces than for lacunar infarcts, as shown in Figure 15.18c.

15.8.2 Classification Scheme

A neural network with six features was employed for distinguishing between lacunar infarcts and enlarged Virchow–Robin spaces. A three-layer neural network, consisting of six input units, two hidden units, and one output unit, was used. The number of hidden units was determined empirically. The input data for the neural network were the six features determined in the previous section. The neural network generates a decision boundary that optimally partitions the feature space into the two classes, that is, lacunar infarcts and enlarged Virchow–Robin spaces. The output value of the neural network indicates the likelihood of occurrence of the lacunar infarct. For training and testing of the neural network, the leave-one-out method was employed. To evaluate the classification performance, ROC analysis was used; the AUC value was 0.945. The sensitivity and specificity of detection of lacunar infarcts were 93.3% (83/89) and 75.0% (15/20), respectively. The results indicate that this computerized method may be useful for the classification of lacunar infarcts and enlarged Virchow–Robin spaces in T_1 and T_2-weighted images.

15.8.3 Fusion Image of T_2-Weighted Image and MRA

MRA images acquired with 3 T MR scanner can visualize blood flow inside small vessels. Therefore, a fusion image of a T_2-weighed image and an MRA may be useful for distinction

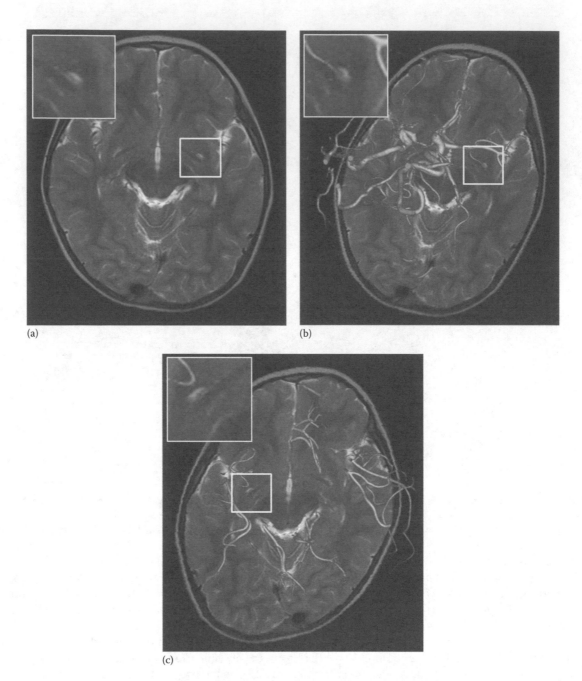

Figure 15.19   Illustration of fusion image of T_2-weighted image and MRA. (a) T_2-weighted image. (b) Fusion image in the bottom-to-top direction. (c) Fusion image in the top-to-bottom direction. (From Uchiyama, Y. et al., *IFMBE Proc.*, 126, 2009.)

between lacunar infarcts and enlarged Virchow–Robin spaces (Uchiyama et al. 2009). Because enlarged Virchow–Robin spaces are formed by atrophy of the tissue surrounding a cerebral artery, blood flow inside the small artery can be observed in these images. However, in the case of lacunar infarct, blood flow is absent. Figure 15.19 illustrates a fusion image of a T_2-weighed image and an MRA, which were acquired with a 3 T MR scanner. In the fusion image, blood flow is clearly visible in the lesion, facilitating the identification of the lesion as an enlarged Virchow–Robin

space. To enerate the fusion image, we determined the location of 2D T_2-weighted images in the 3D MRA image using an image registration technique. In this method, a similarity measure was employed based on the pixel values of the T_2-weighted image and the voxel values of the slice image along the body axis of the 3D MRA image. The vessel regions in MRA image were segmented using the thresholding and region-growing techniques, described in Section 15.2.1. Volume rendering was then used to generate the fusion image.

15.9 CONCLUSIONS

A number of CAD schemes have been developed for the detection and/or classification of cerebrovascular diseases. Observer performance studies indicated that computer output helps radiologists improve their diagnostic accuracy. Therefore, CAD schemes will be useful in assisting radiologists in their assessment of cerebrovascular diseases on MR images.

REFERENCES

Arimura, H., Q. Li, Y. Korogi, T. Hirai, H. Abe, Y. Yamashita et al. 2004. Automated computerized scheme for detection of unruptured intracranial aneurysms in three-dimensional MRA. *Academic Radiology* 11:1093–1104.

Arimura, H., Q. Li, Y. Korogi, T. Hirai, S. Katsuragawa, Y. Yamashita et al. 2006. Computerized detection of intracranial aneurysms for three-dimensional MR angiography: Feature extraction of small protrusions based on a shape-based difference image technique. *Medical Physics* 33:394–401.

Bokura, H., S. Kobayashi, and S. Yamaguchi. 1998. Discrimination of silent lacunar infarction from enlarged Virchow-Robin spaces on brain magnetic resonance imaging: Clinicopathological study. *Journal of Neurology* 245:116–122.

Fogelholm, R., J. Hernesniemi, and M. Vapalahti. 1993. Impact of early surgery on outcome after aneurysm subarachnoid hemorrhage: A population-based study. *Stroke* 24:1649–1654.

Fujita, H., Y. Uchiyama, T. Nakagawa, D. Fukuoka, Y. Hatanaka, T. Hara et al. 2008. Computer-aided diagnosis: The emerging of three CAD systems induced by Japanese health care needs. *Computer Methods and Programs in Biomedicine, Review*, 92(3):238–248.

Gao, X., Y. Uchiyama, X. Zhou, T. Hara, T. Asano, and H. Fujita. 2011. A fast and fully automatic method for cerebrovascular segmentation on time-of-flight (TOF) MRA image. *Journal of Digital Imaging* 24(4):609–625.

Hayashi, H., Y. Masutani, T. Matsumoto, H. Mori, A. Kunimatsu, O. Abe et al. 2003. Feasibility of a curvature-based enhanced display system for detecting cerebral aneurysms in MR angiography. *Magnetic Resonance in Medical Science* 2:29–36.

Hirai, T., Y. Korogi, H. Arimura, S. Katsuragawa, M. Kitajima, M. Yamura et al. 2006. Intracranial aneurysms at MR angiography: Effect of computer-aided diagnosis on radiologists' detection performance. *Radiology* 237:605–610.

Kakeda, S., Y. Korogi, H. Arimura, T. Hirai, S. Katsuragawa, T. Aoki et al. 2008. Diagnostic accuracy and reading time to detect intracranial aneurysms on MR angiography using a computer-aided diagnosis system. *AJR* 190:459–465.

Kobayashi, S., K. Kondo, and Y. Hata. 2006. Computer-aided diagnosis of intracranial aneurysms in MRA images with case-based reasoning. *IEICE Transactions on Information and Systems* E89-D(1):340–350.

Kobayashi, S., K. Okada, H. Koide, H. Bokura, and S. Yamaguchi. 1997. Subcortical silent brain infarction as a risk factor for clinical stroke. *Stroke* 28:1932–1939.

Li, Q., S. Sone, and K. Doi. 2003. Selective enhancement filters for nodule, vessels, and airway walls in two- and three dimensional CT scan. *Medical Physics* 30:2040–2051.

Nakayama, R., Y. Uchiyama, K. Yamamoto, R. Watanabe, and K. Namba. 2006. Computer-aided diagnosis scheme using a filter bank for detection of microcalcification clusters in mammograms. *IEEE Transactions on Biomedical Engineering* 53:273–283.

Shintani, S., T. Shiigai, and T. Arinami. 1998. Silent lacunar infarction on magnetic resonance imaging (MRI): Risk factors. *Journal of Neurological Science* 160:82–86.

Uchiyama, Y., H. Ando, R. Yokoyama, T. Hara, H. Fujita, and T. Iwama. 2005. Computer-aided diagnosis scheme for detection of unruptured intracranial aneurysms in MR angiography. *Conference of Proceedings of IEEE Engineering in Medicine and Biology*, Shanghai, IEEE, 2005:3031–3034.

Uchiyama, Y., T. Asano, T. Hara, H. Fujita, H. Hoshi, T. Iwama et al. 2009. CAD Scheme for differential diagnosis of lacunar infarcts and normal Virchow-Robin spaces on brain MR images. *IFMBE Proceedings*, Munich, Springer, 126–128.

Uchiyama, Y., X. Gao, T. Hara, H. Fujita, H. Ando, H. Yamakawa et al. 2008a. Computerized detection of unruptured aneurysms in MRA images: Reduction of false positives using anatomical location feature. *SPIE Proceedings* 6915: 69151Q-1–69151Q-8.

Uchiyama, Y., T. Kunieda, T. Asano, H. Kato, T. Hara, M. Kanematsu et al. 2008b. Computer-aided diagnosis scheme for classification of lacunar infarcts and enlarged Virchow-Robin spaces in brain MR image. *Conference of Proceedings of IEEE Engineering in Medicine and Biology*, Vancouver, IEEE, 3908–3911.

Uchiyama, Y., M. Yamauchi, H. Ando, R. Yokoyama, T. Hara, H. Fujita et al. 2006. Automated classification of cerebral arteries in MRA images and its application to maximum intensity projection. *Conference Proceedings of IEEE Engineering in Medicine and Biology*, New York, IEEE, 4865–4868.

Uchiyama, Y., R. Yokoyama, H. Ando, T. Asano, H. Kato, H. Yamakawa et al. 2007a. Computer-aided diagnosis scheme for detection of lacunar infarcts on MR image. *Academic Radiology* 14:1554–1561.

Uchiyama, Y., R. Yokoyama, T. Asano, H. Kato, H. Yamakawa, H. Ando et al. 2007b. Improvement of automated detection method of lacunar infarcts in brain MR images. *Conference Proceedings of IEEE Engineering in Medicine and Biology*, Lyon, IEEE, 1599–1602.

Vermeer, S.E., M. Hollander, E. J. Dijk, A. Hofman, P. J. Koudstaal, and M. M. Breteler. 2003. Silent brain infarcts and white matter lesions increase stroke risk in the general population: The Rotterdam scan study. *Stroke* 34:1126–1129.

Wardlaw, J. M., P. M. White. 2000. The detection and management of unruptured intracranial aneurysms. *Brain* 123:205–221.

Yamauchi, M., Y. Uchiyama, R. Yokoyama, T. Hara, H. Fujita, H. Ando et al. 2007. Computerized scheme for detection of arterial obstruction in brain MRA images. *SPIE Proceedings* 6514:65142C-1–65142C-9.

Yang, X., DJ. Blezek, LT. Cheng, WJ. Ryan, DF. Kallmes, and BJ Erickson. 2011. Computer-aided detection of intracranial aneurysms in MR angiography. *Journal of Digital Imaging* 24:86–95.

Yokoyama, R., X. Zhang, Y. Uchiyama, H. Fujita, T. Hara, X. Zhou et al. 2007. Development of an automated method for detection of chronic lacunar infarct regions on brain MR images. *IEICE Transactions on Information and Systems* E90-D(6):943–954.

Chapter 16

Detection of Pulmonary Embolism

Chuan Zhou and Heang-Ping Chan

CONTENTS

16.1 INTRODUCTION

Pulmonary embolism (PEs) is a common and potentially fatal condition associated with significant morbidity and mortality in untreated patients. Prompt and accurate diagnosis of PEs has been shown to greatly influence patient outcome (Dalen and Alpert 1975; Price 1976). Computed tomographic pulmonary angiography (CTPA) has been reported to be an effective means for the clinical diagnosis of PEs (Remy-Jardin et al. 1992; Diffin et al. 1998; Rubin et al. 1998; McCollough and Zink 1999; Stein 1999; Ghaye 2001; Raptopoulos and Boiselle 2001; Schoepf et al. 2002a). CT has advantages over conventional pulmonary angiograms and ventilation/perfusion (V/Q) scan because of its direct imaging of the blood clot, better interobserver agreement, greater accuracy, and possibility to explain patient's sign and symptoms (Remy-Jardin et al. 1992; Rubin et al. 1998; McCollough and Zink 1999; Stein et al. 2006). The main limitation of single-detector spiral CT has been the detection of small peripheral emboli (Goodman et al. 1995; Drucker et al. 1998; Perrier et al. 2001; Schoepf et al. 2004; Schoepf and Costello 2004) and the isolated subsegmental emboli (Stein 1999). The main reason for inadequate detection of PEs in these small vessels is partial volume effects and cardiac and respiratory motions (Ghaye 2001). Although the clinical significance of small PEs has not been established, small PEs may produce significant morbidity in patients with underlying cardiorespiratory disease (Diffin et al. 1998) and may indicate a risk for the recurrence of more significant emboli among stable patients. Studies (Hull et al. 1994; Oser et al. 1996; Patriquin et al. 1998) also indicated that the presence of peripheral PEs may be an indicator for current deep vein thrombosis, thus potentially heralding more severe embolic events. In addition, it is important to estimate the total burden of pulmonary vascular clots in patients with acute PEs to determine proper therapy and to improve patient outcome (Bankier et al. 1997; Qanadli et al. 2001; Wood et al. 2002; Mastora et al. 2003; Araoz et al. 2003; Wu et al. 2004). Figure 16.1 shows examples of PEs visualized on CTPA images.

The advent of multidetector computed tomography (MDCT) offers the possibility of detecting subtle PEs in subsegmental arteries (Ghaye 2001; Schoepf et al. 2002a; Coche et al. 2003; Patel et al. 2003; Schoepf et al. 2004; Schoepf and Costello 2004). The improved visibility results in substantially higher detection rates for subsegmental PEs,

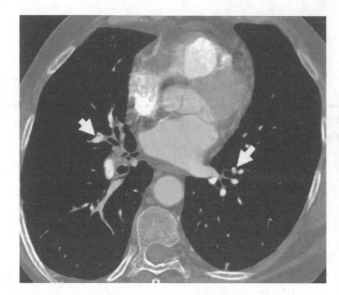 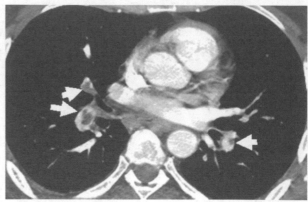

Figure 16.1 Examples of PEs visualized on CTPA images. The PEs identified by radiologists were marked by white arrows.

especially for obliquely oriented vessels, and better agreement among readers (Ghaye 2001; Raptopoulos and Boiselle 2001; Schoepf et al. 2002a). However, a thin-section MDCT study of PEs routinely produced 500–600 transverse images to cover the chest (Schoepf and Costello 2004). Radiologists have to visually track the vessels down to the sixth-order branches of subsegmental pulmonary arteries, adjust window setting and window level to see the small peripheral vessels, and use multiplanar function to justify suspicious artifacts. It is more difficult to review subsegmental small vessels not only because of the large number of these vessels but also because of their lower conspicuity due to partial volume effects (Schoepf et al. 2004). False negatives (FNs, missed diagnosis) are not uncommon because of the complexity of the images and the large number of vessels to be tracked in each case. As shown in the latest results of the PIOPED II study (Sostman et al. 2004; Stein et al. 2006), even with the use of MDCT, the sensitivity was moderate (83% at a specificity of 96%), suggesting that CTPA may not be sufficient as a stand-alone procedure for PEs screening. With CT venography (CTV) added to CTPA, the sensitivity increased to 90% with a specificity of 95%. A combination of CTPA and CTV may be more promising for PEs screening (Stein et al. 2006), but it increases costs and radiation risk.

Computer-aided detection (CAD) may be a viable approach for assisting radiologists in this demanding task and reducing the chance of missing PEs (Ko and Naidich 2004; Schoepf and Costello 2004). With advanced computer vision techniques, the computer may be trained to automatically track the pulmonary vessels, distinguish the arteries from the veins, detect suspicious PEs locations by searching along the arteries, and finally alert the radiologists to the regions of interest (ROIs) for suspicious PEs. If CAD can

improve the sensitivity and specificity for the detection of small peripheral emboli with CTPA, it may reduce unnecessary workup with other diagnostic procedures or help select proper treatment options.

Automated detection of PEs on CT images is a challenging area of computer vision application. This area has not attracted the interest of the CAD community until recently. Masutani et al. (2002) developed a computerized method for PEs detection based on volumetric image analysis. They selected 19 (11 positive and 8 normal) cases from 30 clinical cases, excluding the cases for which the definition of truth or *gold standard of detection* was difficult. One radiologist marked 21 thrombi with a volume greater than 10 mm³ in the 11 positive cases. Their system could detect 100% and 85% of the 21 thrombi with 7.7 and 2.6 FPs/case, respectively, when the PEs volume was between 16 and 64 mm³. Of the 143 FPs for all cases, 92% were related to soft tissues such as lymphoid tissue surrounding vessels. They did not describe the characteristics of the thrombi, such as the percentage of occlusion by the PEs, and how the PEs distributed in segmental and subsegmental arteries, which would reveal the degree of subtlety of the PEs in the study. With only 21 PEs samples, it is impossible to represent the large varieties of PEs that may be encountered in clinical images.

Schoepf et al. (2002b) evaluated the performance of a commercial system (ImageChecker CT, R2 Technology, Inc.) for PEs detection on CT scans. They obtained a sensitivity of 91% and 66%, respectively, for 130 PEs in the segmental and 150 PEs in the subsegmental pulmonary arteries from 15 cases, where the reference standard on the presence of PEs was determined by two radiologists. Although they used a relatively large number of samples of PEs in their study and achieved a reasonable sensitivity, they did not describe the FP rates at these sensitivities. Again, no analysis of the characteristics of the true PEs was given except for the numbers of PEs present in segmental and subsegmental arteries. Das et al. (2003) used the same commercial system to conduct a similar study with a larger dataset that contained 33 cases with 186 segmental and 120 subsegmental PEs. The system achieved a sensitivity of 88% for segmental and 78% for subsegmental PEs with 4 FPs/case. In a study by Digumarthy et al. (2006) using the same commercial system, 39 consecutive patients with high clinical suspicion were included with criteria of good contrast opacification, absence of significant motion artifacts, and pulmonary disease. The reference standard included 270 PEs in arteries greater than 4 mm in diameter. The CAD system detected 92% of the PEs at an average FP rate of 2.8 per case. Jeudy et al. (2006) again evaluated the same commercial system using a dataset of 22 cases. A total of 251 PEs were identified as reference standard, including 188 in the segmental and 63 in the subsegmental arteries. They reported a sensitivity of 80% for the segmental PEs and 76% for the subsegmental PEs at an FP rate of 1.8 per case. Das et al. (2006) evaluated a different commercial system (CAD prototype version 5, Siemens Medical, Malvern, PA, USA) using a dataset of 45 cases. Twenty-nine cases were found to have a total of 213 PEs in all vessel levels. The CAD system detected 82% of the PEs at a median FP rate of three per case.

Zhou et al. (2005) developed an automated vessel segmentation and PEs detection system for CTPA images (Zhou et al. 2003a,b, 2004, 2005, 2007a) and conducted several studies to evaluate the performance of the system. The reference standards were provided by thoracic radiologists who identified PEs locations, estimated the percent diameter occlusion, and rated the conspicuity of each embolus. If a contiguous PEs volume occluded more than one branch of arteries, radiologist virtually split the PEs volume according to the branching of the artery by marking the PEs segment in each branch as a separate PEs. In a recent study (Zhou et al. 2009), they used independent datasets of 128 CTPA scans to evaluate the performance of the CAD system, of which 59 and 69 CTPA cases were retrospectively collected from the patient files at the University of Michigan (UM) and the prospective investigation of pulmonary embolism diagnosis (PIOPED) II clinical trial. Extensive lung parenchymal or pleural diseases were present in 22/59 UM and 26/69 PIOPED datasets. A total of 595 and 800 PEs were identified in the artery branches by experienced radiologists in the UM and PIOPED datasets, respectively. The detection performance was assessed by free-response receiver operating characteristic (FROC) analysis. The FROC analysis indicated that the PEs detection system could achieve an overall sensitivity of 80% at 18.9 FPs/case for the PIOPED cases when the LDA classifier was trained with the UM cases. The test sensitivity with the UM cases was 80% at 22.6 FPs/cases when the LDA classifier was trained with the PIOPED cases.

We are developing computer vision techniques for the automated detection of PEs on CTPA images. In our recent studies (Zhou et al. 2007b, 2009), we have developed a prototype system for PEs detection using multiscale vessel segmentation and vessel tree construction, parallel multi-prescreening method for suspicious PEs detection, and linear discriminant analysis (LDA) classifier for false-positive (FP) reduction. The performance of our method was evaluated on two relatively large independent datasets to demonstrate the feasibility of our methods in PEs detection and the robustness of our method in independent cases.

16.2 AUTOMATIC CONSTRUCTION OF PULMONARY VESSEL TREE IN CTPA IMAGES

Because PEs occurs only inside pulmonary vessels, segmentation and tracking of vessels constitute the fundamental steps to limit the search space for identifying ROIs that contain suspicious PEs. Many of the published vessel segmentation and tracking methods provided accurate results in 2D or 3D images for vascular structures in the retina, brain, and liver, etc. However, few studies have been conducted for segmentation, tracking, and reconstruction of the pulmonary vessel tree on CTPA images because the pulmonary vessels are more complicated compared to the vessels in other parts of the body in several aspects: widely distributed CT values, large variations of vessel sizes ranging from 1 to 20 mm, and the complicated branching structures.

Multiscale filtering has been used for the segmentation of curvilinear or tubular structures in 3D medical images (Lorenz et al. 1997; Frangi et al. 1998; Kanazawa et al. 1998; Krissian et al. 2000; Aylward and Bullitt 2002; Li et al. 2003; Bülow et al. 2004; Shikata et al. 2004) that share a common approach: the images are convolved with 3D Gaussian filters at multiple scales, and the eigenvalues of the Hessian matrix at each voxel are analyzed in terms of a response function to determine the shape of the local structures in the image. The eigenvalues for the voxels that correspond to a linear structure would be different from those that correspond to a planar structure, blob, noise, or no structure. The response of the enhancement filter reaches its maximum when the scale of the filter matches the size of the local structures. The local structures can then be extracted using the local maxima (Aylward and Bullitt 2002). Other efforts in vessel segmentation and tracking include hysteresis thresholding (Masutani et al. 2001), region growing (Higgins et al. 1996; Rubin et al. 1998), statistical modeling and matching methods (Blanks et al. 1999; Chung and Noble 1999) using a priori knowledge provided by radiologists, direction field–based segmentation and detection (Kutka and Stier 1996), and deformable model approaches (McInerney and Terzopoulos 2000;

Lorigo et al. 2001) in which an initial surface estimate is deformed iteratively to optimize an energy criterion so that the model boundary is extended to the vessel wall as a so-called minimal surface. However, for the PEs diagnosis task, it is difficult to track or segment vessel structures in 3D volume using conventional methods because pulmonary vessels cannot be accurately segmented and continuously tracked if they are largely or totally obstructed by PEs. The problem becomes even more difficult if the PEs appears to be connected to its surrounding lymphoid tissues due to partial volume effect, which can easily cause leaking to the soft tissues during vessel segmentation.

16.2.1 Vascular Structure Enhancement

The conventional multiscale 3D filters are limited to specific structures of interest because their filter response functions are defined explicitly (Lorenz et al. 1997; Kanazawa et al. 1998; Frangi et al. 1998; Krissian et al. 2000; Aylward and Bullitt 2002; Li et al. 2003; Shikata et al. 2004). For example, a filter designed to enhance tubular structures cannot enhance the vessel bifurcation, which forms a blob-like structure when the vessel splits into two or more branches, thus causing a gap between the vessel branches. Similarly, a filter designed to enhance blob-like structure cannot enhance tubular structures. We therefore designed a new multiscale 3D filter using the eigenvalues of the Hessian matrix to enhance all vascular structures including vessel bifurcations and to suppress nonvessel structures such as the lymphoid tissue surrounding the vessels (Zhou et al. 2007b).

Let $I(\vec{r})$ be a 3D image with voxels at points $\vec{r} = (x, y, z)$; its Taylor series approximation up to second order for three variables about a point $\vec{r} = \vec{a}$ is

$$I(\vec{r}) \approx I(\vec{a}) + \nabla I(\vec{a})^T (\vec{r} - \vec{a}) + \frac{1}{2}(\vec{r} - \vec{a})^T \nabla^2 I(\vec{a})(\vec{r} - \vec{a}), \quad (16.1)$$

where $\nabla I(\vec{a})$ is the gradient and $\nabla^2 I(\vec{a})$ is the Hessian matrix H at point $\vec{a}$, given by the second-order partial derivatives of the image $I(\vec{r})$:

$$\nabla^2 I(\vec{r}) = \begin{bmatrix} I_{xx}(\vec{r}) & I_{xy}(\vec{r}) & I_{xz}(\vec{r}) \\ I_{yx}(\vec{r}) & I_{yy}(\vec{r}) & I_{yz}(\vec{r}) \\ I_{zx}(\vec{r}) & I_{zy}(\vec{r}) & I_{zz}(\vec{r}) \end{bmatrix}. \quad (16.2)$$

To enhance local structures of variable sizes, the partial second derivatives of $I(\vec{r})$ in the Hessian matrix can be calculated by convolving $I(\vec{r})$ with the partial second derivatives of Gaussian filters with variable standard deviation σ, for example,

$$I_{xx}(\vec{r}; \sigma) = \left(\frac{\partial^2 G(\vec{r}; \sigma)}{\partial x^2} \right) \times I(\vec{r}). \quad (16.3)$$

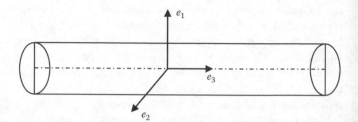

Figure 16.2   An ideal tubular structure and its eigenvectors.

The Hessian matrix H describes the second-order local intensity variations around each point of a 3D structure. Let the eigenvalues of H be $\lambda_1, \lambda_2, \lambda_3$ ($|\lambda_1| > |\lambda_2| > |\lambda_3|$) and their corresponding eigenvectors be e_1, e_2, e_3, respectively. The eigenvector e_1 corresponding to the largest eigenvalue λ_1 represents the direction along which the second derivative is maximum, and λ_1 gives the maximum second derivative value. For an ideal tubular structure in 3D volume, as shown in Figure 16.2 and summarized in Table 16.1, the voxels at the centerline of the tube will be signaled by λ_3 being approximately zero, and λ_1 and λ_2 of larger magnitudes. Similarly, for an ideal sphere, the three eigenvalues $\lambda_1, \lambda_2, \lambda_3$ will be equal at the center of the sphere. Analyzing the second derivatives using eigenvalues thus has an intuitive explanation that the three eigenvalues play an important role in discriminating structures of different shapes. However, the studies of Sato et al. (2000), Lorenz et al. (1997), and Li et al. (2003) make use of only two eigenvalues in their 3D line filters for vessel enhancement. Based on an analysis of the three eigenvalues, Frangi et al. (1998) combined three measurements to define a vesselness response function for vessel enhancement. Two measurements were designed as two geometric ratios, one for the discrimination between a blob-like structure and a tubular or plate-like structure, and the other for the discrimination between a tubular and a plate-like structure. The third measurement was designed to measure the contrast of the structures. Three parameters have to be trained to control the sensitivity of the line filter to the three measurements in their study.

Based on the characteristics of the three eigenvalues of the Hessian matrix, we developed a new multiscale response function $R(\vec{r}; \sigma_s; \lambda_1, \lambda_2, \lambda_3)$ to enhance all vascular structures including vessel bifurcations and to suppress

TABLE 16.1   CHARACTERISTICS OF THE EIGENVALUES OF HESSIAN MATRIX CORRESPONDING TO STRUCTURES OF DIFFERENT SHAPES IN 3D VOLUME

Tubular Structure	Blob-Like (Sphere) Structure	Plate-Like Structure
$|\lambda_3(r)| \approx 0$	$|\lambda_3(r)| \approx |\lambda_2(r)| \approx |\lambda_1(r)|$	$|\lambda_2(r)| \approx |\lambda_3(r)| \approx 0$
$|\lambda_1(r)| \approx |\lambda_2(r)| >> |\lambda_3(r)|$	$|\lambda_3(r)| > 0$	$|\lambda_1(r)| >> |\lambda_2(r)|$

nonvessel structures such as the lymphoid tissue surrounding the vessels:

$$R(\vec{r};\sigma_s;\lambda_1,\lambda_2,\lambda_3)$$

$$= \begin{cases} \dfrac{(|\lambda_1|+|\lambda_2|)}{2}\exp\left(-\left|\dfrac{|\lambda_1|}{\sqrt{\lambda_1^2+\lambda_2^2+\lambda_3^2}}-c\right|\right), & \lambda_1,\lambda_2,\lambda_3<0; \\ \\ 0, & \text{otherwise,} \end{cases}$$

$$(16.4)$$

where $\lambda_1,\lambda_2,\lambda_3$ ($|\lambda_1|>|\lambda_2|>|\lambda_3|$) are Hessian eigenvalues at voxel $\vec{r}=(x,y,z)$ in a 3D image, σ_s is the standard deviation of the Gaussian kernel at scale s, and c is a constant. The negativity of the eigenvalues is due to the fact that the vascular structures are brighter than the background in the CTPA images and occupy a relatively small volume.

The constant c plays an important role in the enhancement of both the tubular and blob-like structures in Equation 16.4. As summarized in Table 16.1, for a branch of the vessels that has tubular structure, $|\lambda_1| \approx |\lambda_2|$, $|\lambda_1| >> |\lambda_3|$, and $|\lambda_3| \approx 0$. The response R_C of tubular structures can be approximated as

$$R_C \approx \frac{2|\lambda_1|}{2}\exp\left(-\left|\frac{|\lambda_1|}{\sqrt{2\lambda_1^2}}-c\right|\right)=\alpha|\lambda_1|, \qquad (16.5)$$

where $\alpha=\exp\left(-\left|\dfrac{1}{\sqrt{2}}-c\right|\right)$.

Similarly, for the vessel bifurcation that forms a blob-like structure when the vessel splits into two or more branches, $|\lambda_1| \approx |\lambda_2| \approx |\lambda_3|$. The response R_B of blob-like structures can be approximated as

$$R_B \approx \frac{2|\lambda_1|}{2}\exp\left(-\left|\frac{|\lambda_1|}{\sqrt{3\lambda_1^2}}-c\right|\right)=\beta|\lambda_1|, \qquad (16.6)$$

where $\beta=\exp\left(-\left|\dfrac{1}{\sqrt{3}}-c\right|\right)$.

The lymphoid tissues surrounding the pulmonary vessels generally are plate-like structures with $|\lambda_1|>>|\lambda_2|$ and $|\lambda_2| \approx |\lambda_3| \approx 0$:

$$R_P \sim \frac{|\lambda_1|}{2}\exp\left(-\left|\frac{|\lambda_1|}{\sqrt{\lambda_1^2}}-c\right|\right)=\kappa|\lambda_1|, \qquad (16.7)$$

where $\kappa=\dfrac{1}{2}\exp(-|1-c|)$.

The largest eigenvalue $|\lambda_1|$ of a plate-like structure is usually much smaller than the largest eigenvalue of a tubular or a blob-like structure at the same scale if the size of the local structure of the lymphoid tissue is larger than that of vascular structure; the response function R_P is therefore even smaller.

The value of α is at its maximum of 1 when $c=1/\sqrt{2}=0.7071$ and β is at its maximum of 1 when $c=1/\sqrt{3}=0.57735$. The maximum of κ is only 0.5 when $c=1$. To maximize the differences of R_C and R_B from R_P, the value of c should be set to between 0.57 and 0.71. For example, if c is chosen to be 0.64, both R_C and R_B can be as high as $0.94|\lambda_1|$ and R_P will be low at $0.35|\lambda_1|$. Considering the real situation in medical images that vascular structures are not an ideal cylinder or sphere, c was set to 0.7 in our study.

16.2.2 Vessel Segmentation at Multiscales

The pulmonary vascular structures within the lung regions have sizes over a wide range. To adapt the 3D enhancement filter response to cover the various sizes, a widely used method to integrate multiscale responses is to calculate the second-order partial derivatives of the 3D image $I(\vec{r})$ in the Hessian matrix by convolving $I(\vec{r})$ with the second-order partial derivatives of Gaussians having variable standard deviations (Lorenz et al. 1997; Frangi et al. 1998; Sato et al. 1998; Wink et al. 2004). By adjusting the standard deviations of the Gaussian kernels, the local structures with a specific range of sizes can be enhanced by combining the local maxima of the filter response at multiple scales.

In order to have a fair comparison of the responses among multiple scales, the filter responses have to be first normalized (Lindeberg 1998). The maximum response among the multiple scales can then be selected as the optimal filter response that matches the vessel size. To achieve this, a normalization parameter γ can be incorporated in Equation 16.2 when calculating the Hessian matrix H of image $I(r)$ at scale s, and Equation 16.2 can be rewritten as

$$\nabla^2 I(\vec{r},s)=s^\gamma\begin{bmatrix} I_{xx}(\vec{r}) & I_{xy}(\vec{r}) & I_{xz}(\vec{r}) \\ I_{yx}(\vec{r}) & I_{yy}(\vec{r}) & I_{yz}(\vec{r}) \\ I_{zx}(\vec{r}) & I_{zy}(\vec{r}) & I_{zz}(\vec{r}) \end{bmatrix}. \qquad (16.8)$$

Similarly, the second-order partial derivatives can be calculated as a convolution with the corresponding derivatives of Gaussians, for example,

$$I_{rr}(\vec{r};s)=s^\gamma\left(\frac{\partial^2 G(\vec{r};s)}{\partial x^2}\right)*I(\vec{r}). \qquad (16.9)$$

The normalization factors were determined in previous studies by using Gaussian-shape models for the ideal step edge, plate, line, and blob structures (Krissian et al. 2000; Sato et al. 2000; Li et al. 2003). However, the normalization factors estimated from the idealized models of the structures do not work well for real structures in clinical images according to our experimental observations.

In a given local volume that contains some vascular structures, the response function in Equation 16.4 may enhance the vascular structures to different degrees at different scales. The voxels with a high response value indicate that there is an enhanced vessel and its size matches the given filter scale, whereas the voxels with a low response value may belong to a suppressed structure such as lymphoid tissue or a vessel of a size that does not match the filter size. The expectation-maximization (EM) segmentation algorithm is applied to the volume containing the response values to segment the vessels by extracting the high response voxels and setting all low response voxels to zero at this single scale. To integrate the segmented vessels at all scales, the simplest way is to unite all the segmented voxels on all scales. However, this will lose the vessel size information that is useful in the analysis of vessel structures for PEs detection and other applications. We therefore designed a hierarchical integration scheme to combine the segmented vessels at all scales and retain their size information. We assume that the sizes of the largest and smallest vessels that are expected to be extracted correspond to filter scales from S_{Max} down to S_{Min} ($S_{Max} > S_{Min}$). The process of integrating the segmented structures at multiple scales begins from the maximum scale S_{Max} down to the minimum scale S_{Min}. Let the EM segmented vascular structure at scale S_k, ($k = $ Min,..., Max) be $T(x, y, z; S_k)$ at voxel (x, y, z) in the 3D volume of response values. The segmented $V(x, y, z)$ is integrated recursively as follows:

1. First segmentation at scale S_{Max}

$$V(x,y,z) = \begin{cases} S_{Max}, & \text{if } T(x,y,z;S_{Max}) > 0; \\ 0, & \text{otherwise.} \end{cases}$$

2. For scale $S_k = S_{Max-1}$ down to S_{Min}
   If $V(x, y, z) = 0$, then,

$$V(x,y,z) = \begin{cases} S_k, & \text{if } T(x,y,z;S_k) > 0; \\ 0, & \text{otherwise.} \end{cases}$$

The voxels in the integrated volume will be the first nonzero segmented voxels and labeled as the scale value $S_k(k = $ Min,...,Max) when going from the larger segmented vascular structure down to the smaller structure, thus recursively incorporating the smaller segmented structures to the integrated volume. In our study, this process is performed for 12 scales ($\sigma = 1,2,...,12$), corresponding to a vessel size ranging approximately from 2 to 24 mm in diameter. The voxels in the integrated volume thus have values $V(x, y, z) \in [0,12]$.

Figure 16.3 shows an example of the responses of our 3D multiscale vessel enhancement filter at different scales and the segmented vessels and structures of different sizes.

The example demonstrates that the multiscale filter can selectively enhance the vessels that match the given filter scale, and the enhanced vessels can be segmented correctly using EM analysis algorithm.

16.3 PARALLEL MULTI-PRESCREENING OF SUSPICIOUS PULMONARY EMBOLISM

PEs can exist anywhere within the arteries, from the main pulmonary artery to the subsegmental arteries and smaller, over which the radius of the arteries may change from over 10 mm to less than 2 mm. The percentage of observable PEs occlusion on the CT images ranges widely from 100% to 5%. It is difficult to use one single method to effectively detect all PEs because of the large variations of the characteristics of the PEs in the patient population. We developed a multiprescreening scheme to identify VOI that contained suspicious PEs (Zhou et al. 2009). In this study, two independent prescreening methods were developed to search for suspicious PEs locally and globally in parallel in the constructed pulmonary arterial tree. The scale information of the vessels was simultaneously recorded, and each voxel of a vessel was labeled by the scale value when the vessel tree was reconstructed using our multiscale segmentation and integration methods (Zhou et al. 2007b). The labeled scale of each voxel therefore provided the approximate local vessel size information from which the size of the search region was estimated, for example, the cubic VOI along the segmented vessels for local search (method 1 described here in the following text) and the vessel tree stratified to different scale ranges for multiscale global search (method 2 described later). The suspicious objects detected by each prescreening method were added to a candidate pool subjected to subsequent FP reduction. For overlapped objects resulted from the two prescreening methods, only the largest object would be chosen as candidate.

16.3.1 Local Search for the Transition Regions Containing Both Normal and PEs Occluded Vessel

This prescreening method is based on the properties of partial or complete filling defects within the lumen of the contrast-enhanced pulmonary arteries. The partial filling defect is often manifested as an area with lower CT values located at the marginal or intravascular central region that is surrounded by a variable amount of contrast material that exhibits higher CT values. Complete filling defect often results in an entire arterial section having low CT values. We developed an EM segmentation–based prescreening method to search for the regions containing partial filling defect and the transition regions between normal arterial section and section of

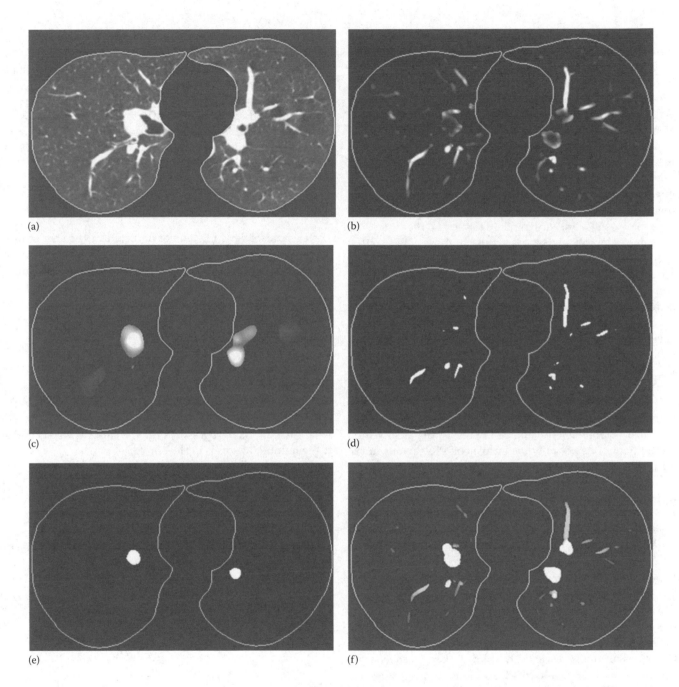

Figure 16.3   Example of vessel segmentation at different scales. (a) CT volume after lung region extraction (only one slice is shown for demonstration), (b) output of the response function at a scale corresponding to vessels of about 6 mm in diameter, (c) output of the response function at a scale corresponding to vessels of about 14 mm in diameter, (d) and (e) segmentation of (b) and (c) using EM segmentation method, and (f) the vessel image after combining the segmentation results from all scales by the hierarchical integration scheme (the gray values, ranging from 0 to 12, indicates that the voxels were segmented at different scales that corresponded to different vessel sizes).

complete filling defect in a local region as follows. After vessel segmentation and reconstruction, a local cubic VOI was formed to enclose several slices of a single branch of the vessel tree. The VOI was centered at a given point along the vessel centerline extracted based on the morphological *hit-and-miss*

transform. The size of the cubic VOI was determined by the labeled scale information of the vessel region, as described earlier. The local search method was based on the assumption that there were two classes of voxels in the local region: one class belonged to the contrast-filled vessel, and the other

PEs and/or lymphoid tissues. A 3D adaptive EM segmentation was applied to the segmented vessel within the VOI to separate the two classes of voxels. With the assumption as a priori knowledge, two Gaussians with equal variances were evenly placed across the gray-level histogram of the local voxels as the initial estimates. After several iterations, the EM algorithm found the optimally fitted Gaussians to the histogram. If there was no PEs or lymphoid tissue in the local volume, the two Gaussian distributions on the histogram might overlap and merge. The EM segmentation would therefore output only one class of voxels: the contrast-filled vessel regions. Otherwise, the EM would output two classes: region of suspicious PEs and/or lymphoid tissue and the vessel. The CT value of lymphoid tissue is similar to those of PEs so that they cannot be separated in EM segmentation. The PEs candidates will be further analyzed in the feature classification step to reduce the FPs such as lymphoid tissue. The VOI would be moved by centering the VOI at each point along the centerline, with its size adapted to each local vessel region, until the entire vessel was screened by the EM segmentation.

16.3.2 Multiscale Adaptive Thresholding for Global Search in the Vessel Tree

Because of the assumption that there were two classes in the local volume when using EM analysis, the local search method could detect only the suspicious PEs regions in the local volume that contained both normal and abnormal vessel segments. However, a significant PEs can occlude an artery by a large percentage, for example, >80%, and extend farther beyond the local volume. A local volume at the transition region may contain only very few contrast-filled voxels. The EM segmentation of the local search method may output one class of voxels that will be labeled as normal vessel. The PEs of large occlusion thus may be missed by local search method. We developed a global search method to overcome the earlier limitation. Because the contrast flows from the central toward the peripheral and smaller arteries, the CT values have different ranges at different arterial levels. For example, the CT values in small arteries may be lower than those in larger arteries, thus, the CT value of PEs-occluded larger artery may be close to those of normal small arteries. To detect the PEs at different levels of arteries, we developed an adaptive multiscale detection method (Zhou et al. 2007a) to search for PEs in vessels of different sizes. Because the vessel tree was reconstructed using our multiscale segmentation and integration methods (Zhou et al. 2007b), each voxel of a segmented vessel was labeled by the scale information. The vessels were stratified to different ranges of scales as illustrated in Figure 16.4. Note that the vessels were not stratified at every single scale; the vessel voxels labeled by a specified range of scales were grouped to one stratified vessel structure. PEs prescreening

was performed separately in each stratified vessel structure using an EM segmentation to identify suspicious PEs objects. Assume that there were two classes of voxels in the stratified vessel structure: voxels in contrast-filled vessel region, and voxels of PEs and/or lymphoid tissue region. If there is no soft tissue or PEs, then EM analysis will find one Gaussian distribution. Otherwise, EM algorithm will output two separate Gaussian distributions: contrast-filled vessel region and PEs and/or lymphoid tissue region.

16.4 FALSE-POSITIVE REDUCTION

For each suspicious PEs object detected in the earlier prescreening step, nine features were extracted. The accurate identification of a true PEs is based on the depiction of partial or complete filling defect within the lumen of the contrast-enhanced pulmonary arteries. We designed the following nine features to describe the filling defects for a detected suspicious PEs object:

(f_1) Average CT value of the detected object ($AvgO$)

$$AvgO = \frac{\sum_i^n x(i)}{n}, \tag{16.10}$$

where $x(i)$, $i = 1,...,n$ represents the CT value of voxel i and n is the number of voxels in the object.

(f_2) Dominant CT value of the detected object (DIO)

$$DIO = \arg\max_x H(x), \tag{16.11}$$

where

$H(x)$ is the histogram of CT values of the detected object and x is the CT value

DIO is the CT value with the largest histogram $H(x)$

(f_3), (f_4) Maximum (MaxScale) and mean (MeanScale) scales of the voxels of the detected object:

$$MaxScale = \overset{n}{\underset{i}{Max}}[S(i)], \tag{16.12}$$

$$MeanScale = \frac{\sum_i^n S(i)}{n}, \tag{16.13}$$

where $S(i)$ is the scale value of the ith voxel of the object. The voxels were labeled when the arterial tree was reconstructed using our multiscale segmentation and integration methods (Zhou et al. 2007b).

(f_5) Number of slices that enclose the detected object (NumSlice).

(f_6) Volume of the detected object ($VolO$).

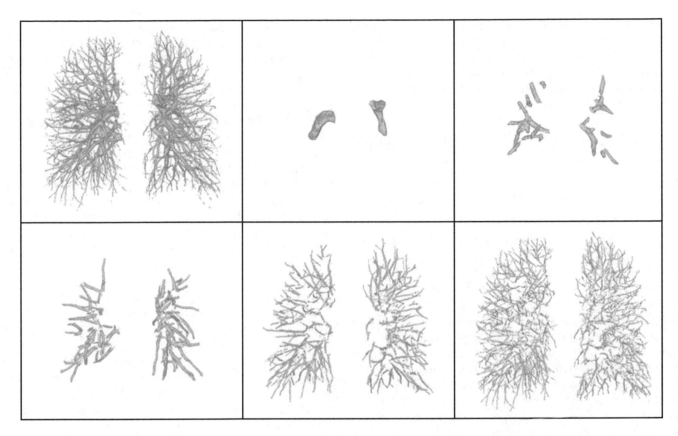

Figure 16.4   Vessel tree stratification. The computer-constructed vessel (top-left) was stratified to multiple levels in terms of the scales (approximately related to the vessel sizes) derived from our vessel segmentation and integration method. The diameters of vessels were stratified from large to small (as shown from left to right, top to bottom).

(f_7), (f_8), (f_9) Three features that describe the difference in CT values between the detected object and the surrounding vessel (ID_1) and the nonvessel background (ID_2 and ID_3) are extracted as follows.

Let $S(i)$ be the labeled scale value of voxel i in the segmented vessel tree and $h(x)$ represent the CT value histogram of voxels for which their labeled scale values $S(i)$ are $MaxScale -2 \leq S(i) \leq MaxScale$; the feature ID_1 is defined as

$$ID_1 = \frac{\underset{x}{\arg\max}\, h(x)}{DIO}, \qquad (16.14)$$

where DIO is the feature f_2, dominant intensity of the detected object.

For a detected object O, a morphological dilation with a structuring element that has a diameter about the equivalent radius of the object is used to enlarge the object to about two times that of the original object O so that the surrounding nonvessel background of object O is enclosed. Let $AvgIn$ denote the average CT value of the voxels of object O and $AvgOut$ the average CT value of the voxels in the nonvessel background surrounding object O (outside

of object O but inside of enlarged object EO); the features ID_2, ID_3 are defined as

$$ID_2 = \frac{AvgIn}{AvgOut}, \qquad (16.15)$$

$$ID_3 = \frac{(AvgIn)^2}{AvgOut}. \qquad (16.16)$$

Our previous studies of CAD for breast and lung cancers indicated that linear or nonlinear combination of a number of features can be very effective in reducing FPs (Chan et al. 1994, 1995a, 1997; Way et al. 2006). In this study, we investigated the feasibility of training an LDA classifier with stepwise feature selection to remove the prescreened objects that were substantially different from the true PEs and generalizing the trained classifier to a relatively large independent test dataset. The details of the implementation of LDA classifier with stepwise feature selection method for CAD applications can be found in our previous studies (Chan et al. 1995b; Sahiner et al. 1999).

Briefly, LDA is a well-established technique (Lachenbruch 1975; Tatsuoka 1988) to find the linear combination of features that best separate two or more classes of data. For a two-class problem, the linear discriminant function is formulated as a weighted sum of a set of selected features as input predictor variables:

$$D = a_0 + \sum_{i-1}^{n} a_i X_i, \quad (16.17)$$

where

n is the number of selected feature variables

X_i are the values of the feature variables

a_i are coefficients (or weights) estimated from the input data during training such that the separation between the distributions of the discriminant scores, D, of the two classes is a maximum. To select the best set of features as input variables (Norusis 1993; Chan et al. 1995b; Sahiner et al. 1999), we used a stepwise procedure to identify the useful features from the available input feature pool using a forward inclusion and backward removal process. The significance of the change in a feature selection criterion, which was chosen to be the Wilks lambda (ratio of the within-class sum of squares to the total sum of squares of the two class distributions), when a new feature is entered or when an included feature is removed is determined based on F-statistics.

16.5 PERFORMANCE EVALUATION FOR PEs DETECTION

We used an overlap criterion to determine whether a detected object was true positive (TP) or FP. A computer-detected object was scored as TP when it overlapped with a reference standard PEs by greater than a threshold T. The overlap ratio was defined as Jaccard coefficient (or Jaccard index) (Jaccard 1912):

$$\text{Overlap} = \frac{VolO \cap VolR}{VolO \cup VolR}, \quad (16.18)$$

where

$VolO$ is the volume of the detected object

$VolR$ is the volume of the reference standard

The threshold was chosen to be 10% in this study. The performance of the LDA classifier was evaluated by ROC analysis. The detection performance was assessed by FROC analysis.

The methods for the determination of ground truth or the criteria for establishing reference standard for the training and testing samples, as well as the methods for scoring the true lesions and FPs, affect the apparent performance of a CAD system. The criterion that the detected object intersects with a reference standard, without a threshold, was used for scoring a true PEs (TP) in most reported studies (Buhmann et al. 2007; Maizlin et al. 2007; Schoepf et al. 2007), while other studies (Masutani et al. 2002; Engelke et al. 2007) did not mention the scoring method. In our study, we also used an overlap criterion to determine whether a detected object was TP or FP. But a detected object could be scored as TP only when it overlapped with a reference standard by greater than a threshold T, instead of intersecting with any voxel of the reference standard. Using the union of the detected object volume and the reference standard PEs volume and imposing an overlap threshold can avoid scoring a detected object as a TP when its size is too large or too small compared with the size of the reference standard. Figure 16.5 illustrated examples of situations of overlap between a detected object and a reference standard. Using our TP scoring criterion, if the overlap threshold was set to a certain value, for example, 10% as in this study, although there was a large overlap compared with the region of either the reference standard ([a] and [b]) or the detected object ([c] and [d]), the detected object in (a)–(d) was still scored as FP. Only the object in (e) could be scored as a TP. However, if the criterion was set to be any intersection between the detected object and the reference standard (equivalent to threshold of >0%), which was commonly used in reported studies (Buhmann et al. 2007; Maizlin et al. 2007; Schoepf et al. 2007), all objects (a)–(e) would be counted as TP. In an extreme case, for example, if the entire vessel was segmented as a detected object, any PEs in the vessel would be counted as TP, resulting in overly optimistic estimate of sensitivity for algorithms that tended to mark long sections of vessels as detected objects.

Because the task of PEs detection is to alert radiologists to the locations suspected of having PEs, the CAD mark indicating a detected PEs location should be close to the true PEs. However, the CAD mark location depends on the accurate volume segmentation of the detected PEs. If the CAD mark was placed at the center of the detected object, for an elongated object as shown in Figure 16.5a and b, the CAD mark would be too far from the true PEs. Furthermore, in our study, for a contiguous volume of PEs that occluded more than one level of arteries and branches of arteries at the same level, the radiologists virtually split the single PEs volume by marking the PEs segment in each branch as a separate PEs. Figure 16.5f shows an example of a contiguous PEs split into three pieces. A detected object had overlap with all three PEs in Figure 16.5g and h. However, the detected object in (g) would not be scored as a TP if its overlap with all three PEs was less than the threshold. Although the object in (h) has large overlap with PEs #1 and could be scored as TP, PEs #2 and #3 would be missed due to overlap below the threshold, resulting in a decrease in the overall sensitivity. In the current study, we chose an overlap threshold of 10%

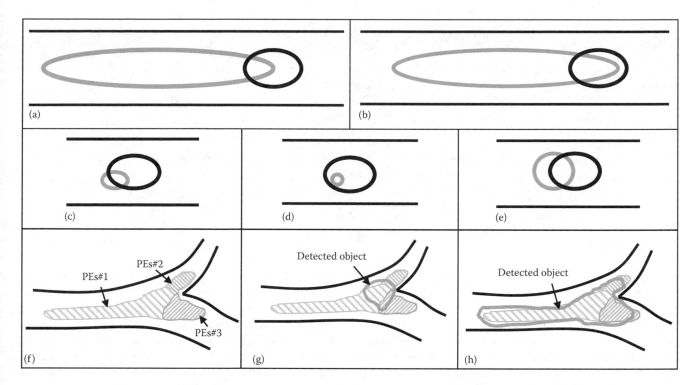

Figure 16.5 Illustration of different situations of overlapping between a computer-detected object (gray) and reference standards (dark [a]–[e] or gray with hatched [f]–[h]) located in a segmented vessel (two parallel lines in dark).

to determine whether a detected object was a TP or FP. This may be somewhat arbitrary, but no standardization of scoring method has been established to date. The determination of reference standard, scoring methods and criterion, and the methods for the presentation of the CAD marks to radiologists are very important issues for CAD development, comparison, and implementation in clinical practice and warrant further investigations in future studies.

16.6 RESULTS

16.6.1 Materials

With the approval of our Institutional Review Board (IRB), 59 inpatient CTPA PEs-positive cases were retrospectively collected from the patient files at the UM. The images were acquired with GE multidetector CT scanners, 120–140 kVp, 300–600 mAs, reconstructed at 1.25 mm slice thickness. Of the 59 cases, 16, 3, 34, and 6 cases were acquired with a 4-, 8-, 16-, and 64-slice CT scanner, respectively. Of the 59 cases, 22 had extensive lung parenchymal and/or pleural disease. With access permission, 69 CTPA PEs-positive cases were randomly selected from the dataset collected in PIOPED II trial, a multicenter, prospective trial supported by the National Institutes of Health and the National Heart, Lung, and Blood Institute. For the UM cases, PEs locations were marked by three experienced thoracic radiologists

on a computer graphical user interface (GUI) developed in our laboratory. The PEs locations in the PIOPED cases were also marked by our radiologists with reference to the documented diagnosis in the PIOPED study. The GUI has functions allowing the radiologist to cine-page through the CT slices, scroll in and out of individual arteries, adjust window setting, and zoom to improve visualization. The radiologists marked the PEs location in every artery where it was present. For a contiguous volume of PEs that occluded more than one level of the arteries and branches of arteries at the same level, the radiologists virtually split the single PEs volume by marking the PEs segment in each branch as a separate PEs. For each PEs, radiologist marked the approximate location of its center and the starting and ending slices of the PEs segment with a cursor, identified the anatomical level of the artery (trunk, main, lobar, segmental, and subsegmental), measured the diameter of the artery with an electronic ruler, and visually estimated the percentage of PEs occlusion in the artery. To generate a volume of the PEs, we developed a semiautomatic computer tool to segment the PEs voxels within the radiologist-marked PEs VOI using a supervised region-growing method (Adams and Bischof 1994; Chang and Li 1994; Castleman 1996; Mehnert 1997).

Radiologists manually marked 595 and 800 PEs in the UM and PIOPED datasets, respectively. Table 16.2 shows the distributions of PEs identified in the two datasets according to their major artery location and the percentage of

TABLE 16.2   REFERENCE STANDARD PEs IDENTIFIED BY RADIOLOGISTS BY ARTERY LEVEL AND PERCENT ARTERIAL OCCLUSION

Dataset	Percent Occlusion (%)	Proximal PEs, # (%)	Subsegmental PEs, # (%)	All PEs, # (%)
59 UM cases	≤20	52 (8.7)	33 (5.6)	85 (14.3)
	20–80	170 (28.6)	94 (15.8)	264 (44.4)
	≥80	128 (21.5)	118 (19.8)	246 (41.3)
	All occlusion	350 (58.8)	245 (41.2)	595
69 PIOPED cases	≤20	53 (6.7)	33 (4.1)	86 (10.8)
	20–80	279 (34.9)	153 (19.1)	432 (54.0)
	≥80	186 (23.3)	96 (12.0)	282 (35.3)
	All occlusion	518 (64.8)	282 (35.2)	800

arterial occlusion. These marked locations were used as the reference standard for algorithm development and evaluation. The PEs occlusion in the datasets ranged from 5% to 100%. Of the 595 PEs identified in UM cases, 245 (41%) and 350 (59%) PEs were located in subsegmental arteries and the more proximal arteries, respectively. Of the 800 PEs identified in the PIOPED cases, 282 (35%) and 518 (65%) PEs were located in the subsegmental and more proximal arteries, respectively.

16.6.2   Results

Two independent dataset including 59 UM and 69 PIOPED CTPA PEs cases were used for the performance evaluation of our method in PEs detection. An LDA classifier with stepwise feature selection was trained with the 59 UM cases, and the performance of the trained classifier was evaluated on the 69 PIOPED cases, and vice versa.

Table 16.3 shows the A_z values for the training and test sets, standard deviations, and the number of features selected when the LDA classifier was trained with the UM or the PIOPED cases. Figure 16.6 shows the test FROC curves for the independent dataset when the classifier was trained with UM cases and PIOPED cases, respectively. These curves represent the performance of our PEs detection system for all PEs with a range of 5%–100% occlusion and

for all CTPA examinations in each dataset including those with extensive parenchymal or pleural disease. The FROC analysis indicated that the overall performance of our PEs detection system could achieve a test sensitivity of 80% at 18.9 FPs/case for the PIOPED cases when the LDA classifier was trained with the UM cases. The test sensitivity with the UM cases was 80% at 22.6 FPs/cases when the LDA classifier was trained with the PIOPED cases.

The detection performance depended on the arterial level where the PEs was located and on the percentage of occlusion. Figure 16.7 shows the test FROC curves stratified for PEs located at two arterial levels (subsegmental arteries and proximal arteries) with different percentages of occlusion (≤20%, 20%–80%, and ≥80%). As expected, the FROC curves indicated that the sensitivity was lower for PEs in the subsegmental arteries than those in the more proximal arteries, and was lower for PEs with less percent occlusion. Figure 16.8a through e shows examples of computer-detected TP PEs with different occlusion to the arteries, FPs, and FN (missed) PEs. Figure 16.9 shows the dependence of the test FROC curves for the UM cases on the overlap thresholds when the LDA classifier was trained with the PIOPED cases. The FROC curves indicated that the best performance was achieved using an overlap threshold of $T > 0\%$. The performance increased when the overlap threshold decreased.

TABLE 16.3   Az VALUE OF TRAINING AND TEST SET AND CORRESPONDING STANDARD DEVIATION (SD), THE NUMBER OF FEATURES SELECTED AS THE INPUT TO LDA CLASSIFIERS WHEN TRAINED WITH UM AND PIOPED CASES, RESPECTIVELY

Dataset	Training Az	SD of Training Az	Test Az	SD of Test Az	Number of Selected Features
Train in PIOPED cases, test on UM cases	0.855	0.009	0.877	0.008	5 $(f_1, f_3, f_4, f_5, f_7)$
Train in UM cases, test on PIOPED cases	0.881	0.008	0.851	0.009	6 $(f_1, f_3, f_4, f_5, f_8, f_9)$

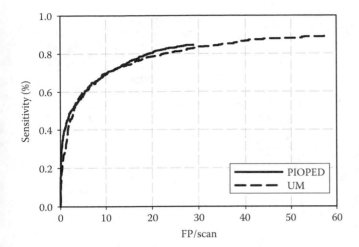

Figure 16.6 The test FROC curves for PIOPED and UM cases, when the LDA classifier was trained with UM cases and PIOPED cases, respectively.

16.7 CHALLENGES IN PEs DETECTION AND DISCUSSIONS

Although the development of CAD systems for PEs detection in CTPA is still at an early stage (Chan et al. 2008), recent studies (Buhmann et al. 2007; Maizlin et al. 2007; Marten and Engelke 2007; Schoepf et al. 2007) indicate that CAD is useful in improving performance for PEs diagnosis and can help radiologists as a second opinion. Automated detection of PEs in CTPA scans is challenging. The difficulty of computerized PEs detection is not only because of the large volume of data but also because of the complexity of the images and the partial volume effect, motion, or other imaging conditions. The performance of a CAD system also depends strongly on the characteristics of the PEs such as their size, percentage of arterial occlusion by PEs, and the diameter of the artery involved.

Few research groups have participated in the development of CAD systems for PEs detection to date. Most of the studies have only evaluated systems developed by commercial companies and reported preliminary results using relatively small sets of case samples. For example, two recent studies (Bouma et al. 2009; Park et al. 2011) used 11 and 19 cases to evaluate their developed CAD system for PEs detection. It is expected that the performance of a CAD system will depend strongly on the characteristics of PEs, such as their size distributions; percentage of occlusion by PEs to an artery, the diameter of the artery being occluded, or patient conditions, such as whether there are other significant pulmonary diseases; and the quality of CT scans, such as the degree of contrast filling and motion artifacts. However, the criteria for the determination of PEs in the reference standards were not clearly defined in most studies. These factors would have to be taken into consideration or a common dataset is used if a meaningful comparison among the performance of different systems is desired.

To develop a CAD system, one of the most challenging tasks is to collect a sufficiently large dataset for training and testing the computer algorithms. The collected cases should be representative of patient population, and the reference truth of the lesion should be well defined. For the clinical CTPA PEs cases, there is no equivalent to biopsy-proven *ground truth* as to whether PEs are present or absent in a given artery. In our study, experienced thoracic radiologists provided the reference standard for PEs by manually marking PEs locations and providing the relevant information such as the size of the PEs, percentage of the PEs arterial occlusion, and the anatomic level of the artery occluded. Because a PEs can extend to multiple branches down to multiple levels of artery, to evaluate the performance of our CAD system at different levels of the arteries, our radiologists virtually split a single volume of PEs into volumes according to the branching of the artery by marking the PEs segment in each branch as a separate PEs. The sensitivity of a CAD algorithm for individual PEs in a case can be treated, in a way, as the collective evaluation of the sensitivity of PEs of different degrees of occlusion and conspicuity that may occur in many PEs cases. Therefore, in the developmental process of a CAD system, it is useful to evaluate the sensitivity for the detection of individual PEs. This will also increase the number of individual PEs for training the CAD system far beyond the number of CTPA cases available because many cases have multiple PEs. The splitting of PEs volume allows us to evaluate the performance of the CAD system at different arterial levels. However, it will also reduce the apparent sensitivity of the CAD system because a nonsplit PEs extending from large to small arteries can be counted as a TP if any part of the PEs is detected, whereas the same PEs split into different arterial branches may generate several FNs if the split PEs in the small arteries are missed. Nevertheless, before a large dataset of PEs cases that contains a sufficiently large number of single PEs located at different levels of the pulmonary tree can be collected, the PEs splitting method may be a good alternative to estimate detection performance at different arterial levels and to alleviate the problem of a limited dataset.

CAD may be a viable approach for assisting radiologists in this demanding task and reducing the chance of missing PEs (Ko and Naidich 2004; Schoepf and Costello 2004). With advanced computer vision techniques, the computer may be trained to automatically track the pulmonary vessels, distinguish the arteries from the veins, detect suspicious PEs locations by searching along the arteries, and finally alert the radiologists to the ROIs for suspicious PEs. If CAD can improve the sensitivity and specificity for the detection of small peripheral emboli with CTPA, it may reduce unnecessary workup with other diagnostic procedures or provide more accurate information for selecting treatment options.

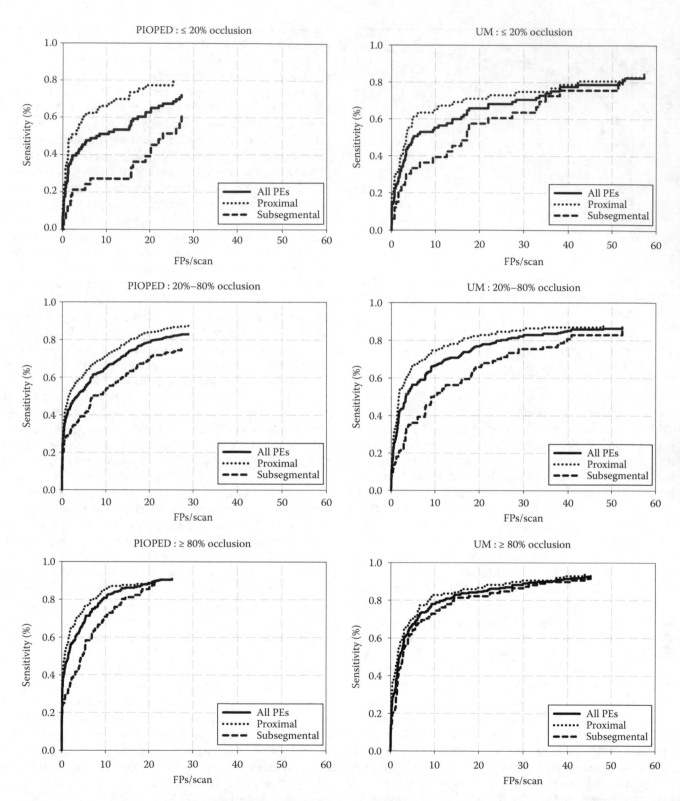

Figure 16.7 The test FROC curves stratified for PEs located at two arterial levels (subsegmental arteries and proximal arteries) and with different percentages of occlusion (≤20%, 20%–80%, and ≥80%). The left and right columns are test results for the PIOPED and UM cases, respectively.

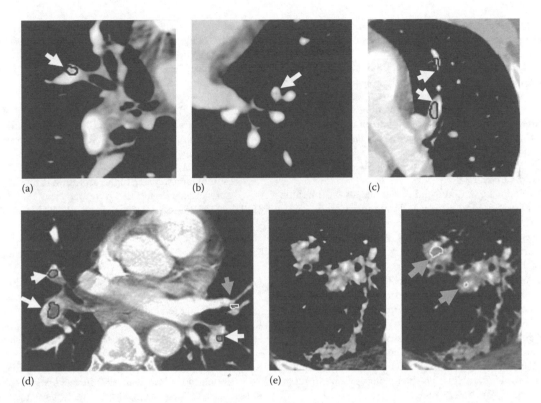

Figure 16.8 Examples of the computer-detected PEs with different occlusions, FP and FN PEs. A TP PEs was enclosed by a black contour and marked by a white arrow, an FP was enclosed by a white contour and marked by a gray arrow, and an FN was marked by a white arrow without contour. Image (a) a TP subsegmental PEs with 30% occlusion, (b) an FN subsegmental PEs with 15% occlusion, (c) two TP PEs with 90% occlusion that were split from the segmental (lower) to the subsegmental level (upper). (d) Three TP PEs were detected, three lobar PEs (top-left, bottom-left, and bottom-right) with 95%, 60%, and 40% occlusion, respectively. The FP in (d) was caused by partial volume effect between a lobar and a subsegmental artery. The two FPs in (e) were caused by extensive lung pleural disease.

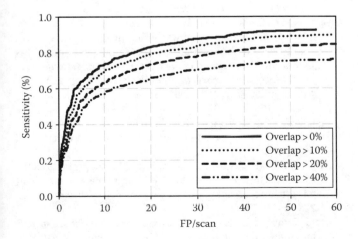

Figure 16.9 Dependence of test FROC curves for UM cases on the overlap thresholds to score detected objects as TP or FP when the LDA classifier was trained with the PIOPED cases.

REFERENCES

Adams, R. and L. Bischof. 1994. Seeded region growing. *IEEE Trans PAMI* 16 (6):641–647.

Araoz, P.A., M.B. Gotway, R.L. Trowbridge et al. 2003. Helical CT pulmonary angiography predictors of in-hospital morbidity and mortality in patients with acute pulmonary embolism. *J Thorac Imaging* 18 (4):207–216.

Aylward, S. and E. Bullitt. 2002. Initialization, noise, singularities, and scale in height ridge traversal for tubular object center-line extraction. *IEEE Trans Med Imag* 21 (2):61–75.

Bankier, A.A., K. Janata, D. Fleischmann et al. 1997. Severity assessment of acute pulmonary embolism with spiral CT: Evaluation of two modified angiographic scores and comparison with clinical data. *J Thorac Imag* 12:150–158.

Blanks, R.G., M.G. Wallis, and R.M. Given-Wilson. 1999. Observer variability in cancer detection during routine repeat (incident) mammographic screening in a study of two versus one view mammography. *J Med Screen* 6:152–158.

Bouma, H., J.J. Sonnemans, A. Vilanova, and F.A. Gerritsen. 2009. Automatic detection of pulmonary embolism in CTA images. *IEEE Trans Med Imag* 28 (8):1223–1230.

Buhmann, S., P. Herzog, J. Liang et al. 2007. Clinical evaluation of a computer-aided diagnosis (CAD) prototype for the detection of pulmonary embolism. *Acad Radiol* 14 (6):651–658.

Bülow, T., C. Lorenz, and S. Renisch. 2004. A general framework for tree segmentation and reconstruction from medical volume data. *Med Image Comput Computer Assist Intervent MICCAI.* 3216:533–540.

Castleman, K.R. 1996. *Digital Image Processing.* Prentice Hall Press, Upper Saddle River, NJ.

Chan, H.P., L.M. Hadjiiski, C. Zhou, and B. Sahiner. 2008. Computer-aided diagnosis of lung cancer and pulmonary embolism in computed tomography—A review. *Acad Radiol* 15 (5):535–555.

Chan, H.P., B. Sahiner, R.F. Wagner, and N. Petrick. 1997. Classifier design for computer-aided diagnosis in mammography: Effects of finite sample size. *Med Phys* 24:1034–1035.

Chan, H.-P., D. Wei, M.A. Helvie et al. 1995b. Computer-aided classification of mammographic masses and normal tissue: Linear discriminant analysis in texture feature space. *Phys Med Biol* 40:857–876.

Chan, H.P., D. Wei, K.L. Lam et al. 1995a. Classification of malignant and benign microcalcifications by texture analysis. *Med Phys* 22:938.

Chan, H.P., D. Wei, L.T. Niklason et al. 1994. Computer-aided classification of malignant/benign microcalcifications in mammography. *Med Phys* 21:875.

Chang, Y.L. and X. Li. 1994. Adaptive image region-growing. *IEEE Trans Image Proces* 3 (6):868–872.

Chung, A. and J.A. Noble. 1999. Statistical 3D vessel segmentation using a Rician distribution. *Int Conf Med Image Comput Computer Assist Intervent* 1679:82–89.

Coche, E., F. Verschuren, A. Keyeux et al. 2003. Diagnosis of acute pulmonary embolism in outpatients: Comparison of thin-collimation multi–detector row spiral CT and planar ventilation-perfusion scintigraphy. *Radiology* 229:757–765.

Dalen, J.E. and J.S. Alpert. 1975. Natural history of pulmonary embolism. *Prog Cardiovas Dis* 17:257–270.

Das, M., M. Salganicoff, A. Bakai et al. 2006. Computer-aided detection of pulmonary embolism: Assessment of sensitivity with regard to vessel segments. Paper read at RSNA, at Chicago, IL.

Das, M., A.C. Schneider, U.O. Schoepf et al. 2003. Computer-aided diagnosis of peripheral pulmonary emboli. Paper read at *RSNA 2003*, November 30–December 5, 2003, at Chicago, IL.

Diffin, D.C., J.R. Leyendecker, S.P. Johnson, R.J. Zucker, and P.J. Grebe. 1998. Effect of anatomic distribution of pulmonary emboli on interobserver agreement in the interpretation of pulmonary angiography. *Am J Roentgenol* 171:1085–1089.

Digumarthy, S., C. Kagay, A. Legasto et al. 2006. Computer-aided detection (CAD) of acute pulmonary emboli: Evaluation in patients without significant pulmonary disease. Paper read at *RSNA*, at Chicago, IL.

Drucker, E.A., S.M. Rivitz, and J.O. Shepard. 1998. Acute pulmonary embolism: Assessment of helical CT for diagnosis. *Radiology* 209:235–241.

Engelke, C., S. Schmidt, A. Bakai, F. Auer, and K. Marten. 2007. Computer-assisted detection of pulmonary embolism: Performance evaluation in consensus with experienced and inexperienced chest radiologists. *Eur Radiol* 18 (2):298–307.

Frangi, A.F., W.J. Neissen, K.L. Vincken, and M.A. Viergever. 1998. Multiscale vessel enhancement filtering. *Med Image Comput Computer Assist Intervent* 1496:130–137.

Ghaye, B. 2001. Peripheral pulmonary arteries: How far in the lung does multi-detector row spiral CT allow analysis? *Radiology* 219:629–636.

Goodman, L.R., J.J. Curtin, and M.W. Mewissen. 1995. Detection of pulmonary embolism in patients with unsolved clinical and scintigraphic diagnosis: Helical CT versus angiography. *Am J Roentgenol* 164 (6):1369–1374.

Higgins, W.E., W.J.T. Spyra, R.A. Warwoski, and E.L. Ritman. 1996. System for analyzing high-resolution three dimensional coronary angiograms. *IEEE Trans Med Imag* 15:377–385.

Hull, R., G.E. Raskob, J.S. Ginsberg et al. 1994. A noninvasive strategy for the treatment of patients with suspected pulmonary embolism. *Arch Intern Med* 154:289–297.

Jaccard, P. 1912. The distribution of the flora in the alpine zone. *New Phytologist* 11 (2):37–50.

Jeudy, J., T. Flukinger, and C. White. 2006. Evaluation of pulmonary embolism using an automated computer-aided detection tool. Paper read at *RSNA*, at Chicago, IL.

Kanazawa, K., Y. Kawata, N. Niki et al. 1998. Computer-aided diagnosis for pulmonary nodules based on helical CT images. *Computer Med Imag Graphics* 22:157–167.

Ko, J.P. and D.P. Naidich. 2004. Computer-aided diagnosis and the evaluation of lung disease. *J Thorac Imag* 19 (3):136–155.

Krissian, K., G. Malandain, N. Ayache, R. Vaillant, and Y. Trousset. 2000. Model-based detection of tubular structures in 3D images. *Computer Vision Image Understand* 80:130–171.

Kutka, R. and S. Stier. 1996. Extraction of line properties based on direction fields. *IEEE Trans Med Imag* 15 (1):51–58.

Lachenbruch, P.A. 1975. *Discriminant Analysis.* New York: Hafner Press.

Li, Q., S. Sone, and K. Doi. 2003. Selective enhancement filters for nodules, vessels, and airway walls in two- and three-dimensional CT scans. *Med Phys* 30 (8):2040–2051.

Lindeberg, T. 1998. Feature detection with automatic scale selection. *Int J Comp Vision* 30 (2):77–116.

Lorenz, C., I.C. Carlsen, T.M. Buzug, C. Fassnacht, and J. Weese. 1997. A multi-scale line filter with automatic scale selection based on the Hessian matrix for medical image segmentation. *Proceedings of the First International Conference on Scale-Space Theory in Computer Vision*, Utrecht, the Netherlands, July 2–4, 1997, Springer Berlin Heidelberg, pp. 152–163.

Lorigo, L.M., O.D. Faugeras, W.E.L. Grimson et al. 2001. CURVES: Curve evolution for vessel segmentation. *Med Image Anal* 5:195–206.

Maizlin, Z.V., P.M. Vos, M.B. Godoy, and P.L. Cooperberg. 2007. Computer-aided detection of pulmonary embolism on CT angiography: Initial experience. *J Thorac Imag* 22 (4):324–329.

Marten, K. and C. Engelke. 2007. Computer-aided detection and automated CT volumetry of pulmonary nodules. *Eur Radiol* 17:888–901.

Mastora, I., M. Remy-Jardin, P. Masson et al. 2003. Severity of acute pulmonary embolism: Evaluation of a new spiral CT angiographic score in correlation with echocardiographic data. *Eur Radiol* 13:29–35.

Masutani, Y., H. Macmahon, and K. Doi. 2001. Automated segmentation and visualization of the pulmonary vascular tree in spiral CT angiography: An anatomy-oriented approach based on tree-dimensional image analysis. *J Computer Assist Tomogr* 25 (4):587–597.

Masutani, Y., H. MacMahon, and K. Doi. 2002. Computerized detection of pulmonary embolism in Spiral CT angiography based on volumetric image analysis. *IEEE Trans Med Imag* 21 (12):1517–1523.

McCollough, C.H. and F.E. Zink. 1999. Performance evaluation of a multi-slice CT system. *Med Phys* 26:2223–2230.

McInerney, T. and D. Terzopoulos. 2000. T-snake: Topology adaptive snakes. *Med Image Anal* 4 (2):73–91.

Mehnert, A. 1997. An improved seeded region growing algorithm. *Pattern Recogn Lett* 18:1065–1071.

Norusis, M.J. 1993. *SPSS for Windows Release 6 Professional Statistics.* Chicago, IL: SPSS, Inc.

Oser, R.F., D.A. Zuckerman, F.R. Gutierrez, and J.A. Brink. 1996. Anatomic distribution of pulmonary emboli at pulmonary angiography: Implications for cross sectional imaging. *Radiology* 199:31–35.

Park, S.C., B.E. Chapman, and B. Zheng. 2011. A multistage approach to improve performance of computer-aided detection of pulmonary embolisms depicted on CT images: Preliminary investigation. *IEEE Trans Biomed Eng* 58 (6):1519–1527.

Patel, S., E.A. Kazerooni, and P.N. Cascade. 2003. Pulmonary embolism: Optimization of small pulmonary artery visualization at multi-detector row CT. *Radiology* 227 (2):455–460.

Patriquin, L., R. Khorasani, and J.F. Polak. 1998. Correlation of diagnostic imaging and subsequent autopsy findings in patients with pulmonary embolism. *Am J Respir Crit Care Med* 171:347–349.

Perrier, A., N. Howarth, D. Didier et al. 2001. Performance of helical computed tomography in unselected outpatients with suspected pulmonary embolism. *Annal Int Med* 135 (2):88–97.

Price, D.G. 1976. Thoughts on immediate care—Pulmonary embolism. Prophylaxis diagnosis and treatment. *Anaesthesia* 31:925–932.

Qanadli, S.D., M.E. Hajjam, A. Vieillard-Baron et al. 2001. New CT index to quantify arterial obstruction in pulmonary embolism: Comparison with angiographic index and echocardiography. *Am J Roentgenol* 176:1415–1420.

Raptopoulos, V. and P.M. Boiselle. 2001. Multi-detector row spiral CT pulmonary angiography: Comparison with single-detector row spiral CT. *Radiology* 221:606–613.

Remy-Jardin, M., J. Remy, L. Wattinne, and F. Giraud. 1992. Central pulmonary thromboembolism: diagnosis with spiral volumetric CT with the single-breath-hold technique-comparison with pulmonary angiography. *Radiology* 185:381–387.

Rubin, G.D., D.S. Paik, P.C. Johnston, and S. Napel. 1998. Measurements of the aorta and its branches with helical CT. *Radiology* 206 (3):823–829.

Sahiner, B., H.P. Chan, N. Petrick, R.F. Wagner, and L.M. Hadjiiski. 1999. Stepwise linear discriminant analysis in computer-aided diagnosis: The effect of finite sample size. *Proc SPIE—Med Imag* 3661:499–510.

Sato, Y., S. Nakajima, N. Shiraga et al. 1998. Three-dimensional multi-scale line filter for segmentation and visualization of curvilinear structures in medical images. *Med Image Anal* 2 (2):143–169.

Sato, Y., C.F. Westin, A. Bhalerao et al. 2000. Tissue classification based on 3D local intensity structures for volume rendering. *IEEE Trans Visual Computer Graphics* 6 (2):160–180.

Schoepf, U.J. and P. Costello. 2004. CT angiography for diagnosis of pulmonary embolism: State of the art. *Radiology* 230:329–337.

Schoepf, U.J., S.Z. Goldhaber, and P. Costello. 2004. Spiral computed tomography for acute pulmonary embolism. *Circulation* 109 (18):2160–2167.

Schoepf, U.J., N. Holzknecht, T.K. Helmberger et al. 2002. Subsegmental pulmonary emboli: Improved detection with thin-collimation multi-detector row spiral CT. *Radiology* 222:483–490.

Schoepf, U.J., A.C. Schneider, M. Das et al. 2007. Pulmonary embolism: Computer-aided detection at multidetector row spiral computed tomography. *J Thorac Imag* 22 (4):319–323.

Schoepf, U.O., M. Das, A.C. Schneider et al. 2002. Computer-aided detection (CAD) of segmental and subsegmental pulmonary embolism on 1-mm multidetector-row CT (MDCT) studies (abstr). *Radiology* 225(p):384.

Shikata, H., E.A. Hoffman, and M. Sonka. 2004. Automated segmentation of pulmonary vascular tree from 3D CT images. *Proc SPIE Med Imag 2004* 5369:107–116.

Sostman, H.D., P.D. Stein, A. Gottschalk et al. 2004. Results of the NIH/NHLBI PIOPED II study: Is spiral CT the best and only test for suspected pulmonary embolism? RSNA 2004, November 28–December 3 RSNA Program Book 2004:55.

Stein, P.D. 1999. Reassessment of pulmonary angiography for the diagnosis of pulmonary embolism: Relation of interpreter agreement to the order of the involved pulmonary arterial branch. *Radiology* 210:689–691.

Stein, P.D., S.E. Fowler, L.R. Goodman et al. 2006. Multidetector computed tomography for acute pulmonary embolism. *New England J Med* 354 (22):2317–2327.

Tatsuoka, M.M. 1988. *Multivariate Analysis, Techniques for Educational and Psychological Research*, 2nd edn. New York: Macmillan.

Way, T.W., L.M. Hadjiiski, B. Sahiner et al. 2006. Computer-aided diagnosis of pulmonary nodules on CT scans: Segmentation and classification using 3D active contours. *Med Phys* 33 (7):2323–2337.

Wink, O., W.J. Niessen, and M.A. Viergever. 2004. Multiscale vessel tracking. *IEEE Trans Med Imag* 23 (1):130–133.

Wood, K.E., L. Visani, and M. De Rosa. 2002. Major pulmonary embolism: Review of a pathophysiologic approach to the golden hour of hemodynamically signification pulmonary embolism. *Chest* 121:877–905.

Wu, A.S., J.A. Pezzullo, H.J. Cronan, D.D. Hou, and W.W. Mayo-Smith. 2004. CT pulmonary angiography: Quantification of pulmonary embolus as a predictor of patient outcome—Initial experience. *Radiology* 230 (3):831–835.

Zhou, C., H.P. Chan, L.M. Hadjiiski et al. 2007. Automated detection of pulmonary embolism (PE) in computed tomographic pulmonary angiographic (CTPA) images: Multiscale hierarchical expectation-maximization segmentation of vessels and PEs. *Proc SPIE* 6514:2F1–2F8.

Zhou, C., H-P. Chan, S. Patel et al. 2004. Computerized Detection of Pulmonary Embolism in 16-slice Computed Tomographic Pulmonary Angiography (CTPA) images. RSNA 2004, November 28-December 3: 350.

Zhou, C., H.P. Chan, S. Patel et al. 2005. Preliminary investigation of computer-aided detection of pulmonary embolism in 3D computed tomographic pulmonary angiography (CTPA) images. *Acad Radiol* 12:782–792.

Zhou, C., H-P. Chan, B. Sahiner et al. 2009. Computer-aided detection of pulmonary embolism in computed tomographic pulmonary angiography (CTPA): Performance evaluation with independent data sets. *Med Phys* 36 (8):3385–3396.

Zhou, C., H.P. Chan, B. Sahiner et al. 2007. Automatic multiscale enhancement and hierarchical segmentation of pulmonary vessels in CT pulmonary angiography (CTPA) images for CAD applications. *Med Phys* 34 (12):4567–4577.

Zhou, C., L.M. Hadjiiski, S. Patel, H.P. Chan, and B. Sahiner. 2003a. Computerized detection of pulmonary embolism in 3D computed tomographic (CT) images. RSNA 2003, Chicago, November 30–December 5:51–51.

Zhou, C., L.M. Hadjiiski, B. Sahiner et al. 2003b. Computerized detection of pulmonary embolism in 3D computed tomographic (CT) images: Vessel tracking and segmentation techniques. *Proc SPIE* 5032:1613–1620.

Chapter 17

Detection of Eye Diseases

Chisako Muramatsu and Hiroshi Fujita

CONTENTS

17.1 INTRODUCTION

According to a WHO report, in 2002, the estimated number of people with blindness worldwide was about 37 million (Resnikoff et al. 2004). Since adults 50 years of age and older account for more than 82% of all blind people, the current prevalence is expected to increase with the aging of the population. The leading cause of blindness is cataracts, which account for approximately 50% of cases. Other main causes include glaucoma, age-related macular degeneration (AMD), corneal opacities, and diabetic retinopathy (DR). In developed countries, glaucoma is the second leading cause of vision loss after AMD. While blindness is unavoidable with AMD, for other diseases, known effective strategies for elimination, screening, and early treatment are critical for the prevention of total blindness.

In a clinical visit, ophthalmologists generally examine the condition of a patient's eye through an ophthalmoscope. While ophthalmoscopy is simple, low cost, and versatile, it is a real-time examination, and the images cannot be stored. Therefore, for screening, diagnostic records, and longitudinal comparisons, retinal fundus photography is frequently and widely used. In reading retinal fundus images, physicians must look for various signs of abnormalities. However, both the number of qualified professionals and their time are limited. To reduce physicians' workload and improve diagnostic efficiency, computer-aided diagnosis of retinal fundus images can be helpful, especially in screening exams in which a large number of normal images are obtained (Fujita et al. 2008). Computerized analysis can also be useful for quantitative measurements of various diagnostic parameters for consistent assessment and follow-up examinations.

17.2 DETECTION OF NORMAL STRUCTURES IN RETINAL FUNDUS IMAGES

The retinal fundus is the only part of the body where blood vessels can be directly observed. A retinal fundus photograph is obtained using a specialized camera system that illuminates the retinal fundus through the pupil and uses a flash of light reflected from the fundus to obtain an image. Figure 17.1a shows a rough sketch of an eye cross section. Retinal blood vessels enter the eyeball through the optic nerve head (ONH) and run inside the retinal nerve layer. Usually, there are four pairs of large arteries and veins extending from the ONH to the upper and lower nasal sides and the upper and lower temporal (ear) sides. The ONH is shaped like a pit as a result of the entering nerve fibers. The state of this dent, called a cup, and the rim constituted by the nerve fibers are important for the diagnosis of glaucoma. The main structures observed in a retinal fundus image include the retinal blood vessels; the ONH, also called the optic disk; and the fovea (Figure 17.1b).

The major purposes for screening by retinal fundus examinations include, but are not limited to, the assessment of hypertensive changes, the diagnosis of DR, and the diagnosis of glaucoma. To detect these diseases, it is important to first identify or segment normal structures, such as blood vessels, the ONH, and fovea, because they can serve as landmarks for image processing and are occasionally sources of false positives in the detection of pathologic lesions. In fact, most of the previously reported CAD schemes include algorithms for detecting these normal structures.

17.2.1 Public Databases for Retinal Image Analysis

There have been numerous studies on the detection and segmentation of the ONH and retinal blood vessels. Many of these studies utilize public databases, such as the Structured Analysis of the Retina (STARE) and the Digital Retinal Images for Vessel Extraction (DRIVE) databases. The STARE database, which is the oldest, is often used for the evaluation of ONH localization and vessel segmentation algorithms. Some of the images contain pathologic lesions, which make the tasks challenging. The DRIVE database may be the most widely used and cited of all public retinal databases. The comparison results from some algorithms published by different groups are presented on the website (Niemeijer et al. 2004). The MESSIDOR database, which includes 1200 images, is the largest database. It provides retinopathy and macular edema grades for each image; however, their locations are not specified. The Retinopathy Online Challenge (ROC) project was organized for the automatic detection of microaneurysms. The database provides 50 training cases with a reference standard, and 50 test cases without. Using this database, an algorithm competition was held at the CAD Conference of SPIE Medical Imaging 2009. There are several other databases available for the development and comparison of computer algorithms, and they are listed in Appendix 17.A. The relatively early availability of these public retinal fundus image databases compared to other medical images may have promoted CAD research.

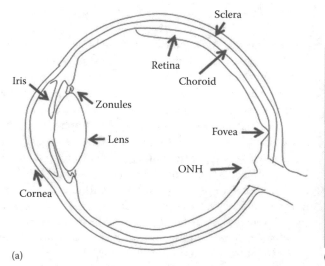

(a)

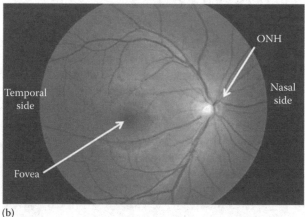

(b)

Figure 17.1   (a) A rough sketch of a cross section of an eye. (b) A retinal fundus photograph of a right eye.

17.2.2 Detection and Segmentation of Optic Nerve Head

A number of groups have been investigating automated methods for the detection and segmentation of ONHs. The ONH has an oval shape where large vessels converge, and it appears as a bright region on a retinal fundus image. On the basis of these characteristics, many detection algorithms utilize pixel thresholding techniques, and some algorithms use the information of vessel orientation. For segmentation, edge information is often used along with techniques such as Hough transformation and deformable models. While it is not difficult for a human to identify the ONH, automatic detection can eliminate the need for manual intervention during preprocessing for other tasks. On the other hand, automatic segmentation results can be used for shape analyses, such as the automatic measurement of disk areas and diameters.

In general, relevant preprocessing is carried out before detecting and segmenting the ONH in most CAD schemes. Some common preprocessing tasks include smoothing operation for noise reduction and/or the removal of small bright lesions, morphological closing operation for vessel removal, luminosity or contrast normalization (linear contrast enhancement), and illumination equalization (background correction) to compensate for uneven brightness, which generally decreases toward the field of view (FOV) borders. To exclude the region outside the FOV from the analysis, a mask image can be created simply by applying the thresholding technique with supplemental morphological closing. Occasionally, mirroring or FOV extension is performed to eliminate the edge effect.

A retinal fundus image generally consists of three color components, red, green, and blue (RGB). Based on the bright characteristic of the ONH, green is a popular color plane used for ONH detection because the red component may sometimes saturate, and the blue component does not provide much information other than noise. Another frequently used component is the luminance, or intensity, of the hue–saturation–luminance/intensity (HLS or HSI) representation, which is convertible from the RGB space. Some studies have employed Lab space (Osareh et al. 2002; Kande et al. 2009). Three color (RGB) planes can be processed independently, and the results can be combined to obtain maximal information (Carmona et al. 2008).

17.2.2.1 ONH Localization

Automated detection of the ONH is relatively straightforward for normal cases; however, it can be difficult in cases with pathologic lesions. In normal cases, one can look for the brightest circular region of a certain size. However, in abnormal cases, other bright lesions, such as exudates, may also be detected, the ONH may be occluded by pathologic lesions, or the ONH boundary may become unclear. To overcome such difficulties, a variety of schemes have been proposed for ONH detection. Although the ONH region is generally bright in retinal fundus images, large vessels coming into the ONH appear dark.

On the basis of this observation, the region with the highest variation in brightness can be considered as the probable location of the ONH (Sinthanayothin et al. 1999). Another strategy is to search for a bright circular region. The edges are detected and used in template matching (Lalonde et al. 2001) or Hough transformation (Chrastek et al. 2004; Aquino et al. 2010; Zhu et al. 2010) in order to locate and/or segment circular objects. In addition, the blood vessel network is an important feature for locating the ONH. The convergence of vessels (Hoover and Goldbaum 2003) and their orientation (Foracchia et al. 2004; Youssif et al. 2008) can indicate the origin of major vessel arches (vertex of parabolas), where the ONH lies. For these approaches, retinal blood vessels must be detected and thinned. The positional relationship between normal structures may be nontrivial information in the search for their locations. The fovea is located on or near the axis of the vessel parabola with its vertex at the ONH at a distance of about twice the diameter of the ONH. Such information can be used to create a probability or reliability map (Perez-Rovira and Trucco 2008).

In many cases, several pieces of information regarding the brightness, blood vessels, and their positional relationship are combined to make the ultimate decision. These features can be used to create probability maps, which would be combined with the prior probability map based on the location of the ONH in training cases, and the posterior probability map suggests the likeliest position (Tobin et al. 2007). In another method, these data are entered into a statistical learning machine, namely, the k-nearest neighbor (kNN) regressor (Devroye et al. 1996), in order to estimate the distances of each pixel to the ONH and fovea (Niemeijer et al. 2009). The pixel with the shortest distance to the ONH is determined as the point of interest after smoothing. Some of these studies have been evaluated using common databases, thus facilitating comparison of their results (Perez-Rovira and Trucco 2008; Zhu et al. 2010).

Most, if not all, of the computer algorithms introduced earlier have achieved high sensitivity rates (above 90%) for ONH detection. Accurate segmentation of the ONH can be even difficult for humans in cases where the ONH is titled or peripapillary chorioretinal atrophy (PPA) is present. In fact, intra- and inter-reader variations are known to exist, although much smaller than those for cup segmentation (Tielsch et al. 1988; Verma et al. 1989). In our experience, the agreement of disk segmentation between readers in terms of the ratio of the region of intersection to the region of union ranged from 0.90 to 0.94 (Muramatsu et al. 2011b). This small but significant variation may make consistent evaluation of the segmentation results difficult, due to the absence of a concrete gold standard.

17.2.2.2 ONH Segmentation

Several research groups have proposed automated schemes for segmentation of the ONH. The common procedure is to first detect the approximate location of the ONH, followed by a precise segmentation. In one study, the bright region with a prespecified range of areas is roughly extracted, and then after suppressing major vessels with a closing operation, the ONH is segmented using the watershed method (Walter and Klein 2001). In another study, the optic nerve region is transformed to a polar coordinate system, and an optimal path corresponding to the ONH border is searched using a cost function based on edge strength, texture, and smoothness constraints (Merickel et al. 2006). A model-based approach can be used to extract normal structures (Li and Chutatape 2004). Landmarks are placed on the border of the ONH and on a large vessel inside the ONH, and the size and orientation of the ONH are adjusted by matching these points to those of the model created with training cases.

A popular strategy is the use of deformable models such as Snakes (Osareh et al. 2002; Xu et al. 2008), circular deformable model (Lowell et al. 2004), level set method (Wong et al. 2008), or another deformable model (Kande et al. 2009). In these methods, the plausible outline is determined by energy optimization, which is generally based on edge strength and smoothness. When employing a deformable model, the initialization may strongly influence the final results. One group proposed a method using genetic algorithm (GA; Carmona et al. 2008), in which probable edge points, called hypothesis points, where the brightness drops radically are first searched radially, and the GA determines the ellipse that includes the largest number of hypothesis points. A pixel classification method was investigated by the

same research group (Abramoff et al. 2007) that proposed the pixel regression method for ONH detection. In this method, the pixels around the ONH region are classified as rim, cup, and background by using the kNN classifier and Gaussian filter bank features.

Authors have compared three different methods: the Snakes active contour model and two pixel classification methods using fuzzy c-means (FCM) clustering and a neural network (NN; Muramatsu et al. 2011b). In this study, the approximate location of the ONH is determined by selecting the center of a region with a maximum area that satisfies the circularity criterion after applying a percentile thresholding method. Edge detection is performed by applying the Canny edge detector on the *blood-vessel-erased* image, which will be described in the next section. For Snakes, the ONH contour is determined by energy minimization based on edge information and contour smoothness. For FCM and NN, images features, such as the original pixel values, the pixel values in surrounding pixels, the contrast, and edge information, are used. These methods were evaluated using separate datasets obtained by two camera systems. In this study, the active contour model and the NN-based method achieved slightly better performance than the FCM-based method, although the difference was very small. The results from the three methods are shown in Figure 17.2.

The results of computer algorithms are often evaluated by comparison with manual contours. Current computerized segmentation schemes work fairly well for normal cases with decent image quality; however, it seems that accurate segmentation of low contrasted ONHs and ONHs with PPA still remains a subject for future investigation.

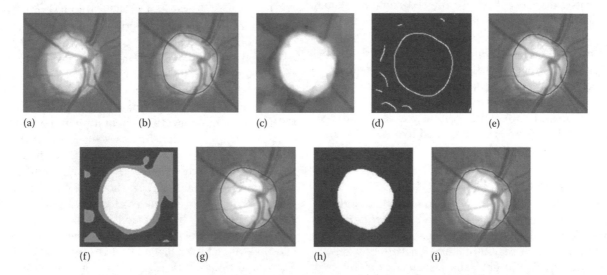

(a)   (b)   (c)   (d)   (e)

(f)   (g)   (h)   (i)

Figure 17.2 Results of ONH segmentation by the three methods. (a) Original image, (b) manual outline by an ophthalmologist, (c) red channel image of the *blood-vessel-erased* image, (d) edge image, (e) outline by the Snakes method, (f) pixel classification result by the FCM method, (g) outline by the FCM method, (h) pixel classification result by the NN method, and (i) outline by the NN method.

17.2.3 Segmentation of Retinal Blood Vessels

As mentioned earlier, the retinal blood vessels can be observed in retinal fundus images without the use of a contrast agent. Although fluorescence images can be obtained with a contrast agent to better visualize capillaries and microaneurysms, they are not routinely utilized. In fundus photographs, blood vessels appear dark and decrease in caliber size from the ONH periphery toward the macula region and the edge of the FOV. Normally, arteries are slightly narrower and lighter red than the collateral veins. In principle, automated segmentation schemes for retinal vessels may be similar to the vessel segmentation methods in angiography and other segmentation algorithms for linear objects.

There have been numerous studies aimed at retinal vessel segmentation in fundus images, and it is still an active research topic. The fundamental procedures include preprocessing of images, vessel enhancement by various filters, and the final determination of vessel regions. Because the green component of RGB images gives the highest contrast for blood vessels, the majority of the computerized schemes utilize green-channel images. In rare cases, red-free images and other color representations are used. The preprocessing techniques include a smoothing operation for noise reduction, contrast normalization, and illumination equalization, which are also employed in ONH segmentation. One preprocessing technique that may be distinctive for the vessel segmentation is a morphological opening operation to reduce the effect of the central light reflex (Marin et al. 2011). Although the profile of a vessel is generally Gaussian shaped, when a flash of light is reflected by the blood, the central part may appear brighter than the vessel walls. This effect, called the central light reflex, can potentially cause some parts of vessels to be misdetected. A morphological opening with a small kernel size may remove these centerlines.

Many variations in filters, vessel models, and other operators are applied for the enhancement or segmentation of blood vessels. Some of these can be grouped as top-hat filters (Condurache and Aach 2006; Mendonca and Campilho 2006; Marin et al. 2011), Gabor filters (Chen and Tian 2008), matched filters with Gaussian profiles (Sofka and Stewart 2006; Al-Rawi et al. 2007; Wu et al. 2007; Kande et al. 2010b; Villalobos-Castaldi et al. 2010), line operators (Mendonca and Campilho 2006; Perfetti et al. 2007; Farnell et al. 2008), and Hessian-based operators (Condurache and Aach 2006). A top-hat filter can enhance a signal that is smaller than the filter element. A popular filter shape is a circle with a diameter larger than that of the thickest vessel. However, this filter would also enhance round objects. Other filters, such as Gabor filters, Gaussian filters, and line filters, are intended to selectively enhance tube-like objects. To enhance vessels of various sizes, filters with multiple sizes in different orientations must be applied. In many studies, the filters are rotated in 12 different directions every 15°. In order to reduce computational costs, a specific direction can be selected in advance by calculating the derivative or the Hessian matrix (Wu et al. 2007; Chen and Tian 2008). Although vessels with different sizes can be enhanced simultaneously with the Hessian-based approach, the edges are also enhanced. In such cases, the presence of parallel edges in which the gradients are in opposite directions is used to distinguish between vessels and edges (Cai and Chung 2006; Sofka and Stewart 2006; Salem et al. 2007). Derivative-based methods are also used to detect ridges, and as a result, the centerline pixels of vessels are determined (Staal et al. 2004; Garg et al. 2007; Salem et al. 2007). Using the centerlines, vessel regions can be segmented by the region growing method, or features can be determined, which are then used in the classification step.

When vessel-like structures are enhanced by filtering, vessel segmentation can be achieved by simply applying a threshold (Al-Rawi et al. 2007; Perfetti et al. 2007; Anzalone et al. 2008; Farnell et al. 2008) or using clustering methods, such as an FCM clustering (Kande et al. 2010). In other studies, features were determined based on the filter output and/or the original images, which were then employed for classifying vessel pixels and nonvessel pixels using various classifiers, such as kNN (Staal et al. 2004), SVM (Ricci and Perfetti 2007), NN (Marin et al. 2011), Bayesian classifier (Soares et al. 2006), and hysteresis classifier, which is a combination of two linear classifiers (Condurache and Aach 2006).

Using thresholding and pixel classification methods, part of a vessel may be missed. One simple way to fill these gaps is a morphological operation; however, when the gaps are large, they cannot be successfully filled. Instead, because all vessels must be connected to the large vessels near the ONH, various vessel-tracing schemes have been proposed. In some methods, several seed points are selected on pixels with a high likelihood of a vessel, and then the vessels can be traced in the likely direction (Delibasis et al. 2010), or eight neighbor pixels may be tested for their vessel likeliness (Vlachos and Dermatas 2010). In another method, first, a strict threshold is applied, and then in the tracked local window, a less strict threshold is selected (Cai and Chung 2006). In this way, low-contrast vessels can be detected without a large increase in false-positive detection.

Authors of this chapter have also attempted to perform the segmentation of blood vessels as a part of various CAD schemes, which will be introduced in the later sections. The presence of blood vessels can be an obstacle for both the detection of pathologic lesions and segmentation of the ONH. In these cases, blood vessels are detected by the use of the top-hat filter, and pixels corresponding to the vessels are interpolated by the surrounding retinal pixels to create a *blood-vessel-erased* image (Nakagawa et al. 2008). In the method for vessel diameter measurement, a modified method based on a combination of the top-hat filter and the double ring filter is used to improve the sensitivity and specificity when segmenting large vessels (Muramatsu et al. 2011a).

For the evaluation of computerized segmentation, receiver operating characteristic (ROC) analysis is often used. Because most of pixels in retinal fundus images constitute nonvessel pixels (generally more than 85%), the performance, in terms of area under the curve, appears to be relatively high (above 0.90). Other indices include measures of overlap in vessel pixels, such as the fraction of pixels correctly identified as vessel (sensitivity) or the ratio of the area of intersection to the area of union. In the evaluation, manual segmentation results are considered the gold standard. However, the manual segmentation process is a time-consuming and difficult task due to the low contrast of tiny vessels. In addition, vessel walls are often diffused making it difficult to determine the exact borderlines. Segmentation can vary depending on the reader, since one reader may trace further down to very thin peripheral vessels than others. As a result, inter-reader variation can be seen to some extent in manual segmentation results. In fact, the accuracy of segmentation, based on the pixel-wise sensitivity and specificity, by a second observer in the DRIVE database is 0.95, with a κ statistic value of 0.76. Many studies of retinal vessel segmentation schemes have utilized public databases for comparative evaluation and because of the availability of the gold standard. The results of some earlier studies can be visually compared and tabulated on the DRIVE website.

17.3 COMPUTERIZED DIAGNOSIS OF GLAUCOMA IN RETINAL FUNDUS IMAGES

Glaucoma is the second leading cause of vision loss in the world, and it is expected to affect about 80 million people in the year 2020 (Quigley and Broman 2006). Because of its slow progressive nature, many patients are unaware of this visual disturbance until the disease reaches an advanced stage. In a population-based prevalence survey of glaucoma in Tajimi, Japan, it was found that 93% of examinees who had primary open-angle glaucoma were previously undiagnosed (Iwase et al. 2004). Early detection of glaucomatous changes is the key to minimizing the chance of significant visual disability. Glaucoma is generally diagnosed by a combination of several tests, which may include ophthalmoscopy, intraocular pressure measurement, visual field testing, retinal fundus photography, Heidelberg retinal tomography (HRT), scanning laser ophthalmoscopy, and

optical coherence tomography (OCT). A retinal fundus photograph is often obtained as a diagnostic record not only for glaucoma but also for other eye diseases. In addition, it can sometimes be used in internal medicine. Because of its relatively simple procedure and low cost, it is well suited for screening examinations.

17.3.1 Detection of Retinal Nerve Fiber Layer Defect

One of the earliest signs of glaucoma are retinal nerve fiber layer defects (NFLDs), which can be observed as dark striations extending from the ONH. There have been several studies about the analysis of NFL using different image modalities, such as fundus photography, scanning laser polarimetry, and OCT. However, to the authors' knowledge, only a few studies have reported the computerized detection and quantification of NFLDs in retinal fundus images. Because retinal fundus photography is widely used, computerized analysis of NFL on fundus photographs could be very informative.

In the earliest study, NFL striation measurement was attempted by comparing the variation in pixel values across the NFL to that along the NFL (Peli et al. 1989). Another group proposed quantification of NFL based on the intensity profile around the ONH. The thickness of the NFLD was measured by taking the first derivative of the intensity profile upon locating its borders (Lee et al. 2004). Texture analysis of NFL may be useful for the detection of cases with NFLD. Using the texture features from the gray level run length matrix, normal eyes and eyes with NFLD were classified by linear discriminant analysis (LDA; Yogesan et al. 1998). The use of other texture features based on the Markov random field was suggested, which was found to be potentially useful for classifying regions of NFLD in glaucoma patients and regions of NFL in normal patients; however, the distinction between defected and nondefected regions in glaucoma patients was more difficult (Kolar and Vacha 2009).

A computerized detection method for NFLDs based on image transformation and Gabor filtering has been investigated (Muramatsu et al. 2010). To facilitate NFLD detection, the images are transformed such that the NFLDs, which are shaped like curved bands or fans in the original images, appear relatively straight. The approximate directions of the nerve fibers in a fovea-centered image are modeled by a set of elliptic lines with respect to the ONH center, and an image transformation is performed that is similar to a polar transformation. After brightness correction, the vertically oriented Gabor filters are applied to enhance NFLDs, and the NN is employed for the classification of candidate regions based on some simple image features. This series of procedures is illustrated in Figure 17.3.

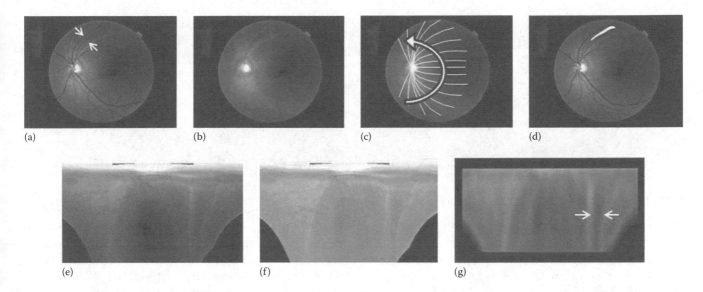

Figure 17.3 An illustration of the NFLD detection method. (a) Original image with arrows specifying an NFLD, (b) the blood-vessel-erased image, (c) elliptic lines approximating the directions of nerve fibers, (d) the computerized detection result, (e) the transformed image, (f) the brightness-corrected image, and (g) the filtered image with arrows indicating the NFLD.

In earlier studies, small numbers of cases (less than 15 cases) were used in the evaluation (Peli et al. 1989; Yogesan et al. 1998; Lee et al. 2004). In one study, glaucoma cases with NFLD and normal cases were classified with 80%–90% accuracy (Yogesan et al. 1998). Sampled regions of interest were analyzed in two studies; the determined feature was moderately correlated (approximately 0.6) with the disease grading by two observers in one study (Peli et al. 1989), whereas defected regions and normal regions sampled from 30 cases were distinguished with 96% accuracy in another (Kolar and Vacha 2009). In our study, a sensitivity of 90% with 1.0 false positive per image was achieved in 81 cases with NFLDs and 81 cases without NFLDs (Muramatsu et al. 2010). Further investigations are expected for the analysis of retinal nerve fibers.

17.3.2 Analysis of Optic Nerve Head

Another major sign of glaucoma is deformation of the ONH. The ONH is generally shaped like a pit where the retinal nerves and blood vessels leave the fundus. When optic nerves are damaged, the rim becomes thin, and the cup enlarges, as shown in Figure 17.4. In general, this deformation, known as cupping in early glaucoma, is more likely to be observed in the inferior and superior parts of the ONH. Therefore, cup–disk diameter ratio (CDR), especially in the vertical direction, as shown in Figure 17.4, is considered an index for the diagnosis of glaucoma (Gloster and Parry 1974). However, in clinical practice, cup and disk diameters are rarely quantitatively measured due to the limited time for diagnosis. In addition, because of the difficulty in

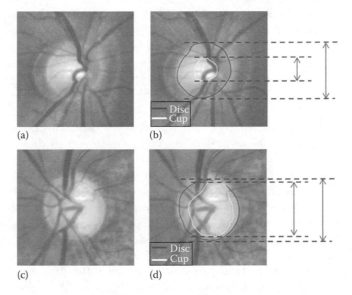

Figure 17.4 The comparison of the normal and glaucomatous ONHs. (a) Normal ONH, (b) the cup and disk outlines by an ophthalmologist, (c) glaucomatous ONH, and (d) the manual outlines.

identifying the cup border in retinal fundus images, intra- and inter-reader variations are not small. Figure 17.5 shows the outlines of cup and disk determined by three expert ophthalmologists. Although the three ophthalmologists agree that this patient has glaucoma, the CDRs based on these outlines range from 0.81 to 0.94. Therefore, computerized measurement of CDR may facilitate consistent diagnosis and longitudinal comparisons while saving ophthalmologists' time.

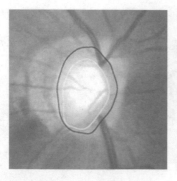 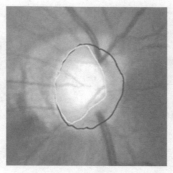 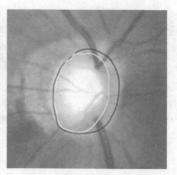

Figure 17.5   Manual outlines of cup and disk by three ophthalmologists.

17.3.2.1   Determination of CDR on Plain Photograph

Despite the difficulty in determining cup boundaries on retinal fundus images, a few research groups have investigated computerized methods for measuring CDRs. Using red and green color planes for disk and cup, respectively, closing and opening operations were applied for smoothing edges and removing some white lesions, and the CDR was determined by measuring the remaining areas using a simple thresholding technique (Nayak et al. 2009). In another study, the level set method was applied to the green plane, and the cup region was determined by fitting an ellipse to the convex points on the output (Zhang et al. 2009). These methods utilize the fact that the cup regions appear brighter than the rim regions. When ophthalmologists read images, they also take into account the vessel directions and their bending points. By detecting the retinal vessels and identifying their kinks inside the optic disk, the cup contour may be determined (Wong et al. 2010).

Because the determination of cup borders is difficult, especially on the temporal side, due to the absence of clear edges and the sparseness of reference vessels, a method for estimating the CDR using the pixel value profiles in the vertical direction was proposed (Hatanaka et al. 2010). After automated determination of the disk outline, several vertical profiles near the center of the disk were obtained from the blood-vessel-erased images. These profiles were averaged and smoothed to reduce the effect of noise, and the cup border points were determined on the basis of the second derivative of the profile. The vertical profiles for normal and glaucomatous cases are shown in Figure 17.6.

17.3.2.2   Determination of CDR on Stereo Photographs

As mentioned earlier, determination of the cup boundary in a plain photograph is difficult even for well-trained ophthalmologists. Therefore, to capture the 3D structure of the ONH, stereo imaging was suggested. Stereo retinal fundus cameras have been marketed by several companies.

Using these devices, a pair of images focused on the ONH, generally with a narrow optic angle, is obtained simultaneously or with an instant delay. Some computerized methods have been proposed for determining CDR in stereo images. In one study, stereo disparities were determined by calculating the cross-correlation in edge-enhanced images. The cup and disk contours were determined semi-automatically based on iso-disparity contours (Corona et al. 2002). Another group investigated two matching methods, including cross-correlation and minimum feature difference, for disparity determination (Xu et al. 2008). In their method, the disk contour was determined using a deformable model, and then the cup margin was located at a prespecified depth from the disk margin. As introduced earlier, the regions of the cup, rim, and background (retina) were determined by the pixel classification method on stereo images by another group (Abramoff et al. 2007). In addition to the color-based features, stereo disparity features were included for the classification, and the CDR was determined by counting the numbers of pixels in the cup and rim groups.

The cross-correlation for the disparity measurement was also utilized by another group (Nakagawa et al. 2008). The disk region was determined using one image of the pair that was imaged first, and then the corresponding region in the other image was extracted by global matching based on the cross-correlation. An apparent disparity due to the patient's motion can be disregarded by this procedure, so that the *real* disparity due to depth remains. The depths were determined at every four pixels by locating the corresponding points with local cross-correlation. Figure 17.7 shows a depth map reconstructed using this method and the corresponding HRT image. The cup outline was determined by searching for the maximum gradient points in radial directions in the depth map.

Same as the evaluation of disk segmentation, cup segmentation results and CDR measurement are often evaluated in comparison with the manual contours and measurements provided by ophthalmologists. The reported correlation coefficient for the performance of

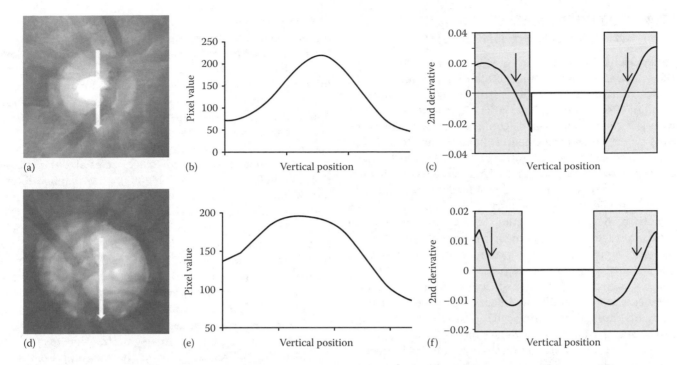

Figure 17.6 The vertical pixel value profiles of the ONHs. Cases with (a) normal and (d) glaucomatous ONHs, (b, e) the smoothed profiles of (a) and (d), and (c, f) the second derivatives of (b) and (e) in effective regions (shaded regions) with the selected cup margin locations indicated by arrows.

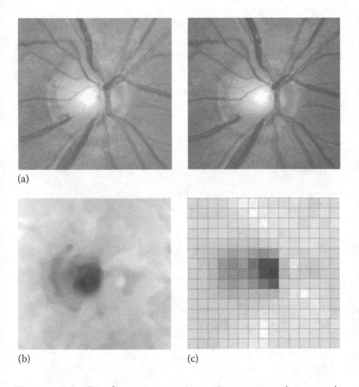

Figure 17.7 Depth reconstruction using a stereo image pair. (a) A stereo image pair, (b) the depth map reconstructed by the cross-correlation-based method, and (c) the HRT image.

the computerized measurement of the CDRs in comparison to the manual measurements ranged from 0.67 to 0.93. In contrast, the performance for the classification of glaucomatous and nonglaucomatous eyes based on CDRs in terms of AUC was approximately 0.8–0.9. However, these results were evaluated by the use of proprietary databases with different numbers of cases, different fractions of glaucoma cases, and a variety of image characteristics, which makes the comparison difficult. In our experience, it is more difficult to determine cup outlines in nonglaucomatous eyes than in glaucomatous eyes, even for ophthalmologists, because nonglaucomatous eyes tend to have sloping cups, while glaucomatous eyes have cups that are likely to have sharp edges. The establishment of a gold standard may be a common problem in CAD research. For depth measurement, data from another modality, such as HRT, may be used as a reference. For glaucoma diagnosis, the results of visual field testing would be considered the gold standard; however, some glaucoma cases may not exhibit cupping. Other image findings and risk factors for glaucoma include disk hemorrhage, shifting of blood vessels, and the presence of PPA, and some of these have been incorporated into the computerized analysis. As more glaucoma diagnosis studies are reported, common databases for the evaluation of computerized schemes are expected to be established.

17.4   COMPUTERIZED DIAGNOSIS OF DIABETIC RETINOPATHY

Patients with diabetes are at considerable risk of developing DR, which is a leading cause of blindness in adults in the United States. Although the prevalence is decreasing as a result of efforts to reduce the risks, the number of patients with severe eye impairment could be further reduced by early detection and treatment. DR can be largely classified into two stages: nonproliferative retinopathy, which can be characterized by the presence of microaneurysms, hemorrhages, and hard exudates, and proliferative retinopathy, in which the microvascular abnormality progresses and the growth of new vessels occurs. Similar to glaucoma, in the early stage, patients often have no symptoms. Although the early signs, such as the presence of microaneurysms and hemorrhages, can be detected more easily with fluorescein angiograms, the use of fluorescein images is limited because they require an injection of a contrast media. Therefore, annual screening with retinal fundus imaging can be effective for the early detection of DR.

A large number of studies on the computerized detection of DR-related lesions and the diagnosis of DR on retinal fundus images can be found in the literature. A comprehensive review of the algorithms for DR detection can also be found (Winder et al. 2009). Many of these studies used relatively large numbers of data, some of which was obtained from large screening programs, indicating the high prevalence of the disease and the interest in this topic. The computerized schemes focus on the two types of lesions as shown in Figure 17.8: red lesions, including microaneurysms and hemorrhages, and white lesions, including the hard exudates and soft exudates, also called cotton wool spots.

A common strategy for detecting red lesions includes the detection of blood vessels, which tend to be the sources of false positives. Similar techniques are used for detecting the red and white lesions, the difference being whether bright areas with high pixel values or dark areas with low pixel values are on the target. Some of the techniques used for detecting the red and white lesions include the top-hat transformation, which was originally proposed for fluorescein angiograms (Spencer et al. 1996; Dupas et al. 2010), region growing (Cree et al. 1997; Usher et al. 2003; Singalavanija et al. 2006; Nagayoshi et al. 2009), template matching (Singalavanija et al. 2006; Bae et al. 2011), adaptive thresholding (Garcia et al. 2009), and matched filtering (Kande et al. 2010a). One group employed template matching in wavelet-transformed images to simplify the parameters of the template that was the Gaussian function model for microaneurysms (Quellec et al. 2008). Based on the insight that a large number of false positives appear to be nearby blood vessels, two classifiers, one for candidates near vessels and one for the others, with different sets of features were used for false-positive reduction (Nagayoshi et al. 2009). Another group proposed a red and white lesion detection method based on the image subtraction technique, in which the differences between the rough and detailed images created by the smoothing filters with different sizes are highlighted (Hatanaka et al. 2008).

Machine learning techniques have been employed by a number of groups. An image is divided into grids, and these regions of interest are classified as background (retina), vessel, exudates, and hemorrhages by use of an artificial neural network (ANN; Gardner et al. 1996). Another group employed the kNN for the classification of pixels as normal background and candidate pixels, which were then clustered using region growing to form candidate lesions (Niemeijer et al. 2005, 2007). ANN was also used for the classification of a case as normal or DR using image features extracted from the whole image (Nayak et al. 2008). In other studies,

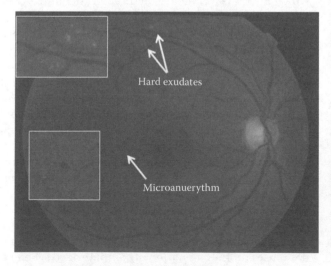

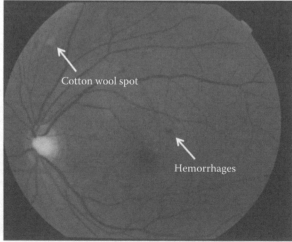

Figure 17.8   Examples of red and white lesions.

a radial basis function NN and support vector machines (SVMs) were used to classify the true lesions and false positives (Usher et al. 2003; Acharya et al. 2009; Garcia et al. 2009; Kande et al. 2010).

In majority of the algorithms, the green plane of the color images was used because of its high contrast in DR-related lesions. In one study, intensity and hue in the HSI space were employed as features for coarse segmentation by FCM clustering, which was then followed by fine segmentation using morphological operations (Sopharak et al. 2009).

In one of the earlier studies, measurement of the exudates was attempted (Phillips et al. 1993). A multithresholding technique was applied to identify large bright exudates and small lower-intensity exudates, and then the results were compared with the manually extracted regions in terms of their overlap, rather than just detection. Generally, in the field of CAD, when the centers of a detected area and the reference lesion are close or when their overlap is large, it is considered a true detection. Conversely, other detected regions are counted as false positives. Because of their shape and appearance, it may be difficult to evaluate the detection performance for hard exudates compared to other types of lesions that can be counted and the center of which can be more easily determined. It is unclear how the sensitivity of hard exudates should be determined. In some studies, the case sensitivity in terms of the *detection of at least one lesion* criterion is employed. This criterion is also applied to determining DR cases and normal cases, such that a case with at least one red or white lesion detected is considered a DR case.

Another issue in the evaluation of the algorithms is that the identification of red lesions, especially the microaneurysms, may be difficult and susceptible to inter-reader variability. Manual identification by multiple readers is desirable to increase the reliability of the gold standard. In some studies, the computer performance is evaluated in terms of lesion-based sensitivity, whereas in others, the case-based sensitivity for distinguishing between DR and non-DR cases is employed. In some studies, the cases are classified into normal and different stages of DR based on the number of lesions detected.

For the detection of DR, the reported lesion-based sensitivities range from about 75% to 95%, whereas the case-based sensitivities can be as high as 100%, with specificities ranging from 46% to 87%. However, these results were evaluated on different databases and, therefore, cannot be compared. To facilitate their comparison, the ROC database was provided, and an algorithm contest for the detection of microaneurysms was held at the 2009 CAD Conference of SPIE Medical Imaging. Brief descriptions of the algorithms developed by the participating groups and their results can be found in the literature (Niemeijer et al. 2010b). The results in terms of the FROC curve are not very high, indicating the difficulty of the cases included. The evaluation of the methods on a common database is desirable and could promote the research. However, the development of a high-quality open database is not easy and would require a great deal of effort.

17.5 COMPUTERIZED DIAGNOSIS OF HYPERTENSIVE RETINOPATHY AND ARTERIOSCLEROSIS

As discussed earlier, the noninvasive visualization of vasculatures is possible through retinal fundus examination, which allows for the detection of arteriolar narrowing and vessel occlusions. Studies have reported the association of retinal microvascular abnormalities with stroke and coronary heart disease, which are major clinical problems (Wong et al. 2001; McClintic et al. 2010). When the retina is damaged as a result of hypertension, hypertensive retinopathy is diagnosed, which may cause visual disturbance and vision loss. One early sign of hypertensive changes is arteriolar narrowing, and as the disease progresses, hemorrhages and hard and soft exudates can also be observed. Arteriosclerosis is considered a main cause of the vessel occlusions. Arteriosclerotic retinopathy may not damage vision, but it is a hazardous sign of arteriosclerosis in the entire body. In retinal fundus images, an early sclerotic change can be seen as arteriovenous crossing phenomena, followed by silver- and copper-wire arteries (Scheie 1953).

17.5.1 Measurement of Arteriolar-to-Venular Diameter Ratio

Arteriolar narrowing in retinal fundus images is generally assessed by the arteriolar-to-venular diameter ratio (AVR). For the evaluation of arteriolar narrowing, the idea of *equivalent central retinal artery width*, the formula of which is based on the widths of vessel branches and their parent trunk, is first proposed (Parr and Spears 1974). Simplified versions of this formula for arteries and veins, namely, the central retinal artery equivalent (CRAE) and the central retinal vein equivalent (CRVE), are later introduced (Hubbard et al. 1999), which are further revised using each of the six largest arteries and veins (Knudtson et al. 2003). The ratio of CRAE and CRVE is often employed for the measurement of AVR on ONH-centered images, as shown in Figure 17.9a. Conversely, in regular macula-centered fundus images, the ratio of the diameters of a major artery and vein pair running side by side each on the upper and lower temporal sides has been recommended in the guideline in Japan (Figure 17.9b). In either case, the measurement is made around the ONH, from a ¼- or ½- to a 1-disk diameter from

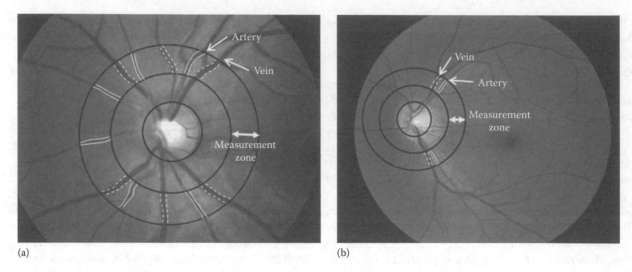

(a)   (b)

Figure 17.9 Selection of arteries and veins for the measurement of AVR in (a) an ONH-centered image and (b) a macula-centered image.

the ONH margin. Recently, a study reported a comparable association for this measurement with cardiovascular risk factors using an extended zone up to a two-disk diameter (Cheung et al. 2010).

Several semi-automated methods for the measurement of AVR have been proposed in which operators manually identified the vessels of interest. Subsequently, the diameters were calculated on the basis of the standard deviation, σ, of fitted Gaussian curves (Gao et al. 2000), the full-width at half maximum of the profile (Pederson et al. 2000), or the edges of vessel walls detected by the Sobel operator (Pakter et al. 2005). Other studies also proposed the use of Gaussian models. An amplitude-modified second-order Gaussian filter is used for the detection and measurement of retinal vessels (Gang et al. 2002). A difference-of-Gaussians model, in which a smaller Gaussian curve is subtracted from a larger one, is used for vessels with light reflex (Lowell et al. 2004). In these studies, vessel widths were determined as a function of σ, or by the second derivative of the model; however, the AVR was not measured.

For the fully automated measurement of AVR, the determination of vessel walls as well as the detection and selection of retinal vessels is required. In addition, the identification of the ONH and the determination of its diameter are often necessary for the selection of the measurement zone. As described in the earlier sections, numerous studies on the automated segmentation of retinal vessels and the ONH have been proposed. Some of these groups have investigated the automated measurement of AVR. After the retinal vessels and the ONH are extracted, the vessels were classified into arteries and veins using a feature characterizing the central reflex, and those with diameters greater than 45 µm were selected for the estimation of AVR (Tramontan et al. 2008). Another group investigated several

classifiers for the classification of arteries and veins, namely, kNN, SVM, LDA, and quadratic discriminant analysis, and the six widest arteries and veins were selected for AVR measurement (Niemeijer et al. 2010a). Another method that does not require vessel detection is proposed (Nam et al. 2009). Using a circular intensity profile at a distance from the ONH, the valleys, which correspond to dark pixels, are classified into arteries and veins according to their shapes, and the vessels larger than a prespecified value are used for AVR calculation.

A method for determining the AVR on macula-centered images was proposed (Muramatsu et al. 2011a). The ONH is segmented and fitted by an ellipse to select the measurement zone. After detecting the vessels, they are partitioned to segments at the bifurcations and intersections, and these segments are classified into arteries and veins using a linear classifier with the color and contrast features. Two pairs of arteries and veins in the upper and lower temporal regions are selected by a set of rules based on vessel orientation and thickness.

The performance of the automated AVR measurement is compared to those manually or semi-manually determined measurements using open software (IVAN; the University of Wisconsin in Madison, United States), and the high correlations (about 0.9) among the computer estimates and the references were reported. For the accurate measurement of the AVR, acquisition of high-resolution images of reasonable quality is essential.

17.5.2 Detection of Arteriovenous Crossing Phenomenon

The arteriovenous crossing phenomenon (AVCP), also called arteriovenous nicking, is the state in which a vein that is constricted by a stiffened artery appears narrower at an artery–vein (AV) crossing. Although there are many studies on automated retinal vessel segmentation and analysis, to our knowledge, in the literature, there is no study focused on the detection of AVCP. Authors have been investigating an automated method for the detection of the AVCP in retinal fundus images (Hatanaka et al. 2009). Our approach consists of the detection of retinal vessels, the detection of AV crossings, and the measurement of venous diameters at two points, one in the vicinity of the crossing and another at a distance from the crossing. After the retinal vessels are segmented by using a double ring filter or the other techniques, a ring filter with radius r is scanned to search for points where more than four vessels cross the perimeter of the ring. If more than four vessels are present, the vessels are paired by checking locations across the perimeter. The two pairs of vessels are classified as an artery pair and a vein pair on the basis of the pixel values in the red and green components. Finally, two diameters of the veins are measured, one of which is represented by the minimum diameter between the crossing point and $1/2r$, and the other is represented by the average diameter between $1/2r$ and the perimeter of the ring. In our study, the presence of AVCP is suspected if the ratio of the diameters is less than 0.8. The performance of the computerized scheme in terms of crossing detection and AVCP detection is currently not very high, due in part to the lack of a high-quality database; therefore, improvement is expected in the future.

17.6 EMERGING TOPIC: COMPUTER ANALYSIS OF OPTICAL COHERENCE TOMOGRAPHY

In recent years, OCT has been used frequently in ophthalmology examinations. As a result, it has gained much interest in the research community. With OCT, a cross-sectional view of the retina can be obtained, allowing for the quantitative measurement of retinal nerves and the detection of macular holes and the other macular pathologies. There are only a few studies related to CAD on OCT at present; however, the number is expected to increase in the future.

An automated layer segmentation technique was proposed and tested on a small number of OCT cases (Lu et al. 2010). By detecting retinal blood vessels using an iterative polynomial smoothing technique, the retinal layers are divided into vessel and nonvessel sections. On the basis of variation across the boundaries, the borders of the nonvessel sections are detected, and the layers are classified into five retinal layers. Another group investigated an image

registration method using probabilistic modeling using an expectation–maximization algorithm for the alignment of successive OCT scans, which potentially reduces measurement variability and facilitates longitudinal assessment (Zhu et al. 2011).

Using spectral domain OCT, which provides a high-quality 3D image as a result of its faster acquisition and high resolution, investigators proposed an automated scheme for the segmentation of the optic cup and neural canal opening (NCO), which may correspond to the disk margin in fundus photographs (Hu et al. 2010). In this method, layer surfaces are first segmented on the original image, and a projection image, similar to a fundus photograph, is created by taking some thin layers. By transforming the image into polar coordinates and using it as the cost function, the NCO and cup boundaries are segmented. They reported a relatively high correlation of 0.85 for the CDR when comparing the algorithm to the reference standard.

17.7 CONCLUSION

Retinal examination using retinal fundus images can be effective for the early diagnosis of glaucoma, DR, and hypertensive retinopathy, and it has the potential to reduce the number of patients who suffer vision loss. Fundus photographs are frequently obtained at ophthalmology visits and in certain screening programs. Computer analysis of the retinal images may assist ophthalmologists and other physicians in fast, consistent, and accurate reading of the images. Many studies have been reported on automated segmentation of the ONH and retinal blood vessels. Using these basic algorithms, investigators have proposed the integrated schemes for the diagnosis of the eye diseases. Although the performances reported for ONH and vessel detections are relatively high, some improvements are expected for disease detection and quantification schemes. Investigations of new algorithms for OCT and multimodality approaches may be interesting future topics.

APPENDIX 17.A: PUBLIC DATABASES FOR RETINAL IMAGE ANALYSIS

In this table, concise information about the public databases (some require a registration before downloading) is provided: (a) research groups; (b) website; (c) the number of images; (d) image resolution; (e) image format; and (f) supplemental files, that is, the gold standard.

Structured Analysis of the Retina (STARE; Hoover et al. 2000; Hoover and Goldbaum 2003)	a. The University of California, San Diego and others b. http://www.ces.clemson.edu/~ahoover/stare c. 81 (for ONH detection), 21 (for vessel segmentation) d. 700 × 605 e. Portable pixmap f. Vessel images for 20 cases
Digital Retinal Images for Vessel Extraction (DRIVE; Staal et al. 2004)	a. Utrecht University, the Netherlands b. www.isi.uu.nl/Research/Databases/DRIVE/ c. 40 (20 training cases, 20 test cases) d. 565 × 584 e. TIFF f. Vessel images
Online Retinal Image Archive (ARIA)	a. Royal Liverpool University Hospital Trust and University of Liverpool, UK b. www.eyecharity.com/aria_online.html c. Multiple images from over 100 patients d. 768 × 576 e. JPEG f. Vessel images, ONH outlines, and fovea locations for most images
Retinal Vessel Image set for Estimation of Widths (REVIEW; Al-Diri et al. 2008)	a. The University of Lincoln, UK b. http://reviewdb.lincoln.ac.uk c. 14 full images, two regions of interest d. 1360 × 1024, 2160 × 1440, or 3584 × 2439 (full images) e. JPEG or BMP f. 5066 vessel profiles measured on 193 vessel segments
Standard Diabetic Retinopathy Databases calibration levels 0 and 1 (DIARETDB0, DIARETDB1)	a. Lappeenranta University of Technology, University of Kuopio, and University of Joensuu in Finland b. http://www2.it.lut.fi/project/imageret c. 130 (DB0), 110 (DB1) d. 1500 × 1152 e. PNG f. Presence of retinopathy signs (DB0), fused annotation images of retinopathy lesions marked by four observers (DB1)
Methodes d'Evaluation de Systemes de Segmentation et d'Indexation Dediees a l'Ophtalmologie Retinienne (MESSIDOR)	a. Program partners in France b. http://messidor.crihan.fr/download-en.php c. 1200 d. 1440 × 960, 2240 × 1488, or 2304 × 1536 e. TIFF f. Retinopathy and macular edema grades, and manual ONH contours by separate research group (Aquino et al. 2010)
Retinopathy Online Challenge (ROC)	a. The University of Iowa and others b. webeye.ophth.uiowa.edu/ROC/var.1/www/ c. 100 (50 training cases, 50 test cases) d. Ranging from 768 × 576 to 1394 × 1392 e. JPEG f. Microaneurysm locations (training cases only)
Hamilton Eye Institute Macular Edema Dataset (HEI-MED; Giancardo et al. 2011)	a. The University of Tennessee, Oak Ridge National Laboratory, and the Universite de Bourgogne b. http://vibot.u-bourgogne.fr/luca/heimed.php c. 169 d. 2196 × 1958 e. JPEG f. Bright lesion location (e.g., exudates, cotton wool spots, and drusen)

Friedrich-Alexander University of Erlangen-Nuremberg	a. Friedrich-Alexander University b. www5.cs.fau.de/en/research/data/fundus-images c. 45 d. 3504 × 2336 e. JPEG f. Vessel images

REFERENCES

Abramoff, M.D., W.L.M. Alward, E.C. Greenlee et al. 2007. Automated segmentation of the optic disc from stereo color photographs using physiologically plausible features. *Invest. Ophthalmol. Vis. Sci.* 48:1665–1673.

Acharya, U.R., C.M. Lim, E.Y.K. Ng, C. Chee, and T. Tamura. 2009. Computer-based detection of diabetes retinopathy stages using digital fundus images. *Proc. Inst. Mech. Eng.* 223:545–553.

Al-Diri, B., A. Hunter, D. Steel, M. Habib, T. Hudaib, and S. Berry. 2008. REVIEW—A reference data set for retinal vessel profiles. In: *Conference Proceedings of the IEEE Engineering in Medicine and Biology Society*, Vancouver, British Columbia, Canada, pp. 20–24.

Al-Rawi, M., M. Qutaishat, and M. Arrar. 2007. An improved matched filter for blood vessel detection of digital retinal images. *Comput. Biol. Med.* 37:262–267.

Anzalone, A., F. Bizzarri, M. Parodi, and M. Storace. 2008. A modular supervised algorithm for vessel segmentation in red-free retinal images. *Comput. Biol. Med.* 38:913–922.

Aquino, A., M.E. Gegundez-Arias, and D. Marin. 2010. Detecting the optic disc boundary in digital fundus images using morphological, edge detection, and feature extraction techniques. *IEEE Trans. Med. Imaging* 29:1860–1869.

Bae, J.P., K.G. Kim, H.C. Kang, C.B. Jeong, K.H. Park, and J.M. Hwang. 2011. A study on hemorrhage detection using hybrid method in fundus images. *J. Digit. Imaging* 24:394–404.

Cai, W. and A.C.S. Chung. 2006. Multi-resolution vessel segmentation using normalized cuts in retinal images. In: *MICCAI 2006, LNCS*, Copenhagen, Denmark, Vol. 4191, pp. 928–936.

Carmona, E.J., M. Rincon, J. Garcia-Feijoo, and J.M. Martinez-de-la-Casa. 2008. Identification of the optic nerve head with genetic algorithms. *Artif. Intell. Med.* 43:243–259.

Chen, J. and J. Tian. 2008. Retinal vessel enhancement based on directional field. *Proc. SPIE Med. Imaging* 6914:191422-1–191422-8.

Cheung, C.Y.L., W. Hsu, M.L. Lee et al. 2010. A new method to measure peripheral retinal vascular caliber over an extended area. *Microcirculation* 17:495–503.

Chrastek, R., M. Skokan, L. Kubecka et al. 2004. Multimodal retinal image registration for optic disk segmentation. *Methods Inform. Med.* 43:336–342.

Condurache, A.P. and T. Aach. 2006. Vessel segmentation in 2D projection images using a supervised linear hysteresis classifier. In: *International Conference on Pattern Recognition* Hong Kong, China, pp. 343–346.

Corona, E., S. Mitra, M. Wilson et al. 2002. Digital stereo image analyzer for generating automated 3-D measures of optic disc deformation in glaucoma. *IEEE Trans. Med. Imaging* 21:1244–1253.

Cree, M.J., J.A. Olson, K.C. McHardy, P.F. Sharp, and J.V. Forrester. 1997. A fully automated comparative microaneurysm digital detection system. *Eye* 11:622–628.

Delibasis, K.K., A.I. Kechriniotis, C. Tsonos, and N. Assimakis. 2010. Automatic model-based tracing algorithm for vessel segmentation and diameter estimation. *Comput. Methods Prog. Biomed.* 100:108–122.

Devroye, L., L. Gyorfi, and G. Lugosi. 1996. *A Probabilistic Theory of Pattern Recognition*. New York: Springer-Verlag.

Dupas, B., T. Walter, A. Erginay et al. 2010. Evaluation of automated fundus photograph analysis algorithms for detecting microaneurysms, haemorrhages and exudates, and of a computer-assisted diagnostic system for grading diabetic retinopathy. *Diab. Metab.* 36:213–220.

Farnell, D.J.J., F.N. Hatfield, P. Knox et al. 2008. Enhancement of blood vessels in digital fundus photographs via the application of multiscale line operators. *J. Franklin Inst.* 345:748–765.

Foracchia, M., E. Grisan, and A. Ruggeri. 2004. Detection of optic disc in retinal images by means of a geometrical model of vessel structure. *IEEE Trans. Med. Imaging* 23:1189–1195.

Fujita, H., Y. Uchiyama, T. Nakagawa et al. 2008. Computer-aided diagnosis: The emerging of three CAD systems induced by Japanese health care needs. *Comput. Methods Prog. Biomed.* 92:238–248.

Gang, L., O. Chutatape, and S.M. Krishnan. 2002. Detection and measurement of retinal vessels in fundus images using amplitude modified second-order Gaussian filter. *IEEE Trans. Biomed. Eng.* 49:168–172.

Gao, X.W., A. Bharath, A. Stanton, A. Hughes, N. Chapman, and S. Thom. 2000. Quantification and characterization of arteries in retinal images. *Comput. Methods Prog. Biomed.* 63:133–146.

Garcia, M., C.I. Sanchez, J. Poza, M.I. Lopez, and R. Hornero. 2009. Detection of hard exudates in retinal images using a radial basis function classifier. *Annals Biomed. Eng.* 37:1448–1463.

Gardner, G.G., D. Keating, T.H. Williamson, and A.T. Elliott. 1996. Automatic detection of diabetic retinopathy using an artificial neural network: A screening tool. *Br. J. Ophthalmol.* 80:940–944.

Garg, S., J. Sivaswamy, and S. Chandra. 2007. Unsupervised curvature-based retinal vessel segmentation. In: *International Symposium on Biomedical Imaging*, Arlington, VA, pp. 344–347.

Giancardo, L., T.P. Kamowski, Y. Li, K.W. Tobin, and E. Chaum. 2011. Automatic retinal exudates segmentation without a manually labeled training set. In: *IEEE International Symposium on Biomedical Imaging* Chicago, IL, pp. 1396–1400.

Gloster, J. and D.G. Parry. 1974. Use of photographs for measuring cupping in the optic disc. *Br. J. Ophthalmol.* 58:850–863.

Hatanaka, Y., T. Nakagawa, Y. Hayashi, T. Hara, and H. Fujita. 2008. Improvement of automated detection method of hemorrhages in fundus images. In: *Conference Proceedings of the IEEE Engineering in Medicine and Biology Society*, Vancouver, British Columbia, Canada, pp. 5429–5432.

Hatanaka, Y., A. Noudo, C. Muramatsu et al. 2010. Vertical cup-to-disc ratio measurement for diagnosis of glaucoma on fundus images. *Proc. SPIE Med. Imaging* 7624:76243C-1–76243C-8.

Hatanaka, Y., C. Muramatsu, T. Hara, and H. Fujita. 2009. Automatic arteriovenous crossing phenomenon detection on retinal fundus images. *Proc. SPIE Med. Imaging.* 7963:79633V-1–79633V-8.

Hoover, A. and M. Goldbaum. 2003. Locating the optic nerve in a retinal image using the fuzzy convergence of the blood vessels. *IEEE Trans. Med. Imaging* 22:951–958.

Hoover, A., V. Kouznetxova, and M. Goldbaum. 2000. Locating blood vessels in retinal images by piecewise threshold probing of a matched filter response. *IEEE Trans. Med. Imaging* 19:203–210.

Hu, Z., M.D. Abramoff, Y.H. Kwon, K. Lee, and M.K. Garvin. 2010. Automated segmentation of neural canal opening and optic cup in 3D spectral optical coherence tomography volumes of the optic nerve head. *Invest. Ophthalmol. Vis. Sci.* 51:5708–5717.

Hubbard, L.D., R.J. Brothers, W.N. King et al. 1999. Methods for evaluation of retinal microvascular abnormalities associated with hypertension/sclerosis in the atherosclerosis risk in communities study. *Ophthalmology* 106:2269–2280.

Iwase, A., Y. Suzuki, M. Araie, et al. 2004. The prevalence of primary open-angle glaucoma in Japanese The Tajimi Study. *Ophthalmol.* 111:1641–1648.

Kande, G.B., T.S. Savithri, and P.V. Subbaiah. 2010a. Automatic detection of microaneurysms and hemorrhages in digital fundus images. *J. Digit. Imaging* 23:430–437.

Kande, G.B., P.V. Subbaiah, and T.S. Savithri. 2009. Feature extraction in digital fundus images. *J. Med. Biol. Eng.* 29:122–130.

Kande, G.B., P.V. Subbaiah, and T.S. Savithri. 2010b. Unsupervised fuzzy based vessel segmentation in pathological digital fundus images. *J. Med. Syst.* 34:849–858.

Knudtson, M.D., K.E. Lee, L.D. Hubbard et al. 2003. Revised formulas for summarizing retinal vessel diameters. *Curr. Eye Res.* 27:143–149.

Kolar, R. and P. Vacha. 2009. Texture analysis of the retinal nerve fiber layer in fundus images via Markov Random Fields. In: *IFMBE Proceedings*, Munich, Germany, Vol. 25/XI, pp. 247–250.

Lalonde, M., M. Beaulier, and L. Gagnon. 2001. Fast and robust optic disk detection using pyramidal decomposition and Hausdorff-based template matching. *IEEE Trans. Med. Imaging* 20:1193–1200.

Lee, S.Y., K.K. Kim, J.M. Seo et al. 2004. Automated quantification of retinal nerve fiber layer atrophy in fundus photograph. In: *Conference Proceedings of the IEEE Engineering in Medicine and Biology Society*, San Francisco, CA, pp. 1241–1243.

Li, H. and O. Chutatape. 2004. Automated feature extraction in color retinal images by a model based approach. *IEEE Trans. Biomed. Eng.* 51:246–254.

Lowell, J., A. Hunter, D. Steel, A. Basu, R. Ryder, and R.L. Kennedy. 2004. Measurement of retinal vessel widths from fundus images based on 2-D modeling. *IEEE Trans. Med. Imaging* 23:1196–1204.

Lu, S., C.Y. Cheung, J. Liu, J.H. Lim, C.K. Leung, and T.Y. Wong. 2010. Automated layer segmentation of optical coherence tomography images. *IEEE Trans. Biomed. Eng.* 57:2605–2608.

Marin, D., A. Aquino, M.E. Gegundez-Arias, and M. Bravo. 2011. A new supervised method for blood vessel segmentation in retinal images by using gray-level and moment invariants-based features. *IEEE Trans. Med. Imaging* 30:146–158.

McClintic, B.R., J.I. McClintic, J.D. Bisognano, and R.C. Block. 2010. The relationship between retinal microvascular abnormalities and coronary heart disease: A review. *Am. J. Med.* 123:374e1–374e7.

Mendonca, A.M. and A. Campilho. 2006. Segmentation of retinal blood vessels by combining the detection of centerlines and morphological reconstruction. *IEEE Trans. Med. Imaging* 25:1200–1213.

Merickel, M.B., X. Wu, M. Sonka, and M. Abramoff. 2006. Optimal segmentation of the optic nerve head from stereo retinal images. *Proc. SPIE Med. Imaging* 6243:61433B-1–61433B-2.

Muramatsu, C., Y. Hatanaka, T. Iwase, T. Hara, and H. Fujita. 2011a. Automated selection of major arteries and veins for measurement of arteriolar-to-venular diameter ratio on retinal fundus images. *Comput. Med. Imaging Graph.* 35:472–480.

Muramatsu, C., Y. Hayashi, A. Sawada et al. 2010. Detection of retinal nerve fiber layer defects on retinal fundus images for early diagnosis of glaucoma. *J. Biomed. Opt.* 15:016021-1–016021-7.

Muramatsu, C., T. Nakagawa, A. Sawada et al. 2011b. Automated segmentation of optic disc region on retinal fundus photographs: Comparison of contour modeling and pixel classification methods. *Comput. Methods Prog. Biomed.* 101:23–32.

Nagayoshi, H., Y. Hiramatsu, H. Sako, M. Himaga, and S. Kato. 2009. Detection of fundus lesions using classifier selection. *IEICE Trans. Inform. Syst.* E92D:1168–1176.

Nakagawa, T., T. Suzuki, Y. Hayashi et al. 2008. Quantitative depth analysis of optic nerve head using stereo retinal fundus image pair. *J. Biomed. Opt.* 13:064026-1–064026-10.

Nam, H.S., J.M. Hwang, H. Chung, and J.M. Seo. 2009. Automated measurement of retinal vessel diameters on digital fundus photographs. In: *IFMBE Proceedings*, Munich, Germany, Vol. 25/XI, pp. 277–280.

Nayak, J., R. Acharya, P.S. Bhat, N. Shetty, and T.C. Lim. 2009. Automated diagnosis of glaucoma using digital fundus images. *J. Med. Syst.* 33:337–346.

Nayak, J., P.S. Bhat, R. Acharya, C.M. Lim, and M. Kagathi. 2008. Automated identification of diabetic retinopathy stages using digital fundus images. *J. Med. Syst.* 32:107–115.

Niemeijer, M., M.D. Abramoff, and B. van Ginneken. 2009. Fast detection of the optic disc and fovea in color fundus photographs. *Med. Image Anal.* 13:859–870.

Niemeijer, M., J.J. Staal, B. van Ginneken, M. Loog, and M.D. Abramoff. 2004. Comparable study of retinal vessel segmentation methods on a new publicly available database. *Proc. SPIE Med. Imaging* 5370:648–656.

Niemeijer, M., B. van Ginneken, and M.D. Abramoff. 2010a. Automatic determination of the artery-vein ratio in retinal images. *Proc. SPIE Med. Imaging* 7624:76240I-1–76240I-10.

Niemeijer, M., B. van Ginneken, M.J. Cree et al. 2010b. Retinopathy online challenge: Automatic detection of microaneurysms in digital color fundus photographs. *IEEE Trans. Med. Imaging* 29:185–195.

Niemeijer, M., B. van Ginneken, S.R. Russell, M.S.A. Suttorp-Schulten, and M.D. Abramoff. 2007. Automated detection and differentiation of drusen, exudates, and cotton-wool spots in digital color fundus photographs for diabetic retinopathy diagnosis. *Invest. Ophthalmol. Vis. Sci.* 48:2260–2267.

Niemeijer, M., B. van Ginneken, J. Stall, M.S.A. Suttorp-Schulten, and M.D. Abramoff. 2005. Automatic detection of red lesions in digital color fundus photographs. *IEEE Trans. Med. Imaging* 24:584–592.

Osareh, A., M. Mirmehdi, B. Thomas, and R. Markham. 2002. Comparison of colour spaces for optic disc localization in retinal images. In: *Proceedings of the International Conference on Pattern Recognition*, Quebec City, Canada, pp. 743–746.

Pakter, H.M., E. Ferlin, S.C. Fuchs et al. 2005. Measuring arteriolar-to-venous ratio in retinal photography of patients with hypertension: Development and application of a new semi-automated method. *Am. J. Hypertens.* 18:417–421.

Parr, J.C. and G.F.S. Spears. 1974. General caliber of the retinal arteries expressed as the equivalent width of the central retinal artery. *Am. J. Ophthalmol.* 77:472–477.

Pederson, L., M. Grunkin, B. Ersball et al. 2000. Quantitative measurement of changes in retinal vessel diameter in ocular fundus images. *Pattern Recogn. Lett.* 21:1215–1223.

Peli, E., T.R. Hedges III, and B. Schwartz. 1989. Computer measurement of retinal nerve fiber layer striations. *Appl. Opt.* 28:1128–1134.

Perez-Rovira, A. and E. Trucco. 2008. Robust optic disc location via combination of weak detectors. In: *Conference Proceedings of the IEEE Engineering in Medicine and Biology Society*, Vancouver, British Columbia, Canada, pp. 3542–3545.

Perfetti, R., E. Ricci, D. Casali, and G. Costantini. 2007. Cellular neural networks with virtual template expansion for retinal vessel segmentation. *IEEE Trans. Circuits Syst. II* 54:141–145.

Phillips, R., J. Forrester, and P. Sharp. 1993. Automated detection and quantification of retinal exudates. *Graefe's Arch. Clin. Exp. Ophthalmol.* 231:90–94.

Quellec, G., M. Lamard, P.M. Josselin, G. Cazuguel, B. Cochener, and C. Roux. 2008. Optimal wavelet transform for the detection of microaneurysms in retinal photographs. *IEEE Trans. Med. Imaging* 27:1230–1241.

Quigley, H.A. and A.T. Broman. 2006. The number of people with glaucoma worldwide in 2010 and 2010. *Br. J. Ophthalmol.* 90:262–267.

Resnikoff, S., D. Pscolini, D. Etya'ale et al. 2004. Global data on visual impairment in the year 2002. *Bull. World Health Organ.* 82:844–851.

Ricci, E. and R. Perfetti. 2007. Retinal blood vessel segmentation using line operators and support vector classification. *IEEE Trans. Med. Imaging* 26:1357–1365.

Salem, A.S., N.M. Salem, and A.K. Nandi. 2007. Segmentation of retinal blood vessels using a novel clustering algorithm (RACAL) with a partial supervision strategy. *Med. Biol. Eng. Comput.* 45:261–273.

Scheie, H.G. 1953. Evaluation of ophthalmoscopic changes of hypertension and arteriolar sclerosis. *AMA Arch. Ophthalmol.* 49:117–138.

Singalavanija, A., J. Supokavej, P. Bamroongsuk et al. 2006. Feasibility study on computer-aided screening for diabetic retinopathy. *Jpn. J. Ophthalmol.* 50:361–366.

Sinthanayothin, C., J.F. Boyce, H.L. Cook, and T.H. Williamson. 1999. Automated localization of the optic disc, fovea, and retinal blood vessels from digital colour fundus images. *Br. J. Ophthalmol.* 83:902–910.

Soares, J.V.B., J.J.G. Leandro, R.M. Cesar, H.F. Jelinek, and M.J. Cree. 2006. Retinal vessel segmentation using the 2-D Gabor wavelet and supervised classification. *IEEE Trans. Med. Imaging* 25:1214–1222.

Sofka, M. and C.V. Stewart. 2006. Retinal vessel centerline extraction using multiscale matched filters, confidence and edge measures. *IEEE Trans. Med. Imaging* 25:1531–1546.

Sopharak, A., B. Uyyanonvara, and S. Barman. 2009. Automatic exudate detection from non-dilated diabetic retinopathy retinal images using fuzzy c-means clustering. *Sensors* 9:2148–2161.

Spencer, T., J.A. Olson, D.C. McHardy, P.F. Sharp, and J.V. Forrester. 1996. An image-processing strategy for the segmentation and quantification of microaneurysms in fluorescein angiograms of the ocular fundus. *Comput. Biomed. Res.* 29:284–302.

Staal, J.J., M.D. Abramoff, M. Niemeijer, M.A. Viergever, and B. van Ginneken. 2004. Ridge based vessel segmentation in color images of the retina. *IEEE Trans. Med. Imaging* 23:501–509.

Tielsch, J.M., J. Katz, H.A. Quigley, N.R. Miller, and A. Sommer. 1988. Intraobserver and interobserver agreement in measurement of optic disc characteristics. *Ophthalmology* 95:350–356.

Tobin, K.W., E. Chaum, V.P. Govindassamy, and T.P. Karnowski. 2007. Detection of anatomic structures in human retinal imagery. *IEEE Trans. Med. Imaging* 26:1729–1739.

Tramontan, L., E. Grisan, and A. Ruggeri. 2008. An improved system for the automatic estimation of the arteriolar-to-venular diameter ratio (AVR) in retinal images. In: *Conference Proceedings of the IEEE Engineering in Medicine and Biology Society*, Vancouver, British Columbia, Canada, pp. 20–24.

Usher, D., M. Dumskyj, M. Himaga, T.H. Williamson, S. Nussey, and J. Boyce. 2003. Automated detection of diabetic retinopathy in digital retinal images: A tool for diabetic retinopathy screening. *Diab. Med.* 21:84–90.

Verma, R., G.L. Spaeth, W.C. Steinmann, and L.J. Katz. 1989. Agreement between clinicians and an image analyzer in estimating cup-to-disc ratios. *Arch. Ophthalmol.* 107:526–529.

Villalobos-Castaldi, F.M., E.M. Felipe-Riveron, and L.P. Sanchez-Fernandez. 2010. A fast, efficient and automated method to extract vessels from fundus images. *J. Vis.* 13:263–270.

Vlachos, M. and F. Dermatas. 2010. Multi-scale retinal vessel segmentation using line tracking. *Comput. Med. Imaging Graph.* 34:213–227.

Walter, T. and J.C. Klein. 2001. Segmentation of color fundus images of the human retina: Detection of the optic disc and the vascular tree using morphological technique. *Int. Symp. Med. Data Anal.* 2199:282–287.

Winder, R.J., P.J. Morrow, I.N. McRitchie, J.R. Bailie, and P.M. Hart. 2009. Algorithms for digital image processing in diabetic retinopathy. *Comput. Med. Imaging Graph.* 33:608–622.

Wong, D.W.K., J. Liu, J.H. Lim et al. 2008. Level-set based automatic cup-to-disc ratio determination using retinal fundus images in ARGALI. In: *Conference Proceedings of the IEEE Engineering in Medicine and Biology Society*, Vancouver, British Columbia, Canada, pp. 2266–2269.

Wong, D.W.K., J. Liu, N.M. Tan et al. 2010. Enhancement of optic cup detection through an improved vessel kink detection framework. *Proc. SPIE Med. Imaging* 7624:762439-1–762439-8.

Wong, T.Y., R. Klein, D.J. Couper et al. 2001. Retinal microvascular abnormalities and incident stroke: The atherosclerosis risk in communities study. *Lancet* 358:1134–1140.

Wu, C., G. Agam, and P. Stanchev. 2007. A hybrid filtering approach to retinal vessel segmentation. In: *IEEE International Symposium on Biomedical Imaging*, Washington, DC, Arlington, VA, pp. 604–607.

Xu, J., H. Ishikawa, G. Wollstein et al. 2008. Automated assessment of the optic nerve head on stereo disc photographs. *Invest. Ophthalmol. Vis. Sci.* 49:2512–2517.

Yogesan, K., R.H. Eikelboom, and C.J. Barry. 1998. Texture analysis of retinal images to determine nerve fibre loss. In: *International Conference on Pattern Recognition*, Brisbane, Queensland, Australia, pp. 1665–1667.

Youssif, A.R., A.Z. Ghalwash, and A.R. Ghoneim. 2008. Optic disc detection from normalized digital fundus images by means of a vessels' direction matched filter. *IEEE Trans. Med. Imaging* 27:11–18.

Zhang, Z., J. Liu, N.S. Cherian et al. 2009. Convex hull based neuro-retinal optic cup ellipse optimization in glaucoma diagnosis. In: *Conference Proceedings of the IEEE Engineering in Medicine and Biology Society*, Minneapolis, MN, pp. 1441–1444.

Zhu, H., D.P. Crabb, P.G. Schlottmann, G. Wollstein, and D. Garway-Heath. 2011. Aligning scan acquisition circles in optical coherence tomography images of the retinal nerve fibre layer. *IEEE Trans. Med. Imaging* 30:1228–1238.

Zhu, X., R.M. Rangayyan, and A.L. Ells. 2010. Detection of the optic nerve head in fundus images of the retina using the Hough transform for circles. *J. Digit. Imaging* 23:332–341.

Chapter 18

Detection and Diagnosis of Prostate Cancer in MR

Pieter Vos, Geert Litjens, and Henkjan Huisman

CONTENTS

18.1 INTRODUCTION

Prostate cancer is the most commonly diagnosed cancer and the second leading cause of cancer death in men. The growth of the population and, more importantly, the aging population is a major cause of the high number of prostate cancer cases and will continue to contribute to increase the cancer burden. For that reason, there is an ongoing debate whether screening for prostate cancer should be performed.

Prostate cancer mortality using current diagnostic tools can be reduced, but at the cost of too many biopsies and overtreatment. Prostate cancer is currently diagnosed using prostate-specific antigen (PSA) testing and systematic ultrasound (sysUS) biopsy. The common PSA test misses 15% of cancers and causes false alarm in 65%–75% of the normal cases, resulting in many unnecessary biopsies. The poor specificity results from elevated PSA levels at benign conditions such as prostatitis or benign prostatic hyperplasia (BPH). Furthermore, sysUS biopsies after PSA testing miss at least 20% of cancers and undergrade the cancers in 50% of the cases. The uncertainty of the tumor aggressiveness leads to overtreatment. Using PSA + sysUS biopsy as screening tool can reduce 25% of prostate cancer mortality (Schröder et al. 2009). However, the amount of unnecessary biopsies and overtreatment is considered too large to justify screening.

Magnetic resonance (MR) imaging in a screening setting can help reduce the number of biopsies and overtreatment, making prostate cancer screening a more viable option. Prostate MR has been shown to be very sensitive and, more importantly, very specific in the detection of aggressive prostate cancers (Fütterer et al. 2006, Haider et al. 2007, Tanimoto et al. 2007, Puech et al. 2009, Kitajima et al. 2010). A prostate MR after a PSA test can help in three ways. Firstly, it will help reduce unnecessary biopsies by having a high negative predictive value. Secondly, it will increase the detection rate by being able to accurately localize the cancer, allowing for fewer, better targeted biopsies (Hambrock et al. 2011). Thirdly, it will help reduce overtreatment by being able to correctly establish the aggressive part of the cancer. A biopsy targeted at the most aggressive part will result in a better assessment of the cancer aggressiveness (Hambrock et al. 2011), which will result in a better informed decision for a subsequent treatment plan. Furthermore, indolent prostate cancer can then be more confidently monitored without intervention. Prostate MR interpretation is however difficult and time consuming and prone to error under high-volume reading conditions.

Prostate MR computer-aided diagnosis (CADe) will become mandatory for high-volume sensitive reading in a screening scenario. In this chapter, we will first present a short overview of prostate MR to understand the issues involved. Next, the current research in various parts of the CADe pipeline is summarized.

18.2 MULTIPARAMETRIC PROSTATE MR

To understand prostate MR, first some basic anatomy is described. The prostate is normally a relatively small organ in the pelvis. It is located between the pelvic bones, in front of the rectum and below the bladder. Figure 18.1 shows a schematic drawing of the pelvis and its different structures. The prostate in elderly men mainly comprises two distinct parts: the peripheral zone (PZ) and transition zone (TZ) (Figure 18.2). The majority of prostate cancers originate in the PZ (70%–80%) and TZ (10%–20%).

Prostate MR achieves the best performance when it is done multiparametric (Sciarra et al. 2011) and in 3D. The MR study should comprise at least T2-weighted, diffusion-weighted imaging, dynamic contrast–enhanced T1-weighted MRI (DCE-MRI), and/or spectroscopic (MRS) imaging series. This will result in several 3D and 4D volumes: T2-weighted, apparent diffusion coefficient (ADC), DCE-derived, and metabolic maps. Each MR parameter depicts different aspects of the prostate, and the combined evaluation produces the best diagnostic performance. The following two sections will give some information on T2-weighted, ADC, and DCE-derived prostate MR.

T2-weighted MR imaging provides high-resolution details of prostate anatomy (Figure 18.3a). A high-signal-intensity homogeneous PZ is clearly distinguished from the inhomogeneous TZ. Low-signal areas in the PZ are indicative of cancer, yet other benign abnormalities may induce these as well. The TZ area is more difficult to interpret due to the presence of BPH.

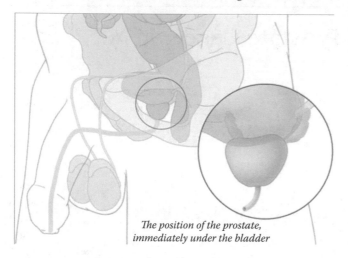

The position of the prostate, immediately under the bladder

Figure 18.1 A schematic drawing of the male pelvis in which several anatomical structures are indicated.

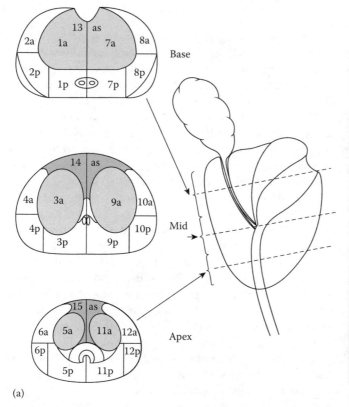

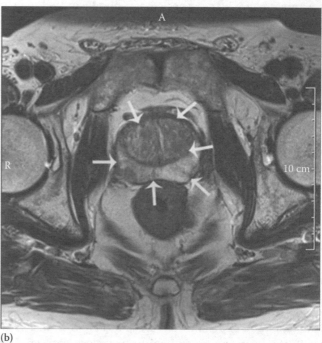

Figure 18.2 (a) Schematic drawing of the prostate, comprising three axial slices and a sagittal projection of the prostate. The white sections in the axial slices represent the peripheral zone and the gray sections the transition zone. (From Dickinson, L. et al., *Eur. Urol.*, 59, 477, 2011, http://dx.doi.org/10.1016/j.eururo.2010.12.009.) (b) Transversal T2-weighted MRI slice. The gray lower arrows indicate the peripheral zone, and the white upper arrows the transition zone.

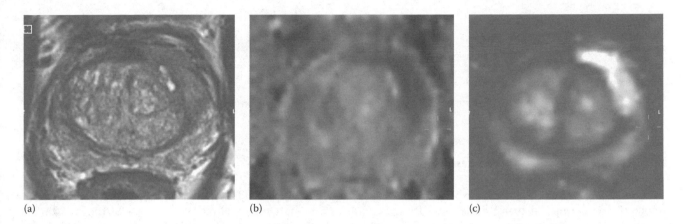

(a) (b) (c)

Figure 18.3 Example multiparametric MR images of a prostate cancer patient: (a) T2-weighted image, (b) ADC map (note a hypodense area indicative of tumor), and (c) pharmacokinetic (PK) parameter map Ktrans (note the large, bright highly perfused area confirming the presence of tumor).

ADC MR maps local diffusivity of protons, which is high in the water-rich ductal environment. Relatively low ADC values are indicative of cancer (Figure 18.3b), because of the pathological increase of malignant cell density and concomitant decrease in glandular lumen volume. Absolute ADC intensity has been shown to inversely correlate with aggressiveness allowing to differentiate indolent from aggressive cancers. Interpretation of ADC in the TZ is more complex.

DCE MR provides information about tissue perfusion and vascular permeability by monitoring contrast agent uptake in repeated T1-weighted images (Figure 18.3c). Tumor physiology often differs from normal tissue in its high vascularity, an increased capillary permeability, and an increased interstitial space due to hypertension. As a result, DCE uptake curves in tumor are often stronger, rise more rapidly, and show stronger decay or washout (Padhani et al. 2000, Huisman et al. 2001, van Engeland et al. 2003, Noworolski et al. 2005, Kozlowski et al. 2006). The uptake curves are commonly summarized in basic curve shape parameters (e.g., peak, slope), resulting in DCE maps, that are displayed as color-coded transparent overlays. A disadvantage of these curve shape parameters is that they show strong dependence on the arterial input function (AIF). Pharmacokinetic (PK) modeling with adequate AIF estimation is required for optimal performance (Vos et al. 2008). Multiple studies have shown the benefit of using PK parameters as additional information to the traditional T2-weighted images to diagnose prostate cancer (Fütterer et al. 2006, Haider et al. 2007, Puech et al. 2009).

Recent MR studies applied in a screening setting show that multiparametric MR has good diagnostic accuracy. Tanimoto et al. (2007) showed on 83 cases with PSA > 4 that multiparametric MR@1.5 T (T2-weighted + ADC + DCE) could achieve an accuracy of 86%. Kitajima

et al. (2010) using 3.0 T showed an improvement to 90%. Vilanova et al. (2001) got similar results as Tanimoto et al., but when including PSA, they reached an accuracy of 95%! New larger studies are under preparation by various groups.

18.3 COMPUTER-AIDED DETECTION

Prostate MR computer-aided detection (CADe) will become important in a screening scenario. Screening radiologists need to be able to quickly read many multiparametric prostate MRs with high specificity to find only the few cases that contain an actionable lesion. For screening to be really effective, aggressive cancers need to be detected at an early stage to provide ample opportunity for successful treatment, requiring a need to target the smaller cancers (2–5 mm) as well. CADe thus needs to be robust, automatic, and embedded in reading workstations that allow fast viewing of multiparametric MR. Current commercial prostate MR CADe tools do not offer such facility. DynaCad (InVivo), VividLook (iCAD), and 4DTissue (Siemens) offer interactive computerized tools with DCE analysis, multiparametric MR viewing, and structured reporting, but they are not automatic, are time-consuming, and have no CADe. CADe methods for prostate MR are only just starting to receive attention in the scientific literature, and as a consequence, adequate solutions for various parts of the CADe pipeline are lacking or at a performance level that is too low to be applicable in a clinical setting. In this section, we will summarize the current state of prostate MR CADe in the literature.

18.3.1 Prostate CADe Pipeline

In Figure 18.4, a typical CADe pipeline is presented for detecting prostate cancer. First the organ of interest, the prostate,

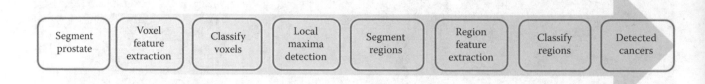

Figure 18.4   General pipeline for prostate cancer CADe methods.

is segmented, after which voxel features are calculated. Voxel classification is performed using these voxel features, and subsequently local maxima are detected on the resultant likelihood map. These local maxima are used as seed points for region segmentation. For each of the regions, new features describing the finding are extracted that are used to drive a second classifier to compute the likelihood of cancer. At the end of the CADe pipeline, a threshold is applied to prompt only regions with a sufficiently high likelihood. The next subsections will provide an overview for each of the CADe steps.

18.3.2 Automatic Prostate Segmentation

Automatic prostate segmentation in MR images is a topic of increasing interest. All studies agree in that it is a difficult task to robustly find and delineate the prostate. Challenges include similar intensity profiles with surrounding organs, its relative small size in the male pelvis, a lack of well-defined edges in the apex and base, the presence of imaging artifacts due to air in the rectum and inhomogeneities of the magnetic field, and finally the large anatomical variability between subjects.

Multiobject segmentation methods are currently the only option to robustly and automatically find as well as delineate the prostate. Single-object methods (e.g., active shape models, active appearance models, Markov random field models) by definition model only the prostate itself and often focus on a single MR parameter (Tsai et al. 2003, Pasquier et al. 2007, Liu et al. 2009a, Makni et al. 2009, Toth et al. 2011). These methods are all semiautomatic and require manual initialization to find the prostate in the complex pelvic MR. Automatic multiobject segmentation studies do exist (Tsai et al. 2004, Klein et al. 2008, Martin et al. 2010, Chen et al. 2011, Litjens et al. 2011b). The key advantage of a multiobject approach is that organs/structures with low-contrast can be accurately segmented when nearby well-defined organs/structures are taken into account. We will briefly discuss two multiobject approaches that have been applied to prostate MR: atlas-based methods and parametric deformable multimodel methods.

Atlas-based multiobject segmentation methods have gained strong popularity for segmenting pelvic MR images.

Klein et al. (2008) described a nonrigid registration-based atlas matching technique to segment the prostate and obtained a median dice similarity coefficient (DSC) of around 0.85 on a dataset of 20 healthy volunteers, which was later improved slightly in Langerak et al. (2010) by using an atlas selection method. Martin et al. (2010) extended the atlas-based segmentation with a spatially constrained deformable model, which on their data showed a DSC improvement from 0.80 to 0.84. Segmentation errors occur in those studies that are too dissimilar to any of the abdominal studies in the atlas set. The large anatomical variation between subjects necessitates a large atlas set, which causes the atlas-based methods to become very computationally intensive. For example, bladder and rectum filling causes large anatomic variability even for the same patient. It is difficult to define a sufficient atlas set that captures all of these variations. Examples of multiobject atlas-based method were presented by Litjens et al. (2012) and Makni et al. (2011).

Parametric deformable model segmentation methods use parametric multiobjects models, where each object is representative of an anatomical element (e.g., prostate, bladder, rectum). An example object model is a deformable super-ellipsoid (Gong et al. 2004). The model parameters describe each individual object's shape and multivariate appearance (e.g., T2 and ADC appearance) and the relations between all the objects (e.g., position of prostate relative to the bladder). The parametric model is fitted to an MR study by minimizing a cost function that combines multivariate appearance similarity and constraints from a population model. An application of such a method was shown in Litjens et al. (2011b). They constructed a parametric multiobject multivariate (PAMMO) model using ellipsoids and explicit object relations. Although being very simple, their pilot PAMMO implementation showed a fast and robust method that obtained a DSC of 0.78 on a dataset of 35 prostate cancer patients.

18.3.3 Initial Voxel-Based Detection

The voxels in the prostate are further analyzed by computing various voxel features driving a classifier to determine a likelihood of malignancy for each voxel.

Several approaches exist in the literature, which will be considered in the next paragraphs.

Some studies use only a single MR parameter classification (Madabhushi et al. 2005, Weber et al. 2007, Kim et al. 2008, Viswanath et al. 2008, Vos et al. 2008, Puech et al. 2009). However, combining information from multiple different MR parameters has been shown to be more successful (Chan et al. 2003, de Lange et al. 2009, Liu et al. 2009b, Ozer et al. 2010, Vos et al. 2010, Tiwari et al. 2011). For example, Langer et al. (2009) performed a logistic regression on quantitative T2, ADC maps, and DCE-MRI-derived maps. Liu et al. (2009b) used a Markov random fields model to detect prostate cancer using information from T2-weighted, ADC, and DCE-MRI, whereas Vos et al. (2010) and Ozer et al. (2010) used a supervised support vector machine to perform the classification using quantitative T2, DWI, and DCE-MRI.

Texture features are used by experienced prostate MR radiologists in the detection of prostate cancer. Automatic texture-based feature analysis has, however, seen only limited application in the automated detection of prostate cancer. Lv et al. (2009) explored the use of fractal on T2-weighted images. Similar work on fractal analysis was performed by Lopes et al. (2011). Madabhushi et al. (2005) explored statistical and gradient features extracted from T2-weighted images and classified them using a Bayesian classifier. In addition, Tiwari et al. (2011) investigated the use of Gabor features in the context of prostate cancer detection and combined them with spectroscopy information. Vos et al. (2012) demonstrated the additional value of detecting blob-like textures using a multiscale blobness feature filter (an example is demonstrated in Figure 18.5).

This feature exploits scale-space characteristics to quantify the likeness of image regions to blobs, which works especially well in the PZ of the prostate.

Another important aspect is that prostate cancer differs in appearance depending on the zone as presented by Hoeks et al. (2011) and Viswanath et al. (2012). This has been recently investigated in a CADe study that showed that two separate classifiers, one for each zone, outperformed a single whole prostate detector approach (Litjens et al. 2011a). This warrants further refinement of segmentation methods.

18.3.4 Region Segmentation

Initial detections result from scanning the voxel-based likelihood map for maxima above a certain threshold. These detections are often not very specific. The likelihood map will show many obvious (to radiologists) false positives. To reduce these false positives, the regions defined by these initial detections are segmented to allow further analysis. The segmentation also entails merging of several initial detections within the same region.

Quite a few published CADe pipelines try to segment the cancerous regions by further processing of the initial voxel likelihood image. Some papers do this in the same step as the initial classification, where the trained classifier is combined with spatial regularization, for example, Markov random fields (Liu et al. 2009b). Other approaches include conditional random fields (Artan et al. 2010) and using binary classifier predictions obtained using graph-embedding (Tiwari et al. 2011).

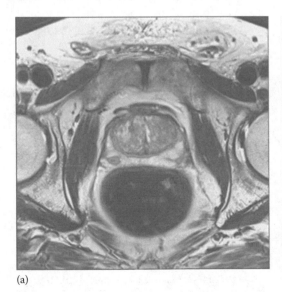
(a)

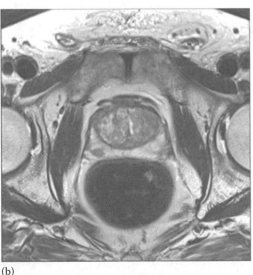
(b)

Figure 18.5 **(See color insert.)** Demonstration of using blobness as a feature to detect prostate cancer. (a) Response of a multiscale blobness filter on the peripheral zone in a T2 MR image. (b) The image represents the same filter, but the response is restricted to the transition zone. A cancer is present in the left side of the images within the peripheral zone. These images show that such a feature is able to distinguish cancer from normal tissue.

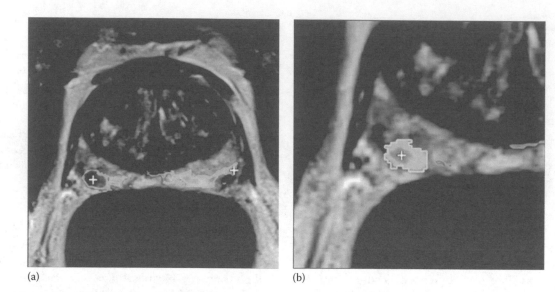

(a)

(b)

Figure 18.6   (See color insert.) (a) The output (+) of a local maxima detection on the initial likelihood map (color overlay), (b) the results (yellow solid outline) of a bounded region-growing segmentation using the local maximum as a seed point.

In a more regular computer-aided detection approach, one would like to segment candidate regions individually for further processing. Only very few papers have been published that include this approach in a complete prostate MR CADe system (Litjens et al. 2011b, Vos et al. 2012). They segment the individual candidate regions by first performing local maxima detection on the initial likelihood map. Then, a bounded region-growing approach is used to segment the lesion. An example is shown in Figure 18.6.

18.3.5 Region Classification

The segmented regions after the initial detection stage are analyzed further to try to reduce the number of false positives of the initial detector. One of the advantages at this stage is that we can handle and compute many more features for each region besides the voxel-based features. The voxel feature statistics are readily available. Contrast between the lesion and its environment could be determined. Finally, shape- and boundary-based features can be included in this classification, for example, volume, circularity, and boundary diffusivity (Litjens et al. 2012).

A second classifier is trained to respond with a region-based cancer likelihood. The aim of this second classifier is to reduce false positives that were incorrectly identified at the initial stage. This second classifier is trained on the set of initially detected regions and should respond with a high likelihood in these regions that correctly identify a prostate cancer. Again, a threshold is applied to set the CADe system to respond with regions that are highly predictive of prostate cancer at a low number of false positives.

18.4 CONCLUSION

The challenge to introduce CADe in the clinical workflow with a prostate cancer screening environment is enormous. The lack of standardized sequences and objective quantitative features are important obstacles for prostate MR CADe to become widely available. Furthermore, to become successful in a clinical environment, the intended CADe system should be fully automated, robust to the large population variation, and fast enough for a typical screening production of say 30–40 cases a day. As of today, there is no commercial prostate CADe system available that fulfills the mentioned requirements.

Although prostate MR CADe is starting to emerge as a research topic and several parts of the CADe pipeline have been investigated, as of yet no fully automatic CADe is currently available for the clinical practice. Future research is required on all areas of the CADe pipeline. CADe research can benefit from the currently starting clinical prostate MR screening trials on a general population of men.

REFERENCES

Artan, Y., Haider, M. A., Langer, D. L., van der Kwast, T. H., Evans, A. J., Yang, Y., Wernick, M. N., Trachtenberg, J., and Yetik, I. S. (2010). Prostate cancer localization with multispectral MRI using cost-sensitive support vector machines and conditional random fields, *IEEE Transactions on Image Processing* **19**, 2444–2455. http://dx.doi.org/10.1109/TIP.2010.2048612.

Chan, I., Wells, W., Mulkern, R. V., Haker, S., Zhang, J., Zou, K. H., Maier, S. E., and Tempany, C. M. C. (2003). Detection of prostate cancer by integration of line-scan diffusion, T2-mapping and T2-weighted magnetic resonance imaging; a multichannel statistical classifier, *Medical Physics* **30**, 2390–2398.

Chen, S., Lovelock, D. M., and Radke, R. J. (2011). Segmenting the prostate and rectum in CT imagery using anatomical constraints, *Medical Image Analysis* **15**, 1–11. http://dx.doi.org/10.1016/j.media.2010.06.004.

deLange, E. E., Altes, T. A., Patrie, J. T., Battiston, J. J., Juersivich, A. P., Mugler, J. P., and Platts-Mills, T. A. (2009). Changes in regional airflow obstruction over time in the lungs of patients with asthma: Evaluation with 3He MR imaging, *Radiology* **250**, 567–575. http://dx.doi.org/10.1148/radiol.2502080188.

Dickinson, L., Ahmed, H. U., Allen, C., Barentsz, J. O., Carey, B., Fütterer, J. J., Heijmink, S. W. et al. (2011). Magnetic resonance imaging for the detection, localisation, and characterisation of prostate cancer: Recommendations from a European consensus meeting, *European Urology* **59**, 477–494. http://dx.doi.org/10.1016/j.eururo.2010.12.009.

Fütterer, J. J., Heijmink, S. W. T. P. J., Scheenen, T. W. J., Veltman, J., Huisman, H. J., Vos, P., Hulsbergen-van de Kaa, C. A., Witjes, J. A., Krabbe, P. F. M., Heerschap, A., and Barentsz, J. O. (2006). Prostate cancer localization with dynamic contrast-enhanced MR imaging and proton MR spectroscopic imaging, *Radiology* **241**, 449–458. http://dx.doi.org/10.1148/radiol.2412051866.

Gong, L., Pathak, S. D., Haynor, D. R., Cho, P. S., and Kim, Y. (2004). Parametric shape modeling using deformable superellipses for prostate segmentation, *IEEE Transactions on Medical Imaging* **23**, 340–349. http://dx.doi.org/10.1109/TMI.2004.824237.

Haider, M. A., van der Kwast, T. H., Tanguay, J., Evans, A. J., Hashmi, A.-T., Lockwood, G., and Trachtenberg, J. (2007). Combined T2-weighted and diffusion-weighted MRI for localization of prostate cancer, *American Journal of Roentgenology* **189**, 323–328. http://dx.doi.org/10.2214/AJR.07.2211.

Hambrock, T., Somford, D. M., Huisman, H. J., van Oort, I. M., Witjes, J. A., Hulsbergen-van de Kaa, C. A., Scheenen, T., and Barentsz, J. O. (2011). Relationship between apparent diffusion coefficients at 3.0-T MR imaging and Gleason grade in peripheral zone prostate cancer, *Radiology* **259**, 453–461. http://dx.doi.org/10.1148/radiol.11091409.

Hoeks, C. M. A., Barentsz, J. O., Hambrock, T., Yakar, D., Somford, D. M., Heijmink, S. W. T. P. J., Scheenen, T. W. J. et al. (2011). Prostate cancer: Multiparametric MR imaging for detection, localization, and staging, *Radiology* **261**, 46–66. http://dx.doi.org/10.1148/radiol.11091822.

Huisman, H. J., Engelbrecht, M. R., and Barentsz, J. O. (2001). Accurate estimation of pharmacokinetic contrast-enhanced dynamic MRI parameters of the prostate, *Journal of Magnetic Resonance Imaging* **13**, 607–614.

Kim, H. J., Li, G., Gjertson, D., Elashoff, R., Shah, S. K., Ochs, R., Vasunilashorn, F., Abtin, F., Brown, M. S., and Goldin, J. G. (2008). Classification of parenchymal abnormality in scleroderma lung using a novel approach to denoise images collected via a multicenter study, *Academic Radiology* **15**, 1004–1016.

Kitajima, K., Kaji, Y., Fukabori, Y., Yoshida, K., Suganuma, N., and Sugimura, K. (2010). Prostate cancer detection with 3 T MRI: Comparison of diffusion-weighted imaging and dynamic contrast-enhanced MRI in combination with T2-weighted imaging, *Journal of Magnetic Resonance Imaging* **31**, 625–631. http://dx.doi.org/10.1002/jmri.22075.

Klein, S., van der Heide, U. A., Lips, I. M., van Vulpen, M., Staring, M., and Pluim, J. P. W. (2008). Automatic segmentation of the prostate in 3D MR images by atlas matching using localized mutual information, *Medical Physics* **35**, 1407–1417.

Kozlowski, P., Chang, S. D., Jones, E. C., Berean, K. W., Chen, H., and Goldenberg, S. L. (2006). Combined diffusion-weighted and dynamic contrast-enhanced MRI for prostate cancer diagnosis—Correlation with biopsy and histopathology, *Journal of Magnetic Resonance Imaging* **24**, 108–113. http://dx.doi.org/10.1002/jmri.20626.

Langer, D. L., van der Kwast, T. H., Evans, A. J., Trachtenberg, J., Wilson, B. C., and Haider, M. A. (2009). Prostate cancer detection with multi-parametric MRI: Logistic regression analysis of quantitative T2, diffusion-weighted imaging, and dynamic contrast-enhanced MRI, *Journal of Magnetic Resonance Imaging* **30**, 327–334. http://dx.doi.org/10.1002/jmri.21824.

Langerak, T. R., van der Heide, U. A., Kotte, A. N. T. J., Viergever, M. A., van Vulpen, M., and Pluim, J. P. W. (2010). Label fusion in atlas-based segmentation using a selective and iterative method for performance level estimation (SIMPLE), *IEEE Transactions on Medical Imaging* **29**, 2000–2008. http://dx.doi.org/10.1109/TMI.2010.2057442.

Litjens, G., Barentsz, J., Karssemeijer, N., and Huisman, H. (2012). Automated computer-aided detection of prostate cancer in MR images: From a whole-organ to a zone-based approach, *SPIE Medical Imaging*, 83150G-83150G-6.

Litjens, G., Barentsz, J. O., Karssemeijer, N., and Huisman, H. (2011a). Zone-specific automatic computer-aided detection of prostate cancer in MRI, *IEEE Transactions on Medical Imaging* **33**(5), 1083–1092.

Litjens, G., Vos, P., Barentsz, J., Karssemeijer, N., and Huisman, H. (2011b). Automatic computer aided detection of abnormalities in multi-parametric prostate MRI, in: *Medical Imaging, Proceedings of the SPIE*, Vol. 7963.

Liu, X., Langer, D. L., Haider, M. A., der Kwast, T. H. V., Evans, A. J., Wernick, M. N., and Yetik, I. S. (2009a). Unsupervised segmentation of the prostate using MR images based on level set with a shape prior, in: *Conference Proceedings of the IEEE Engineering in Medicine and Biology Society*, Minneapolis, MN, pp. 3613–3616. http://dx.doi.org/10.1109/IEMBS.2009.5333519.

Liu, X., Langer, D. L., Haider, M. A., Yang, Y., Wernick, M. N., and Yetik, I. S. (2009b). Prostate cancer segmentation with simultaneous estimation of Markov random field parameters and class, *IEEE Transactions on Medical Imaging* **28**, 906–915. http://dx.doi.org/10.1109/TMI.2009.2012888.

Lopes, R., Ayache, A., Makni, N., Puech, P., Villers, A., Mordon, S., and Betrouni, N. (2011). Prostate cancer characterization on MR images using fractal features, *Medical Physics* **38**, 83–95.

Lv, D., Guo, X., Wang, X., Zhang, J., and Fang, J. (2009). Computerized characterization of prostate cancer by fractal analysis in MR images, *Journal of Magnetic Resonance Imaging* **30**, 161–168. http://dx.doi.org/10.1002/jmri.21819.

Madabhushi, A., Feldman, M., Metaxas, D., Tomaszewski, J., and Chute, D. (2005). Automated detection of prostatic adenocarcinoma from high-resolution ex vivo MRI, *IEEE Transactions on Medical Imaging* **24**, 1611–1625. http://eutils.ncbi.nlm.nih.gov/entrez/eutils/elink.fcgi?cmd=prlinks&dbfrom=pubmed&retmode=ref&id=16350920.

Makni, N., Iancu, A., Colot, O., Puech, P., Mordon, S., and Betrouni, N. (2011). Zonal segmentation of prostate using multispectral magnetic resonance images, *Medical Physics* **38**, 6093. http://dx.doi.org/10.1118/1.3651610.

Makni, N., Puech, P., Lopes, R., Dewalle, A. S., Colot, O., and Betrouni, N. (2009). Combining a deformable model and a probabilistic framework for an automatic 3D segmentation of prostate on MRI, *International Journal of Computer Assisted Radiology and Surgery* **4**, 181–188. http://dx.doi.org/10.1007/s11548-008-0281-y.

Martin, S., Troccaz, J., and Daanenc, V. (2010). Automated segmentation of the prostate in 3D MR images using a probabilistic atlas and a spatially constrained deformable model, *Medical Physics* **37**, 1579–1590.

Noworolski, S. M., Henry, R. G., Vigneron, D. B., and Kurhanewicz, J. (2005). Dynamic contrast-enhanced MRI in normal and abnormal prostate tissues as defined by biopsy, MRI, and 3D MRSI, *Magnetic Resonance in Medicine* **53**, 249–255. http://dx.doi.org/10.1002/mrm.203743.

Ozer, S., Langer, D. L., Liu, X., Haider, M. A., van der Kwast, T. H., Evans, A. J., Yang, Y., Wernick, M. N., and Yetik, I. S. (2010). Supervised and unsupervised methods for prostate cancer segmentation with multispectral MRI, *Medical Physics* **37**, 1873–1883.

Padhani, A. R., Gapinski, C. J., Macvicar, D. A., Parker, G. J., Suckling, J., Revell, P. B., Leach, M. O., Dearnaley, D. P., and Husband, J. E. (2000). Dynamic contrast enhanced MRI of prostate cancer: Correlation with morphology and tumour stage, histological grade and PSA, *Clinical Radiology* **55**, 99–109. http://dx.doi.org/10.1053/crad.1999.0327.

Pasquier, D., Lacornerie, T., Vermandel, M., Rousseau, J., Lartigau, E., and Betrouni, N. (2007). Automatic segmentation of pelvic structures from magnetic resonance images for prostate cancer radiotherapy, *International Journal of Radiation Oncology, Biology, Physics* **68**, 592–600. http://dx.doi.org/10.1016/j.ijrobp.2007.02.005.

Puech, P., Potiron, E., Lemaitre, L., Leroy, X., Haber, G.-P., Crouzet, S., Kamoi, K., and Villers, A. (2009). Dynamic contrast-enhanced-magnetic resonance imaging evaluation of intraprostatic prostate cancer: Correlation with radical prostatectomy specimens, *Urology* **74**, 1094–1099. http://dx.doi.org/10.1016/j.urology.2009.04.102.

Schröder, F. H., Hugosson, J., Roobol, M. J., Tammela, T. L. J., Ciatto, S., Nelen, V., Kwiatkowski, M. et al. (2009). Screening and prostate-cancer mortality in a randomized European study, *New England Journal of Medicine* **360**, 1320–1328. http://dx.doi.org/10.1056/NEJMoa0810084.

Sciarra, A., Barentsz, J., Bjartell, A., Eastham, J., Hricak, H., Panebianco, V., and Witjes, J. A. (2011). Advances in magnetic resonance imaging: How they are changing the management of prostate cancer, *European Urology* **59**, 962–977. http://dx.doi.org/10.1016/j.eururo.2011.02.034.

Tanimoto, A., Nakashima, J., Kohno, H., Shinmoto, H., and Kuribayashi, S. (2007). Prostate cancer screening: The clinical value of diffusion-weighted imaging and dynamic MR imaging in combination with T2-weighted imaging, *Journal of Magnetic Resonance Imaging* **25**, 146–152. http://dx.doi.org/10.1002/jmri.20793.

Tiwari, P., Viswanath, S., Kurhanewicz, J., Sridhar, A., and Madabhushi, A. (2011). Multimodal wavelet embedding representation for data combination (MaWERiC): Integrating magnetic resonance imaging and spectroscopy for prostate cancer detection, *NMR in Biomedicine* **25**(4), 607–619. http://dx.doi.org/10.1002/nbm.1777.

Toth, R., Bloch, B. N., Genega, E. M., Rofsky, N. M., Lenkinski, R. E., Rosen, M. A., Kalyanpur, A., Pungavkar, S., and Madabhushi, A. (2011). Accurate prostate volume estimation using multi-feature active shape models on T2-weighted MRI, *Academic Radiology* **18**, 745–754. http://dx.doi.org/10.1016/j.acra.2011.01.016.

Tsai, A., Wells, W., Tempany, C., Grimson, E., and Willsky, A. (2004). Mutual information in coupled multi-shape model for medical image segmentation, *Medical Image Analysis* **8**, 429–445. http://dx.doi.org/10.1016/j.media.2004.01.003.

Tsai, A., Yezzi, A., Wells, W., Tempany, C., Tucker, D., Fan, A., Grimson, W. E., and Willsky, A. (2003). A shape-based approach to the segmentation of medical imagery using level sets, *IEEE Transactions on Medical Imaging* **22**, 137–154. http://dx.doi.org/10.1109/TMI.2002.808355.

van Engeland, S., Snoeren, P., Hendriks, J., and Karssemeijer, N. (2003). A comparison of methods for mammogram registration, *IEEE Transactions on Medical Imaging* **22**, 1436–1444.

Vilanova, J. C., Comet, J., Capdevila, A., Barceló, J., Dolz, J. L., Huguet, M., Barceló, C., Aldomà, J., and Delgado, E. (2001). The value of endorectal MR imaging to predict positive biopsies in clinically intermediate-risk prostate cancer patients, *European Radiology* **11**, 229–235.

Viswanath, S., Bloch, B. N., Genega, E., Rofsky, N., Lenkinski, R., Chappelow, J., Toth, R., and Madabhushi, A. (2008). A comprehensive segmentation, registration, and cancer detection scheme on 3 tesla in vivo prostate DCE-MRI, *Medical Image Computing and Computer-Assisted Intervention* **11**, 662–669.

Viswanath, S. E., Bloch, N. B., Chappelow, J. C., Toth, R., Rofsky, N. M., Genega, E. M., Lenkinski, R. E., and Madabhushi, A. (2012). Central gland and peripheral zone prostate tumors have significantly different quantitative imaging signatures on 3 tesla endorectal, in vivo T2-weighted MR imagery, *Journal of Magnetic Resonance Imaging*. http://dx.doi.org/10.1002/jmri.23618.

Vos, P. C., Barentsz, J. O., Karssemeijer, N., and Huisman, H. J. (2012). Automatic computer-aided detection of prostate cancer based on multiparametric magnetic resonance image analysis, *Physics in Medicine and Biology* **57**, 1527–1542. http://dx.doi.org/10.1088/0031-9155/57/6/1527.

Vos, P. C., Hambrock, T., Barentsz, J. O., and Huisman, H. J. (2010). Computer-assisted analysis of peripheral zone prostate lesions using T2-weighted and dynamic contrast enhanced T1-weighted MRI, *Physics in Medicine and Biology* **55**, 1719–1734. http://dx.doi.org/10.1088/0031-9155/55/6/012.

Vos, P. C., Hambrock, T., van de Kaa, C. A. H., Fütterer, J. J., Barentsz, J. O., and Huisman, H. J. (2008). Computerized analysis of prostate lesions in the peripheral zone using dynamic contrast enhanced MRI, *Medical Physics* **35**, 888–899.

Weber, C., Zechmann, C. M., Kelm, B. M., Zamecnik, P., Hendricks, D., Waldherr, R., Hamprecht, F. A., Delorme, S., Bachert, P., and Ikinger, U. (2007). Comparison of the accuracy of manual and automatic evaluation of MR spectra in prostate carcinoma, *Urologe A* **46**, 1252. http://dx.doi.org/10.1007/s00120-007-1488-1.

Chapter 19

Detection of Bone Metastasis in Bone Scan

Junji Shiraishi

CONTENTS

19.1 INTRODUCTION

Bone scintigraphy is the most frequent examination among various diagnostic nuclear medicine procedures. According to an UNSCEAR (2008) report, which included the results of a comprehensive survey of radiology practice worldwide, bone scintigraphy accounted for 33.6% of all diagnostic nuclear medicine procedures for the period 1997–2007 in the specific country group of health care level I in which a country has more than 1 physician per 1000 population (Figure 19.1). Bone scans are commonly used for the imaging of new bone formation that may occur due to the presence of almost any skeletal pathology and for demonstrating increased and/or decreased gamma ray emissions localized to the site of bone abnormalities by use of the radioisotope of technetium-99m methylene diphosphonate (MDP) hydroxymethane diphosphonate (HDP). Thus, the bone scan has been applied as an initial procedure for

identifying several disorders such as skeletal metastases, osteosarcoma, osteomyelitis, and nondisplaced fractures. In addition, bone scans are often repeated regularly for the same patient who requires monitoring for identifying several disorders such as skeletal metastases, primary bone tumors, and osteomyelitis.

The sensitivity of bone scan examinations for the detection of bone abnormalities has been considered to be very high; however, it is still difficult to detect very subtle lesions and time consuming to identify multiple lesions such as bone metastases of prostate and breast cancers. Furthermore, when the patient has a previous image available, it is difficult to detect subtle changes between two successive abnormal bone scans because of variations in patient conditions, the accumulation of radioisotopes during each examination, and the image quality of gamma cameras. Therefore, a computerized scheme that can assist

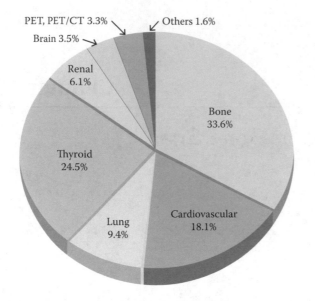

Figure 19.1 Frequency of bone scans in diagnostic nuclear medicine procedures.

radiologists in the detection of subtle bone abnormalities and/or quantification of interval changes in successive bone scans would be useful by reducing the interpretation time and by quantifying the extent of an increase or a decrease in the radioisotope uptake between two different bone scans.

19.2　TEMPORAL SUBTRACTION TECHNIQUE IN NUCLEAR MEDICINE

The development of the temporal subtraction method originated with chest radiographs (Kano et al. 1994, Ishida et al. 1999). The method employed a nonlinear image-warping technique for reducing registration artifacts in temporal subtraction images of two successive chest radiographs. The clinical usefulness of the temporal subtraction method for two sequential chest images was demonstrated by observer study (Difazio et al. 1997, Kakeda et al. 2002). In addition to the application to chest images, the temporal subtraction methods were introduced into successive chest computed tomography (CT) (Abe et al. 2004) and brain MRI images (Ilkko et al. 2004).

Note that the clinical utility of the temporal subtraction method is particularly efficient when the same radiological examination is performed frequently for one patient, so that there is a higher likelihood for patients to have more than two sequential images for the interpretation. Therefore, bone scintigraphy was very appropriate for applying the temporal subtraction method to detect interval changes between successive bone scans. Shiraishi et al. (2007b) developed a temporal subtraction scheme for the detection

of interval changes in successive whole-body bone scans as well as a computer-aided diagnostic (CAD) scheme for the detection of interval changes in successive bone scans.

19.2.1　Imaging Property of Bone Scan Images

In the nuclear medicine technique, the patient is injected (usually into a vein in the arm or hand, occasionally the foot) with a small amount of radioactive material such as 600 MBq of technetium-99m-MDP and then scanned with a gamma camera, a device sensitive to the radiation emitted by the injected material. Two-dimensional projections of scintigraphy may be enough, but in order to view small lesions (<1 cm) especially in the spine, single photon emission computed tomography (SPECT) imaging technique may be required. In the United States, most insurance companies require separate authorization for SPECT imaging.

In bone scintigraphy, about half of the radioactive material is localized by the bones. The more active the bone turnover, the more radioactive material will be seen. Some tumors, fractures, and infections show up as areas of increased uptake. The area with increased uptake is called a *hot lesion*. In contrast, others can cause decreased uptake of radioactive material. The area with decreased uptake is called a *cold lesion*. Not all tumors are easily seen on the bone scan. Some lesions, especially lytic (destructive) ones, require positron emission tomography for visualization. In 2–4 h after injection, about half of the radioactive material leaves the body through kidneys and bladder in urine. Therefore, the patient is injected with the radioisotope and returns in 2–4 h for imaging. Note that anyone having a study should empty their bladder immediately before images are taken.

Image acquisition takes from 30 to 70 min, depending on if SPECT images are required. If the physician wants to evaluate for osteomyelitis (bone infection) or fractures, then a three-phase bone scan is performed where the first- and second-phase images are taken immediately after the initial injection with a 20–30 min interval. The patient then returns in 2–3 h for additional images (third phase). Sometimes late images are taken at 24 h after injection.

Most of computer workstations for bone scintigrams included image viewers for displaying and archiving bone scan images with appropriate grayscales; original count data for each pixel were adjusted automatically by use of histogram analysis or min–max value of pixel data. However, as is common in whole-body bone scintigrams, residual radioactive urine in the bladder and/or a leakage at the injection site has caused extremely high intensities on bone scan images, even though the automated adjustment was applied. These high intensities frequently prevent a proper display of bone scan images of clinical interest as shown in Figure 19.2.

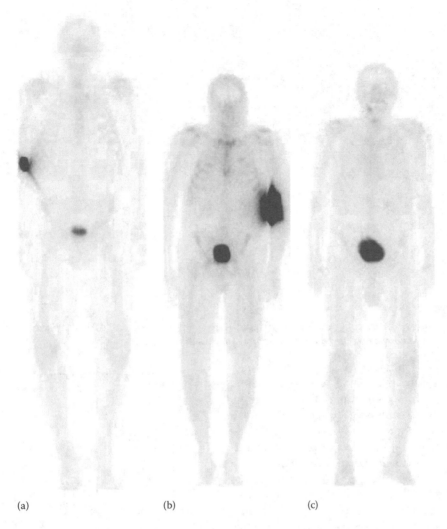

(a)   (b)   (c)

Figure 19.2   Examples of inappropriately adjusted bone scan images with extremely high intensities due to a leakage at the injection site (a, b) and residual radioactive urine in the bladder (c).

19.2.2   Normalization and Initial Matching of Bone Scan Images

In order to avoid receiving a negative influence from the extremely high intensities due to residual radioactive urine in the bladder and/or a leakage at the injection site, a computerized scheme for normalizing gray scale of bone scan images was attempted (Shiraishi et al. 2007b). In this computerized scheme, the original gray scale (16 bit) of each of the raw image data was converted to the images with 10-bit gray scale by use of a histogram analysis for removal of areas with extremely high intensities. In this gray-scale conversion method, the pixel values in the upper 0.2% and 98% of the area under the histogram of the original raw image data were linearly mapped to 1023 and 0, respectively, in the bone scan image. Figure 19.3 shows an example of posterior views of (a) original raw image data and (b) density-adjusted

image, which is applied to the computerized scheme. The dynamic range of pixel values in the input image was generally decreased from the raw image data by use of this conversion method, such that the contrast of clinical interest in the input image was increased.

When two or more gamma cameras are used for bone scintigram in one medical department, the raw image data sometimes had different pixel sizes for different gamma cameras. Therefore, it is important to confirm that the pixel size for all images is identical or has small differences for subtracting each other. In general, <20% of errors in pixel size would be negligible in the low-resolution images of whole-body bone scans.

In addition to the effect of high intensities caused by urine and/or leakage at the site of injection, high intensities for bone abnormalities occasionally affect the optimization

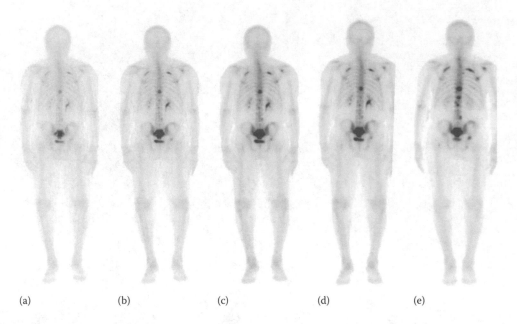

(a)   (b)   (c)   (d)   (e)

Figure 19.3   Posterior views of (a) original raw, (b) density-adjusted, (c) normalized, and (d) density/size-matched images of previous image. They are matched to (e) current image to provide temporal subtraction image.

of the gray scale of bone scan images. For example, normal bone structures represented relatively low pixel values in the abnormal bone scan images compared with those in the normal bone scan images. In order to reduce the effect of high-intensity lesions on bone scan images for optimization of the gray scale, an average pixel value of normal bone structures could be used to normalize the gray scale of each image (Shiraishi et al. 2007b). In this gray-scale normalization, a multiple thresholding method for the area under the histogram of the input image was applied to identify initially a number of high-intensity regions, which included all abnormal lesions and some normal areas. Once a number of high-intensity regions were identified, the average pixel values for all of these regions by a multiple thresholding method were analyzed in order to determine the transition point that corresponds to the threshold value for distinguishing between abnormal lesions and normal areas (i.e., normal bone structures) with very high intensities. With this method, all identified areas were sorted first based on the order (ranking) of their average pixel values.

Figure 19.4 shows the relationship between the rank order of identified areas and the average pixel values for the posterior view of the bone scan image illustrated in Figure 19.3. The transition point was determined based on a large change in the average pixel values between the group of abnormal lesions and the group of normal areas. Note that the variation in the average pixel values in normal areas is relatively small. The mean (P) of the average pixel values of five identified normal areas, whose average pixel values were immediately below the transition point, was used. The pixel values in a normalized image were determined by

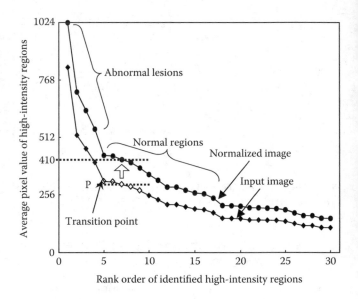

Figure 19.4   Relationship between the rank order and the average pixel values of high-intensity regions on posterior-view bone scan image before and after normalization.

the product of a normalization factor (F) and the original pixel value of an input image. The F value was determined by k/P, where k was selected empirically as 358 (35% of the maximum gray scale of 1024) for the anterior view and 410 (40% of the maximum gray scale of 1024) for the posterior view. Figure 19.3 shows posterior views of (b) an input image and (c) a normalized image.

In the next step, after gray scale in each image was normalized, the previous image was matched to the current image in terms of the image size, orientation, and gray scale, in order to minimize the difference between the two images for visual comparison and for the application of a nonlinear image-warping technique for obtaining the temporal subtraction image. The horizontal profiles of the previous and the current image were used for determining the top and bottom positions, and the midline of the body projections, and then the magnification/minification and the orientation of the previous image were made to match those of the current image.

The gray scale of the previous image was matched to that of the current image by the analysis of the correlation between the average pixel values of the corresponding small regions of interest (ROIs: 16 × 16 matrix size) in the two images. Figure 19.5 shows the relationship between the average pixel values in the previous and the current images, which were shown in Figure 19.3. Initially, a regression line for the relationship between the average pixel values in the previous and the current images was estimated, and then the pixel values of the previous image were converted linearly by use of the slope and the intersection that were obtained from the estimated regression line. Figure 19.3 shows posterior views of (c) the normalized image and (d) the matched image of the previous scan, which should be compared to (e) the normalized image of the current posterior view. In order to neglect large differences due to actual

interval changes, some ROIs were excluded for this normalization process when the difference in the average pixel value between the two ROIs in the previous and the current images was more than 50% of the average value of the ROI in the current image. This is because some ROIs included actual interval changes, so that the correlation in the average pixel values between such ROIs would be very low.

19.2.3 Nonlinear Image-Warping Technique

For reducing misregistration artifacts in the subtraction image, a nonlinear image-warping technique, which was originally developed for the contralateral subtraction technique in chest radiographs (Li et al. 2000), was employed and was modified for bone scan images. Such artifacts may be due to the difference in patient conditions, patient positioning, and the equipment used for examinations.

19.2.3.1 Global Matching between the Previous and Current Images

The purpose of global matching is to register the previous and current images approximately, so that the subsequent local matching and image-warping technique, described later, can provide improved subtraction images and can also be more efficient. In order for saving computational time, the matrix sizes of the previous and current images were reduced initially by 50% by using a subsampling technique. All of the processing steps in the global matching are then applied to the reduced image only.

The global matching technique shown here is based on multiple small ROIs distributed over the entire 2D image space. In the previous image, many template ROIs 20 × 20 in size are determined, and in the current image, many search area ROIs of the size 44 × 108 were determined. The center of a template ROI in the previous image is equal to the center of the corresponding search area ROI in the current image. The distance between the adjacent ROIs is 10 pixels for the templates and the search areas. Please note that the search area is a rectangle, because the possible shift value in the vertical direction is generally much larger than that in the horizontal direction.

For a given shift vector, a template can be shifted by the shift vector and a corresponding region inside the search area is determined. In addition, the cross-correlation between the shifted template and the corresponding region inside the search area can be determined. For each of all possible shift vectors, the similarity between the previous and current images is defined as the sum of correlation values between all shifted templates and the corresponding regions in the search areas. The shift vector with the maximum correlation value (similarity) between the previous and current images is determined as the *optimal* shift vector for the two images. This optimal shift vector is then

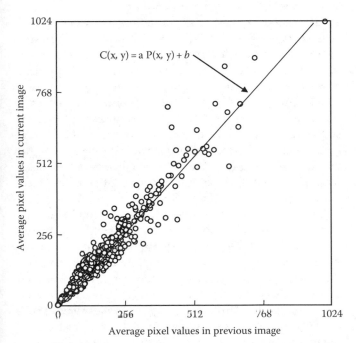

Figure 19.5 Relationship between average pixel values of ROIs in the previous and current images. The slope a and the intersection b were estimated from the correlation of the pixel values of the previous image (P(x, y)) and the pixel values of the current image (C(x, y)).

multiplied by two and is used to shift the full-size previous image so that the two images match approximately.

However, the previous image may be slightly scaled and/or rotated relative to the current image. To take this factor into our global matching, 15(5 × 3) scaled and rotated versions of the previous image with five scaling factors (0.9, 0.95, 1.0, 1.05, 1.1) and three rotation angles (−1°, 0°, 1°) were produced. Among the 15 transformed versions of the previous image, the one providing the largest similarity with the current image is selected and is employed in the subsequent processing.

19.2.3.2 Matching Legs between the Previous and Current Images

After the global matching, the two images are registered approximately. However, the corresponding legs in the two images are often still far from each other in the horizontal direction. This makes the matching of the legs in the two images very difficult and makes the legs the main source of misregistration artifacts. To address this problem, a simple technique was attempted to match the legs approximately in the two images as described later in this chapter.

Initially, the body of patient in the two images is delineated by use of a thresholding segmentation technique. The threshold is determined empirically such that the total area of the object pixels in the segmented image (with a value of 1) is equal to 65% of the image size. The subsequent processing steps in this section are restricted to the segmented binary image unless otherwise stated. Please note that the segmentation result did not need to be very accurate for the approximate matching of legs. Finally, all isolated objects are labeled, and only one with the largest area is retained. This largest object corresponds to the body of a patient. In addition, a subregion in the segmented images that contains the lower 35% (in height) of the body is determined. For example, if the height of the body is 800 pixels, then the height of the subregion, which is located at the bottom of the body, is 800 × 0.35 = 280 pixels.

Registration of the leg is started on the left side of the two images. It can be right leg or left leg depending on whether the bone scan is acquired on the anterior or posterior side. To determine the leg on the left, the left 55% of the earlier-mentioned subregion is retained and the right 45% of the subregion is removed. In the remaining left region, all isolated objects are labeled again, and the largest one is retained. The largest object corresponds to the leg on the left. The central line (known as medial line or skeleton in computer vision) of the leg is determined by identifying the central point of object pixels in each row of the subregions. The shift value in the horizontal direction for each row is defined as the displacement of the two central points for the row in the two images. Please note that only the horizontal

shift value is used because the legs in the two images are generally away from each other in the horizontal direction.

Once the shift values for each row of the subregions are determined, a three-point average smoothing method is used 100 times to smooth the shift values. The smoothed shift values are then used for shifting the leg on the left in the previous image. A technique similar to that described earlier is used for shifting the legs on the right of the two images so that they can match. The only difference is now to retain the right 55%, instead of the left 55%, of the subregion, in which the leg on the right will be included.

19.2.3.3 Local Image Matching and Warping by Use of an Elastic Matching Technique

The local image-matching and -warping technique tries to register accurately the two images that are roughly matched by use of global matching and leg matching. The technique consists of three steps. The first step is the automatic selection of many template ROIs in the previous image and many search area ROIs in the current image. For applying this technique to whole-body bone scans, which usually has a matrix size of 256 × 1024 for one image, the matrix sizes of the template ROIs and the search area ROIs are determined with 12 × 12 and 24 × 24, respectively. The distance between the adjacent ROIs is 8 pixels. Therefore, there is 33.3% and 66.7% overlap between two adjacent template ROIs and two adjacent search area ROIs, respectively.

The second step is the determination of cross-correlation values between template ROIs and the corresponding search area ROIs for measuring their similarities. A shift vector indicates a shift in the location of a template ROI (12 × 12 pixels) to be matched with a corresponding local region (12 × 12 pixels) included in the search area ROI (24 × 24 pixels), and a correlation value indicates the extent of the similarity between the shifted template and the corresponding region of the search area. An array of correlation values for a given template ROI with all possible shift vectors is obtained for iteratively determining the final shift vector by the application of the elastic matching technique (Li et al. 2000).

The third step is the determination of final shift vectors for the template ROIs by use of the elastic matching technique. The elastic matching technique iteratively updates the shift vectors by taking into account the cross-correlation values and the consistency and/or smoothness between adjacent shift vectors. Therefore, the elastic matching technique iteratively changes the current shift vector for each ROI according to two measures. The first measure, or the internal energy, is to examine the consistency (smoothness) of the local shift vectors, which is given here by the squared sum of the first and the second derivatives over the local shift vectors. The smoother the local shift vectors, the smaller the internal energy will be. The second measure, or the external energy, is equal to the negative value of the cross-correlation value, so that a shift vector with a large correlation value provides a small external energy. The local energy for a given template ROI is thus defined as the weighted sum of the internal and external energies.

The objective for the elastic matching technique is to minimize the total energy over the entire image, which is given by the sum of the local energies for all template ROIs. The initial shift vector for each ROI can be selected arbitrarily, and in this study, it was taken to be the one with the maximum correlation value. The shift vectors are then updated by use of a greedy algorithm. At a specific iteration, the shift vector for a template ROI is assumed to be represented by a 2D vector (dx, dy). With the greedy algorithm, the new shift vector for the template ROI at the next iteration is selected as the one with the minimum local energy among $(2N + 1) \times (2N + 1)$ possible shift vectors, that is, the $(2N + 1) \times (2N + 1)$ combinations of $(2N + 1)$ X-shift values $\{dx - N, dx - N + 1, ..., dx + N - 1, dx + N\}$ and $(2N + 1)$ Y-shift values $\{dy - N, dy - N + 1, ..., dy + N - 1, dy + N\}$. For bone scan images, N was determined empirically to be 4. This procedure is applied to each of the template ROIs for an iteration of update of the shift vectors and is repeated several times over the entire image until no more than 1% of shift vectors in all ROIs are updated.

Once the final shift vectors for all ROIs were obtained, a bilinear interpolation technique was employed for the determination of the shift vectors for all pixels over the entire previous image. The interpolated shift vectors were then used to warp the previous image. Finally, the warped previous image was subtracted pixel-by-pixel from the original image to provide the temporal subtraction image. In order to indicate both hot and cold regions in the temporal subtraction image, the base pixel value of 256 (25% of the maximum gray scale) was added to the subtraction image. Figure 19.6 shows posterior views of (a) the matched image and (b) the warped image of the previous scan, which was subtracted from (c) the current scan to provide (d) the temporal subtraction image.

19.3 COMPUTERIZED DETECTION OF INTERVAL CHANGES ON TEMPORAL SUBTRACTION IMAGES

Potential clinical utility of temporal subtraction images for successive whole-body bone scan is not only displaying subtraction images but utilized for computerized detection of interval changes. For developing the computerized scheme, 58 pairs of successive whole-body bone scans were selected with several inclusion criteria determined by two experienced radiologists as follows: (1) at least one abnormal finding in either view, (2) a maximum number of 20 interval changes, and (3) one image pair per patient.

In order to determine a *gold standard* for the development of computerized scheme, independent identifications of interval changes, which were provided by the two radiologists, are used.

The computerized scheme for the detection of interval changes shown here included four steps: (1) an initial identification of candidates for interval changes, (2) image feature extraction of candidates for interval changes, (3) removal of some false positives by use of a rule-based test, and (4) display of the computer output for identified interval changes. Two types of interval changes, for hot and cold lesions, are identified separately by use of the same techniques, but with different parameters. In addition, all of the procedures in the computerized scheme are carried out separately for each view, and the overall performance for the detection of interval changes is evaluated based on the number of *gold standard* interval changes included in each case. Note that, in the temporal subtraction images, hot lesions appear as dark areas, whereas cold lesions appear as light areas. Therefore, hot-lesion images are created by the elimination of cold lesions, that is, by changing the pixel values in cold lesions to the base pixel value of 256. On the other hand, cold-lesion images are created by reversing the pixel values in the temporal subtraction image such that cold legions appeared as dark areas and hot lesions as light areas. Then, cold-lesion images are obtained by the elimination of light areas in the same way as that used for hot-lesion images.

19.3.1 Initial Identification of Interval Changes

Candidates for interval changes in each view are identified initially by use of a multiple thresholding technique for hot-lesion-enhanced and cold-lesion-enhanced images, which are obtained from the hot-lesion and cold-lesion images, respectively. The pixel values of the hot-lesion-enhanced image are obtained from the same location of the hot-lesion image if the original pixel values in the previous image are >30, which can be considered as the threshold pixel value for distinguishing hot lesions from both background noise and normal bone structures. In the same way, the pixel values of the cold lesions are obtained if the original pixel values in the current images are >30. The gray scales of the hot-lesion-enhanced and the cold-lesion-enhanced images are normalized linearly by use of the upper 5% and 85% of the area under the histogram of pixel values included in the image. In addition, a Gaussian filter is applied to the images normalized as described earlier in order to reduce some remaining noise in the image.

The multiple-gray-level thresholding technique can be applied sequentially for identifying candidates of interval changes, by use of the area under the histogram of the lesion-enhanced image with an increment of 2%, until the threshold pixel value became <512 or the percentage of

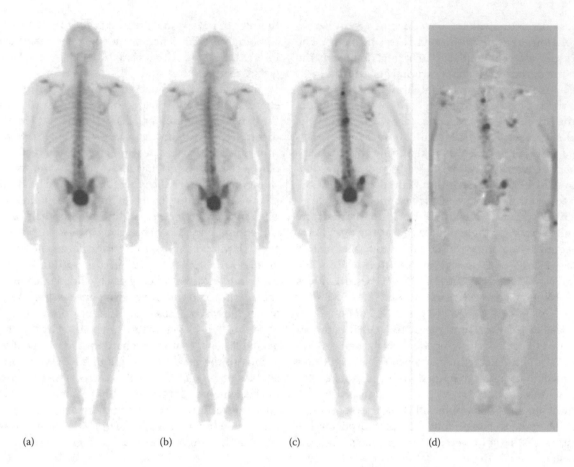

(a)   (b)   (c)   (d)

Figure 19.6   Examples of (a) normalized and matched previous image, (b) nonlinear warped image obtained from matched image corresponding to (c) normalized current image, and (d) temporal subtraction image obtained by subtraction of (b) the previous image from (c) the current image.

the area became 66% of the total area. Initial candidates of interval changes are identified if (1) the centroid of the candidate, which is called an island here and is derived by multiple-gray-level thresholding, is not overlapped with the candidates identified in the previous threshold levels, and (2) the effective diameter of the island is >3.0 and <200.0 mm. In order for determining the contour of each candidate, a region-growing technique with a seed point over the centroid of the identified island can be applied.

19.3.2   Feature Extraction and Selection

In the process of initial identification, a number of image features can be obtained based on the contour of an island in the hot-lesion/cold-lesion-enhanced image, such as the (1) threshold value (%) at the initial identification level, (2) sequential order of the candidate among all of the candidates detected initially, (3) effective diameter, (4) circularity, (5) irregularity, (6) normalized vertical location, (7) contrast value obtained by the difference between the maximum and minimum pixel values within the island,

(8) average pixel value within the island, (9) standard deviation of pixel values within the island, and (10) difference in the pixel value between the inside and outside regions of the island.

If the nonlinear image-warping technique does not work successfully for matching two images, misregistration artifacts may occur in the temporal subtraction image, with some false positives for interval changes. Therefore, in addition to the 10 initial image features, 4 image features (the contrast, average pixel value, standard deviation of the pixel value, and the difference between the inside and outside regions) can be obtained from the warped previous image and also from the current image at the locations of identified candidates in order to examine the pixel values and image features in the original images.

19.3.3   False-Positive Reduction

A rule-based scheme for the removal of a number of false positives is also applied in each view. A number of image feature pairs are determined for both hot and cold lesions by use of a 2D linear discriminant analysis (LDA) method. The 2D LDA method is first trained by use of all of the 58 case pairs and then is tested by use of the same case pairs.

Finally, all interval changes identified in each view and also in either hot or cold lesions are combined. Because some lesions had high intensities for both anterior and posterior views, one lesion (i.e., one truth) can be identified in both views or in either view. Therefore, an interval change is considered to be a true positive when the lesion is identified in either view, even if the truth is marked in both views by the radiologists. The interval change is considered to have been detected correctly, that is, to be a true-positive detection, when the distance between the truth location identified by the radiologists and the centroid of the region of the identified interval change is <20 mm.

19.3.4 Performance Evaluation for Detection of Interval Changes

The overall sensitivity in the detection of 107 *gold standard* interval changes, including both hot and cold lesions, in the 58 successive bone scan pairs was 95.3%, with 5.78 false positives per view. The sensitivity and false positives per view in each view and in each type (hot/cold) of lesion were 95.5% and 3.79 for hot lesions on anterior views, 91.7% and 0.72 for cold lesions on anterior views, 88.2% and 6.21 for hot lesions on posterior views, and 94.1% and 1.78 for cold lesions on posterior views. However, the computer performance shown here was obtained with the same training and test cases. Therefore, performance of this CAD scheme should be evaluated with little bias by use of a validated approach such as the jackknife method or the round-robin method.

19.4 OBSERVER STUDIES FOR INTERVAL CHANGES IN SUCCESSIVE WHOLE-BODY BONE SCANS

In order for evaluating the usefulness of temporal subtraction images obtained from two successive whole-body bone scans, an observer performance study was conducted (Shiraishi et al. 2007a) by use of a jackknife free-response receiver operating characteristic (JAFROC) analysis method (Chakraborty and Berbaum 2004). In this observer study, 20 pairs of successive whole-body bone scans were randomly selected from a total of 58 bone scintigram cases, which were used for the development of the computerized temporal subtraction technique for successive whole-body bone scans as described

in the previous section. Each scan included both posterior and anterior views obtained simultaneously by use of a set of two gamma cameras placed face to face. Based on the two radiologists' agreement on both the location and the type of each lesion, 72 *gold standard* interval changes among the 20 pairs were determined. Seventy-two *gold standard* interval changes included 64 hot lesions (uptake was increased when compared with the previous scan or a new uptake was found in the current scan) and 8 cold lesions (uptake decreased or disappeared) for anterior and/or posterior views. For each case, lesions that could be identified in both views were counted as a single *gold standard*. The average number of interval changes for the 20 pairs was 3.6 (range: 0–11); 3 of the 20 pairs had no interval change even if all cases included one or more abnormalities in at least one view. In addition, another 5 cases were selected from the original 58 cases to be used as a training set for the observer performance study.

The JAFROC analysis has been proposed for estimating statistically significant differences between modalities when location issues are relevant. The JAFROC analysis is based on a free-response receiver operating characteristic (FROC) paradigm and accounts for reader variation (Chakraborty and Berbaum 2004). Conventional ROC analysis is of limited value for this kind of application because only one signal can be used per case and the location of the signal cannot be taken into account in the evaluation (Zheng et al. 2005), whereas FROC analysis allows one to evaluate radiologists' performance in diagnosing medical images by using multiple responses, each with information on the confidence level and location (Chakraborty and Winter 1990). Because all cases used in this observer study had abnormal lesions and only three of these cases contained no interval changes (i.e., negative cases), method 1 of JAFROC was applicable to this observer study.

Five radiologists, including three attendings and two residents, participated in the observer study. All of the radiologists were trained to interpret bone scans and/or had clinical experience in nuclear medicine radiology.

The observer study was organized into two reading sessions separated by an interval of at least 2 weeks. In the first session, without temporal subtraction images, the previous and current images were shown to the radiologist, and then he or she marked lesion locations on the current images and provided confidence ratings on potential interval changes by observing the previous images. In the second session, temporal subtraction images were shown together with the modified previous and current images.

During the observer study, a radiologist identified the most likely location of an interval change by clicking the left button of the mouse and provided a probability (likelihood) of an interval change on a bar displayed in a dialog window next to the clicking point. The levels reported on the bar ranged from *definitely change* at the right end and *probably no change* at the left end. Each radiologist repeated this procedure until he or she could not observe any additional possible interval changes between the images and then moved to the next case. The radiologists were allowed to change the window level and width of each image on the LCD monitor.

The radiologists were not informed that a reading time was being measured during the observer study in order to reduce possible sources of bias in the evaluation. Only in the training session the *gold standards* were indicated on the monitor after the radiologists' final decision.

Figure 19.7 shows the average FROC curves for all radiologists, which compared the radiologists' performance with regard to the sensitivity for the detection of interval changes at the specific false-positive level (i.e., 2.0 false positives per case) without and with temporal subtraction images. For these FROC data, the average figure-of-merit values for all radiologists increased to a statistically significant degree, from 0.508 without the temporal subtraction images to 0.613 with the images (p = 0.035).

The mean reading time per case was reduced significantly from 134 to 91 s (p = 0.004) by use of the temporal subtraction image. In addition, the reading time for each radiologist was reduced significantly for four of the five radiologists, with more than a 20% reduction in reading times.

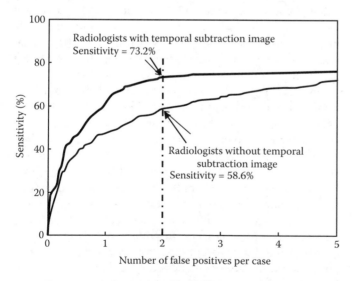

Figure 19.7 Average FROC curves for the five radiologists' performance in the detection of interval changes in 20 successive whole-body bone scans without and with temporal subtraction images.

19.5 PROSPECTIVE CLINICAL STUDY FOR EVALUATING THE CLINICAL UTILITY

The observer study for demonstrating the usefulness of temporal subtraction images in terms of the reduction of reading time and improvement in diagnostic accuracy for identifying interval changes (Shiraishi et al. 2007a) was followed by a prospective clinical study for evaluating the clinical utility of temporal subtraction images in successive whole-body bone scans (Shiraishi et al. 2011).

19.5.1 Construction of Image Server System for Prospective Clinical Study

A temporal subtraction image server is the key for the prospective clinical study, because all images in the clinical situation are usually managed with a picture archiving and communication system (PACS). The temporal subtraction image server in this study was developed for including five special functions: (1) an automated image-retrieval system for searching the most recent whole-body bone scan images in PACS, (2) an automated image-conversion system for converting several types of image formats into raw image data with a 256 × 1024 matrix size, (3) an automated temporal subtraction image production system, (4) a computer interface for displaying and evaluating temporal subtraction images together with the routine diagnosis by use of the PACS, and (5) an automated data-archiving system by securing patient identification.

In this clinical study, the radiologist first determined whether consent from each patient was given or not. If consent was obtained, temporal subtraction images were prepared automatically by the temporal subtraction server by entering the patient ID in the computer. It took 5–10 min for computing temporal subtraction images in each case.

In the standard reading without temporal subtraction images, the radiologist made his or her initial decision regarding bone scan scintigrams by using a standard PACS viewer (Stentor) as usual and dictated the findings (or reviewed with a resident to dictate). At this step, the radiologist did not sign/finalize his or her report until he or she had viewed the temporal subtraction images. Following the standard reading, the radiologist was required to read the case again along with the temporal subtraction images immediately after the completion of the initial reading if the temporal subtraction images were available for viewing. In cases where the temporal subtraction images were not immediately available following the initial clinical read, the radiologist was allowed to review them at his or her earliest convenience. During the second reading with the temporal subtraction images, the radiologist referred to his or her original assessments in order to confirm his or her impression from the temporal subtraction images.

Immediately after the second reading, in order to evaluate the clinical utility of temporal subtraction images, the radiologist was asked a question concerning the overall utility of temporal subtraction images by using a discrete five-point scale (i.e., extremely beneficial, somewhat beneficial, no utility, somewhat detrimental, and extremely detrimental). In addition, the overall utility was evaluated and graded with a number of reasons such as "change in impression," "increase/decrease in confidence," "change in findings," or "the potential to increase/reduce the reading time." It should be noted that the radiologists were asked to identify only the interval changes related to malignant lesions that were visible on the original images viewed with the use of the standard PACS; they did not include other interval changes considered due to benign etiology such as osteoarthritis and fractures. In addition, when the radiologist provided any responses except for "no utility," he or she was asked to mark the positions of the relevant interval changes (if he or she found them because of the use of temporal subtraction images) and to select one of five reasons. Among the five reasons, three are related to characteristics of marked interval changes (new bone lesion, change in bone lesion, or soft-tissue change), and two are related to whether a case has interval changes or no interval change. Moreover, in order to estimate the utility of temporal subtraction images in terms of actual clinical actions, the radiologist was also asked again whether the use of temporal subtraction images changed his or her original impression in the report. However, in order for the radiologist to change the original report following a review of the temporal subtraction images, he or she was asked to confirm his or her judgment by using the clinical PACS for viewing the original bone scans as well as static images of lesions of interest.

In order to confirm that the changes in the impression made during the prospective study were not adversely affected by the use of temporal subtraction images, a consensus was made for all corresponding cases retrospectively by a panel of two radiologists who specialized in nuclear medicine.

19.5.2 Diagnostic Utility of Temporal Subtraction Images

The prospective study was performed between November 22, 2006, and November 30, 2008, in the University of Chicago Hospitals. We had 256 consenting patients of whom 143 had one or more pairs of whole-body bone scans available for temporal subtraction images. For the 143 patients with consent, there were 304 pairs of bone scans. We obtained temporal subtraction images successfully in 292 (96.1%) pairs and failed to produce temporal subtraction images in

12 pairs. There was 1 pair of whole-body bone scans available for temporal subtraction images in 69 patients, 2 pairs for 28, 3 for 26, 4 for 9, and 5 or more for 11 (n = 304). The average number of pairs available for temporal subtraction images per patient was 2.1, and the maximum number of pairs was 8 during the period of our prospective study. We failed to produce temporal subtraction images for 12 pairs of successive bone scans because of (1) missing raw image data for a previous examination (7 pairs), (2) inadequate imaging condition (3 pairs), and (3) improper positioning of the patients (arms up or prone position) (2 pairs).

Radiologists' subjective ratings for the clinical utility of temporal subtraction images applied to the 292 pairs of successive bone scans in this prospective study indicated that temporal subtraction images were considered as "extremely beneficial (n = 24)" or "somewhat beneficial (n = 223)" in 247 (84.6%) pairs of successive bone scans, whereas they were considered as having "no utility" in 44 pairs and as "somewhat detrimental" in only one pair. There was no case considered "extremely detrimental."

For 247 temporal subtraction images for pairs of successive bone scans, which were considered as "extremely beneficial" or "somewhat beneficial," major reasons for radiologists' positive feedback were "temporal subtraction image increased radiologist's confidence in his or her original assessment" (102: 41.3%) and "temporal subtraction image increased radiologist's confidence for no change in successive scans" (89: 36.0%). In addition, the radiologists changed the final impression of their initial report in 18 pairs of successive bone scans (6.2%). All changes made by use of temporal subtraction images were retrospectively confirmed as "correct responses" by the consensus of two expert radiologists. Figure 19.8 shows one example that was considered as "extremely beneficial" in the prospective study because the radiologist's confidence in his or her original assessment was increased by the use of temporal subtraction images.

19.6 CONCLUSION

In order for the detection of bone metastases in bone scan images, the temporal subtraction techniques would be the most effective and realistic way to apply. The usefulness of temporal subtraction images in successive whole-body bone scans has been demonstrated in terms of its clinical utility in the prospective clinical study as well as the reduction of reading time in the observer study. The temporal subtraction image could, with negligible detrimental effects, be used as a *second opinion* for radiologists to detect interval changes due to bone metastases in successive whole-body bone scans, and thus it could increase their accuracy, speed, and confidence in the interpretation of whole-body bone scans.

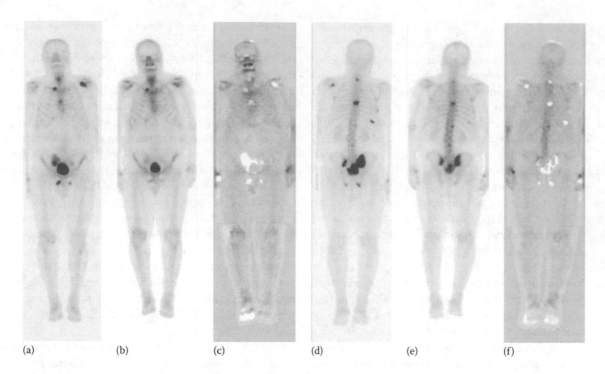

(a)   (b)   (c)   (d)   (e)   (f)

Figure 19.8   Metastatic evaluation in a 73-year-old man with prostate carcinoma. The initial bone scan demonstrated multiple metastases. The follow-up scan was initially interpreted as improvement of all lesions. However, the temporal subtraction images revealed a subtle increasing focus at T12 suspicious for progression of disease at this site: (a) anterior view previous image, (b) anterior view current image, (c) anterior view temporal subtraction image, (d) posterior view previous image, (e) posterior view current image, and (f) posterior view temporal subtraction image.

REFERENCES

Abe, H., T. Ishida, J. Shiraishi, F. Li, S. Katsuragawa, S. Sone, H. MacMahon, and K. Doi. 2004. Effect of temporal subtraction images on radiologists' detection of lung cancer on CT: Results of the observer performance study with use of film computed tomography images. *Acad. Radiol.* 11:1337–1343.

Chakraborty, D.P. and K.S. Berbaum. 2004. Observer studies involving detection and localization: Modeling, analysis, and validation. *Med. Phys.* 31:2313–2330.

Chakraborty, D.P. and L.H. Winter. 1990. Free-response methodology: Alternate analysis and a new observer-performance experiment. *Radiology* 174:873–881.

Difazio, M.C., H. MacMahon, X.W. Xu, P. Tsai, J. Shiraishi, S.G. Armato, 3rd, and K. Doi. 1997. Digital chest radiography: Effect of temporal subtraction images on detection accuracy. *Radiology* 202:447–452.

Ilkko, E., K. Suomi, A. Karttunen, and O. Tervonen. 2004. Computer-assisted diagnosis by temporal subtraction in postoperative brain tumor patients: A feasibility study. *Acad. Radiol.* 11:887–893.

Ishida, T., S. Katsuragawa, K. Nakamura, H. MacMahon, and K. Doi. 1999. Iterative image warping technique for temporal subtraction of sequential chest radiographs to detect interval change. *Med. Phys.* 26:1320–1329.

Kakeda, S., K. Nakamura, K. Kamada, H. Watanabe, H. Nakata, S. Katsuragawa, and K. Doi. 2002. Improved detection of lung nodules by using a temporal subtraction technique. *Radiology* 224:145–151.

Kano, A., K. Doi, H. MacMahon, D.D. Hassell, and M.L. Giger. 1994. Digital image subtraction of temporally sequential chest images for detection of interval change. *Med. Phys.* 21:453–461.

Li, Q., S. Katsuragawa, and K. Doi. 2000. Improved contralateral subtraction images by use of elastic matching technique. *Med. Phys.* 27:1934–1942.

Shiraishi, J., D. Appelbaum, Y. Pu, R. Engelmann, Q. Li, and K. Doi. 2011. Clinical utility of temporal subtraction images in successive whole-body bone scans: Evaluation in a prospective clinical study. *J. Digit. Imaging* 24:680–687.

Shiraishi, J., D. Appelbaum, Y. Pu, Q. Li, L. Pesce, and K. Doi. 2007a. Usefulness of temporal subtraction images for identification of interval changes in successive whole-body bone scans: JAFROC analysis of radiologists' performance. *Acad. Radiol.* 14:959–966.

Shiraishi, J., Q. Li, D. Appelbaum, Y. Pu, and K. Doi. 2007b. Development of a computer-aided diagnostic scheme for detection of interval changes in successive whole-body bone scans. *Med. Phys.* 34:25–36.

UNSCEAR. 2008. Report to the general assembly, with scientific annexes. *United Nations Scientific Committee on the Effects of Atomic Radiation*, New York.

Zheng, B., D.P. Chakraborty, H.E. Rockette, G.S. Maitz, and D. Gur. 2005. A comparison of two data analyses from two observer performance studies using Jackknife ROC and JAFROC. *Med. Phys.* 32:1031–1034.

Chapter 20

Integration of CAD and PACS

Brent J. Liu, Anh Le, and H.K. Huang

CONTENTS

20.1 NEED FOR CAD–PACS™ INTEGRATION

One of the ultimate goals of PACS-based computer-aided detection and diagnosis (CAD) is to integrate CAD results into daily clinical practice as a second reader to aid the radiologist's diagnosis of medical images (Doi 2007, Huang and Doi 2007). CAD relies on the images and related information from Picture Archiving and Communication System (PACS) to improve its accuracy, while PACS benefits from the CAD results online and available at the PACS workstation (WS). Currently, these two technologies remain as two separate independent systems with only minimal system integration. In order to fully achieve the ultimate goal of PACS-based CAD through system integration, it requires certain basic ingredients from Health Level 7 (HL7) standard for textual data, Digital Imaging and Communications in Medicine (DICOM) standard for images, and Integrating the Healthcare Enterprise (IHE) workflow profiles together with the Health Insurance Portability and Accountability Act (HIPAA)-compliant requirements. The key components from the DICOM standard include DICOM structured reporting (DICOM-SR). Likewise, the IHE workflow profiles that need to be utilized include the IHE Key Image Note (KIN), Simple Image and Numeric Report (SIR), and postprocessing workflows (PWFs). These topics with a specific soup-to-nuts CAD example are presented in this chapter.

20.2 FOUR APPROACHES OF CAD–PACS INTEGRATION

Conceptually, integration of CAD with DICOM PACS can have four approaches. In the first three described later in this text, the CAD is connected directly to the PACS, while the fourth approach is to use a CAD server to connect with the PACS (Huang 2007, 2008, 2010). For all four approaches,

CAD software (Doi 2007) can be implemented within a stand-alone CAD WS, a CAD server, or integrated in a PACS WS as PACS-based CAD.

20.2.1 PACS/Modality Push, CAD WS Performs Detection

In this approach, either the imaging modality or the PACS will push images to the CAD WS, which performs the detection. Figure 20.1a illustrates the steps of integration. The user must have knowledge of which imaging studies are to be pushed to the CAD WS. This method involves either the PACS server or the imaging modality, and the CAD WS. A DICOM C-store function must be installed in the CAD WS.

The major disadvantage to this approach is that the particular studies must be selected and manually pushed to the CAD WS for processing. In addition, once the results are generated, they reside only on the CAD WS.

20.2.2 CAD WS Q/R and Performs Detection

In this approach, the CAD WS performs both query and retrieve (Q/R) and then the detection. This method involves

only the PACS server and the CAD WS. Again, the user must have knowledge of which imaging studies are to be retrieved to the CAD WS. The function of the PACS server is almost identical to that of the last method. The only difference is that in the last method, the user must push the imaging studies from either the PACS server or directly from the imaging modality, whereas in this method, the CAD WS performs the Q/R. Consequently, DICOM Q/R functionality must be installed in the CAD WS. Figure 20.1b describes the steps.

Although the CAD WS can directly Q/R from the PACS to obtain the particular image study for processing, the workflow is still manual and a disadvantage. In addition, once the results are generated, they reside only on the CAD WS.

20.2.3 PACS WS with Integrated CAD Software

The third approach is to install the CAD software directly within the PACS WS. This approach eliminates all components in the CAD system and relies on the PACS WS to connect to the PACS. However, it involves a complex integration and mutual deeper knowledge of two software applications (e.g., CAD and PACS WS) from two different manufacturers. Because of this,

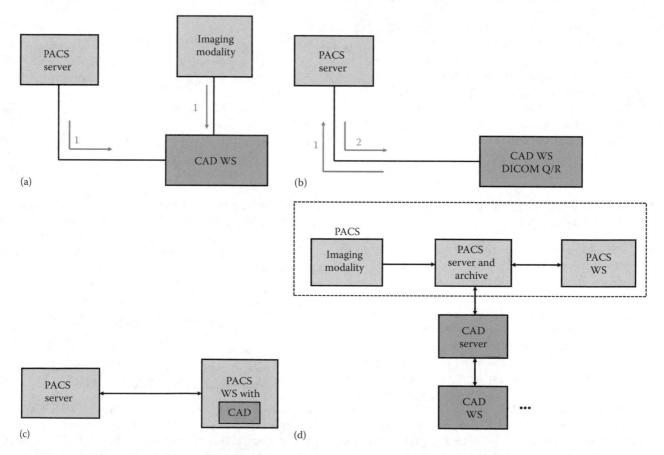

Figure 20.1 Four methods of integrating CAD with DICOM PACS. (a) PACS/Modality Push, CAD WS performs detection. (b) CAD WS query/retrieve and performs detection. (c) PACS WS has the CAD software integrated. (d) Integration of CAD server with PACS.

the third approach is usually a scenario in which the PACS manufacturer acquires and integrates the CAD software into the PACS WS. Figure 20.1c shows the steps involved.

Most of the CAD components can be eliminated, which is an advantage. However, the major disadvantage is that the CAD must be integrated directly with PACS, which requires the CAD manufacturer to work closely with the PACS manufacturer, or vice versa, to open up the software, which rarely happens due to the competitive market.

20.2.4 Integration of CAD Server with PACS

In this method, the CAD server is connected to the PACS server. The CAD server is used to perform Q/R automatically or manually as well as the CAD processing. It contains a separate database for the storage of CAD data and images. The CAD results can be viewed either remotely with a CAD WS or on the same hardware as the PACS WS if the CAD server supports a web-based client for display or directly within the PACS WS application. Figure 20.1d describes the steps involved.

This is the most ideal and practical approach to a CAD–PACS integration as the CAD server can automatically manage the clinical workflow of image studies to be processed, archive CAD results back to PACS for the clinicians to review on PACS WS, and eliminate the need for both CAD and PACS manufacturers to open up their respective software platforms for integration.

Currently, several PACS and CAD manufacturers have successfully integrated their CAD applications within the PACS

operations utilizing one of the four approaches described earlier, but these applications are either in a CAD-specific WS or in a closed PACS operation environment using proprietary software. For example, in mammography, CAD has become an integral part of a routine clinical assessment of breast cancer in many hospitals and clinics across the United States and abroad. Unfortunately, this is not the norm as the overall value and effectiveness of CAD for other clinical applications are compromised by the inconvenience of a stand-alone CAD WS or server that limits how the CAD data are accessed and viewed within daily clinical practice. Table 20.1 shows a brief summary overview of the four approaches and their features, advantages, and disadvantages.

20.3 UTILIZATION OF DICOM AND IHE FOR CAD–PACS INTEGRATION

In order to integrate CAD and PACS more efficiently, certain key components from the DICOM (1999) standard for images and IHE (2008) workflow profiles are needed in order to comply with HIPAA requirements. Specifically, these are DICOM-SR and IHE KIN, SINR, and PWF (Le et al. 2009, Zhou et al. 2007). These will be described in more detail in the following sections.

20.3.1 DICOM Structured Reporting

DICOM-SR is the standardization of SR documents within the clinical imaging environment (DICOM 2008). In clinical practice, the use of structured forms for reporting is beneficial in reducing the ambiguity of natural language format reporting by enhancing the precision, clarity, and value of the clinical document. In addition, SR documents record observations made for an imaging-based diagnostic or interventional procedure, particularly information that describes or references images, waveforms, or specific regions of interest. DICOM-SR was introduced in 1994, and Supplement 23 was adopted by the DICOM Committee in 1999 for clinical reports. Since then, the DICOM Committee has ratified more than 12 supplements to define specific SR document templates, two of which relate to capturing CAD results. These templates are the Mammography CAD SR (Supplement 50, 2000), which allows for presentation and storage of CAD results including ACR's BI-RADS™ reporting structure and detected findings such as calcifications and masses, and the Chest CT CAD SR (Supplement 65, 2001), which also supports presentation and storage of detected findings.

The DICOM-SR object is considered part of the DICOM information object definitions and services for storage and transmission similar to the DICOM image object. Figure 20.2 provides a simplified version of the DICOM model of the real world showing where DICOM-SR object resides. The most important part of an SR object is the content, which is an SR

TABLE 20.1 SUMMARY OVERVIEW OF THE ADVANTAGES AND DISADVANTAGES OF THE FOUR APPROACHES TO CAD–PACS INTEGRATION

CAD–PACS Integration Approach	Advantages	Disadvantages
PACS WS Q/R, CAD WS detect	Simple integration; CAD WS requires only DICOM C-store.	Study will not be processed at CAD WS unless manually pushed.
CAD WS Q/R and detect	Simple integration; CAD must support DICOM Q/R.	Study will not be processed at CAD WS unless manually Q/R.
PACS WS with CAD SW	Integrated workflow w/ PACS WS.	Complex integration requires PACS manufacturer to install CAD SW in PACS WS.
CAD server with PACS	Automatic integrated workflow w/PACS WS.	Simpler integration—no need to install CAD SW in the PACS WS.

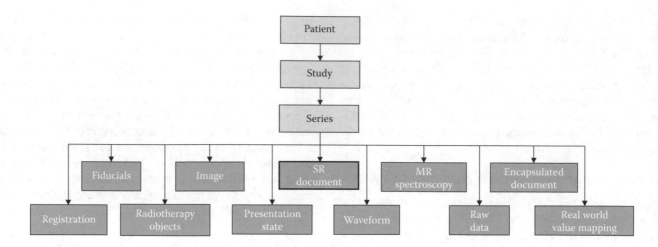

Figure 20.2 DICOM-SR objects in the DICOM model of the real world. The SR document outlined in bold is located in the DICOM data model, which is at the same level as the DICOM image.

template that consists of different design patterns for various applications. CAD results with images, graphs, overlays, annotations, and text can be translated into an SR template designed for this application. The data in the specific template can be treated as a DICOM object stored in the worklist of the data model (see Figure 20.2 box outlined in bold). Likewise, it can be displayed for review by a DICOM-compliant PACS WS that supports DICOM-SR display functionality. In order to display the results, the original images from which the CAD results were generated are required so that the CAD results can be overlaid onto the images and are achieved through the DICOM image reference object. The SR display function can link and download these images from the PACS archive and display them on the PACS WS.

20.3.2   IHE Profiles

IHE profiles address the integration needs of healthcare sites and IT products through a common language and how they interact with each other in clinical scenarios. They provide implementation paths for communications and security standards in DICOM and HL7 W3C to streamline workflow. Three such IHE (2008) profiles are relevant for CAD–PACS integration:

1. KIN profile: Allows users to flag images as significant (for referring, for surgery, etc.) and add a note to explain the content
2. SINR profile: Specifies how diagnostic radiology reports (including images and numeric data) are created, exchanged, and used
3. PWF profile: Provides a worklist, status, and result tracking for post-acquisition processing tasks, such as CAD or volumetric (3D) image processing

20.4   SOLUTION FOR CAD–PACS INTEGRATION: THE CAD–PACS TOOLKIT

Currently, there is no solution that utilizes HL7 and DICOM standards together with IHE profiles described previously to provide a fully integrated CAD–PACS workflow. The following section describes a software toolkit that will allow CAD manufacturers to integrate with PACS not only for improving workflow efficiency but also for CAD results query and knowledge discovery in the future.

20.4.1   Current CAD Workflow

Figure 20.3 depicts the PACS environment, including an RIS, Modality, PACS server, and PACS WS, and a CAD WS/server (blue box) that is outside the realm of PACS. Usually, these two systems are disjoint as described previously as one of the four approaches to CAD–PACS. Currently, when an image is needed for CAD processing, the workflow steps are as follows with corresponding numerals and black-colored lines in Figure 20.3:

1. An imaging study is ordered through RIS that requires CAD postprocessing. A technologist acquires the imaging study at the modality, and the original images are manually sent to the PACS server and then the radiologist can view the imaging study at the PACS WS.
2. A technologist or radiologist then transmits the original images from the PACS server or PACS WS to CAD WS/server for processing. The CAD results are stored within the CAD domain, since the CAD WS or server is a closed system and clinicians need

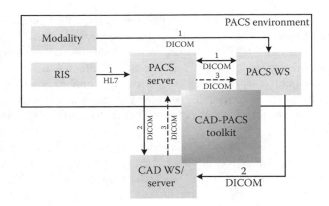

Figure 20.3 CAD workflow in the PACS environment with the CAD–PACS toolkit.

to physically go to the CAD WS to view results. There are current available solutions including a specialized WS that integrates the imaging study and the CAD results. However, these specialized WSs are not true PACS WSs.

20.4.2 Concept of the CAD–PACS Toolkit

CAD–PACS is a software toolkit that was developed in-house at the Image Processing and Informatics Laboratory (IPILab), Department of Biomedical Engineering, University of Southern California. It utilizes the HL7 standard for textual information; DICOM standard for various types of data formats, including images, waveforms, graphics, overlays, and annotations; and IHE workflow profiles described in the previous sections for the integration of CAD results within the PACS workflow (Le et al. 2009). From Figure 20.3, with the integration of the CAD–PACS toolkit, workflow step 3 with dashed-line arrows is described as follows:

1. The CAD–PACS toolkit, which can integrate with the PACS server, PACS WS, and the CAD server/ WS together via the DICOM standard and IHE

profiles, sends the CAD results to the PACS server for archiving and the PACS WS for viewing and query/retrieve original images from PACS server to PACS WS to be overlaid with the CAD results. In addition, it can automatically pass images directly from the PACS server or PACS WS to the CAD WS for processing.

This CAD software toolkit is modularized, and its components are flexible and can be installed in five different configurations: (1) CAD WS, (2) CAD server, (3) PACS WS, (4) PACS server, or (5) a mix of the previous four configurations. A CAD manufacturer would be more comfortable with the first two approaches because there is very little collaboration needed for the PACS software, which is too complex for most CAD manufacturers. On the other hand, a PACS manufacturer would prefer the latter three approaches for integrating in-house or acquired CAD solutions.

20.4.3 Infrastructure of the CAD–PACS Toolkit

The CAD–PACS toolkit has three editions: DICOM–SC™, first edition; DICOM–PACS–IHE™, second edition; and DICOM–CAD–IHE™, third edition. There are five software modules: i-CAD-SC™, i-CAD™, i-PPM™, Receive-SR™, and Display-SR™. Each edition contains some or all of the software modules. Figure 20.4 shows the overall architecture of the toolkit.

The toolkit is classified into three editions for different levels of PACS integration requirements. The first edition converts a simple screen capture output, and the CAD data are not stored for future use. The second edition is for full CAD–PACS integration requiring elaborate collaboration between the CAD developer and the PACS manufacturer. The third edition does not require the elaborate integration efforts of the two parties. The use of the CAD–PACS toolkit is sufficient, which favors the independent CAD

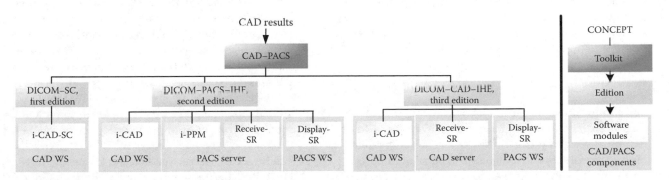

Figure 20.4 The infrastructure of the CAD–PACS integration toolkit. Right: The four-level CAD–PACS integration toolkit. (From Le, A. et al., *Int. J. Comp. Asst. Rad. Surg.*, 4, 317, 2009.)

manufacturer. The following briefly describes the five software modules (Le et al. 2009):

1. i-CAD-SC module creates the screenshots for any CAD application results, converts it to a DICOM Secondary Capture object, and sends it to the PACS server for storage.
2. i-CAD module resides in the CAD WS and provides key functionality for CAD–PACS integration, including DICOM-SR object creation and archival, query/retrieval of images for CAD processing, and communication with the i-PPM module.
3. i-PPM module resides in the PACS server and provides functions to schedule and track the status of CAD postprocessing tasks in the CAD–PACS workflow. This module is also used as a supplement for PACS manufacturers that do not support postprocessing management but needs to be DICOM and IHE-compliant for CAD–PACS integration.
4. Receive-SR module resides in the PACS server and performs the functions of archiving and query/retrieval of DICOM-SR objects from the PACS server.
5. Display-SR module resides in the PACS WS. This module is used when PACS does not support DICOM-SR C-Store SCU and C-Find as well as displaying DICOM-SR objects. The module is developed as a web server with DICOM-SR C-Store and C-Find features to allow for the greatest flexibility for implementation.

20.5 UTILIZATION OF THE CAD–PACS TOOLKIT: A USE CASE

In this section, we provide a step-by-step use case to integrate a CAD application with PACS. The CAD application is an automatic bone age assessment (BAA) of children using a hand-and-wrist radiograph. We will first describe the CAD application, its clinical evaluation and implementation, and finally, its integration with PACS using the CAD–PACS toolkit. For simplicity, we will use the third edition CAD–PACS toolkit to implement the use case (Huang et al. 2011).

20.5.1 Bone Age Assessment of Children

BAA is a clinical procedure in pediatric radiology to evaluate the stage of skeletal maturity based on a left hand and wrist radiograph through bone growth observations. The determination of skeletal maturity (*bone age*) plays an important role in diagnostic and therapeutic investigations of endocrinological abnormality and growth disorders of children.

In clinical practice, the most commonly used BAA method is to match a left hand and wrist radiograph against the Greulich & Pyle (G&P) atlas, which contains a reference set of normal standard hand images collected in 1950s with subjects exclusively from middle- and upper-class Caucasian populations. The atlas has been used for BAA around the world for more than 50 years (Greulich and Pyle 1959).

Over the past 30 years, many studies have raised questions regarding the appropriateness of using the G&P atlas for BAA of contemporary children especially considering the ethnic diversity and environmental factors (Huang 2010). Therefore, a digital hand atlas (DHA) with normal children collected in the United States along with a CAD BAA method has been developed as a means to verify the accuracy of using the G&P atlas to assess today's children's bone age (Gertych et al. 2007). The DHA consists of eight categories, where each category contains 19 age groups. The 19 age groups comprised of one group for subjects younger than 1 year and 18 age groups at 1-year intervals for subjects aged 1–18 years with as even as possible case distribution. The total number of cases (1390) is distributed as follows for the eight categories: 167 Asian girls, 167 Asian boys, 174 African-American girls, 184 African-American boys, 166 Caucasian girls, 167 Caucasian boys, 183 Hispanic girls, and 182 Hispanic boys. At least two pediatric radiologists verified the normality and chronological age for each case. In addition, the bone age of the child was assessed based on the G&P atlas matching method for each case (Zhang et al. 2009).

20.5.2 Evaluation of BAA CAD in Laboratory and Clinical Settings

In order to evaluate the BAA CAD system, it needs to be integrated to PACS. The integration is evaluated first in a laboratory setting, followed by the clinical environment. The laboratory setup mimics the clinical workflow as shown in Figure 20.5 with the following four steps:

1. Once the hand image is acquired by computed radiography (CR), digital radiography (DR), or film scanner, the digital image is sent to the PACS server. The radiologist sitting at the PACS WS manually queries and retrieves the hand image from PACS and displays it on the monitors, or the study can be automatically pushed to the PACS WS.
2. The modality/PACS server also automatically sends a second copy of the hand image to the BAA CAD server, which generates the BAA CAD results.
3. The BAA CAD server sends the CAD results to the PACS WS. The radiologist reviews both the image and BAA CAD results on the PACS WS.

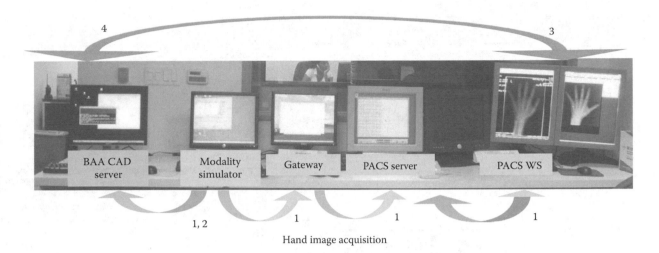

Figure 20.5 Clinical workflow diagram of the BAA CAD system in the laboratory environment using the PACS simulator. (From Zhou, Z. et al., An educational RIS/PACS simulator. InfoRAD exhibit, *Radiology Society of North America 88th Scientific Assembly and Annual Meeting*, Chicago, IL, December 1–6, 2002, p. 753.) See text for descriptions of the workflow steps.

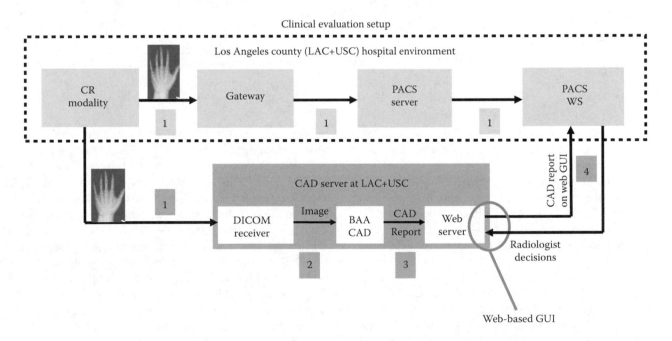

Figure 20.6 BAA CAD system in clinical environment. The diagram depicts the workflow implemented in LAC+USC (Los Angeles County) Hospital with the clinical PACS and the CAD server. See text for descriptions of workflow steps.

4. Diagnosis from the radiologist assisted by CAD results is sent back to the CAD server for storage and future analysis.

After laboratory validation, the BAA CAD system is installed in a clinical environment for evaluation. In this example, the clinical environment is located at the Radiology Department of Los Angeles County Hospital (LAC+USC), where the CAD server can access the PACS and CR images. The clinical workflow shown in Figure 20.6 is similar to the laboratory workflow and is as follows:

1. CR sends a copy of the hand image to the web-based CAD server located in the radiology reading room. The PACS WS also receives a copy of the image from the PACS server under normal clinical operations.

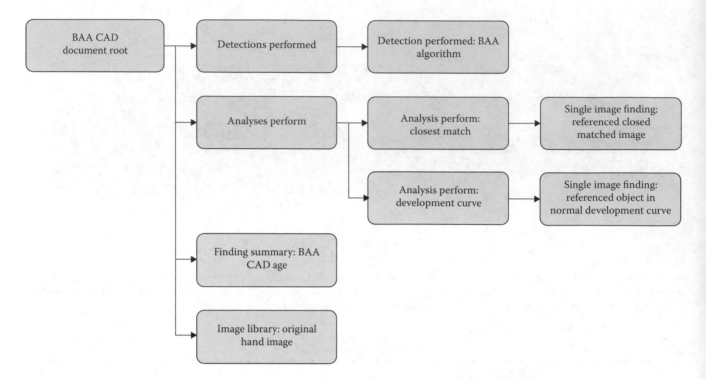

Figure 20.7   DICOM-SR template for BAA CAD. The SR template is designed based on the types of output radiologists are required to review.

2. The CAD server receives the image, performs the BAA CAD, and records the results in the CAD server database.

3. The CAD server searches the PAC server/WS to locate the original image and link up with the CAD result together with the best-matched image from the DHA in the CAD database and prepares the results for display through a web server.

4. The web-based GUI (graphical user interface) is integrated with the PACS WS and displays the original image and the best-matched image and assists the radiologist to make the final diagnosis with the CAD results. The radiologist's decision is captured within the GUI and stored in the web server for future analysis.

20.5.3   Integration of BAA CAD with PACS Utilizing the CAD–PACS Toolkit

In Section 20.3.1, we presented the concept of a DICOM-SR object and the need for converting CAD results and

report data into a DICOM-SR format in order to provide a standardized solution to display on the PACS WS. Figure 20.7 shows the DICOM-SR template for the BAA CAD. Figure 20.8 left illustrates the first page of the BAA CAD report in DICOM-SR format of Patient 1. To the right is the plot of the bone age (vertical axis) against the chronological age (horizontal axis) of Patient 1 (red dot) within the ±2 standard deviations of the normal cases in the DHA. Figure 20.9 depicts an image page of the CAD SR report of Patient 2 including the original image (left) from which the BAA result was obtained, the G&P atlas best-matched image (middle), and the DHA best-matched image (right). The chronologic age and the CAD-assessed age of Patient 2, and the chronological age of the best-matched image in the DHA are enclosed inside the outlines in the upper right corner. The plot of the CAD assessed bone age of Patient 2 within the ±2 standard deviations of the normal cases in the DHA is shown in the upper right corner. This example shows how the BAA CAD results can be integrated in a standardized DICOM-SR object that can be archived in PACS and displayed on PACS WS. The BAA CAD data can now be queried and mined for future analysis.

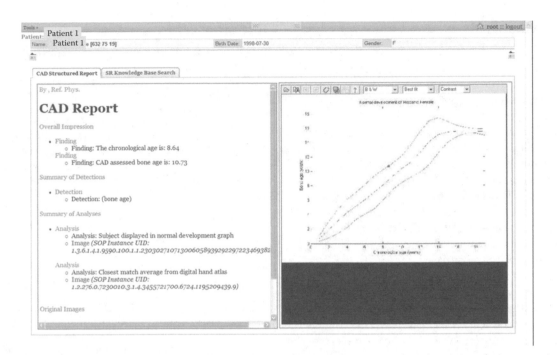

Figure 20.8 Integrating bone age assessment CAD with DICOM-SR. Left: CAD report in DICOM-SR format based on the design of the SR template as shown in Figure 20.7. Right: A component in the DICOM-SR that is a plot of the CAD BAA results of a patient (dot) compared with the normals and ±2 standard deviations in the digital hand atlas.

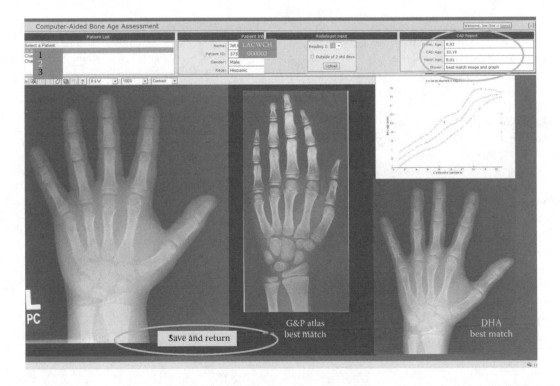

Figure 20.9 BAA CAD clinical evaluation web-based GUI application as shown on the PACS WS. The original image (left), the best-matched G&P atlas image (center), and the best-matched DHA image (right). The best-matched DHA image is obtained by using the CAD age of the patient to search the DHA in the order of race, sex, and age. The image with the closest chronologic age (the best-matched age) is the matched image in the DHA. The chronologic age, BAA bone age, and the matched DHA age are shown at the upper right of the screen within the ellipse. The CAD accessed bone age of the patient compared to the children in the normal range in the DHA is shown in the plot.

20.6 CONCLUSION

In order for CAD to be useful to aid diagnosis/detection, it has to be integrated into the existing clinical workflow. In the case of image-based CAD, the integration is with the PACS daily workflow. We have presented the rationale and methods of CAD–PACS integration with emphasis in PACS workflow profiles using the DICOM standard and IHE workflow profiles.

In the PACS-based workflow approach, the CAD results do not have to reside in the PACS server and storage; instead, they are in the CAD server until the PACS server can eventually support storage of DICOM-SR. PACS images used by the CAD are linked with the CAD results so that both images and CAD results in DICOM format can be displayed on the PACS WS. In this chapter, CAD for the BAA on hand and wrist joint radiographs was presented as a use case for the CAD–PACS toolkit. This use case example demonstrates the advantage of CAD and PACS integration for daily clinical practice. As an example, physicians can assess the bone age of a child using the G&P method. In addition, with the integration of BAA CAD directly into the PACS workflow, the radiologist would have the CAD results as a second reader to assist his/her BAA diagnosis without having to access separate stand-alone WSs and can perform future analysis on key CAD result data in a standardized fashion.

Integration of CAD to PACS clinical workflow has many distinct advantages:

1. PACS technology is mature. Integrating CAD with the PACS can take advantage of the powerful computers and high-speed networks utilized in PACS to enhance the computational and communication power of the CAD.
2. The DICOM-SR and IHE workflow profiles can be readily applied to facilitate the integration of CAD results to PACS WS.
3. PACS-based query/retrieve tools can facilitate CAD users to obtain images and related patient data directly from PACS for CAD algorithm enhancement and execution.
4. CAD–PACS integration results can be directly viewed at the PACS WS together with relevant PACS data.
5. The very large, dynamic, and up-to-date PACS databases can be utilized by CAD to improve its diagnostic accuracy.

REFERENCES

DICOM Standard. Supplement 23: Structured Reporting Object; 1999. http://medical.nema.org/medical/dicom/.

DICOM Standards. 2008. http://medical.nema.org/medical/dicom/.

Doi K. Computer-aided diagnosis in medical imaging: Historical review, current status and future potential. *Computerized Medical Imaging and Graphics* 31(4–5):198–211; 2007.

Gertych A, Zhang A, Sayre J, Pospiech-Kurkowska S, Huang HK. Bone age assessment of children using a digital hand atlas. *Computerized Medical Imaging and Graphics* 31(4–5):322–331; 2007.

Greulich WW, Pyle SI. *Radiographic Atlas of Skeletal Development of Hand Wrist.* Stanford, CA: Stanford University Press, pp. 1–36, 190, 194–195; 1959.

Health Level 7; 2008. http://www.hl7.org/.

Huang HK. *PACS and Imaging Informatics: Basic Principles and Applications,* 2nd edn. Hoboken, NJ: Wiley and Blackwell; 2010.

Huang HK. Tutorial on CAD-PACS integration. *Computer Assisted Radiology and Surgery: CARS,* Berlin, Germany, June 27–30; 2007.

Huang HK. Tutorial on CAD-PACS integration. *Computer Assisted Radiology and Surgery: CARS,* Barcelona, Spain, June 25–28; 2008.

Huang HK, Doi K. CAD and image-guided decision support. *Computerized Medical Imaging and Graphics* 31(4–5):195–197; 2007.

Huang HK, Liu BJ, Le A, Documet J. PACS-based computer-aided detection and diagnosis. *Biomedical Image Processing,* Thomas M. Deserno, Ed., Chapter 18. Berlin, Germany: Springer-Verlag, pp. 455–469; 2011.

IHE 2008. http://www.ihe.net.

Le AHT, Liu B, Huang HK. Integration of computer-aided diagnosis/detection (CAD) results in a PACS environment using CAD–PACS toolkit and DICOM SR. *International Journal of Computer Assisted Radiology and Surgery* 4:317–329; 2009.

Zhang A, Sayre, JW, Vachon L, Liu BJ, Huang HK. Cross-racial differences in growth patterns of children based on bone age assessment. *Journal of Radiology* 290(1):228–235; 2009.

Zhou Z, Law M, Huang HK, Cao F, Liu B, Zhang J. An educational RIS/PACS simulator. InfoRAD exhibit. *Radiology Society of North America 88th Scientific Assembly and Annual Meeting,* Chicago, IL, December 1–6, p. 753; 2002.

Zhou Z, Liu BJ, Le A. CAD-PACS integration tool kit-based on DICOM screen capture (SC) and structured reporting (SR) and IHE workflow profiles. *Journal of Computerized Medical Imaging and Graphics* 31(4–5):346–352; 2007.

Assessment and Clinical Utility of Computer-Aided Detection and Diagnosis

Chapter 21

Methodologies for the Assessment of CAD Systems

Yulei Jiang

CONTENTS

21.1 INTRODUCTION

Computer-aided diagnosis (CAD) refers to an approach to diagnostic practice in which the radiologist in the interpretation of medical images is assisted by a computer, which analyzes the image data with a mathematical algorithm implemented as computer software. Currently, only computer-aided detection (CADe) has been introduced in clinical practice. The goal of CADe is to help radiologists detect cancers or other abnormalities that they might miss without the assistance of CADe. In CADe, the computer identifies a number of possible lesions or abnormalities in the images and presents the results to the radiologist, who then must decide whether the computer detection results are true lesions or true abnormalities or false positives. This chapter discusses several methodological issues for the assessment of the clinical effect of CAD, particularly of CADe.

The assessment of the performance and effect of clinical use of CAD systems is important. CAD is still relatively novel in the long history of clinical practice of modern medicine;

the clinical effect of CAD remains controversial and not fully understood. As a new technology, there are great interests in finding out whether it works as intended—to ascertain its clinical benefit and any other clinical effects. CAD is also unique in that, unlike other imaging technologies when they are novel, CAD does not provide a new kind of image; rather, its effect and benefit depend on the combined system of the radiologist and the CAD computer. This unique characteristic is another reason underscoring the interests in understanding the clinical effect and benefit of CAD. The US Food and Drug Administration (FDA) has a mandate to study the safety and effectiveness of CAD systems as novel medical devices before it issues approval for the marketing of such devices in the United States for clinical use. Therefore, the FDA has a particular interest in the assessment of CAD systems.

The assessment of CAD systems by definition of its intended clinical use encompasses the assessment of the radiologist–CAD–computer system. Assessment of the CAD computer is often the first step, but is not complete by itself. A full assessment of CAD must include the radiologist's use of the CAD device. This assessment of a combined human expert–equipment system is relatively new.

There are many obstacles to accurate assessment of CADe systems. Many issues and nuances must be considered, and some of these are discussed in this chapter. The evaluation of the combined human–computer system presents considerable challenges. Furthermore, because CADe systems are often designed for screening settings, such as screening mammography for breast cancer, it is often an unavoidable necessity to design the assessment study for *small numbers* because of the relative rarity of cancers in the overall patient population undergoing screening. Thus, the statistical consequences of small numbers often must be considered in the assessment of CADe systems. Finally, to isolate the effect of CADe from other confounding factors often presents significant challenges.

In this chapter, we will discuss several types of assessment studies of CADe systems and a few general issues that can confound the assessment of CADe systems. We will first discuss the early demonstration of potential clinical benefit of CADe with the missed-lesion study, then discuss the standalone performance evaluation of the CADe computer by itself, next discuss laboratory observer performance studies, and finally discuss four types of clinical assessment studies: the head-to-head comparison of radiologists' diagnostic performance without the use of CADe vs. their performance with the use of CADe, the histological-control comparison of before and after the clinical introduction of a CADe system, the comparison of the use of CADe with double reading by radiologists, and the randomized controlled clinical trial. We discuss three confounding factors important for the assessment of CADe systems: the statistical issue with small numbers of cancers, the issue and effects of variability in the clinical performance of radiologists, and the issue with expected transient changes in the cancer detection rate as a result of the clinical use of CADe.

21.2 EARLY DEMONSTRATION OF POTENTIAL BENEFIT

In the early stages in the development of CADe systems, there is a critical need to demonstrate the potential of CADe systems. The emphasis here is on *potential*. At this stage, it is not realistic to conduct a full and complete assessment because the CADe systems have not yet been developed maturely and because not enough is known about these systems (e.g., how they might be used clinically) to determine the appropriate evaluation methodology. Yet an early assessment on *potential* is paramount both to justify and to motivate efforts devoted to the development of such systems.

One particularly clever method for this early evaluation is to study missed-lesion cases. That is to use a CADe system—specifically the computer by itself—to analyze a set of clinical cases that contain missed lesions. A case is said to contain a missed lesion if the images of the case contain a lesion, but the lesion was not identified correctly at the time the case was interpreted clinically by a radiologist, and it was determined subsequently and retrospectively that the lesion was indeed present in the image or images. This is a clever approach because, if a CADe computer is able to detect missed lesions, it not only proves that the CADe computer is able to detect lesions, but also proves that the CADe computer is able to detect lesions that radiologists miss. Thus, this study outcome would suggest that the CADe computer might be able to help radiologists detect missed lesions, which is a significant potential clinical benefit.

Clearly, this clever study design can be used to show *potential* clinical benefit but not *actual* clinical benefit. Because the CADe computer has not actually helped radiologists detect missed lesions, it only demonstrates a tantalizing potential for the CADe computer to do so. This study design shows the first of two necessary happenings for CADe to help radiologists detect missed lesions (that the CADe computer is able to detect missed lesions), and it does not show the second necessary happenings (that radiologists respond correctly to what the CADe computer detects and recognize the lesion that they have missed). There are reasons that radiologists may not respond correctly to everything that the CADe computer detects, and those reasons will be discussed later. Yet the missed-lesion study is so crucial in the early development of CADe systems that they are almost a necessary first step in the development of CADe systems. The potential clinical benefit that these studies demonstrate—limited as it is—provides powerful motivation and rationale for the development of CADe systems.

The general idea of a missed-lesion study is straightforward, but to conduct such a study can be a serious undertaking. The general steps are as follows: first, collect a set of cases that contain missed lesions; then, use the CADe computer to analyze these cases; and finally, calculate the true-positive and false-positive detections made by the computer. To collect a large enough number of missed-lesion cases is not easy, because presumably missed lesions are infrequent clinical events. Another reason for this to be difficult is because it is not easy to capture missed lesions (false negatives) from the much large pool of true-negative cases—cases that do not contain the target lesions—both of which are treated the same clinically until the missed lesion becomes evident. Missed-lesion cases are typically identified retrospectively. When a cancer is diagnosed, one can look back in previous images of the same case and see whether the cancer was indeed in the earlier images.

If the cancer was in the previous images, then it is a candidate case of missed lesion. But to decide whether a known cancer is in an image can be truly difficult. Must the cancer be clearly visible, or does a vague shadow that merely suggests something at the location of the cancer differs from its surroundings suffice as a missed lesion? It can be much easier to see a cancer after we know that it is definitely there, but where do we set the bar to judge that someone else has missed the cancer when the images were interpreted—vs. the alternative that what's in the image is not enough for the cancer to be recognized? There are no easy answers to these questions. An accepted practice is to have a panel of expert radiologists review candidate cases and decide, based on their opinion, whether each lesion is a missed lesion—that the clinical radiologist who interpreted the case and did not act on it was reasonably expected to act on it. When the experts disagree, as they often do, a predetermined majority rule can be applied to determine a unique decision for each candidate case.

We mention here in passing another factor that can complicate a missed-lesion study: the determination of whether a CADe computer actually detects a cancer. That is, how close do we require the point of the arrowhead—if that is how CADe computer detection results are indicated—to the center of the cancer to call the CADe computer result a true positive, and how far away does the arrowhead have to be from the edge of the cancer before we call it a false positive? The stakes here are high. If we impose stringent criteria for calling true positives, the estimated sensitivity of the CADe computer (the fraction of cancers detected correctly) will tend to be lower and the false-positive rate of the CADe computer (the number of false-positive computer detections per image or per case) will tend to be higher, because some of the computer detection results (e.g., those that consisted of a part of a cancer and something else—perhaps normal dense tissue) might be scored as a false positive instead of a true positive. If we impose lenient criteria for calling true positives, the estimated sensitivity will tend to be higher and false-positive rate will tend to be lower, but there will be an increased risk for a randomly thrown dart—rather than the targeted detection made by the CADe computer—to hit the cancer and be counted as a true positive. This is a vexing problem not just for a missed-lesion study, but a common issue whenever the results of a CADe computer need to be scored to determine its sensitivity and false-positive rate.

A well-known example of missed-lesion studies is that of Warren Burhenne et al. in 2000 [1]. The study was conducted by an early pioneering commercial company making a CADe device for the detection of clustered microcalcifications and malignant masses in screening mammograms. The study was a key part of the company's submission to the FDA for approval to market the device in the United States. The case materials involved in this study began with 1083 biopsy-proven breast cancers diagnosed at 13 US clinical facilities. A review found 427 of these patients had prior screening mammograms 9–24 months before the cancer diagnosis (mammograms that were thought to be unsuitable for retrospective interpretation for whatever reason was not included in the 427 cases). Of these 427 prior mammograms that a cancer was diagnosed subsequently, the cancer was determined to be visible in 286 (67%) cases. A panel of 20 radiologists who read mammograms in a community-practice setting (who met the Mammography Quality Standard Act, or MQSA, qualification standards) was then assembled to review the 286 cases of prior mammograms, with five radiologists reading any given case, to determine, in their opinion, whether the retrospectively visible cancer was actionable in the prior mammograms. Actionable was defined as Breast Imaging Reporting and Data System (BI-RADS) assessment categories 0 (need additional imaging evaluation), 4 (suspicious abnormality—biopsy should be considered), or 5 (highly suggestive of malignancy—appropriate action should be taken) [2,3]. The investigators decided that if one of five radiologists considered a lesion actionable, then they assessed a 20% probability for that lesion to be actionable; if two of five radiologists considered a lesion actionable, then they assessed a 40% probability for that lesion to be actionable; and so on. This review found 115 actionable cancers in the 427 cancers in prior mammograms (27%), or the 1083 cancers that the study began with (11%)—a relatively low yield of missed-cancer cases. Interestingly, the numbers of cancers in the prior mammograms that were assessed a probability for being actionable of 20%, 40%, etc., were distributed remarkably evenly [1]. An analysis then showed that the CADe computer correctly marked 89 (77%) of the 115 missed cancers in the prior mammograms. The company successfully obtained FDA premarketing approval for this CADe device based in large part on this missed-lesion study.

As a part of the Warren Burhenne study, in estimating the potential benefit of the CADe device on radiologists' false-negative rate, they stated that the use of the CADe device "could have potentially helped reduce this false-negative rate by 77% (89 of 155)" [1]. This estimate assumes that the radiologist who uses the CADe device clinically would correctly act on the computer mark pointing to a missed cancer. But this may not be true. Because the CADe computer also produces false-positive marks, the radiologist will not act on every computer mark. Whether the radiologist will act correctly on a potential missed cancer that the CADe computer detects will depend on whether the radiologist successfully avoids simply dismissing the computer mark as a frivolous false positive and whether the lesion surpasses the radiologist's threshold to take action (to report it as BI-RADS 0, or 4, or 5). Recognizing that missed-lesion studies demonstrate *potential*, rather than *actual*, clinical benefit, the FDA has not granted premarketing approval of other CADe devices on the basis of missed-lesion studies. Instead, the FDA has required other types of studies that demonstrate safety and effectiveness more explicitly.

The missed-lesion studies benefit from a clever study design and are highly effective in motivating early development of CADe systems. Although to conduct this type of study entails nuances and challenges, the study is relatively low cost. The study results are valuable, and these studies are a necessary first step in the evaluation of CADe systems. However, the main weakness of missed-lesion studies is that they demonstrate potential, rather than actual, clinical benefit.

21.3   STANDALONE PERFORMANCE ASSESSMENT

A study of a CADe computer by itself, not involving the radiologist user at all, is sometimes called a standalone study. It differs from a missed-lesion study only in the images and cases that are analyzed in the study: a missed-lesion study focuses on only cases that contain verified missed lesions, whereas a standalone study involves a broader spectrum of cases.

A standalone study is used primarily as a benchmark test of the CADe computer, to assess its performance independently of the radiologist user. There are many reasons why this assessment is needed. For example, before one carries out a study in which radiologists use a CADe system, one needs to know the performance of the CADe computer and inform the radiologists who participate in the study so that they could form a strategy for how to use the CADe system appropriately. One also needs a performance benchmark of a CADe system for reporting it, describing it, marketing it, or promoting it, either in the literature, to the FDA, or to radiologist users. Quality control for commercial CADe systems, both at the time of system installation and thereafter on a routine basis, also requires a convenient way to obtain performance benchmarks of a CADe system (routine quality control of commercial CADe systems is essentially nonexistent at present). Another, particularly interesting, example is CADe computer performance benchmarks as documentation for CADe computer software upgrades. Obviously, the performance benchmarks are needed to document that the performance of the CADe computer has improved after an upgrade, or at a minimum that the performance has not decreased. The FDA—which is required to approve CADe computer upgrades because, for CADe systems, such upgrades can mean either the CADe device remains essentially the same or it becomes a substantially different device or anywhere in between—is particularly interested in the standalone performance of CADe systems as a surrogate

of the CADe system performance in clinical use by radiologists (more on this later).

To conduct a standalone study of a CADe computer is straightforward and similar to missed-lesion studies discussed earlier. The general steps are to collect a set of images and cases, to analyze those images and cases with the CADe computer, and to tabulate the performance of the CADe computer in terms of sensitivity, false-positive rate, and other relevant performance indices. One may want to break down the overall performance benchmark by subset of cases: for example, for malignant masses and for malignant clustered calcifications in mammograms and for different groups of lung nodules differentiated by size. One may also want to break down the overall performance benchmark specifically on what has changed in the CADe computer before and after the software upgrade.

An important consideration for conducting a standalone study is the test images and cases. Ideally, one would want to use a random sample of the cases that the CADe computer will analyze in clinical practice to obtain an unbiased estimate of the computer performance in clinical practice. However, this is often not practical. For screening mammography, the prevalence of breast cancer is approximately 0.5%, or lower. A random sample of screening mammograms implies that cancer cases make up only about 0.5% of the total number of cases. If one wants to study a minimum of 100 cancer cases, then a total of 20,000 cases must be studied. This would have been a highly inefficient study because the uncertainty of the estimated sensitivity will be determined entirely by the 100 cancer cases, even though the study had a total of 20,000 cases. To get around this problem, enrichment of cancer cases is common, which means that to include in a screening mammography study more cancer cases in the test cases than 0.5%. Stratified random sampling is a reasonable alternative to random sampling. With stratified random sampling, one identifies a set of case groups (strata) by some specified characteristics and then samples cases randomly within each stratum while maintaining some predetermined proportions of the number of cases between the various strata. Cancer and noncancer cases can define two strata. Breast masses and clustered calcifications can also define two strata. BI-RADS assessment categories can further be used to define strata. The possibilities are many, and one needs to consider them carefully based on the specifics of the CADe system. It is important to recognize, and remember, that bias in the estimate of CADe computer performance can result from stratified random sampling if the proportions of the strata are too far different from those of clinical practice. For example, too many large and conspicuous cancers could inflate the estimate of sensitivity. Similarly, it is also important to include the entire spectrum of clinical cases in the study, because omission of a group of cases could lead to biased estimate of performance—for example, omission of mammograms of heterogeneously or extremely dense breasts can be expected to lead to underestimation of computer false positives. At the same time, one must also keep the need for inclusion of the full clinical case spectrum in perspective; it may not be a good idea to insist on inclusion of all types of rare cases because rare cases are—after all—rare and biases could also result if rare cases make up too much of the study.

A consequence of the relative ease of a standalone study—compared with other types of studies discussed later—is that it tends to be done repeatedly. Indeed, once a set of test cases is constructed, it is not too hard to run the CADe computer on it and obtain an estimate of the computer performance. It is also easy to run the computer on the set of test cases repeatedly during the research and development process of a CADe system, or whenever a CADe system undergoes software upgrade. However, is it a good idea from a statistical point of view to use a set of test cases repeatedly, or must an entirely new set of test cases be constructed each and every time the performance of a CADe computer needs to be estimated? Constructing new sets of test cases would ensure statistical independence, and therefore validity, in the performance estimates, but at exorbitant costs. Reuse of a fixed set of test cases and tuning the CADe computer algorithm specifically to the fixed test cases would encourage *overtraining* of the CADe algorithm and cause the CADe computer to perform less well on clinical cases at large. There has not been a lot of research on this question. An idea that has gained popularity is to establish an institutional entity that holds a large set of test cases. This entity will provide a service to CAD developers to test their CADe computer on a subset of the reserved test cases and provide feedback to the developer only in broad and general terms of the CADe computer performance. The idea is that by putting test cases into quarantine and creating a firewall between CAD developers and the test cases, one prevents CAD developers from tuning CADe computers specifically to the test cases and, at the same time, reuses the test cases for multiple standalone studies.

The literature has a large number of reports on standalone CADe computer performance studies. These studies are too numerous to cite here, and we refer the reader to other chapters in this book for examples. A standalone study is a good way to demonstrate the merit of novel CADe techniques, methods, and algorithms. However, unfortunately, the information reported in the literature is often incomplete for proper interpretation of the results of standalone studies. In addition to details on the computer performance study, such as those for the commonly used receiver operating characteristic (ROC) analysis [4,5], one should also report full and complete information on the test cases and the criteria that are used to score the computer detection as true positives or false positives. Both of these are important

considerations for a standalone study, and the reader needs this information to properly interpret the results. A consequence of incomplete information in literature reports is that it is very difficult to compare the merits of competing CADe techniques, methods, or algorithms based on the reports alone. In the engineering literature outside of medical imaging, a partial solution to this problem is the availability of a few datasets that are publicly accessible and can be used as a common yardstick by authors. However, this has not proven easily translatable to the medical imaging literature in part because medical images are sensitive to patient-confidentiality issues and are simply not widely accessible.

An advantage of the standalone study of a CADe computer is its relative ease to conduct compared with other types of studies that we discuss in this chapter—once a set of test cases is constructed, which can be a demanding task. However, a disadvantage of the standalone study is that it does not involve the radiologists who will use the CADe computer in clinical practice, and thus the performance estimate is limited to only the CADe computer and generally cannot be easily generalized to the performance of the combined radiologist–CADe computer system. Nevertheless, when the FDA considers a CADe computer software upgrade, it needs to assess the effect that the upgrade produces on the clinical performance of radiologists, in terms of safety and effectiveness of CADe systems as medical devices when used by radiologists. It is not reasonable to require CADe device manufacturers to conduct a study that involves radiologists (this type of study is discussed next) for each and every computer software upgrade, and the FDA instead considers the standalone study of the CADe computer as a surrogate.

21.4 LABORATORY OBSERVER PERFORMANCE STUDIES

The laboratory observer performance study is a common and highly effective method for evaluation of the effectiveness of CADe systems. As its name implies, the study is conducted in a laboratory outside of clinical practice and focuses on the performance of human observers, typically practicing radiologists, who use a CADe system. For evaluation of CADe systems, the study is typically designed to compare observer performance with, against without, the use of the CADe system.

The laboratory observer study is an important method for the evaluation of CADe systems because it is rigorous, can be well controlled, and is practical to conduct. It is the culmination of decades of research on evaluation methodologies and ROC analysis [4–9]. In an observer study that compares two modalities (e.g., CADe vs. no CADe), a group of readers read a set of cases in both modalities to allow the estimation of the ROC curves of the readers for each modality and the differences between those ROC curves. The design of this experiment allows the study findings to be generalized to other readers and other cases at large—the very reason to undertake such a study in the first place [10,11]. By studying a group of readers, this experiment allows the effect of variations in performance between readers to be estimated; similarly, by studying a set of cases, the experiment allows the effect of variations between cases to be estimated; and finally, by having the readers read the cases in both modalities, the experiment allows the effect of variations in the interactions between readers, cases, and modalities (e.g., readers might perform better in easy-to-diagnose cases than in difficult cases; readers may perform better in one modality than the other; and readers may find certain cases easier to diagnose in one modality than the other) to be estimated. By having readers read all cases in both modalities, this experiment maximizes statistical power for the detection of differences in the ROC curves between the two modalities. Thus, this experiment rigorously and efficiently accounts for various sources of variations from readers, cases, and the modalities. Known simply as a *multireader multicase* experiment, a carefully designed laboratory observer study typically involves tens of readers and hundreds of cases and can be carried out in a few months; thus, the laboratory observer study is also practical—more so than many clinical studies described later in this chapter. For all of these reasons, the laboratory observer study is an important vehicle for the FDA as a methodology for the evaluation of safety and effectiveness of CADe systems.

To conduct a laboratory observer study requires considerable preparation and planning. First, a set of study cases with known diagnostic truth must be assembled. This is similar to the construction of case sets in missed-lesion and standalone studies, but the case mix may differ from that of those other types of studies. Because the cases will be read by expert radiologists, the case mix needs to reflect, at least in some ways, the clinical case mix, and images must be prepared for readers to interpret in addition to having digital image files for the CADe computer to analyze. We will discuss this more later. Second, a group of readers must be assembled. Because the objective here is to estimate diagnostic performance of clinical radiologists, readers are ideally selected randomly from the target population of radiologists; one should not, for example, select readers only from among expert radiologists. Third, the study needs to be carefully planned, with specific details such as when a particular reader will read which particular case. Experimental instruments, such as a computer–reader interface to be used for image interpretation and for recording reader-response data, must be prepared. Finally, instructions to readers and

what information of the study is to be provided to the readers must be carefully considered and prepared.

In the most common design of an observer study, every reader reads every case twice, once in each modality. The study is typically carried out by breaking the cases into several smaller sets, with each subset of cases read in a single session, and by breaking the readers into at least two smaller groups. The reading of the cases is then broken into multiple sessions. It is important to take advantage of this opportunity for designing the reading sessions to minimize any potential biases from the study design. For example, for the comparison of two modalities, if one modality is always read before the other, the possibility of a reading-order effect cannot be ruled out. Therefore, to minimize that potential bias, one should design the reading sessions so that roughly half of the cases are read in one modality first and the other half of the cases are read in the other modality first. But the evaluation of a CADe system is an exception to this general idea, because the CADe system is to be used, clinically, only after the radiologist has read the images first. For CADe, a reading-session design in which all readers read all cases without CADe first, and then immediately after with CADe, is appropriate because it reflects how the CADe system will be used clinically. Other potential biases must also be considered; a thorough and excellent discussion is given by Metz [12].

It is obviously important to orient the readers so that they are acquainted with the study before it begins to enable them to employ a consistent strategy in their reading of the cases throughout the study. Because a reader's perception of the case mix—for example, from what he or she sees clinically—can influence the reader's response to cases in the study, and because the case mix in an observer study often differs in some aspect from the clinical case mix, it is a good idea to inform the readers the general characteristics of the study case mix. For example, one may tell readers that the case mix is roughly 30% cancer and 70% no cancer. One should avoid saying that there are exactly 30 cancer and 70 no-cancer study cases, to discourage readers from being tempted to count cancer cases during the study, which may unduly—and possibly negatively—influence his or her performance.

To facilitate the estimation of ROC curves, reader response usually must be in the form of an ordinal confidence rating, for example, the confidence that a breast cancer is present in a mammogram. This rating may be on an ordinal categorical scale (e.g., a five-point scale of 1–5), or on a quasi-continuous scale (e.g., from 0% to 100% with an increment of 1%). In addition, it is useful to collect, separately, an action-type response, for example, whether a reader recommends biopsy. The BI-RADS assessment categories are sometimes used for the action-type response, because the BI-RADS assessment categories, used clinically, are clearly defined in terms of the recommended clinical action to help reduce ambiguities in communicating the radiologist's interpretation of the images to clinicians and to patients. While it is possible for one to make assumptions and to derive action-type data from readers' confidence ratings (e.g., by applying a threshold), the collection of explicit action-type data eliminates such assumption and its associated uncertainty and, at the same time, provides an opportunity to scrutinize the consistency between a reader's confidence ratings and action-type data. (We note in passing here that the BI-RADS assessment categories are not a formally ordinal scale and are not an appropriate instrument for recording reader confidence in an observer performance study of screening mammography—of asymptomatic and apparently healthy women—but can be more easily adapted for an observer performance study of diagnostic mammography—of patients with known suspected abnormality [13].)

Chan, Doi, and colleagues performed one of the earliest laboratory observer performance studies for the evaluation of CADe systems [14]. They showed that CADe was able to improve radiologists' performance in the detection of clustered microcalcifications on mammograms. Their laboratory observer performance studies consisted of 60 single-view mammograms, 30 of which contained a cluster of microcalcifications and 30 of which did not, and 7 attending radiologists and 8 radiology residents as expert observers. Their results in terms of *composite* ROC curves of all of the observers, reproduced in Figure 21.1, showed statistically significant improvement (p < 0.001) in the radiologists' performance in terms of the area under the ROC curve for the detection of clustered

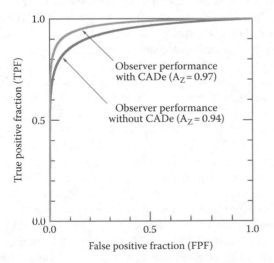

Figure 21.1 ROC curves adapted from the observer performance study of [13] showing statistically significant improvement (p < 0.001) in 15 radiologists' performance in the detection of clustered microcalcifications on mammograms with the assistance of CADe.

microcalcifications on mammograms. Since the publication of this study, many laboratory observer performance studies have been conducted, and here is but a small sample [15–18].

The laboratory observer performance study is a rigorous and well-controlled experiment and can produce definitive and unambiguous assessments of the diagnostic performance of CADe systems and other medical imaging systems. The laboratory observer performance study benefits from decades of research and advances on the theory, methodology, and practice of the fundamentals of signal detection and medical decision making. Although it requires substantial effort and great attention to nuanced details, the laboratory observer performance study is a practical approach for the assessment of CADe systems. Perhaps the most important criticism to the laboratory observer performance study coincides with one of its main strength: because the study is done in the laboratory outside of clinical practice, questions can be raised concerning to what extent observers behave the same in the laboratory experiment as in clinical practice. The appeal of the laboratory observer performance study would increase if its well-established study design can be expanded and new more flexible study designs can be developed.

21.5 CLINICAL ASSESSMENT

In a clinical study, a CADe system is evaluated as a part of clinical practice. An important characteristic of this type of studies—in addition to full involvement of the radiologist in the study in the use of the CADe system—is that patient management occurs during the course of the study. There are several common designs for a clinical CADe study. We will refer to them as the head-to-head comparison, historical-control study, comparison with double readings, and randomized controlled trials.

Clinical studies are important because the goal for the evaluation of a CADe system is to understand its effect, or benefit, in clinical practice. Thus, clinical studies provide a realistic study setting and a direct means to achieve that goal. However, even minimally designed clinically studies are often larger in scale than laboratory observer performance studies. They typically involve more study radiologists, require more patient cases, and take longer to complete. Furthermore, their more straightforward study design generally does not share the same level of efficiency as do laboratory observer performance studies. In addition, as we will discuss later, there are various concerns of potential biases. As a result, the laboratory observer study is more common than large clinical studies. However, the important role of clinical studies for the evaluation of benefits of CADe systems should not be underestimated.

21.5.1   Head-to-Head Comparison

A head-to-head comparison study compares the use of CADe vs. no-CADe on a case-by-case basis. That is, each case is read both without CADe and with CADe. This allows one to identify cases for which the no-CADe and CADe reads are concordant and cases for which the no-CADe and CADe reads yield different findings. After determination through clinical follow-up of the cases that harbor the disease of interest, this allows one to identify the cases for which the no-CADe read yields the correct diagnosis and the cases for which the CADe read yields the correct diagnosis. It is especially appealing here to be able to pinpoint the specific cases that the use of CADe benefits the radiologist—by changing an incorrect diagnosis into a correct diagnosis, as well as cases that the use of CADe affects the diagnosis detrimentally.

A head-to-head comparison study requires each and every case to be read twice in clinical practice. Thus, it takes careful planning to conduct such a study. Dedicated study radiologists must be identified: will every radiologist in a clinical practice participate as study radiologists, or will only specific individuals participate? Similarly, will all clinical cases be treated as a part of the study, or only a subset of them? The length of the study, and the statistical power of the study, will be determined in part by the number of study radiologists and the number of study cases. A reasonably efficient clinical workflow must be developed to facilitate the repeat reads, which typically would entail a radiologist reading a case without the use of CADe first, formally recording his or her findings, then reading the case again with the use of CADe, and formally recording his or her findings again. One way to formally record findings is to dictate the clinical report, which means that there needs to be a mechanism to accept two reports for each case: the no-CADe report and the with-CADe report. The clinical action for cases that CADe findings differ from no-CADe findings must also be decided before the study begins, and this decision can affect the extent to which the study is able to determine the true diagnosis for cases of discordant findings (because the true diagnosis can be determined immediately only in cases for which a definitive diagnostic action such as biopsy is taken).

Because each and every case will be read twice, a head-to-head comparison study tends to be small in the number of cases and in the number of readers. Consequently, the studies may suffer from a lack of statistical power. This problem is exacerbated for low-prevalence diseases such as in breast cancer screening where the cancer prevalence is around 0.5%. Questions on the performance of the study radiologists can also be raised. Because the study radiologist anticipates the assistance of the CADe device immediately after his or her interpretation of the images, will the radiologist be less vigilant in his or her own interpretation than his or her normal practice otherwise, or will the radiologist be more vigilant in his or her interpretation to compete with the CADe device? The head-to-head comparison study does not have a build-in mechanism to control for these potential factors that could lead to bias. However, these questions are also not unique to the head-to-head comparison study and can be raised in general with regard to the clinical use of CADe systems.

Freer and Ulissey published a well-known study that assessed the effect of a CADe device on the interpretation of screening mammograms in a community breast center [19]. Their study spanned 12 months and encompassed 12,860 screening mammograms. The two radiologists (authors) interpreted all mammograms with the aid of a CADe system. Each mammogram was initially interpreted without the assistance of the CADe system, followed immediately by a reevaluation of areas marked by the CADe system. Data were recorded after each interpretation to estimate the effect of CADe on the recall rate, positive predictive value (PPV) for biopsy, cancer detection rate, and stage of malignancies at the time of cancer detection. They reported the following observed effects of use of the CADe system compared with their performance without the use of CADe: (1) an increase in recall rate from 6.5% to 7.7%; (2) no change in the PPV for biopsy at 38%; (3) an increase in the number of cancers detected of 19.5%, for eight additional cancers detected; and (4) an increase in the proportion of early stage (stage 0 and stage 1) malignancies from 73% to 78%. Of the 12,860 screening mammograms, the radiologists recalled 830 patients without the aid of CADe (6.5% recall rate), and an additional 156 patients were recalled attributable to CADe, for a total of 986 patients recalled (7.7% recall rate). Of these, 107 patients underwent biopsy attributable to the radiologists' interpretations without CADe, and additional 21 patients underwent biopsy attributable to CADe, for a total of 128 patients who underwent biopsy. Of these, 41 cancers were diagnosed attributable to the radiologists' interpretation without CADe (38% PPV), and additional 8 cancers were diagnosed attributable to CADe (19.5% = 8/41), for a total of 49 cancers diagnosed (38% PPV). Of these cancers, 30 found by the radiologists without CADe were stage 0 or stage 1 (73% = 30/41), and an additional eight cancers attributable to CADe were stage 0 or stage 1 (78% = 38/49). This excellently executed study illustrates, of a head-to-head comparison study, the considerable effort required of a small number of radiologists (two) to interpret a large number of cases (12,860) to identify a small number of cancers detected attributable to the use of CADe (eight), and the ability to identify these cancers specifically.

The head-to-head comparison study is particularly appealing in its ability to allow one to pinpoint the cases that the use of a CADe system helps radiologists make correct clinical diagnoses. However, because each and every case will be read twice in routine clinical practice, constraints on the size of the study in terms of the number of study cases and the number of study radiologists may cause the study to lack in statistical power. Questions can be raised with regard to the performance of the study radiologists and the benefit of CADe systems derived from their performance: whether the study radiologists are more, or less, vigilant in their own interpretation without the assistance of the CADe system can potentially bias the observed benefit of the CADe system. These questions are relevant to the head-to-head comparison study as well as clinical use of CADe systems in general.

21.5.2 Historical-Control Comparison

A historical-control study of the clinical use of a CADe system compares clinical practice performance before and after the CADe system begins to be used clinically. The objective is to determine the incremental effect when a CADe system is first introduced into clinical practice. This type of studies can be of great interest when a new technology is introduced into clinical practice. It rapidly establishes a snapshot of the potential benefits and other effects of the new technology, and can be quite influential to motivate early adopters of the new technology.

To conduct a historical-control study of a new CADe system generally requires the participation of an entire group of radiologists at a clinical practice and requires the practice to routinely maintain a record of a set of performance metrics. By the time the decision is made to adopt the new CADe system, and to conduct a historical-control study, the time to conduct the control-arm study likely has already been passed, because the length of that study might be more than a few months, and perhaps a year or more. Thus, this type of study is suited for clinical practice groups that are able to collect practice performance data on a regular basis. Unfortunately, ROC analysis is not amenable as a performance metric in this type of study, because it is not easy to determine sensitivity and specificity, or the diagnostic *truth* for cases, on a routine basis in clinical practice. Instead, some other readily measurable metrics need to be used. Common choices of performance metrics for breast cancer screening include the cancer detection rate (the number of cancers detected per 1000 imaging studies) and the recall rate (the number of studies with abnormal findings that require additional imaging study as a fraction of all screening studies). These measures can be calculated from routine clinical practice data, and do not require dedicated follow-ups. However, unlike sensitivity and specificity, the information that these two measures provide is neither complete nor strictly complementary for the purpose of diagnostic performance evaluation. Once these decisions are made and the new CADe system is introduced to the clinical

practice, the study then proceeds as routine and with careful recordkeeping to document the performance of the clinical practice. At the end of the study, the performance data are compared between the historical-control arm before the CADe system was introduced and the CADe study arm after the CADe system was introduced. It may be necessary to exclude some initial data of CADe use from the analysis to account for the study radiologists' *learning curves*, which may not accurately reflect their performance in the use of the CADe system.

Although the objective of a historical-control study is to determine the incremental effect of the use of a CADe system, it is not easy to isolate that effect. Anything else that has also changed between the historical-control-arm study time period and the CADe arm study time period will contribute to the observed incremental change in performance together with the use of the CADe system. Have there been changes in patient demographics—perhaps due to insurance payment change or health organization's recommendation change? Have there been new radiologists entering the practice, veteran radiologists leaving the practice? Have there been changes in the practice pattern of radiologists— for example, relatively inexperienced radiologists gaining experience over time? Have there been changes in the imaging equipment, imaging protocol, image quality, and radiation dose? All of these, and more, could play a role in the observed change in diagnostic performance, and it can be difficult to isolate their individual effects. Furthermore, the effect detected in a historical-control study may be that of a transient nature if it takes longer than the CADe arm study period for the use of the CADe system to achieve equilibrium (see Section 21.6.3).

Gur and colleagues conducted a historical-control study that assessed changes in screening mammography recall rate and cancer detection rate after the introduction of a CADe system into a clinical radiology practice in an academic setting [20]. Their study spanned 2000, 2001, and 2002 and encompassed mammograms interpreted by 24 radiologists. The control arm of the study encompassed 56,432 screening mammograms interpreted without the aid of CADe, whereas the study arm encompassed 59,139 screening mammograms interpreted with the aid of CADe after the CADe system was used consistently in their clinical practice. They reported similar recall rates and cancer detection rates without and with the assistance of CADe. The recall rate was 11.39% (6430 recalls) without and 11.40% (6741 recalls) with the assistance of CADe (p = 0.96). The cancer detection rate was 3.49 (197 cancers detected) without and 3.55 (210 cancers detected) with the assistance of CADe per 1000 screening mammograms (p = 0.68). They concluded that the introduction of CADe into their clinical practice was not associated with statistically significant changes in recall rate and cancer detection rate. This study illustrates the sheer size that a historical-control study can accomplish, and controversy regarding this study illustrates complications in the interpretation of the results of a historical-control study [21,35].

An advantage of the historical-control study is that it can be scaled up relatively easily into large studies, due in part to its straightforward study design. Another advantage is that by positioning in time precisely at the initial introduction of a novel technology, the study can provide a rapid and timely snapshot of the benefit and effect of a new medical imaging system. A disadvantage of the historical-control study is that it can suffer from various biases and confounding effects, and thus may be limited in its ability to ascertain the effect of the novel medical technology. Another disadvantage is that the historical-control study is best suited for the initial introduction of a new medical technology but is more difficult to monitor the effect of the technology as it matures in clinical practice.

21.5.3   Comparison with Double Reading by Radiologists

Double reading is a practice in which each and every case is read by two radiologists. The motivation for this practice is that, to the extent that every radiologist will inadvertently miss some cancers, two radiologists are likely to miss different cancers. Thus, by having two radiologists read each and every case, fewer cancers will be missed than if a single radiologist reads the cases. This is similar to the reasoning behind CADe except that in CADe, a computer serves the role of the second radiologist. It is therefore natural to compare CADe against double reading by two radiologists.

Double reading by two radiologists is common in European clinical practice, whereas it is much less practiced in the United States. Double reading by two radiologists has considerable economic costs because two radiologists must review each and every case, but subspecialty radiologists are not an abundant resource in medical practice. Although CADe also has considerable economic costs associated with the research and development of the system, it may cost less in the long run compared with double reading by two radiologists. Thus, it is natural to ask how one radiologist reading with the aid of a CADe system compares with double reading by two radiologists. If a radiologist aided by a CADe system produces similar diagnostic performance as double reading by two radiologists, then the CADe system can be an alternative to double reading by two radiologists. While double reading by two radiologists shares much in common with CADe, there appears to be better acceptance of double reading, at least in Europe,

without having had as much call for clinical evaluation of benefits and effects as for CADe. Double reading is also more flexible than CADe; for example, double reading can be combined with a variety of arbitration approaches to cases that the readings of the two radiologists are discrepant. For CADe, the one radiologist usually makes the final decision, in part because large numbers of marks produced by the CADe computer—most of which are false positives—make it impractical to scrutinize those marks systematically. Thus, the question is generally whether CADe can produce diagnostic performance similar to that of double reading by two radiologists.

While it is possible to conduct comparison studies of double reading and single reading with the use of CADe in the setting of laboratory observer performance experiment, it is more common that such studies are done at least in part in the clinical setting. For example, if double reading is practiced clinically, then a set of consecutive cases can be identified and read retrospectively in an experiment setting by a single reader with the use of CADe. Alternatively, prospective trial can be designed to compare double reading and single reading with the use of CADe on the same patients. In principle, double reading and single reading with the use of CADe can be compared on two different sets of patient cases, but with reduced statistical power, compared with the study designs involving matched cases between the two reading conditions. Common clinical performance metrics can be compared, such as the cancer detection rate, recall rate, sensitivity, specificity, and PPV.

Gilbert et al. conducted a prospective trial to determine whether the performance of a single reader using a CADe system would match the performance achieved by two readers [22]. Their trial was designed to show equivalence. The trial included 31,057 women undergoing routine screening for breast cancer by film mammography at three centers in England. The women were randomly assigned by a ratio of 1:1:28 to one of (a) double reading by two readers, (b) single reading by one reader plus CADe, or (c) both double reading by two readers and single reading by one reader plus CADe. They reported a total of 227 cancers detected in 28,204 women assigned to the (c) group. Of these cancers, double reading detected 199 cancers (87.7%) and single reading plus CADe detected 198 cancers (87.2%). The recall rate was 3.4% for double reading and 3.9% for single reading plus CADe (p < 0.001). They estimated that sensitivity, specificity, and PPV were 87.7%, 97.4%, and 21.1%, respectively, for double reading, and 87.2%, 96.9%, and 18.0%, respectively, for single reading plus CADe. They concluded that single reading plus CADe could be an alternative to double reading by two readers and could improve the rate of cancer detection from screening mammograms read by a single reader.

Comparing CADe with double reading by two radiologists is a clinically relevant approach to the assessment of clinical benefit and effect of CADe. If the use of CADe yields similar clinical results as double reading by two radiologists, then the economic savings from the use of CADe over the long run makes CADe an attractive alternative to double reading by two radiologists. However, ascertainment of the clinical performance of double reading and comparison with that of CADe are by no means easy, just as ascertainment of the clinical performance of CADe and no-CADe. Because double reading by two radiologists is common in clinical practice in Europe, comparison studies of CADe and double readings tend to originate from Europe.

21.5.4 Randomized Controlled Trial

The randomized, controlled clinical trial is a workhorse for medical research, especially for the evaluation of therapeutic agents and procedures. In a randomized controlled trial, a patient cohort is randomly assigned to either a control group or a study group. The random assignment of the group membership ensures that the control-group and study-group patient cohorts are similar in number and characteristics. The two patient groups are then treated identically except for what is being studied, thus ensuring that any difference observed between the two groups of patients comes from what is being studied. If a randomized controlled trial were to be conducted to evaluate CADe, then patients who enroll in the trial would be assigned randomly to either a study group or a control group. For patients in the study group, radiologists would read their images with the CADe system, and for patients in the control group, radiologists would read their image without the CADe system. Diagnostic performance measures estimated from the study-group patients and from the control-group patients would then be compared.

No randomized controlled clinical trial of a CADe system has been done. Because current CADe systems are designed to help detect cancers in a screening setting, a randomized controlled clinical trial of CADe will be necessarily large—and larger than a trial of the screening imaging test. The Digital Mammography Imaging Screening Trial enrolled over 49,500 patients [23]. The trial is large because breast cancer has a prevalence of only approximately 0.5% in the patient population. A similar trial for CADe will require even more patients because the target effect of CADe is the detection of missed cancers, which by definition have prevalence much lower than 0.5%. Therefore, to conduct a randomized control trial of breast cancer screening with CADe is not practical.

21.5.5 Observational Studies

Observational studies are an epidemiological and statistical method. They are in contrast with the clinical experiments and trials that we have discussed so far in that an observational study has no control over the assignment of any patient that enters the study group (CADe in our context) or the control group (no-CADe in our context). Rather, the observational study relies solely on observations of typically large numbers of patients—some satisfy the *study* condition (CADe) and others satisfy the *control* condition (no-CADe)—and draws inferences on possible reasons for differences between the study (CADe) and control (no-CADe) groups. For example, if one is able to collect all screening mammogram interpretation data from a number of US states, then one could separate patients in these data into two groups: one that patient mammograms were read with CADe and the other that patient mammograms were read without the use of CADe. One could then make comparisons between the two patient groups and make inferences about CADe: for example, one could compare the cancer detection rate, and the recall rate, between the two groups. Clearly, such a comparison is meaningful only if one were confident that *all else is equal*, because any other difference between the two groups would give rise to the possibility of incorrect inference. Imagine a simplistic situation—for the sake of argument—that the study (CADe) patients had an average age of 45, whereas the control (no-CADe) patients had an average age of 65. Then, if a possible observation of lower cancer detection rate in the study (CADe) patients compared with the control (no-CADe) patients is interpreted as an effect of CADe, then that inference would be erroneous because it is well known that the incidence of breast cancer increases with age. The age differences in this simplistic and hypothetical scenario are a confounding factor and are likely responsible for giving rise to the erroneous inference. Investigators of observational studies go to great length to control for known confounding factors. However, insofar, as it is not possible to eliminate all confounding factors, observational studies are not reliable resources of factual statements of clinical efficacy, but they can provide useful *real-world* clinical information (e.g., regarding the use of CADe).

Fenton and colleagues published two large observational studies [24,25]. We refer the reader to their original publications for study details because these studies involved complex methodological details and data modeling. These authors concluded that the use of CADe "is associated with reduced accuracy of interpretation of screening mammograms," "with decreased specificity but not with improvement in the detection rate or prognostic characteristics of invasive breast cancer"—strong conclusions given that these are observational studies. Not surprisingly, these studies are controversial on grounds of both study methodologies and result interpretation [26–32].

21.6 CONFOUNDING FACTORS AND METRIC OF ASSESSMENT

21.6.1 Statistical Issues with Small Numbers

The clinical use of CADe systems is to help radiologists minimize missed cancers. To achieve this objective, a CADe system must be used by radiologists in each and every case, but they can only help radiologists in the small number of cancer cases that radiologists miss had the CADe system not been used. This means that to detect the clinical benefit of CADe systems, one will necessarily deal with small numbers and their statistical consequences. This can be a difficult proposition. Consider breast cancer screening, for example, the cancer prevalence in an average risk and asymptomatic patient population is about 0.5%, which is a small number. Of these, let us assume that radiologists miss about 20% [33], and let us assume that the use of a CADe system helps radiologist avoid half of the misses, which would be 10%. Thus, we would expect to see the benefit of the CADe system in 0.05% of all screening cases, which is a really small fraction. This works out to be 5 missed cancers detected because of CADe in 10,000 cases or 500 missed cancers detected in 1,000,000 cases. It means that in any given study or for any particular clinical practice, to encounter missed cancers that are detected because of CADe will be rare, but on a larger—regional or nation—scale, the number of missed cancers detected because of CADe could be considerably large. This suggests that the benefit from CADe may be worthwhile, but it will be difficult to ascertain that benefit.

We must not forget that the use of CADe can also have an effect on noncancer cases, which would be to increase the number of false-positive diagnosis—a detrimental effect. In our example of breast cancer screening, because the recall rate of mammography—let us say it is about 10%, lower in many US practices but possibly higher in other US practices and substantially lower in Europe—is much higher than the expected cancer detection rate, it is much easier to notice any change in the recall rate than in the cancer detection rate. This means that if a CADe system has a detrimental effect on causing an increase in false-positive diagnosis, the impact of that effect will be large by virtue of the large number of cases for which the effect impacts, and thus the effect will be easier to notice.

21.6.2 Reader Variability Issues

Variation in diagnostic performance between radiologists is recognized as substantial [34]. Radiologists operate clinically with different levels of diagnostic performance. If it were possible to measure their diagnostic performance with ROC curve estimates, their ROC curves would differ. Even for radiologists who operate on essentially the same ROC curve, their clinical sensitivity and specificity can still differ, depending on where they choose to operate on that ROC curve. These differences in diagnostic performance are evident in variations in the recall rate and, less clearly, in the cancer detection rate between radiologists. However, this variability is all but hidden in routine clinical practice in the United States, in which a single radiologist renders the expert interpretation of a clinical case, as if other radiologists would make the same diagnosis. Nevertheless, variability in the diagnostic performance among radiologists has important clinical consequences and affects the clinical evaluation of CADe.

If this reader variability were absent, it would be much easier to ascertain diagnostic performance of radiologists without the use of CADe and that with the use of CADe, and hence their difference, because such estimates would be the same between different radiologists and the same over time. However, the presence of reader variability makes it more difficult to accurately estimate all of these. Large variance in the diagnostic performance of radiologists without, or with, the use of CADe implies that the estimates of radiologists' performance must be made on a large number of radiologists and a large number of patient cases. Because the variance in the difference in radiologists' diagnostic performance between use and no use of CADe will be greater than the variance in either their diagnostic performance without the use of CADe or their diagnostic performance with the use of CADe, to estimate this difference in clinical diagnostic performance between no-CADe and CADe requires even more radiologists and patient cases. Jiang et al. estimated the magnitude of this effect based on the cancer detection rate data from the Breast Cancer Surveillance Consortium of 510 US radiologists, and their results are shown in Figure 21.2 [33]. These results show that given a postulated large increase in the cancer detection rate of 0.1%, which may well be not realistic because it is roughly 20% of the expected breast cancer prevalence, to observe this large increase in the cancer detection rate in clinical practice is not a certainty. For example, for a practice group of 10 radiologists, there would be a less than 40% chance to observe a statistically significant increase in the cancer detection rate, and there would be a small but as high as close to 20% chance to observe a decrease in the cancer detection rate, even though there was an underlying large increase in the cancer detection rate.

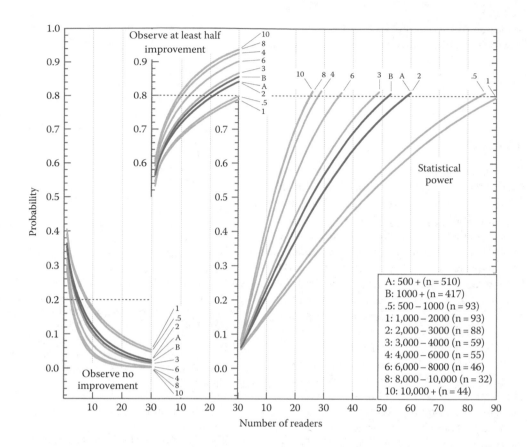

Figure 21.2 Probabilities as a function of the number of readers in a trial for observing, given a postulated increase in one additional cancer detected per 1000 screening mammograms, (left) no additional cancer detected, (middle) one half or more additional cancers detected per 1000 screening mammograms, and (right) statistically significant increase in the cancer detection rate (i.e., statistical power). Correlation of individual reader's cancer detection rates between the two arms of a trial is not included. Variability in the observed single-reader cancer detection rates causes the discrepancies between the postulated and observed changes in the cancer detection rates. Curves are grouped by single-reader total screening mammogram volume; n is the number of readers on whom the calculation was based. Sample sizes refer to half of a two-arm trial. (Reprinted from Jiang et al., *Radiology*, 243, 360, 2007.)

21.6.3 Transient Changes in the Cancer Detection Rate

The cancer detection rate is an oft-used metric of diagnostic performance in clinical studies because it can be readily measured. However, it is not a perfect diagnostic performance measure for the evaluation of the clinical effect of CADe. To see this, consider the oft-made claim of the clinical benefit of CADe—to increase the number of cancers detected. On the surface, this appears to be true, because if CADe helps radiologists avoid missing cancers, then the number of cancers detected must increase. But more thoughts on this will reveal a problem. If CADe use leads to a sustained increase in the number of cancers detected over time, does that mean the total number of cancers—those detected by radiologists plus those detected by the use of CADe, and those not detected—increases? The total number of cancers will likely not change

as a result of CADe use; the additional cancers detected by the use of CADe likely will cause the number of cancers that radiologists detect to reduce because, after potential missed cancers are detected by the use of CADe, they cannot be detected by radiologists again subsequently when the cancer becomes more conspicuous. Cancers not detected due to limitation of the imaging modality might not be detected by the use of CADe, which is based on the same underlying imaging modality. This suggests that there likely will be a transient increase in the cancer detection rate when CADe is introduced into clinical practice, but the cancer detection rate will subsequently stabilize to a level comparable to that before the clinical introduction of CADe, but the use of CADe results in earlier detection of those potential missed cancers. This transient effect, particularly when coupled with the variability between radiologists in their performance and their timing in the adoption of CADe, implies that the benefit of CADe use will not likely manifest in unambiguous changes in the cancer detection rate. Nishikawa et al. modeled this transient effect and analyzed its implications for the evaluation of CADe in detail [35].

21.7 CONCLUSION

It is important to assess the effects and benefits of clinical CADe systems. Evaluation of CADe systems began in the early days of the development of CADe systems. The methodology for such evaluations has evolved substantially and has benefited from decades of research on the methodologies for the evaluation of diagnostic imaging systems in general. Yet, the methodology for the evaluation of CADe systems still faces many challenges today; in particular, it is difficult to conduct clinical assessment studies of CADe systems, and there does not appear to be a clear winner in the study design for a clinical evaluation study of CADe systems. However, as CADe continues to be developed and used clinically, we will undoubtedly learn more about its clinical use, and its true effects and benefits. Much has already been learned about the many issues and nuances that must be considered in the evaluation of CADe systems, some of which are discussed in this chapter. These and what we will learn in the future from clinical experience of the use of CADe will guide us to better develop and use this novel technology.

REFERENCES

1. Warren Burhenne LJ, Wood SA, D'Orsi CJ et al. Potential contribution of computer-aided detection to the sensitivity of screening mammography. *Radiology* 2000;215(2):554–562.
2. D'Orsi CJ, Bassett LW, Berg WA et al. *Breast Imaging Reporting and Data System: ACR BI-RADS-Mammography*, 4th edn. Reston, VA: American College of Radiology, 2003.
3. American College of Radiology (ACR). *Breast Imaging Reporting and Data System (BI-RADSTM)*, 3rd edn. Reston, VA: American College of Radiology, 1998.
4. Metz CE. Basic principles of ROC analysis. *Semin Nucl Med.* 1978;8(4):283–298.
5. Wagner RF, Metz CE, Campbell G. Assessment of medical imaging systems and computer aids: A tutorial review. *Acad Radiol.* 2007;14(6):723–748.
6. Green DM, Swets JA. *Signal Detection Theory and Psychophysics.* New York: John Wiley and Sons, 1966.
7. Lusted LB. Decision-making studies in patient management. *N Engl J Med.* 1971;284(8):416–424.
8. Swets JA, Pickett RM. *Evaluation of Diagnostic Systems: Methods from Signal Detection Theory.* New York: Academic Press, 1982.
9. Swets JA. Measuring the accuracy of diagnostic systems. *Science* 1988;240(4857):1285–1293.
10. Dorfman DD, Berbaum KS, Metz CE. Receiver operating characteristic rating analysis. Generalization to the population of readers and patients with the jackknife method. *Invest Radiol.* 1992;27(9):723–731.
11. Roe CA, Metz CE. Variance-component modeling in the analysis of receiver operating characteristic index estimates. *Acad Radiol.* 1997;4(8):587–600.
12. Metz CE. Some practical issues of experimental design and data analysis in radiological ROC studies. *Invest Radiol.* 1989;24(3):234–245.
13. Jiang Y, Metz CE. BI-RADS data should not be used to estimate ROC curves. *Radiology* 2010;256(1):29–31.
14. Chan HP, Doi K, Vyborny CJ et al. Improvement in radiologists' detection of clustered microcalcifications on mammograms. The potential of computer-aided diagnosis. *Invest Radiol.* 1990;25(10):1102–1110.
15. Kobayashi T, Xu XW, MacMahon H, Metz CE, Doi K. Effect of a computer-aided diagnosis scheme on radiologists' performance in detection of lung nodules on radiographs. *Radiology* 1996;199(3):843–848.
16. Jiang Y, Nishikawa RM, Schmidt RA, Metz CE, Giger ML, Doi K. Improving breast cancer diagnosis with computer-aided diagnosis. *Acad Radiol.* 1999;6(1):22–33.
17. Huo Z, Giger ML, Vyborny CJ, Metz CE. Breast cancer: Effectiveness of computer-aided diagnosis observer study with independent database of mammograms. *Radiology* 2002;224(2):560–568.
18. Chan HP, Sahiner B, Helvie MA et al. Improvement of radiologists' characterization of mammographic masses by using computer-aided diagnosis: An ROC study. *Radiology* 1999;212(3):817–827.
19. Freer TW, Ulissey MJ. Screening mammography with computer-aided detection: Prospective study of 12,860 patients in a community breast center. *Radiology* 2001;220(3):781–786.
20. Gur D, Sumkin JH, Rockette HE et al. Changes in breast cancer detection and mammography recall rates after the introduction of a computer-aided detection system. *J Natl Cancer Inst.* 2004;96(3):185–190.
21. Feig SA, Sickles EA, Evans WP, Linver MN. Re: Changes in breast cancer detection and mammography recall rates after the introduction of a computer-aided detection system. *J Natl Cancer Inst.* 2004;96(16):1260–1261; author reply 1261.
22. Gilbert FJ, Astley SM, Gillan MG et al. Single reading with computer-aided detection for screening mammography. *N Engl J Med.* 2008;359(16):1675–1684.
23. Pisano ED, Gatsonis C, Hendrick E et al. Diagnostic performance of digital versus film mammography for breast-cancer screening. *N Engl J Med.* 2005;353(17):1773–1783.
24. Fenton JJ, Abraham L, Taplin SH et al. Effectiveness of computer-aided detection in community mammography practice. *J Natl Cancer Inst.* 2011;103(15):1152–1161.
25. Fenton JJ, Taplin SH, Carney PA et al. Influence of computer-aided detection on performance of screening mammography. *N Engl J Med.* 2007;356(14):1399–1409.
26. Ciatto S, Houssami N. Computer-aided screening mammography. *N Engl J Med.* 2007;357(1):83; author reply 85.

27. Gur D. Computer-aided screening mammography. *N Engl J Med.* 2007;357(1):83–84; author reply 85.
28. Nishikawa RM, Schmidt RA, Metz CE. Computer-aided screening mammography. *N Engl J Med.* 2007;357(1):84; author reply 85.
29. Ruiz JF. Computer-aided screening mammography. *N Engl J Med.* 2007;357(1):84; author reply 85.
30. Feig SA, Birdwell RL, Linver MN. Computer-aided screening mammography. *N Engl J Med.* 2007;357(1):84; author reply 85.
31. Nishikawa RM, Giger ML, Jiang Y, Metz CE. Re: Effectiveness of computer-aided detection in community mammography practice. *J Natl Cancer Inst.* 2012;104(1):77.
32. Levman J. Re: Effectiveness of computer-aided detection in community mammography practice. *J Natl Cancer Inst.* 2012;104(1):77–78.
33. Jiang Y, Miglioretti DL, Metz CE, Schmidt RA. Breast cancer detection rate: Designing imaging trials to demonstrate improvements. *Radiology* 2007;243(2):360–367.
34. Beam CA, Layde PM, Sullivan DC. Variability in the interpretation of screening mammograms by US radiologists. Findings from a national sample. *Arch Intern Med.* 1996;156(2):209–213.
35. Nishikawa RM, Pesce LL. Computer-aided detection evaluation methods are not created equal. *Radiology* 2009;251(3):634–636.

Clinical Utility of CAD Systems for Breast Cancer

Jocelyn A. Rapelyea and Rachel F. Brem

CONTENTS

22.1 INTRODUCTION

Breast cancer is a leading cause of mortality among North American women regardless of race or ethnicity. Screening and therapy advancements[1,2] lead the charge in the breast cancer mortality decline since 1990.[3] Several recent reports document screening mammography's impact on breast cancer survival. Smith et al.[4] evaluated the clinical presentation and outcome of 6000 Michigan women diagnosed with breast cancer. In this study, mammography detected 65% of breast cancers. The parameters of patient age and cancer stage at the time of diagnosis stratify the patients. In women less than 50 years of age, mammography detected less than half of the breast cancers. The authors note that the screen-detected cancers had favorable prognostic indicators including (1) earlier stage, (2) lower tumor grade, (3) fewer mastectomies (27% with screen-detected cancers vs. 46% with cancers presenting with palpable findings), and (4) less chemotherapy requirements. In fact, the authors conclude that when patients or physicians find cancer on physical examination, it is more often due to advanced cancers that may require mastectomies. Further, in one of largest randomized controlled breast screening trials, Tabar et al. report a 30% decline in mortality when women undergo regular screening mammography.[5]

Detecting cancer with screening mammography is difficult for a number of reasons. First, in a screening population, mammography detects 2–10 cancer in 1000 women.[6] With this low prevalence of disease, it is challenging to identify the cancer. This is further confounded by the marked variability in breast cancer incidence in different populations including those with different age, ethnic composition, and geographic distribution, as all these factors impact a women's risk of developing breast cancer. Further, the prevalence of cancer in a population of women undergoing screening mammography depends on whether it is the patient's initial screen with a prevalence of 5–7 cancers in 1000, which decreases to 2 cancers per 1000 women with subsequent screens due to the ability to detect more subtle changes with comparison examinations.[7] Further, the experience of the interpreting radiologist impacts the detection of cancer with screening mammography. Sickles et al. report a statistically significant higher cancer detection rate among radiologists specialized in breast imaging who detect 6 cancers per 1000 women vs. only 3.4 for general radiologists.[8] What is clear is that numerous factors impact the ability to detect breast cancer with mammography. However, in order to detect early nonpalpable breast cancer with screening mammography, the cancer must be detected, and approaches to optimizing breast cancer detection are needed, hence, the development of computer-aided detection (CADe) to assist the radiologist in improving breast cancer detection.

Breast density significantly impacts the ability to detect breast cancer with a marked reduction in the sensitivity of mammography in women with dense breasts.[9] In a retrospective review of 400,000 women, Mandelson et al.[10] find sensitivity sharply declines from 80% in women with fatty tissue to 30% in women with extremely dense tissue. Detecting cancer in women with dense breasts is further confounded by the fact that breast density is a strong independent risk factor as women with dense breast tissue have a sixfold greater risk in developing interval breast cancers than women who do not have increased breast density. This is due to the complex biological nature of dense breast parenchyma; dense tissue can obscure a mass due to the lack of contrast since both breast parenchyma and breast masses appear white on a mammogram.[10] Clearly, additional tools are needed to improve breast cancer detection with mammography where the goal would be to achieve a higher sensitivity. These issues further demonstrate the need for integrating tools such CADe to assist in improving breast cancer detection.

Human search performance, a fundamental issue in mammographic interpretation where the radiologist must *search* for cancers, is imperfect. We are reminded of this nearly daily when we *search* for something such as our keys, and cannot find them, only to realize after much consternation that they were, in fact, always right in front of us. The reasons the keys were not appreciated are similar to the reasons that cancers may not be perceived when a mammogram is reviewed. When a cancer, which is present is not appreciated, we term this a *miss*, which can result from errors in perception (overlooked mammographic features of subtle findings) or errors in analysis (i.e., interpreting a perceived lesion as benign when it is in fact a cancer). Harvey et al. explored breast cancer misses in a retrospective evaluation and found that in 25%–41%, there was evidence of cancer on the mammogram 1 year prior to the time of diagnosis. Asymmetric densities account for 53% of the cancer misses in the study.[11] Other studies report similar findings.[12] Ikeda et al. identified 172 normal or benign appearing mammographic findings 9–24 months prior to a breast cancer diagnosis. The study finds 54% noncalcified lesions that have densities indistinguishable from normal islands of fibroglandular tissue.[13] So even holding the risk factors of breast density and modality selection constant (SFM vs. FFDM), observational oversights still occur. Doctors are human.

One approach to improved detection of breast cancer is the double reading of mammograms by two radiologists.[14–17] There are two approaches to double interpretation protocols. In the first, both radiologists independently identify areas of concern. All suspicious findings determined by either radiologist trigger additional imaging. In this method, while additional imaging improves the sensitivity and identifies more cancers, the specificity diminishes. Harvey et al. report an increase in sensitivity from 74.4% to 79.4% utilizing double independent interpretation, that is, a 6.3% increase in cancer detection.[18] However, the increased sensitivity came increased recall rate from 11.5% to 14.2%. In the second approach, radiologists independently review the mammogram, but any discrepancies in interpretation are resolved by consensus. Only collectively agreed findings result in patient recall for additional imaging. In the latter method, sensitivity improves, although less than if all findings by both radiologists are treated as actionable as the influence of one radiologist in consensus may result in not recalling a patient for a cancer that was appreciated by the other radiologist. While there are clear advantages of double reading, in practice, it is not economically feasible due to the shortage of radiologists who face high screening volumes with limited staff and the low reimbursement for mammography. Because double reading is time consuming, CADe can act as a surrogate for the additional interpreting radiologists and can improve the overall sensitivity of the screening examination. Many peer-reviewed studies in the literature demonstrate CADe's potential impact on the radiologist's performance and the performance of the mammographic examination. In order to address the challenges of optimally detecting breast cancer with mammography, CADe assists the radiologist with limitations in search performance as well as helps the radiologist overcome the difficulties of detecting cancer in women with dense breasts. The ability of CADe to improve the sensitivity of breast cancer detection in all women with an acceptable impact on recall rate is evident. This chapter will focus on these reports and CADe's positive influence on the performance of mammography in North America.

22.2 COMPARISON OF CADe AND INTERPRETATION OF MAMMOGRAMS BY TWO RADIOLOGISTS (DOUBLE READING)

Multiple studies compare single reading, double reading, and CADe.[19–21] Georgian-Smith[19] finds double reading with either an additional radiologist or CADe detects an increase in the number of cancers but the data did not reach statistical significance. Destounis et al.[20] observe an additional 71% increase in cancer detection using CADe in a group of screening exams over those previously employing radiologist double reading. CADe correctly marks 37 of the 52 actionable findings double read as negative in previous screening years. In this case, the false-negative rate declines by nearly a third, from 31% to 19%. In a large retrospective review of mammograms over a four-year period, Gromet[21] compares the sensitivity, positive predictive value (PPV), and cancer detection rates for three reading methods: (1) single reading with CADe, (2) double reading with two radiologists, and (3) double reading man vs. machine where the performance of a second radiologist is compared to that of CADe. The sensitivity of the first reader notably increases from 81.4% to 88% by adding the second reader. The performance of a single reader with CADe increases sensitivity further to 90.4% with only a moderate increase in the recall rate from 10.2% to 11.9%. The improvement is statistically significant, p < 0.001. Because double reading is time consuming, costly, and requires additional radiologist time, CADe can act as a surrogate for the additional interpreting radiologists and improves overall screening examination sensitivity.

22.3 OVERVIEW OF CADe IN NORTH AMERICA

In 1998, the Food and Drug Administration approved CADe as a second reader for the interpreting radiologist. Approximately three out of four screening mammograms performed in the United States include CADe in the interpretation with an annual direct Medicare cost exceeding $30 million.[22] The CADe device marks regions of interest after the radiologist formulates an initial read. The system minimizes observational oversights while pointing out areas of concern that warrant additional evaluation. Earlier CADe studies were performed prior to the introduction of digital mammography necessitating digitizing analog film screen mammograms to digital data, which would then undergo CADe analysis. Analog screen-film images were digitized with high-resolution digitizers. Once digitized, CADe software algorithms search for masses, calcifications, and architectural distortion. The result is a computer soft copy or paper hard copy that is interpreted with the original mammogram. Later generations of CADe replace this labor-intensive system by integrating CADe software directly into the digital image. In practice, the performance of each CADe system using SFM or FFDM is similar. One study by Wei et al.[23] compares CADe findings from exams using FFDM and SFM obtained in the same patient and finds no statistically significant difference in detecting breast masses.

22.4 STUDIES EVALUATING CADe PERFORMANCE IN SCREEN-FILM MAMMOGRAPHY

Using SFM CADe acquisition methods, many studies assess the performance of CADe along the following parameters: sensitivity, specificity, cancer detection rate, and recall rate. In the first large prospective study in the United States,

Freer and Ulissey[24] evaluate CADe's performance in a screening population of 12,860 women. Their data validate previous retrospective studies that report the positive impact CADe has on breast cancer detection. Freer and Ulissey reveal a dramatic increase of 19.5% in the cancer detection rate (an increase from 3.2 to 3.8 cancers per 1000 women screened). The additional eight cancers CADe identifies are all early stage, 0 or 1. Early cancer detection is critical to saving the lives of women. CADe's ability to detect early-stage cancers is clinically significant and results in sharp reductions of cancer-related morbidity and mortality. While CADe identifies 19% more actionable findings, rise in false-positive findings serve as a setback. Like a detective following a false lead, CADe erroneously marks a suspicious finding as cancer without a cancer presence in the area. In turn, these false-positive findings result in an extremely high (19%) incremental increase in the recall rate of 6.5%–7.7%. Freer and Ulissey's study finds that CADe alone detects 82% of the malignancies, and the radiologist alone detects 84% of the cancers. Together, the radiologist and CADe are 20% better than either one alone.[24]

Birdwell et al.,[25] Morton et al.,[26] and Ko et al.[27] (see Table 22.1) demonstrate similar findings of cancer detection improvement albeit not as high as the 19.5% increase by Freer and Ulissey. These authors[36–38] follow a protocol similar to Freer and Ulissey, which consists of sequential reading of mammography with and without CADe. Birdwell et al.[25] report an incremental increase in two cancers detected, corresponding to a 7.4% increase in the cancer detection rate. Morton et al.[26] the largest out of all the prospective CADe studies report a comparable 7.62% increase in breast cancer detection, a yield of eight additional cancers (total 113 cancers/21,349 screenings) not detected by the radiologist alone. Ko[27] reveals a smaller incremental increase in CADe cancer detection finding two additional cancers, an increase of a more modest 4.7%.

In addition to prospective studies, historical control trials demonstrate the benefits of CADe. In this design, the cancer detection rate prior to the implementation of CADe is compared to the rate of cancer detection following the use of CADe in a clinical practice. Clearly, in this design, CADe is used on a different population of patients. Using historical controls, Cupples et al.[28] reported a 16.1% increase in the cancer detection rate over a period of 2 years and an 8.1% increase in the recall rate. The 16.1% increase in the cancer detection rate includes an even more significant 31.3% increase in the detection of small invasive cancers, those most often associated with improved survival and implying that CADe not only detects more cancers but also smaller cancers as well. Another study by Gur et al.[29] with similar design demonstrated contradictory, although somewhat skewed results. Contrary to most, the authors report

TABLE 22.1   OVERVIEW OF CAD STUDIES IN NORTH AMERICA

References	Type of Study	Total Number	Sensitivity Specificity		Incremental Cancer Detection Rate	Change in Recall Rate	Change in Biopsy Rate
			Outcomes Addressed				
Ko et al.[27]	Prospective	5016 Mammograms	Sensitivity = 94%;↑ 4%		+4.7%	+14.7%	+5.9%
Morton et al.[26]	Prospective Academic	21,349 Mammograms			+7.6%	+9.5%	+8.2%
Birdwell et al.[25]	Prospective Academic	8,682 Mammograms			+7.4%	+9%	+5%
Freer and Ulissey[24]	Prospective Academic	12,860 Mammograms			+19.5%	+18%	+19%
Gromet[21]	Historical review/ retrospective	118,808 Mammograms	Sensitivity = 90.4%; ↑2.7%		+1.9%	+3.9%	*No statistical significant difference in cancer detection rate
Fenton et al.[32]	Historical review/ retrospective	429,345 Mammograms	Sensitivity = 84%;↑3.6%	Specificity = 87.2%; ↓3%	16.1%	+3.1%	+19.7%
Fenton et al.[33]		23,830 Mammograms	Sensitivity = 81.1%; ↑0.4%	Specificity = 91%; ↓0.5%	*Cancer not associated with higher detection rates	+8.9%	
Georgian-Smith et al.[19]	Retrospective	6,381 Mammograms			0%	+6.4%	+10%
Gur et al.[29]	Historical review/ retrospective Community	59,129 Mammograms			+1.7%	+.09%	
Cupples et al.[28]	Historical review/ retrospective Community	19,402 Mammograms			+ 16.1%, *Detection of invasive cancers < 1 cm ↑164%	+ 8.1%	+6.7%
Burhenne et al.[35]	Retrospective multi-institutional	1,083 Mammograms	N/A			Net result: −0.7%	
Brem et al.[36]	Retrospective multi-institutional	930 Mammograms	Sensitivity = 91.4%; ↑21.2%				

a negligible 1.7% improvement in the cancer detection rate. The large confidence interval of CI –11% to +19% reported by the authors limits the ability to understand the implications of the findings. The considerable range diminishes accuracy and power and actually includes the 16.1% reported by Cupples et al.[28] Second and perhaps more importantly, Gur et al. analyzed a subset of 7 out of the 24 radiologists included in this study who interpret a large volume of mammograms (>8000 screening mammograms/year) and found a 3.2% decrease in the cancer detection rate (CI –15% to 9%) with a decrease in the recall rate of −4.9% (CI –21% to 4%). However, Gur did not analyze the impact of CADe on the radiologists with a lower volume of mammography interpretation per year, even though these radiologists constituted the majority of the radiologists in the study, and those who ought to benefit most from CADe. Feig et al.[30] analyzed the impact of CADe on the 17 lower volume radiologists and found that there was, in fact, a statistically significant 19.67% increase in the cancer detection rate with the addition of CADe. Feig's findings are similar to those of Freer and Ulissey who reported a 19% improvement in cancer detection with the use of CADe. Finally, Feig et al. point out yet another flaw in the Gur study using the historical control study design. The low cancer detection rate may be due to the cancer prevalence in the pre-CADe control group vs. cancer in the post-CADe group, which is not controlled in this study. Therefore, even the Gur study, which overall did not demonstrate a statistically significant increase in cancer detection with CADe, did demonstrate a significant increase in cancer detection when radiologists who interpret less than 8000 mammograms per year used CADe.

In a study population of screening and diagnostic mammograms, Dean and Ilvento[31] corroborate other prospective screening studies, noting a 10.8% increase in the cancer detection rate using CADe. The authors site the previously noted finding (Freer and Ulissey) that the cancers that radiologists miss that are detected with CADe are stage 0 and 1 cancers. The authors make note of a learning curve with CADe, which results in improved accuracy as experience with CADe increases specifically the recall rate. During the first 2 months after the introduction of CADe, the recall rate more than doubled from 6.2% to 13.4% (p value <0.0001). However, at the end of the two-year study, the recall rate returns to a level closer to the period prior to the introduction of CADe, that is, a 7.8% recall rate. A similar trend is noted in the study authored by Freer and Ulissey,[24] 6.5%–7.7%.

A controversial study by Fenton et al.[32,33] reported a reduction in the diagnostic performance of screen-film mammography after the introduction of CADe. In this, the largest historical review published to date, which reviews 1.6 million screen-film mammograms from 1998 to 2006 in 25 imaging centers, and a more recent follow-up study (2011); Fenton and colleagues report a reduction in the accuracy of mammography with the use of CADe with film screen mammography. Of note is that Fenton does report an improvement in cancer detection with a concomitant increase in recall rate, resulting in a statically reduced accuracy. However, the primary aim of CADe is to improve cancer detection, which it did. Arguably, the exclusion of digital mammography in the 2011 study, which builds upon the 2007 study, is not consistent with the majority of current CADe software performed in the country (the digitization of film screen mammograms prior to CADe analysis vs. digital CADe). Fenton et al.[33] admit this as a limitation in their study as "digitizing

screen-film exams prior to CADe can potentially introduce noise and effect the performance of this tool."[32] Fenton et al.[32,33] conclude that utilizing CADe decreases screening exam accuracy by having a statistically significant lower specificity and PPV. The higher recall rate translates to a decrease in accuracy. However, some argue that increases in the false positive or recall rate is a cost of cancer detection improvements (Freer and Ulissey).[24] Notably in the study by Fenton et al., CADe increases sensitivity in the detection of early breast cancers such as ductal carcinoma in situ (DCIS), which approached statistical significance. CADe's variable performance in their study may be due to the diverse interpretative skills of the radiologist (the ability to interpret benign from malignant) as well as the differences in the characteristics of the patient population.

Increases in recall rates are challenging for patients as well as for radiologists. Similar to previous prospective and retrospective studies, Fenton et al.[32,33] find recall rates, and false-positive marks increase with the use of CADe. This may be due to the quality of CADe marks (software that is more than 5 years old) or the radiologist's ability to distinguish false-positive marks from actionable marks. Mahoney and Meganathan[34] reviewed false-positive marks from CADe systems Fenton and other prospective studies use. The authors conclude that most false-positive CADe marks are easy to dismiss and should not affect clinical performance. Similarly, Ko et al.[27] note that radiologists in their study dismiss 97% of the 13,719 suspicious CADe findings, with an average of one CADe mark per image. Thus, these studies conclude that the combination of radiologists' interpretive skills and available technology (including CADe) increase cancer detection and sensitivity.[34]

In direct disagreement with Fenton, two large multi-institutional trials[35,36] conclude that CADe significantly improves cancer detection. These retrospective trials collect data from community and hospital facilities in the United States. Thirteen and eighteen facilities participate in the studies by Warren Burhenne et al.[35] and Brem et al.[37] respectively. Both report a significant number of cancers visible on mammograms 9–24 months prior to diagnosis. Warren Burhenne et al. report 67% of 427 cancers visible on mammograms prior to diagnosis, 27% of which are actionable. Similarly, Brem et al. report 47% of 377 cancers visible on mammograms prior to diagnosis, 32% of which are actionable. Like in Fenton et al.,[32,33] screen-film mammograms undergo a digitization prior to CADe analysis. Sixty-five percent of cases benefit from CADe in Brem et al. and 77% in the Warren Burhenne et al. study. Brem et al.[36] report a greater than 21% improvement in the sensitivity of the interpreting radiologist by decreasing the false-negative rate with the use of CADe.

22.5 STUDIES EVALUATING CADe PERFORMANCE IN FULL-FIELD DIGITAL MAMMOGRAPHY

The number of publications in the North American literature evaluating CADe's performance in full-field digital mammography is limited. In a similar protocol to Warren Burhenne et al.[35] and Brem et al.,[37] The and colleagues[38] review the performance of CADe in FFDM images. In a retrospective review of 123 malignancies on both screening and diagnostic exams, CADe detects 94% of the cancers. CADe systems in FFDM compare well to older versions of screen-film CADe systems, 94% vs. 80%–84% (Burhenne and Brem).[35,37] The FFDM CADe system false-positive rate is 2.3 marks per four-image case, comparable to some of the later versions of screen-film CADe in Mahoney and Meganathan.[34] In a comparison of two commercial digital CADe systems, Leon et al.[39] find no difference in the total number of markers between the R2 and iCAD systems, which display 0.55 and 0.52 markers per image, respectively. However, while the R2 CADe markers split evenly between masses and calcifications, the iCAD markers weight heavily toward masses 0.43/image than calcifications, 0.10/image.

In the study by The et al., CADe sensitivity remains consistent across all types of cancers and is not dependent on tumor size.[38] CADe detects 94% of the invasive ductal carcinomas (IDCs), 100% of the invasive lobular carcinomas, and 93% of DCIS. Based on the mammographic appearance, CADe detects both nonspiculated and spiculated masses and 100% of architectural distortions. Detection of asymmetries is more modest, with 75% of asymmetries detected with CADe. Wei et al. also evaluated CADe performance on FFDM and SFM images. Wei finds that FFDM CADe systems achieve higher detection sensitivity than the SFM CADe system at the same false-positive marks per malignant case. The overall performance of their FFDM and SFM CADe systems is similar for the entire data.[23]

Breast density increases the difficulty of finding breast cancer. How does CADe perform in women with different breast densities? In fact, the utility of CADe would increase if the performance were equal in women with dense and nondense breasts. Based on breast density, The and colleagues find that CADe correctly marks 100% of cancers in fatty breasts, 95% of cancers in breasts containing scattered fibroglandular densities, 93% of cancers in heterogeneously dense breasts, and a 60% of cancers in extremely dense breasts. Combining fatty and scattered fibroglandular cases as nondense, CADe has a sensitivity of 96%. When heterogeneously and extremely dense cases combine, CADe in dense breasts has a sensitivity of 90%.[38] CADe in dense and nondense groups shows no statistical significant difference in sensitivity. Brem et al.[40] study the potential impact breast density has on CADe interpretation in screen-film mammography and corroborate that breast density does not have an overall impact in the detection of breast cancer. However, there were more false-positive marks on dense breasts vs. nondense breast tissue, p value = 0.04.

The and colleagues find that CADe detects 93% of cancers manifesting as calcifications, 92% as masses, and 100% as mixed masses and calcifications.[49] Earlier screen-film CADe studies demonstrate similar findings. Warren Burhenne et al.[35] find that CADe correctly marks 906 of the 1083 mammograms, with 99% of the cancers that contain microcalcifications and 75% of the cancers display masses. In addition, in the study by Freer and Ulyssey,[24] CADe correctly marks 100% of the malignant calcifications and 67% of the masses. Historically, CADe performs well in detecting microcalcification and early breast cancers. The results are less favorable for a developing asymmetry or a mass, as surrounding breast tissue obscures findings.

22.6 PERFORMANCE OF CADe BY THE MAMMOGRAPHIC APPEARANCE OF BREAST CANCER

Since radiologists may miss cancers that present as masses more readily than calcifications (Birdwell[12]), it is important to evaluate the performance of CADe with various mammographic appearances of cancer, particularly in its ability to detect masses. In a retrospective review of 273 women with biopsy-proven breast cancer, Brem et al. (Cancer[37]) evaluated CADe performance based on mammographic appearance and histopathology. CADe correctly marks 89% of all cancers, detecting 98% presenting as calcifications, 89% presenting as mixed mass with calcifications, and 84% presenting as masses. This is comparable to Burhenne et al.,[35] who report a 99% sensitivity of CADe in the detection of malignant calcifications and 75% for the detection of a malignant masses.

All studies have demonstrated that CADe is more sensitive in detecting microcalcifications than masses, undoubtedly due to the algorithms used. However, not all calcifications are detected with equal sensitivity. Scott Soo and coworkers reported that CADe performance drops in detecting amorphous calcifications, detecting only 57% of the malignant amorphous calcifications. This is an important finding as a significant number of calcifications recommended for biopsy are amorphous in appearance. Amorphous calcifications represent 34% of the calcifications recommended for biopsy, 20% of which are malignant and another 20% representing high-risk lesions.[41] Berg et al. describe amorphous calcifications as indistinct, with limited conspicuity and difficult to image. Radiologists can overlook amorphous calcifications with Berg approximating 78% of this type of calcification visible only in retrospect and not prospectively.

Therefore, it is critical that further algorithmic development of CADe focuses on those calcifications that are more difficult for the radiologist as well as more challenging for CADe detection, specifically amorphous calcifications. Of note is that in an earlier study by Brem and Schoonjans,[42] the sensitivity of CADe for malignant calcifications is statistically greater than benign calcifications. Further work is needed to evaluate if the calcifications detected with CADe are predominantly malignant, with CADe not detecting the benign calcifications. If so, the morphologic differences of the calcification may help in further CADe by using the objective characteristics used with CADe algorithms to differentiate benign from malignant calcifications.

In assessing the ability of CADe to detect breast masses, Birdwell et al.[25] reported a 7.4% increase in mammographic sensitivity with the addition of CADe. Most studies evaluating CADe and mammographic manifestation of cancer evaluated masses and microcalcification. However, the ability for CADe to detect the third most common mammographic manifestation of cancer, that is, architectural distortion and spiculation,[43] is less promising and is often missed at the time of interpretation.[44] Baker et al. evaluate CAD's ability to detect cancers presenting as architectural distortion. In two commercially available CADe systems, the ability to detect architectural distortion is limited. On average, CADe detects one in five cases of architectural distortion, and in one small study by Vyborny et al.,[44] CADe correctly identifies 86% of the spiculated breast cancers.

CADe sensitivity can vary based on the size of the lesion. In the study by Ellis et al.,[45] all invasive cancers manifesting as masses measuring less than 10 and 20 mm have a CADe sensitivity of 81% and 92%, respectively. Brem et al.[46] (AJR) further stratify mammographic masses manifesting as pure masses and masses with associated calcifications. CADe sensitivity for pure masses was similar to that in Ellis et al.[45] with a range of 81%–91% for masses 1–20 mm in size; however, the value significantly decreases to 75% for masses larger than 20 mm (Brem et al.[46]). Perhaps this is due to the algorithms being developed to detect smaller masses. CADe sensitivity for masses with associated microcalcifications measuring greater than 10 mm and less than 5 mm was 100%, and CADe sensitivity for those masses with associated microcalcifications measuring 6–10 mm in size is 71%. Similarly, Ellis et al.[45] find that 71% of missed cancers utilizing two independent CADe systems (R2 and iCAD) show invasive cancers less than 10 mm in size. The ability of CADe to detect malignancies at a small size and therefore an earlier stage is beneficial for the patient.

Further studies on CAD's performance in detecting the histopathological types of cancer demonstrate that CADe correctly marks a significant number of cancers regardless of the type of cancer. Brem et al. (Cancer[37]) reported that CADe correctly detects 87% of all invasive cancers with 85% sensitivity in the detection of IDCs and 95% sensitivity for invasive lobular carcinomas. Invasive lobular carcinoma is known to be difficult to detect on mammography as the tumor cells create little disruption in the adjacent tissue and the malignant cells form along a linear pattern into the breast parenchyma. Invasive lobular cancer presents more as a subtle asymmetry or architectural distortion[47] and less likely to present as a mass or calcifications. Therefore, mammographic detection can be quite challenging. In an additional study by Evans et al.,[48] the authors evaluate CAD's performance in detecting invasive lobular carcinoma and conclude that CADe correctly marks a high percentage (91%) of invasive lobular carcinomas. The use of CADe increases the likelihood of detecting these difficult breast cancers on screening mammography, a significant contribution when using CADe.

Pai et al.[49] explore CADe performance in the detection of DCIS, the earliest form of breast cancer. In a retrospective review of biopsy-proven cancers evaluating only DCIS, CADe had a sensitivity of 91%. Similar to other prospective and retrospective studies that evaluate mixed cancers of DCIS with invasive breast cancer, Brem et al.[37] demonstrate a sensitivity of 95% for pure DCIS. Interestingly, researchers attribute the detection improvement to CADe's increase in sensitivity for calcifications, a common presentation of DCIS.

22.7 FUTURE OF CADe IN MAMMOGRAPHY

Along with advantages of CADe in the detection of early breast cancer, CADe also increases recall rates as well as biopsies. There are, of course, sensitivity increases coupled with decreased specificity. Reconciling this inverse relationship is difficult where screening exam utility diminishes as the false-positive marks grow. An interesting sequence occurs whereby the higher the number of CADe marks, the higher the detection rate, but with increasing CADe marks per image, the CADe marks become increasingly distracting as well as result in a higher likelihood that the radiologists dismiss the significant CADe prompts. In order to improve the overall accuracy and decrease the false-positive rate of a CADe system, a two-view method has been proposed in which the lesion is marked by CADe only if it is identified in both the craniocaudal and mediolateral mammographic projections.[50] This approach improves accuracy by reducing false-positive marks such as those resulting from the superimposition of normal glandular tissue. Samulski and Karssemeijer[50] believe that the two-view method results in a decrease in pseudo findings related to superimposition of normal glandular tissue and a significant decrease in the false-positive rate.

A CADe system with the ability to incorporate the radiologist's decision-making process into its algorithm also decreases the false-positive rate.[51] Wu et al. examine a CADe system that employs symmetry of the breast parenchymal tissue. The authors' algorithm for CADe detects masses worthy of further analysis and classifies the contralateral mammogram information. This algorithm fuses CAD's evaluation in detecting potential masses and incorporates *symmetry* information from the left and right breasts in order to differentiate symmetric (likely false positive) and asymmetric (likely mass) structures. On the positive side, Wu et al show a statistically significant false-positive rate decrease when utilizing their bilateral algorithm. Unfortunately, the authors admit that miss-registration may occur with poor positioning of the breasts. Any poor positioning negates the potential information gains and results in no change to the false-positive rate.

Recently, digital breast tomosynthesis (DBT) gained FDA approval and is now commercially available. The multiple (number can vary based on the manufacturer) projection-view mammograms of tomosynthesis have the potential to resolve false-positive findings that occur as a result of overlapping normal glandular tissue, particularly in dense breasts. Where 2D mammography and its CADe system are unsuccessful, 3D imaging (tomosynthesis) shows promise. The 3D data allow further analysis of concerning findings such as shape, margin, size, and associate calcifications and its location, which decrease false-positive findings. Tomosynthesis improves specificity of the screening exam by significantly decreasing the recall rate.

The influence of tomosynthesis on breast cancer detection is beyond the scope of this chapter, however, preliminary data on CADe systems for the evaluation of masses on digital tomosynthesis are promising.[52–54] To date, the FDA has yet to approve CADe for tomosynthesis, but many supporting studies are underway. Chan et al. show that CADe is more effective in distinguishing suspicious masses from normal tissue. Key in the study is the prescreening and segmentation of masses. In an additional study, Chan compares CADe performance in automated mass detection using multiple algorithms and finds that accuracy improves when 2D and 3D (tomosynthesis) imaging combine over 3D alone.[53] Conspicuity of a finding is dependent on the 3D imaging acquisition method. Notably, breast tissue slice thickness obscures findings such as cluster calcifications, a concerning finding for malignancy. The clarity of cluster calcifications on 2D imaging vs. 3D DBT method is a question for much larger studies. However, in a small study, Spangler et al.[55] report the ability of conventional two-view digital mammogram surpasses tomosynthesis in detecting and classifying calcifications. The authors conclude that the diagnostic performance of the two modalities is not significantly different based on the area under the curve. Additionally, Kopans et al.[56] investigate the performance of the two different modalities and the clarity of calcifications. The authors conclude that once the presence of calcifications is known, DBT and not two-view digital mammography improves the diagnostic capability and clarity of calcifications. That said, improvements in calcification visualization are secondary to the decrease in structural noise (decrease in the overlap of normal breast tissue).

In an interesting approach to DBT, Kopans et al. employ a multiplanar technique that combines data from many adjacent slices to make a *slab* of data. The stacked slabs of data increase the potential to evaluate cluster calcifications. The authors are quick to state that these results are not reproducible for all types of DBT as techniques in acquisition vary from manufacturer to manufacturer. However, all vendors have, or are developing, both slice and slab approach to reviewing tomosynthesis studies. That said, tomosynthesis does help to discriminate abnormal findings from the surrounding normal fibroglandular tissue. CADe tomosynthesis shows promise in helping decrease the false-positive rate.

The future of CADe not only continues to follow algorithms that aid radiologists but also clarifies and characterizes findings on the scale of benign to malignant. An appropriate label for the future is *computer-aided diagnosis* (CADx) where a system not only aids radiologist in detecting cancer but also characterizes the likelihood of cancer. Clearly, a transition from the binary information on most CADe systems, to the additional information of the likelihood that a lesion with characteristics similar to that being evaluated will enormously aid in the utility of CAD. For example, when a radiologist detects a lesion and the CADe score determines a 5% likelihood of malignancy, it will be evaluated very differently than if the CADe score had a 90% likelihood of malignancy. Currently, both these lesions would be marked, but the transition from a binary to a stratified likelihood of malignancy approach to lesion analysis will greatly aid the radiologist.

In support of the progression from CADe to CADx, many are investigating CAD algorithms that predict a woman's risk of developing a breast cancer based on density alone. Here, studies[57,58] use computerized analysis isolate breast density as an independent cancer risk factor. Computerized analysis provides an objective reproducible assessment that assists not just detection but also diagnosis. In a retrospective review that compares computer-aided mammographic density estimates (MDEST) with estimates made by radiologists, Martin et al.[59] conclude that MDEST are more accurate than the radiologists' visual breast density estimates. In their study, radiologists tend to overestimate breast density by approximately 6%. Some believe a true density analysis should be based on a quantitative approach utilizing volume not just the estimate area of fibroglandular tissue. Kontos et al.[60] analyze breast parenchyma utilizing digital mammography and DBT. The authors conclude that DBT texture analysis correlates stronger with breast density than digital mammography. Others[61] evaluate digital mammograms in women who are at significant risk of developing breast cancer (BRCA 1 and 2 gene mutation carriers) to test the potential pattern of breast parenchyma in the retroareolar region. Since mammograms overlap normal structures such as skin, a true assessment of glandular tissue such subcutaneous skin and deeper parenchymal tissue is not achievable. Knowing that breast cancer risk is impacted by the amount of fibroglandular tissue (density), analysis that targets glandular tissue using DBT is a more accurate way of measuring this important risk factor. Clearly, a quantitative analysis of breast density, and thereby cancer risk, is more accurate than qualitative analysis.

There is an increasing interest in augmenting risk assessment models for breast cancer with measures of breast density. Chen et al.[62] develop a relative risk model for white women by adding many variables of the Gail model 2 (available at http://www.cancer.gov/bcrisktool/) to breast density. In this case, density measures the percentage of the breast area on the craniocaudal view. Attributable risks such as (1) age at the birth of first live child, (2) number of first-degree relatives (mother or sisters) with breast cancer, (3) number of previous benign breast biopsies, and (4) weight are all considered. The average of the density percentages in each breast defines patient mammographic density percentage. The authors' model finds higher risk values over the Gail model for women with a higher percentage of dense breast area. These preliminary data are promising. Adding breast density elevates the discriminatory power of the risk model.

22.8 CADe IN OTHER MODALITIES OF BREAST IMAGING

In some patient populations, the effectiveness of screening mammography is limited.

As we discuss in this chapter, an example of this is women with dense breast tissue. Many radiologists employ ultrasound as the most common supplemental tool used in conjunction with mammography. It is cost effective, is readily available, and characterizes findings that mammography or physical examination does not identify. The American College of Radiology Imaging Network (ACRIN) 6666 trial demonstrates a 28% improvement in cancer detection after the addition of ultrasound to screening mammography in a high-risk population. The combination screen results in a fourfold increase in false-positive findings over mammography alone. However, the improved accuracy of mammography with the addition of ultrasound

yields an impressive supplemental increase of 4.2 cancer per 1000 women screened.[63]

There are a limited number of FDA-approved CADx systems for ultrasound use despite interpreting radiologist performance improvements. The FDA approved the first CADe systems for ultrasound in 2005. Ultrasound CADx, unlike CADe in mammography, is CADx as it does not detect the lesion, but rather analyzes the lesion identified as the region of interest by the radiologist.[64] CADx for breast ultrasound applies ultrasound CADx algorithms to find the edge of a solid mass and then further characterizes it based on individual features such as shape, sharpness, shadowing, and texture.[65] Using ACR BI-RADS Lexicon descriptors, a US CADx algorithm assesses individual features suggesting a BI-RADS category based on the probability of malignancy.

When CADe for mammography is coupled with CADx for ultrasound, Jesneck et al.[66] find an overall improvement in the CAD performance. By using BI-RADS features for both mammography and sonography, the automated classification (linear discriminant analysis, LDA) of CADx matched the radiologist performance with classification. The authors utilized 803 lesions with the first 500 cases used to train the CADx system and the next consecutive 303 cases used to retest the system or the radiologist performance. On the retest dataset, the LDA and radiologists performed with similar negative predictive values 97% vs. 98%, p value = 0.25. In one case in which the LDA and radiologist disagreed, the LDA correctly classified the lesion as benign. The authors conclude, "if the radiologists were to adopt all the recommendations of the computer model, they could substantially increase specificity while maintaining a high sensitivity level" (Jesneck et al. *Radiology*[66]). Other authors[67] have noticed no difference in the specificity with and without the use of CADe but noticed an improvement in the sensitivity with the help of CADx.

Contrast-enhanced breast MRI is complementary to mammography and ultrasound and is now widely used in the United States.[68] This screening tool has the ability to differentiate lesions from adjacent breast tissue as well as image abnormalities in three dimensions. The temporal information or time course of signal intensity within a lesion after the administration of a contrast agent can help in differentiating benign from malignant lesions. Automated computer-generated kinetic assessments and morphologic characteristics of breast lesions enable the radiologist further assessment of a lesion as benign or malignant. Using kinetic information along with morphologic analysis is currently the approach used to characterize MRI-detected breast lesions. Similar to CADe in mammography, MRI CADe helps the radiologist to improve the overall accuracy of the exam.

In a retrospective review, Williams et al.[69] evaluate the sensitivity of computer-aided evaluation in MRI.

Information obtained from the kinetic information is color mapped based on the amount of enhancement after the administration of contrast. Areas that reach a threshold level of enhancement determined by the CADe software algorithm is denoted by a color based on the amount of enhancement on delayed images minus the first projected image postcontrast. The automated color projection image overlay, or *color map*, allows the radiologist to determine if findings are more suspicious. The authors find that the use of MRI CADx helped to improve the discriminant power of benign vs. malignant characteristics compared to the interpretation of the radiologist alone. The improvement was attributed to the addition of computer-aided evaluation. In addition, CADe helped decrease the false-positive rate by correctly demonstrating 23% of benign lesions with no enhancement beyond the threshold level.

The future of CAD MRI will evaluate kinetic and morphologic features of lesions. In a study by Bhooshan et al.,[70] the authors evaluate CAD's ability to automate the kinetic and morphologic characteristics of invasive and noninvasive breast cancers and further discriminate known cancers for the possibility of metastatic and nonmetastatic diseases. This provides an MRI assessment of a prognostic indicator in a known cancer in a reproducible and objective way. Breast cancer that has spread to the lymph nodes has a poor prognosis when compared to cancer that is contained within the breast.[71] Bhooshan identifies trends in the kinetic and enhancement pattern of breast malignancies with DCIS and benign lesions demonstrating lower contrast uptake rates when compared to IDC. All malignant lesions (IDC and DCIS) demonstrate large values in contrast enhancement with a peak in the first or second postcontrast time point. Additionally, IDCs without nodal metastasis and DCIS demonstrate a longer time to peak enhancement even though all cancers peaked at the first or second postcontrast time point. CAD extraction of these objective characteristics has the potential to extend two prognostic tasks: (1) classification of invasive and noninvasive (DCIS) breast cancers and (2) further classification of IDC into positive and negative lymph nodes (Bhooshan et al.[70]). Others have used various characteristics of lesions, including *blooming of lesions* identified with breast MRI to further discriminate lesions. By correlating CAD's prognostic indicators with suspicious findings, CAD will further our detection, understanding, and characterization of breast lesions.

22.9   SUMMARY

CADe is now an integral component of most clinical breast practices. In fact, 95% of digital mammography units purchased in the United States are purchased with CADe. With the current iterations of most CADe, there is the ability to detect additional, earlier, and difficult-to-detect breast cancers, which manifest as microcalcification, masses, or combinations of the two. With ongoing developments, CAD will likely further the ability to differentiate benign from malignant lesions by likelihood of malignancy information as well as further the ability to assess a women's risk based on breast density and parenchymal characteristics.

Although CADe has been in clinical use for nearly two decades, it is still clearly in development. As we move from CADe to CADx, we will continue to integrate CAD's additional uses into daily practice.

REFERENCES

1. Berry DA, Cronin KA, Plevritis SK et al. Effect of screening and adjuvant therapy on mortality from breast cancer. *N Engl J Med*. 2005;353(17):1784–1792.
2. Burrell HC, Sibbering DM, Wilson AR et al. Screening interval breast cancers: Mammographic features and prognostic factors. *Radiology* 1996;199:811–817.
3. Surveillance, Epidemiology, and End Results (SEER) Program (www.seer.cancer.gov) SEER Fast Stat Database: Mortality—All COD, Aggregated With State, Total U.S. (1969–2008) <Katrina/Rita Population Adjustment>, National Cancer Institute, DCCPS, Surveillance Research Program, Cancer Statistics Branch, released October 2011. Underlying mortality data provided by NCHS (www.cdc.gov/nchs).
4. Smith DR, Caughran J, Kreinbrink J, Parish GK, Silver SM, Breslin TM, Pettinga JE et al. Clinical presentation of breast cancer: Age, stage, and treatment modalities in a contemporary cohort of Michigan women [abstr]. In: 2011 Breast Cancer Symposium San Francisco. September 8, 2011.
5. Tabar L, Vitak B, Chen T, Yen A, Cohen A, Tot T, Chiu S, Chen S, Fann J, Rossell J, Fohlin H, Smith R, Duffy S. Swedish two-county trial: Impact of mammographic screening on breast cancer mortality during 3 Decades. *Radiology* 2011;260:658–663.
6. Rosenberg R, Yankaskas B, Abraham L, Sickles E, Lehman C, Geller B, Carney P, Kerlidowske K, Buist D, Weaver D, Barlow W, Ballard-Barbash R. Performance benchmarks for screening mammography. *Radiology* 2006;241(1):55–66.
7. Quality determinants of mammography. *Quality Determinants of Mammography Guidelines Panel*. Rockville, MD: United States Department of Health and Human Services, Public Health Service, Agency for Health Care Policy and Research, 1994, pp. 78–86.
8. Sickles EA, Wolverton DE, Dee KE. Performance parameters for screening and diagnostic mammography: Specialist and general radiologists. *Radiology* 2002;224:861–869.
9. Majid A, de Paredes E, Doherty R, Sharma N, Salvador X. Missed breast carcinoma: Pitfalls and pearls. *RadioGraphics* 2003;23:881–895.
10. Mandelson MT, Oestreicher N, Porter PL, White D, Finder CA, Taplin SH, White E. Breast density as a predictor of mammographic detection: Comparison of interval- and screen-detects cancers. *J Natl Cancer Inst* 2000;92(13):1081–1087.

11. Harvey JA, Fajardo LL, Innis CA. Previous mammograms in patients with impalpable breast carcinoma; retrospective vs. blinded interpretation. *Am J Roentgenol* 1993;161:1167–1172.

12. Birdwell R, Ikeda D, O'Shaughnessey K, Sickles E. Mammographic characteristics of 115 missed cancers later detects with screening mammography and the potential utility of computer-aided detection. *Radiology* 2001;219:192–202.

13. Ikeda DM, Birdwell RL, O'Shaughnessey KO, Brenner RJ, Sickles EA. Analysis of 172 subtle findings on prior normal mammograms in women with breast cancer detects at follow-up screening. *Radiology* 2003;226;494–503.

14. Thurfjell E, Lernevall K, Taube A. Benefit of independent double reading in a population-based mammography screening program. *Radiology* 1994;191:241–244.

15. Thurfjell E. Mammography screening: One versus two views and independent double reading. *Acta Radiol* 1994;35:345–350.

16. Anderson E, Muir B, Walsh J, Kirkpatrick A. The efficacy of double reading mammograms in breast screening. *Clin Radiol* 1994;49:248–251.

17. Warren R, Duffy S. Comparison of single reading with double reading of mammograms, and change in effectiveness with experience. *Br J Radiol* 1995;68:958–962.

18. Harvey S, Geller B, Oppenheimer R, Pinet M, Riddell L, Garra B. Increase in cancer detection and recall rates with independent double interpretation of screening. *Am J Roentgenol* 2003;180:1461–1467.

19. Georgian-Smith D, Moore RH, Halpern E, Yeh ED, Rafferty EA, D'Alessandro HA, Staffa M, Hall DA, McCarthy KA, Kopans DB. Blinded comparison of computer-aided detection with human second reading in screening mammography. *Am J Roentgenol* 2007;189:1135–1141.

20. Destounis S, DiNitto P, Logan-Young W, Bonaccio E, Zuley ML, Willison K. Can computer-aided detection with double reading of screening mammograms help decrease the false-negative rate? Initial experience. *Radiology* 2004;232:578–584.

21. Gromet M. Comparison of computer-aided detection to double reading of screening mammograms: Review of 231,221 mammograms. *Am J Roentgenol* 2008;190:850–859.

22. Rao VM, Levin DC, Parker L, Cavanaugh B, Frangos AJ, Sunshine JH. How widely is computer-aided detection used in screening and diagnostic mammography? *J Am Coll Radiol* 2010;7(10):802–805.

23. Wei J, Hakjiiski LM, Sahiner B, Chan H, Ge J, Roubidoux MA, Helvie MA, Zhou C, Wu Y. Computer aided detection systems for breast masses: Comparison of performances on full-field digital mammograms and digitized screen-film mammograms. *Acad Radiol* 2007;14(6):659–669.

24. Freer TW, Ulissey MJ. Screening mammography with computer-aided detection: Prospective study of 12,860 patients in a community breast center. *Radiology* 2001;220:781–786.

25. Birdwell RL, Bandodkar P, Ikeda DM. Computer-aided detection with screening mammography in a university hospital setting. *Radiology* 2005;236:451–457.

26. Morton MJ, Whaley DH, Brandt KR, Amrami KK. Screening mammograms: Interpretation with computer-aided detection-prospective evaluation. *Radiology* 2006;239(2):375–383.

27. Ko JM, Nicholas MJ, Mendel JB, Slanetz PJ. Prospective assessment of computer-aided detection in interpretation of screening mammography. *AJR* 2006;187(6):1483–1491.

28. Cupples TE, Cunningham JE, Reynolds JC. Impact of computer-aided detection in a regional screening mammography program. *Am J Roentgenol* 2005;185:944–950.

29. Gur D, Sumkin JH, Rockette H, Ganott M, Hamkim C, Hardesty L, Poller WR, Shah R, Wallace L. Changes in breast cancer detection and mammography recall rates after the introduction of a computer-aided detection system. *J Natl Cancer Inst* 2004; 96(3):185–190.

30. Feig S, Sickles E, Evans WP, Linver M. Re: Changes in breast cancer detection and mammography recall rates after introduction of a computer-aided detection system (letter). *J Natl Cancer Inst* 2004;96:1260–1261.

31. Dean J and Ilvento CC. Improved cancer detection using computer-aided detection with diagnostic and screening mammography: Prospective study of 104 cancers. *Am J Roentgenol* 2006;187:20–28.

32. Fenton JJ, Taplin SH, Carney PA, Abraham L, Sickles EA, D'Orsi CD, Berns EA, Cutter G, Hendrick E, Barlow WE and Elmore JG. Influence of computer-aided detection on performance of screening mammography. *N Engl J Med* 2007;356:1399–409.

33. Fenton JJ, Abraham L, Taplin SH, Geller BM, Carney PA, D'Orsi C, Elmore JG, Barlow WE; for the Breast Cancer Surveillance Consortium. Effectiveness of computer-aided detection in community mammography practice. *J Natl Cancer Inst* 2011;103:1152–1161.

34. Mahoney MC and Meganathan K. False positive marks on unsuspicious screening mammography with computer-aided detection. *J Digit Imaging* 2011;24:772–777.

35. Warren Burhenne LJ, Wood SA, D'Orsi CJ, Feig SA, Kopans DB, O'Shaughnessy KF, Sickles EA, Tabar L, Vyborny CJ, Castellino RA. Potential contribution of computer-aided detection to the sensitivity of screening mammography. *Radiology* 2000;215:554–562.

36. Brem RF, Baum J, Lechner M, Kaplan S, Souders S, Naul LG, Hoffmeister J. Improvement in sensitivity of screening mammography with computer-aided detection: A multiinstitutional trial. *Am J Roentgenol* 2003;181:687–693.

37. Brem RF, Rapelyea JA, Zisman G, Hoffmeister JW, DeSimio MP. Evaluation of breast cancer with a computer-aided detection system by mammographic appearance and histopathology. *Cancer* 2005;104;931–935.

38. The JS, Schilling KJ, Hoffmeister JW. Friedmann E, McGinnis R, Holcomb RG. Detection of breast cancer with full-field digital mammography and computer-aided detection. *Am J Roentgenol* 2009;192:337–340.

39. Leon S, Brateman L, Honeyman-Buck J and Marshall J. Comparison of two commercial CAD systems for digital mammography. *J Digit Imaging* 2009;22:421–423.

40. Brem RF, Hoffmeister JW, Rapelyea JA, Zisman G, Mohtashomi K, Jindal G, DiSimio MP, Rogers SK. Impact of breast density on computer-aided detection for breast cancer. *Am J Roentgenol* 2005;184:439–444.

41. Berg WA, Arnoldus CL, Teferra E, Bhargavan M. Biopsy of amorphous breast calcifications: Pathologic outcome and yield at stereotactic biopsy. *Radiology* 2001;221:495–503.

42. Brem RG, Schoonjans JM. Radiologist detection of microcalcifications with and without computer-aided detection: A comparative study. *Clin Radiology* 2001;56:150–154.

43. Baker, JA, Rosen EL, Lo JY, Gimenez EI, Walsh r, Scott Soo M. Computer-aided detection (CAD) in screening mammography: Sensitivity of commercial CAD systems for detecting architectural distortion. *Am J Roentgenol* 2003;181:1083–1088.

44. Vyborny CJ, Doi T, O'Shaughnessy KF, Romsdahl HM, Schneider AC, Stein AA. Breast cancer: Importance of spiculation in computer-aided detection. *Radiology* 2000;215:703–707.

45. Ellis RL, Meade AA, Mathiason MA, Willison KM, Logan-Young W. Evaluation of computer-aided detection systems in the detection of small invasive breast carcinoma. *Radiology* 2007;245:88–94.

46. Brem RF, Hoffmeister JW, Zisman G, DeSimio MP, Rogers SK. A computer-aided detection system for the evaluation of breast cancer by mammographic appearance and lesion size. *Am J Roentgenol* 2005;184:893–896.

47. Helvie MA, Paramaguul C, Oberman HA, Adler DD. Invasive lobular carcinoma: Imaging features and clinical detection. *Invest Radiol* 1993;28:202–207.

48. Evans WP, Warren Burhenne LJ, Laurie L, O'Shaughnessey KF, Castellino RA. Invasive lobular carcinoma of the breast: Mammographic characteristics and computer-aided detection. *Radiology* 2002;225:182–189.

49. Pai VR, Gregory NE, Swinford AE, Rebner M. Ductal carcinoma in situ: computer-aided detection in screening mammography. *Radiology* 2006;241:689–694.

50. Samulski M and Karssemeijer N. Optimizing case-based detection performance in a multiview CAD system for mammography. *IEEE Trans Med Imaging* 2011;30(4):1001–1009.

51. Wu Y, Wei J, Hadjiiski LM, Sahiner B, Zhou C, Ge J, Shi J, Zhang Y, Chan H. Bilateral analysis based false positive reduction for computer-aided mass detection. *Med Phys* 2007;34(8):3334–3344.

52. Chan H, Wei J, Sahiner B, Rafferty EA, Wu T, Roubidoux MA, Moore RH, Kopans DB, Hadjiiski LM, Helvie MA. Computer-aided detection system for breast masses on digital tomosynthesis mammograms: Preliminary experience. *Radiology* 2005;237:1075–1080.

53. Chan H, Wei J, Zhang Y, Helvie MA, Moore RG, Sahiner B, Hadjiiski L, Kopans DB. Computer-aided detection of masses in digital tomosynthesis mammography: Comparison of three approaches. *Med Phys* 2008;35(9):4087–4095.

54. Reiser R, Nishikawa M, Giger ML, Wu T, Rafferty EA, Moore RT, Kopans DB. Computerized mass detection for digital breast tomosynthesis directly from the projection images. *Med Phys* 2006;33:482–491.

55. Spangler ML, Zuley ML, Sumkin JH, Abrams G, Ganott MA, Hakim C, Perrin R, Chough DM, Shah R, Gur D. Detection and classification of calcifications on digital breast tomosynthesis and 2D digital mammography: A comparison. *Am J Roentgenol* 2011;196:320–324.

56. Kopans D, Gavenonis S, Halpern E, Moore R. Calcifications in the breast and digital breast tomosynthesis. *Breast J* 2011;16:638–644.

57. Boyd NF, Guo H, Martin L, Stone J, Fishell E, Jong RA, Hislop G, Chiarelli A, Minkin S, Yaffe MJ. Mammographic density and the risk and detection of breast cancer. *N Engl J Med* 2007;356(3):227–236.

58. *Boyd* NF, Byng JW, Jong RA, Fishell EK, Little LE, Miller AB, Lockwood GA, Tritchler DL, Yaffe MJ. Quantitative classification of mammographic densities and breast cancer risk: Results from the Canadian national breast screening study. *J Natl Cancer Inst* 1995;87(9):670–675.

59. Martin KE, Helvie MA, Zhou C, Roubidoux MA, Bailey JE, Paramagul C, Blane CE, Klein KA, Sonnad SS, Chan H. Mammographic density measured with quantitative computer-aided method: Comparison with radiologists' estimates and BI-RADS categories. *Radiology* 2006;240:656–665.

60. Kontos D, Bakic PR, Troxel AB, Conant E, Maidment ADA. Digital breast tomosynthesis parenchymal texture analysis for breast cancer risk estimation: A preliminary study. In: Krupinski EA, ed. *Digital Mammography* (IWDM). Berlin, Germany: Springer-Verlag, 2008:681–688.

61. Huo Z, Giger ML, Olopade OI, Wolverton DE, Weber BL, Metz CE, Zhong W, Cummings SA. Computerized analysis of digitized mammograms of BRCA1 and BRCA2 gene mutation carriers. *Radiology* 2002;225(2):519–526.

62. Chen J, Pee D, Ayyagari R, Graubard B, Schairer C, Byrne C, Benichou J, Gail MH. Projecting absolute invasive breast cancer risk in white women with a model that includes mammographic density. *J Natl Cancer Inst* 2006;98:1215–1226.

63. Berg WA, Blume JD, Cormack JB, Mendelson EB, Lehrer D, Bohm-Velez M, Pisano ED et al., for the ACRIN 6666 Investigators. Combined screening with ultrasound and mammography vs. mammography alone in women at elevated risk of breast cancer. *J Am Med Assoc* 2008;299(18):2151–2163.

64. Stavros A Thomas. New advances in breast ultrasound: Computer-aided detection. *Ultrasound Clin* 2009;4:285–290.

65. Gruszauskas NP, Drukker K, Giger ML, Chang R, Sennett CA, Moon WK, Pesce LL. Breast US computer-aided diagnosis system: Robustness across urban populations in South Korea and the United States. *Radiology* 2009;3:661–671.

66. Jesneck JL, Lo JY, Baker JA. Breast Mass Lesions: Computer-aided diagnosis models with mammographic and sonographic descriptors. *Radiology* 2007;244(2):390–398.

67. Horsch K, Giger ML, Vyborny CJ, Lan L, Mendelson EB, Hendrick RE. Classification of breast lesions with multimodality computer-aided diagnosis: Observer study results on an independent clinical data set. *Radiology* 2006;240(2):357–368.

68. Bassett LW, Dhaliwal SG, Eradat J, Khan O, Farria DF, Brenner RJ, Sayre JW. National trends and practices in breast MRI. *Am J Roentgenol* 2008;191:332–339.

69. Williams TC, DeMartini WB, Partridge SC, Peacock S, Lehman CD. Breast MR Imaging: Computer-aided evaluation program for discriminating benign from malignant lesions. *Radiology* 2007;244:94–103.

70. Bhooshan N, Giger ML, Jansen SA, Li H, Lan L, Newstead GM. Cancerous breast lesions on dynamic contrast-enhanced MR images: Computerized characterization for image-based prognostic markers. *Radiology* 2010;254(3):680–690.

71. Arriagada R, Le MG, Dunant A, Tubiana M, Contesso G. Twenty-five years of follow-up in patients with operable breast carcinoma: Correlation between clinicopathologic factors and the risk of death in each 5-year period. *Cancer* 2006;106:743–750.

Chapter 23

Clinical Utility of CADe for Screening Mammography

A European Perspective

Maureen G.C. Gillan and Fiona J. Gilbert

CONTENTS

23.1 INTRODUCTION

This chapter reviews the clinical utility of computer-aided detection (CADe) systems in the context of screening mammography programs in Europe. Screening mammography in Europe differs considerably from the United States. In the United States, screening is more of an opportunistic than an organized activity and therefore population access is more restricted (Smith-Bindman et al. 2005). Screening is provided in private practice, healthcare organizations, or academic medical centers, whereas in Europe, screening is primarily conducted via organized population-based programs. There are also differences in the age range of women screened, the time interval between mammography examinations, and the assessment methods used to investigate suspicious cases (Smith-Bindman et al. 2005, U.S. Preventive Services Task Force 2009). U.S. physicians are required to read approximately 5- to 10-fold fewer mammograms annually than European readers to fulfill quality assurance (QA) standards, and physicians face higher rates of litigation for missed cancers (Elmore et al. 2003, Fletcher and Elmore 2003, Perry et al. 2006, Smith-Bindman et al. 2005). These factors may partly explain why cancer detection rates are similar in the United States and Europe, but recall and surgical biopsy rates are almost twice as high in the United States. Therefore, the clinical utility of CADe may differ considerably between these two environments.

23.1.1 Principles and Philosophy of Breast Screening

The fundamental concept of a screening test is that early detection of disease, before clinical signs and symptoms are manifest, allows treatment at an earlier stage and may improve the prospects for survival. A population-based screening program targets a largely asymptomatic population. Ideally, a screening test should have a high sensitivity and specificity. Sensitivity measures the proportion of truly positive cases in the preclinical detectable stage in the screened population, and specificity measures the proportion of truly negative, nondiseased cases in the screened population. Population screening provides a number of parameters (e.g., screening attendance of the target population, numbers of screen-detected and interval cancer cases, stage distribution

of cancers, and mortality rates) that can be used to measure the performance of the screening program. It is also important that screening programs are evidence based and respond appropriately to the emergence of new technologies that could improve their performance and reduce mortality.

23.1.2 Organization of Screening in Europe

In the mid-1980s, the results of randomized trials of mammographic screening and their long-term follow-up indicated that a reduction in breast cancer mortality of 25%–30% could be achieved in groups of women invited for screening compared with control groups that received standard care (Blamey et al. 2000, Humphrey et al. 2002, IARC 2002) (Figure 23.1). These data were later substantiated by evidence from outside the research setting in the organized service screening (Gabe and Duffy 2005, Hakama et al. 2008). In 1988, the United Kingdom was one of the first countries in the world to set up a national breast screening program. QA has been fundamental to the UK National Health Service Breast Screening Programme (NHSBSP) and is one of its greatest strengths. A national QA network is organized on a regional basis, and reference centers collate

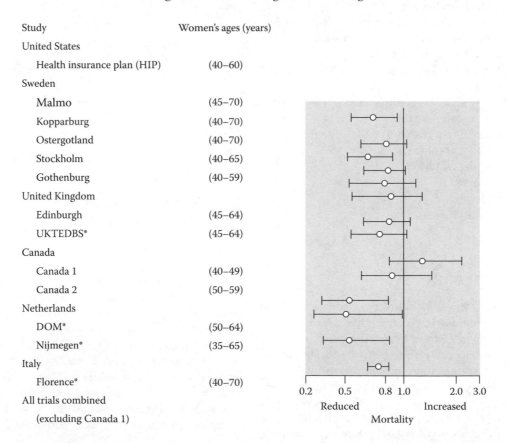

Figure 23.1 Summary of 7–12 years' mortality data from randomized and case–control (*) studies of breast cancer screening. Points and lines represent absolute change in mortality and confidence interval.

performance and outcome data from each screening unit within the region. In addition, three yearly QA inspection visits to each individual unit ensure that professional competence is maintained (Sinnatamby and Britton 2007). Guidelines for good practice, national standards, and targets for all aspects of breast screening, including both staff and equipment, are published by the NHSBSP (NHS Breast Screening Programme, accessed April 12, 2011, http://cancerscreening.nhs.uk/breastscreen). Evidence from commissioned research by the NHSBSP led to improvements in the program, for example, double reading (Blanks et al. 1998) and the implementation of two-view mammography (Wald et al. 1995), and the program continues to evolve in light of ongoing research.

In 2002, a Working Group of the International Agency for Cancer Research (IARC), consisting of 24 experts from 11 countries, concluded that the results of breast screening trials provided sufficient evidence for the efficacy of mammography screening in reducing breast cancer mortality in women 50 and 69 years but only limited evidence of a reduction in mortality for women aged 40–49 years (Armstrong et al. 2007, Larsson et al. 1997). The group also recognized that the effectiveness of national screening programs would vary according to a number of factors including differences in coverage and compliance, technical quality of the mammograms, methods of assessment, and treatment. They concluded that organized programs were more likely to be effective in reducing mortality rates than was the sporadic screening of selected groups of women (IARC 2002). In 2003, the Council of the European Union (EU) adopted recommendations inviting all member states to introduce structured population-based screening programs, and the European Commission produced guidelines to help with the introduction of screening and QA.

According to the EU guidelines (Jons 2006, Perry et al. 2006), mammography screening should involve

- Population-based invitation to all women aged between 50 and 69 every 2 years to have a voluntary breast X-ray paid for by their health insurer
- Blinded double reading of the mammograms with confirmation by a third radiologist if required
- Further diagnostic tests (ultrasound, biopsy, and MRI) to investigate any findings
- Breast specialist radiologists, radiographers (technicians), and pathologists with radiologists required to read at least 5000 mammograms per year
- Strict standards and regular checks on equipment and image quality by independent reference centers

Breast cancer screening (in some form) now exists in 26 of the 27 EU states. Most countries have organized national or regional screening programs, and population register–based invitations ensure that the target population and

entire range of socioeconomic groups are invited at regular intervals with a recommended participation rate of >70% (Perry et al. 2006) (Table 23.1). Most European countries with organized screening report participation rates of >60% of the target population (Anttila et al. 2002, European Cancer Observatory 2011, Holland et al. 2007, Sinnatamby and Britton 2007).

TABLE 23.1   ORGANIZATION OF BREAST SCREENING PROGRAMS IN EUROPE (2007–2008)

Country	Program Type[a]	Year Program Started	Age Range	Recommended Screening Interval for Average-Risk Women	
				Age 40–49	Age 50+
Belgium	NS	2001	50–69	NA	2 years
Czech Republic	N	2002	45–69	2 years	2 years
Denmark	S	1991	50–69	NA	2 years
Finland	N	1986	50–69	NA	2 years
France	N	2003	50–74	NA	2 years
Germany	NS	2005	50–69	NA	2 years
Hungary	N	2002	45–64	2 years	2 years
Iceland	N	1987	40–69[b]	2 years	2 years
Ireland	N	2000	50–64	2 years	2 years
Israel	N	1997	50–74	NA	2 years
Italy	NS	2002	50–69	NA	2 years
Luxembourg	N	1992	50–69	NA	2 years
The Netherlands	N	1989	50–74	NA	2 years
Norway	N	1996	50–69	NA	2 years
Portugal	S	1990	45–69	2 years	2 years
Spain	S	1990	45–69	2 years	2 years
Switzerland	S	1999	50–69	NA	2 years
Turkey	NS	1999	50–69	NA	2 years
United Kingdom	N	1988	50–70	NA	3 years

Sources: Based on data from the International Cancer Screening Network (http://appliedresearch.cancer.gov/icsn/breast/screening.html); Dowling et al., *J. Med. Screen.*, 17, 139, 2010.

NS, National screening policy with state/provincial/regional screening program implementation; S, State/provincial/regional screening and program implementation.

[a] Program types: N, National screening policy with national program implementation.

[b] Women 70+ are not targeted but are eligible to attend.

23.1.2.1 Age Range

As shown in Table 23.1, the age range invited to screening and the screening interval vary across the EU states (European Cancer Observatory 2011), but in general, women aged 50–69 are sent direct mail invitations to attend screening every 2 years or every 3 years in the United Kingdom. In the United Kingdom, screening of women aged 47–73 is currently being phased in, and the National Institute for Health and Clinical Excellence (NICE) has published guidance recommending that women aged 40–49 who have a family history of breast cancer are offered annual mammographic screening (NICE 2010). Screening of younger women (40–49 years) is not common practice in other parts of Europe. In the United States, annual screening mammography was recommended from age 40 and for high-risk women from age 30 years (Lee et al. 2010). However, the United States Preventive Services Task Force (USPSTF) guidelines recently created widespread controversy recently by changing their previous recommendations and delaying the initial screening of asymptomatic women from age 40 to 50 and recommending biennial rather than annual breast cancer screening (Hirsch and Lyman 2011, USPSTF 2009).

23.1.2.2 Screening Mammography

Mammography is performed using either screen film or digital mammography systems with most programs now in the process of converting to digital technology (Dowling et al. 2010). The overall diagnostic accuracy of digital and film mammography is similar (Sala et al. 2009, 2011, Skaane 2009, Vinnicombe et al. 2009) although digital mammography is more accurate in women under 50 years of age and in women with radiographically dense breasts (Pisano et al. 2008, Skaane 2009).

23.1.2.3 Number of Mammographic Views

When screening programs were first established, it was routine practice to obtain only one (mediolateral oblique [MLO]) view of each breast. However, the results of a randomized controlled trial in the United Kingdom showed a 24% increase in cancer detection rates for two-view mammography (MLO and craniocaudal [CC] views) at the first (prevalent) screen (Wald et al. 1995). Two-view mammography for the prevalent screen was introduced as mandatory policy in 1995 and subsequently extended to all screens in the United Kingdom (Given-Wilson and Blanks 1999, Patnick 2004). Most European countries are now using two-view mammography for all screens (Table 23.2).

23.1.2.4 Reading Policy

Double reading compared with single reading of mammograms has been shown to increase the cancer detection rate by between 4% and 14% (Antinnen et al. 1993, Ciatto et al. 2005, Helvie 2007) although this obviously increases the workload for readers. Double reading of mammograms can be performed in several ways. The second reader may be blinded to the first interpretation (blinded double reading) or not (independent or nonblinded double reading). Screening programs also apply different methods for resolving reader disagreements. A woman may be recalled if only one reader considers the mammogram abnormal without discussion with the other reader; mammograms may be interpreted by consensus reading, in which recall occurs only with the agreement of the two readers involved; or reader disagreement may be decided by arbitration by another reader or readers. The use of arbitration or consensus reading has been shown to increase the detection of small invasive cancers (Blanks et al. 1998). Although double reading of mammograms has not been widely adopted in the United States (Yankaskas et al. 2004), it is standard practice in most European countries and a few use a third reader to resolve discordant cases (Table 23.3).

23.1.2.5 Film Readers

In the United Kingdom, in order to reduce the increasing workload of radiologists, the NHSBSP now employs a mix of film readers, all of whom have specialist training in screening mammography. Some are consultant radiologists, and others are radiographers (technicians) specializing in mammography who have trained as screen readers. In the NHSBSP, there are now approximately equal numbers of radiographers and radiologists involved in mammography reading (Sarah Sellars email message to author April 4, 2011).

PERFORMS™ (PERsonal perFORMance in Mammographic Screening) is a voluntary self-assessment test sent out to readers in the NHSBSP to improve their breast cancer detection skills (Gale 2003, Scott and Gale 2006). Each year, a set of new cases of early and difficult signs of mammographic abnormalities are collated from screening centers and circulated to readers. A reader reviews the cases and records their decisions. Readers are given confidential feedback and information on how their performance compares with their peers. No significant difference in performance has been reported between radiologist and nonradiologist readers (Pauli et al. 1996, Scott et al. 2004, Taylor et al. 2005, Van den Biggelaar et al. 2010, Wivell et al. 2003).

23.1.3 Current Review of Effectiveness of Screening

There are several performance indicators (primarily uptake and compliance rates, numbers of screen detected and interval cancers, stage of disease, and breast cancer mortality) that can be used to measure the effectiveness of a screening program. In Europe, population-based mammography screening programs are monitored according to

TABLE 23.2 POLICIES ON NUMBER OF VIEWS AND READING PROTOCOL IN BREAST SCREENING PROGRAMS IN EUROPE (2007–2008)

Country	Number of Views Initial Screen	Subsequent Screens	Double Reading (% Double Read) Initial Screen	Subsequent Screens	Resolution of Discordant Cases
Belgium	2	2	Yes (100%)	Yes (100%)	Third expert
Czech Republic	2	2	No (76%)	No (80%)	Second reader responsible for decision
Denmark	2	1	Yes (100%)	Yes (100%)	Discussion between readers
Finland	2	2	Yes (100%)	Yes (100%)	Discussion between readers
France	2	2	Yes (90%)	Yes (95%)	Discussion between readers
Germany	2	2	Yes (100%)	Yes (100%)	Review by consensus panel or committee
Hungary	2	2	Yes (100%)	Yes (100%)	Discussion between readers
Iceland	2	2	Yes (85%)	Yes (85%)	Woman always recalled
Ireland	2	2	Yes (100%)	Yes (100%)	Discussion between readers
Israel	2	2	No (2%)	No (5%)	
Italy	2	1	Yes	Yes	Third expert
Luxembourg	2	2	Yes (100%)	Yes (100%)	Discussion between readers
The Netherlands	2	1	Yes (100%)	Yes (100%)	Discussion between readers
Norway	2	2	Yes (100%)	Yes (100%)	Other: varies
Portugal	2	2	Yes (100%)	Yes (100%)	Third expert
Spain	2	2	No	No	Other
Switzerland	2	2	Yes (100%)	Yes (100%)	Third expert
Turkey	2	2	Yes	No	Woman always recalled
United Kingdom	2	2	No (99%)	No (99%)	Woman always recalled; discussion between readers, third expert

QA standards and guidelines for all aspects of the screening process. This embraces the screening examination, training and accreditation of healthcare professionals, diagnostic procedures for abnormal results, data collection, notification of results, and evaluation of screening outcome. Much of the success of organized screening programs has been achieved via the use of local and national monitoring of set targets and performance indicators (Klabunde and Ballard-Barbash 2007, Perry et al. 2006). However, individual performance is difficult to monitor since readers will encounter only 30–40 cancer cases in reading 5000 cases per year.

23.1.4 Controversies Surrounding Screening

Evaluation of the reduction in mortality from population-based screening programs is complicated by a number of confounding factors, for example, the time since the screening program was implemented, age range of the screened population, the stage of preexisting disease, and the effect of improved management on patient outcome and survival. Several studies have reported that less than half of the reduction in breast cancer mortality over time can be directly attributed to early detection via screening, and the true contribution of screening on breast cancer mortality remains a topic of great debate due to the methodological variations in how this should be calculated (Berry et al. 2005, Blanks et al. 2000, Kalager et al. 2010).

A related topic that attracts considerable interest and controversy is the issue of overdiagnosis (Puliti and Paci 2009). Improvements in imaging technology have increased the probability of detecting smaller and lower-grade tumors. Overdiagnosis of these slow-growing cancers that in the absence of screening, which might never present clinically during a woman's natural lifetime, can result in patient anxiety and stress and additional healthcare costs due to unnecessary tests and treatment. Estimates of overdiagnosis range from less than 10% of screen-detected cancers to up to 50% (Duffy et al. 2010). One group of Danish researchers that conducted systematic reviews of breast

TABLE 23.3   SUMMARY OF STUDIES COMPARING SINGLE READING AND DOUBLE READING

Study	Year	Form of Double Reading	Sample Size	Screening Age Range	Country	Number of Readers	Reader's Experience (Years)	Study Duration (Months)	Proportional Impact of Double Reading on CDR	Proportional Impact of Double Reading on Recall Rate
Renaud[22]	1991	Arbitration	17,228	50–65	France			12	0.31	−0.19
Pauli[20]	1996	Arbitration	17,202	50–64	United Kingdom				0.06	0.14
Tonita[21]	1999	Arbitration	27,863	50–69	Canada	8		14	0.06	−0.03
Liston[23]	2003	Arbitration	177,167	50–64	United Kingdom	5		84	0.08	0.06
Duijm[19]	2004	Arbitration	65,779	59	Netherlands	8	31 months	30	0.04	−0.07
Anttinen[16]	1993	Consensus	15,457	50–59	Finland	4		15	0.03	−0.34
Williams[17]	1995	Consensus	5,659	50–64	New Zealand	2		18	0.04	−0.06
Brown[18]	1996	Consensus	33,734	50–64	United Kingdom	6		41	0.13	−0.39
Leivo[24]	1999	Mixed	95,423	50–59	Finland			60	0.11	0.32
Ciatto[25]	2005	Mixed	17,7631	50–69	Italy	11		66	0.04	0.19
Anderson[29]	1994	Unilateral	31,146	50–64	United Kingdom	3	3, 14	16	0.06	0.25
Ciatto[26]	1995	Unilateral	18,817	50–69	Italy				0.04	0.14
Seradour[30]	1997	Unilateral	95,967	50–69	France	126		24	0.18	0.25
Deans[28]	1998	Unilateral	257,212	50–64	United Kingdom	18		48	0.13	0.38
Harvey[27]	2003	Unilateral	25,369	>40	United States	7	3, 18	18	0.07	0.08
Georgian-Smith[14]	2007	Unilateral	6,381	Unknown	United States	8	3, 26	22	0.15	0.18
Gromet[15]	2008	Mixed	112,413	54	United States	9	15	48	0.08	0.07

Source: Taylor and Potts, *Eur. J. Cancer*, 44, 798, 2008.

The proportional impact on CDR is $(CDR_{double\ reading} - CDR_{control})/CDR_{control}$. The proportional impact on recall rate is $(RR_{double\ reading} - RR_{control})/RR_{control}$.

screening trials and screening program data questioned the effectiveness of breast screening (Gotzsche and Nielsen 2011, Jorgensen and Gotzsche 2009). They reported evidence of overdiagnosis rates of up to 30% and suggested that screening resulted in no reduction in overall mortality in women and might do more harm than good. The accuracy of their conclusions has been challenged by other researchers (Biesheuvel et al. 2007, Duffy et al. 2010, Puliti and Paci 2009) who argue that most published estimates of overdiagnosis contain multiple sources of bias. The least biased overdetection estimates ranging from −4% to 7.1% for women aged 40–49 years, 1.7% to 54% for women aged 50–59 years, and 7% to 21% for women aged 60–69 years (Biesheuvel et al. 2007).

A screening program will always result in some participants testing positive, although they turn out to be disease-free after further assessment. These false positives constitute one of the inevitable negative side effects of screening. In screening, it is important to find an acceptable balance between sensitivity and specificity. Recall rates must trade off the need to find small cancers with the anxiety caused by recall for potentially unnecessary additional diagnostic procedures. In most European screening programs, between 2% and 5% of screened women are recalled to undergo additional tests before they can be cleared of the suspicion of breast cancer. Further assessment can include additional diagnostic imaging (mammography, ultrasonography, MRI) and invasive procedures (fine-needle aspiration cytology, core-needle biopsy, or open biopsy). European guidelines recommend a target recall rate for further assessment of <5% with an acceptable rate of less than 7% for first screening round and a target recall rate of <3% with an acceptable rate of <5% for subsequent screening rounds (Perry et al. 2006). This contrasts with the United States, where recall rates are approximately twofold higher (Elmore 2003, Schell et al. 2007, Smith-Bindman et al. 2005). In addition to incurring additional healthcare costs, these recalls provoke anxiety and may affect their subsequent attendance at screening attendance (Armstrong et al. 2007, Brewer et al. 2007, Lampic et al. 2001, McCann et al. 2002). Elmore et al. (1998) estimated that, after 10 annual screening mammograms, nearly 24% of U.S. women had had at least one false-positive result with a cumulative risk of approximately 50%, compared with a cumulative risk of 20%–30% in Europe (Castells et al. 2006, Hofvind et al. 2004). These differences are largely attributable to organizational differences in screening practice. In addition, the higher rate of false-positive findings and recommendations for repeat imaging and biopsies in the United States is reflective of its more litigious environment (Elmore et al. 2005).

Along with overdiagnosis and overtreatment, the false-positive mammogram has fuelled the debate over the risks and benefits of breast screening. The difficulty is achieving balanced, evidence-based recommendations for healthcare providers and providing understandable information so that women can make an informed decision on participation (Castells et al. 2006).

23.2 CADe IN SCREENING MAMMOGRAPHY

In a breast screening program, film readers are required to read large volumes of mammograms to detect a relatively small number of cancers (<1.0%). This is a challenging task involving a complex interaction of the reader's visual, perceptual, and cognitive processes and is prone to reader fatigue or distraction (Huynh et al. 1998).

There is also wide variation in the performance level of readers (Anderson et al. 1994, Elmore et al. 1994). Even with experienced readers and a double reading protocol, some cancers are missed at screening due to oversight, and others are dismissed as not requiring any action by the reader (Nodine et al. 1996, 2001). However, retrospective evaluation of these interval cancer cases (cancers diagnosed in the interval between screening rounds) suggests that 16%–27% of cases show evidence of an abnormality on the previous screening mammogram (Astley 2004, Duncan et al. 1998, Saarenmaa et al. 2001, Taylor 2002, Warren Burhenne et al. 2000) with at least 40% of cases having been wrongly dismissed (Bird et al. 1992, Blanks et al. 1999).

CADe systems have been developed to assist mammography film readers by attracting attention to regions with potentially suspicious features. The reader must then decide if the case warrants further assessment. It has been reported that CADe correctly marked 42%–77% of regions prospectively overlooked or dismissed by radiologists that subsequently developed into cancers (Birdwell et al. 2001, Brem et al. 2005, Cho et al. 2010, Ikeda et al. 2004, Warren Burhenne et al. 2000). This potential of CADe systems to reduce observational oversight or misclassification errors raised the possibility that a single reader could match the performance achieved by double reading by using CADe as the second reader. If this was achievable, it could improve the performance of screening centers undertaking single reading and provide an alternative work practice to reduce the workload in screening programs using double reading. There are also reports that CADe increases the detection of small (<1 cm) or early stage lesions (Brem et al. 2005, Cupples et al. 2005, Dean and Ilvento 2006, Freer and Ullisey 2001, Morton et al. 2006, Sadaf et al. 2011, The et al. 2009), which is a key element of earlier treatment and improved survival.

23.2.1   CADe and Reader Type

It has been reported that CADe may have a greater impact on the performance of less experienced readers (Astley et al. 2006, Balleyguier et al. 2005, Van den Biggelaar 2010).

23.2.2   Training

The introduction of CADe into a clinical setting involves a learning curve. A period of reader training is essential for readers to understand how CADe systems perform and gain confidence in integrating the information provided by CADe with their knowledge and experience of mammographic interpretation. In particular, readers need to gain confidence in readily dismissing false prompts (Dean and Ilvento 2006, Ko et al. 2006, Krupinski 2004) but retain their sensitivity in recalling cases where there are visible lesions that have not been marked by CADe (Houssami and Given-Wilson 2007).

One of the options initially suggested for using CADe in screening mammography was as a preselection tool to reduce the number of cases for the human reader to review. Although the sensitivity of the CADe algorithms is very high (~98%), there is poor specificity. In the screening setting, where the majority of cases are normal, most of the CADe marks are "false prompts" requiring virtually all cases to be reviewed by the human reader, leading to increased reading time and workload. In addition, since CADe algorithms have not reached 100%, some malignant cases with no CADe marks would bypass review by a human reader, and cancers would be missed (Lederman et al. 2010). Therefore, based on current CADe algorithm sensitivity and specificity, preselection of cases for human review would not be a feasible option.

23.2.3   CADe Trials in Screening Setting

There has been much debate in the literature regarding the efficacy of CADe in clinical practice. Early published studies comparing single reading and single reading with CADe reported increases in cancer detection rate of up to 19% but increases in recall rate from 6% to 35% (Table 23.4), which would limit its overall effectiveness due to the increased healthcare costs incurred for additional follow-up assessment in addition to the adverse psychological impact. To evaluate the potential contribution of CADe to screening mammography in the European setting requires comparison of single reading with CADe and the recommended practice of double reading.

Bennett et al. reviewed eight European studies that compare single reading with CADe and double reading (Bennett et al. 2006). The main characteristics of the study designs and results are summarized in Table 23.5. Many of the studies used small test sets containing a high proportion of cancer cases that would be unrepresentative of the case mix encountered in screening where only a small number of cancer cases are encountered. In addition, the studies were conducted with a limited number of readers with variable training in the use of CADe (Malich et al. 2006). Therefore, methodological differences limit the validity of much of the published study data in relation to the use of single reading with CADe in the real-life setting of a screening program (Philpotts 2009).

Taylor and Potts used pooled estimates of effect sizes from two meta-analyses (one covering 10 U.S. studies of single reading and single reading with CADe and a second covering 17 studies of single reading and double reading) (3 from the United States) (Taylor and Potts 2008). Double reading significantly improved the cancer detection rate by 10%, and

TABLE 23.4   EVIDENCE ON INCREMENTAL CANCER DETECTION AND RECALL FROM COMBINING CADe WITH A SINGLE READER

Study	Year	Incremental Cancer Detection with CADe (%)	Incremental Recall with CADe (Recall Rate %)
Florence (CSPO) studies[14,15]	2003	85/617 (+13.7%)	245/703 (+35.5%)
Freer and Ulissey[16]	2001	8/41 (+19.5%)	34/344 (+9.8%)
Helvie et al.[17]	2004	1/10 (+10.0%)	57/487 (+11.7%)
Gur et al.[18]	2004	4/206 (+1.9%)	214/1163 (+18.4%)
Khoo et al.[19]	2005	2/61 (+1.3%)	18/372 (+5.8%)
Birdwell et al.[20]	2005	2/27 (+7.4%)	73/887 (+8.2%)
Cupples et al.[21]	2005	17/101 (+16.8%)	164/2100 (+7.8%)
Ko et al.[22]	2006	2/45 (+4.4%)	100/602 (+16.6%)
Morton et al.[23]	2006	8/105 (+ 7.6%)	191/1996 (+9.5%)
Dean et al.[24]	2006	10/104 (+9.6%)	152/590 (+25.7%)

Source: Houssami et al., *J. Med. Imag. Rad. Oncol.*, 53, 171, 2009.

TABLE 23.5   MAIN CHARACTERISTICS OF STUDIES COMPARING SINGLE READING WITH CAD WITH DOUBLE READING

| Paper (First Author) | Year | Test Set | | CAD System | Location |
		Selection of Films/Test Set	Number of Film Sets (% of Cancers) (Type)		
Ciatto[5]	2003	As used in national proficiency test	150 (11) (screen detected)	CADx	Italy
Ciatto[6]	2003	Negate mammograms seeded with the prior negate screening mammograms of interval cancers	120 (26) (interval cancers)	CADx	Italy
Ciatto[7]	2003	As used in a national proficiency test	140 (23) (screen detected)	R2 ImageChecker	Italy
Ciatto[8]	2004	Negate mammograms seeded with the prior negative screening mammograms of interval cancers	120 (26) (interval cancers)	CADx R2 ImageChecker	Italy
Taylor[10]	2004	Within unit: cases where cancer had been missed by at least one reader in the past	120 (37) (screen detected)	R2 ImageChecker (version 2.2)	United Kingdom
Karssemeijer[12]	2003	Nationally—all breast cancers randomly; 125 screen detected and 125 interval cancers plus 250 normal (all with two prev. mammos)	500 (50) (50% interval cancers 5Cft screen detected)	R2 ImageChecker (version 2.0)	Netherlands
Khoo[9]	2005	Within unit: all mammograms taken between March 21, 2003, and January 9, 2005	61,111 (62) (screen detected)	R2 ImageChecker (version 5.0)	United Kingdom
Gilbert[11]	2006	Random sample of films double read in 1996	10,267 (236) (screen detected and interval cancers)	R2 ImageChecker (version 5.0)	United Kingdom

(Continued)

TABLE 23.5 (Continued)   MAIN CHARACTERISTICS OF STUDIES COMPARING SINGLE READING WITH CAD WITH DOUBLE READING

One Reader + CAD	Reading Type		Sensitivity (%)			Specificity		Overall Conclusion
	Double Reading	Single Reading	One Reader + CAD	Double Reading	Single Reading	One Reader + CAD	Double Reading	
Observed	Simulated—recall if one suggests	92.7[a]	97.0	96.0	93.6	89.3	89.4	No statistically significant difference in sensitivity or specificity.
Observed	Simulated—recall if one suggests	32.2	42.1	46.1	33.1	76.1	73.9	No statistically significant difference in sensitivity. Borderline evidence to suggest single reading with CAD is more specific than double reading.
Observed	Simulated—recall if one suggests	85.4	90.6	92.9	83.4	76.5	73.9	No statistically significant difference in sensitivity or specificity.
Observed	Simulated—recall if one suggests	58.6	CAD 70.9 / R2 70.9	79.7	81.9	CAD 70.3 / R2 75.7	71.4	Moderate evidence to suggest double reading is more sensitive than single reading with CAD. No statistically significant difference in specificity.
Observed	Simulated—recall based on decision of third random reader	77.0	80.0	81.0	85.0	86.0	88.0	No statistically significant difference in sensitivity or specificity.
Simulated	Simulated	39.4	Step 42.6 / Linear 46.4	49.9	NK	NK	NK	Strong evidence to suggest that double reading is more sensitive than single reading with CAD (at a false-positive fraction of less than 10%).
Observed	Observed	90.2	91.5	98.4	NA	NA	NA	No statistically significant difference in sensitivity.
Observed	Observed		49.1	42.6		92.3	94.3	Evidence to suggest single reading with CAD is more sensitive than double reading and double reading is more specific than single reading with CAD.

Source: Bennett et al., *Clin. Radiol.*, 61, 1023, 2006.
[a] Calculated for four "expert" radiologists to allow comparability.

TABLE 23.6   META-ANALYSES OF STUDIES COMPARING SINGLE READING WITH (A) DOUBLE READING, (B) DOUBLE READING WITH ARBITRATION, AND (C) SINGLE READING WITH CADe

	Impact on Cancer Detection Rates	Impact on Recall Rates
Double reading	1.10 (1.06–1.14)	1.17 (1.15–1.18)
Double reading with arbitration	1.08 (1.02–1.15)	0.94 (0.92–0.96)
Single reading with CADe	1.04 (0.96–1.13) NS	1.10 (1.09–1.12)

Source: Taylor et al., NHSBSP Equipment Report 0910, 2009.
Results are given as odds ratios with 95% confidence intervals in brackets. An odds ratio of less than 1 indicates that the intervention decreases rates and greater than 1 indicates that the intervention increases rates. A confidence interval that crosses 1 indicates a nonsignificant effect.

double reading using arbitration/consensus for discordant cases increased the cancer detection rate by 8%. Single reading with CADe produced a nonsignificant increase in cancer detection rate of 4%. The effect of reading regimen on recall rate was more complex to analyze since differing recall protocols were employed. For double reading with arbitration, there was a significant reduction in recall rate of 6%, but single reading with CADe significantly increased the recall rate by 10% (Table 23.6). These data suggest that a protocol of double reading with arbitration is superior to single reading with CADe. However, the authors noted that most of the studies included in their meta-analysis were conducted in the United States, where recall rates are almost double those in Europe, although cancer detection rates are similar (Smith-Bindman et al. 2005). Intrinsic differences in the organization and QA implementation that exists in the United Kingdom and other European screening programs (NHS Breast Screening Programme 2005, Perry et al. 2006, Smith-Bindman et al. 2005) compared with the United States make it difficult to judge to what extent single reading with CADe would compare to that of double reading. Furthermore, reviews and meta-analyses of CADe studies have highlighted the limitations of generalizing the applicability of research results to the real-world clinical environment. Reader behavior may differ between "laboratory" studies and prospective studies in a screening setting (Gur et al. 2008, Samulski et al. 2010) since readers may be more (or less) vigilant or alter their decision threshold (Gilbert et al. 2008b, Taylor et al. 2004 a,b). More robust evidence from large-scale prospective randomized trials is required to evaluate the true clinical utility of CADe in the context of a screening program where <1% of cases are true cancer cases. One large U.K. multicenter prospective trial involving 28,723 screening mammograms reported no significant difference in cancer detection rate between single reading with CADe (7.02 per 1000) and double reading (7.06 per 1000), but the recall rate for single reading with CADe (3.9%) was 0.5% higher than that for double reading (3.4%) equivalent to a relative difference of 15% (Gilbert et al. 2008a). These data compare favorably with the pooled estimates predicted by Taylor and Potts (2008). Interestingly,

in the trial, there were 57 discordant recall decisions (29 cases recalled by double reading but not single reading with CADe and 28 cases recalled by the single reader with CADe but not by double reading). This confirms the findings of other published studies that readers are not misled by the absence of a correctly placed CADe mark (Alberdi et al. 2005, Gilbert et al. 2008b, Taylor et al. 2005).

One potential disadvantage of increased cancer detection by CADe relates to tumor biology (Noble et al. 2009, Warren and Eleti 2006). Fenton et al. reported that CADe was associated with an increased detection of ductal carcinoma in situ (DCIS) compared with invasive cancers (Fenton et al. 2007). DCIS represents a spectrum of disease ranging from high-grade disease that can rapidly progress to life-threatening invasive disease to low-grade disease with a long clinical progression to invasive disease (Sanders et al. 2005). Therefore, if CADe increases the proportion of cases diagnosed as DCIS, this could exacerbate the overdiagnosis and overtreatment controversy, challenging screening programs in recent years.

23.2.4   Implementation of CADe

In the United States, despite continued debate over its efficacy, the CADe use in screening mammography almost doubled over the period of 2004–2008, and by 2008, CADe was used in 74% of cases. It has been suggested that this is partly due to the introduction of financial reimbursement for mammograms read with CADe (Rao et al. 2010). However, there is little evidence of any significant use of CADe in European population-based screening programs. This has been attributed to the greater use of double reading and the fact that there is no reimbursement for the use of CADe (Skaane 2009),

23.2.4.1   CADe and Digital Mammography

Several studies have evaluated the performance of CADe in full-field digital mammography (Baum et al. 2002, Brancato et al. 2007, Kim et al. 2006, 2008, Sadaf et al. 2011, Skaane et al. 2007, The et al. 2009, Van den Biggelaar et al. 2010, Yang et al. 2007) with reported sensitivities varying from 78% (Van den Biggelaar et al. 2010) to 96% (Kim et al. 2008).

In centers using film-based mammography, the use of CADe technology is likely to impact on workflow since extra time is required to digitize films prior to CADe algorithm analysis. However, as more centers adopt digital mammography, this will facilitate the clinical utility of CADe. CADe prompts can be viewed directly on the digitally acquired images displayed on a workstation. In addition, using CADe in conjunction with digital mammography systems will allow a temporal comparison of CADe marks on mammograms from a previous screening round with the current screen.

23.2.4.2 Workflow Issues

The practicalities of implementing CADe in a screening program pose other workflow challenges that need to be addressed.

There are now several commercial CADe systems available, but very few studies have conducted a comparison of algorithms on the same case set (Chersevani et al. 2010, Leon et al. 2009).

23.3 BARRIERS TO IMPLEMENTATION

23.3.1 Algorithms

The success of CADe in a screening program depends on high sensitivity, relatively high specificity, and the reader taking appropriate action to CADe markers (Astley 2004, D'Orsi 2001, Zheng et al. 2004). A CADe system with a high false-marker rate is likely to result in reader fatigue and reduced performance and would be unacceptable in a screening program. The selected operating points of the CADe algorithms that determine the threshold for the display of CADe marks must be optimized to balance sensitivity and specificity of detection for both masses and microcalcifications. Current versions of the CADe algorithms operate at a level of one or two false-positive marks per four-view case equating to a few hundred false-positive marks for every true-positive cancer in a screening setting.

In addition to improvements in algorithm performance, a better understanding of the human reader–CADe interaction is required to establish the optimal method of using CADe information to enhance the reader's perception and assessment of an abnormality (Birdwell 2009, Krupinski 2004, Krupinski et al. 2005, Samulski et al. 2010). In clinical practice, the human reader interprets mammograms by combining the information from both (MLO and CC) views of each breast, checking for differences between the two breasts that may indicate a developing lesion and looking for any changes between the current and any previous mammograms.

To improve the accuracy of CADe marking, some research groups are investigating whether the correspondence of CADe marks on areas on two different mammographic views may be more indicative of regions that merit further attention (Cho et al. 2010, Paquerault et al. 2002, Sahiner et al. 2006, van Engeland and Karssemeijer 2007, Wei et al. 2011). In addition, comparison of CADe marked regions on current and prior mammograms could show temporal changes that may indicate lesion development.

23.3.2 Legal Issues

Since misread mammograms are a leading cause of claims against radiologists, often resulting in the highest monetary payouts, there are legal concerns about the role of CADe in breast imaging (Greenberg 2006). This is more of a problem in the United States, where radiologists are faced with a strong incentive to increase sensitivity at the expense of specificity. In contrast, a 10-year review at a Netherlands breast cancer screening program discovered only three medicolegal cases stemming from screening mammography (http://www.auntminnieeurope.com/index.aspx?sec=sup&sub=wom&pag=dis&itemId=604901, accessed April 12, 2011). The impact on CADe on malpractice litigation is uncertain since CADe could potentially be used for or against the reader. The late diagnosis of a cancer, correctly marked by CADe but dismissed by a reader as nonactionable, could be used as evidence of a breach of standard care, despite recognition of the low reliability of CADe marking. In the only appellate court case to date, the absence of CADe marking on a subtle lesion on a mammogram was viewed as reliable supportive evidence that a cancer had not been overlooked (Brenner et al. 2006). In relation to this, if CADe-marked mammograms are to be archived for legal purposes or for temporal comparison with a mammogram from the next screening round, both the unprocessed and processed image files need to be stored since the CADe software analyzes the unprocessed digital images. This means that CADe systems purchased for use with an image archiving system and review workstations from different manufacturers need to comply with the DICOM standards and support Mammography CADe SR class as a Service Class Provider to permit the archiving of CADe data (Taylor et al. 2009).

23.3.3 Cost Effectiveness

The introduction of any new health technology into clinical practice requires accurate estimates of their cost effectiveness to justify whether the benefits are sufficient to justify the substantial financial investment. Very few publications have addressed this aspect of CADe (Guierrerio et al. 2011, Lindfors et al. 2006, Taylor et al. 2005, 2009, 2010). Implementing single reading with CADe across a screening program would involve capital investment in CADe equipment, staff training, and additional health-care costs arising from the higher recall rate. On the other hand, CADe could be potentially cost saving in reading time.

Since most screening programs will be moving to digital mammography in the near future, economic evaluations should be based on digital rather than film screen mammography. The cost of CADe includes the software license for a CADe workstation, the number of workstations required (which will depend on the size of the screening unit and its screening volume per annum), and a maintenance contract to cover software upgrades. If CADe was to be adopted by large-scale screening programs, it is likely that different licensing agreements and discounts may be available for bulk purchase software licenses and maintenance contracts (Taylor et al. 2009, 2010). Other costs that need to be considered are the reader type and reader training and the cost of assessment visits (staff time and any diagnostic tests). Cost savings in reading time by introducing single reading with CADe would be highest if all the cases were read by radiologist readers. However, there is an increasing trend to employ radiographers (technicians) with specialist training in screening mammography as readers (Scott and Gale 2004, Wivell et al. 2003), and Taylor et al. suggested that using radiographers as double readers would be a more cost-effective alternative to single reading with CADe (Taylor et al. 2010). In agreement with previous studies (Lindfors et al. 2006, Taylor et al. 2004, 2005), economic modeling of data from the UK CADET II study (Guerrerio et al. 2011) suggested that CADe would be cost-increasing compared with double reading in all sizes of screening units. Any savings arising from shorter reading time would be offset by the cost of reader training, the cost of CADe, and in particular the increased cost of assessment but with no significant increase in cancer detection rate (Houssami et al. 2009).

23.4 SUMMARY

CADe is intended as a complementary technology in mammography to alert the reader to review features on a mammogram that may have been overlooked. There is considerable variation in the reported level of benefit deriving from the use of CADe, and its contribution to the diagnostic process is not yet clear. Overall, CADe may produce modest increases in the cancer detection rate (sensitivity) of a single reader, but this is largely offset by an increase in the recall rate and associated healthcare costs. The implementation of digital mammography, specific reader training with CADe, refinement of CADe algorithms, and a better understanding of the human reader–CADe interaction may increase the utility of CADe in screening mammography. However, at present, in European breast screening programs, CADe would be considered less effective than the standard practice of double reading.

REFERENCES

Alberdi, E., A. A. Povyakalo, L. Strigini et al. 2005. Use of computer-aided detection (CADe) tools in screening mammography: A multidisciplinary investigation. *British Journal of Radiology* 78:S31–S40.

Anderson, E. D., B. B. Muir, J. S. Walsh, and A. E. Kirkpatrick. 1994. The efficacy of double reading mammograms in breast screening. *Clinical Radiology* 49:248–251.

Antinnen, M., M. Pamilo, M. Soiva, and M. Roiha. 1993. Double reading of mammography screening films—One radiologist or two? *Clinical Radiology* 48:414–421.

Anttila, A., J. Koskela, and M. Hakama. 2002. Programme sensitivity and effectiveness of mammography service screening in Helsinki, Finland. *Journal of Medical Screening* 9:153–158.

Armstrong, K., E. Moye, S. Williams, J. A. Berlin, and E. E. Reynolds. 2007. Screening mammography in women 40 to 49 years of age: A systematic review for the American College of Physicians. *Annals of Internal Medicine* 146:516–526.

Astley, S. M. 2004. Computer-aided detection for screening mammography. *Academic Radiology* 11:1139–1143.

Astley, S. M., S. W. Duffy, C. R. M. Boggis et al. 2006. Mammography reading with computer-aided detection (CADe): Performance of different readers. *Lecture Notes Computing Science* 4046:97–104.

Balleyguier, C., K. Kinkel, J. Fermanian et al. 2005. Computer-aided detection (CADe) in mammography: Does it help the junior or the senior radiologist? *European Journal of Radiology* 54:90–96.

Baum, F., U. Fischer, S. Obenauer, and E. Grabbe. 2002. Computer-aided detection in direct digital full-field mammography: Initial results. *European Radiology* 12:3015–3017.

Bennett, R. L., R. G. Blanks, S. M. Moss. 2006. Does the accuracy of single reading with CADe (computer-aided detection) compare with that of double reading?: A review of the literature. *Clinical Radiology* 61:1023–1028.

Berry, D. A., K. A. Cronin, S. K. Plevritis et al. 2005. Effect of screening and adjuvant therapy on mortality from breast cancer. *New England Journal of Medicine* 353:1784–1792.

Biesheuvel, C., A. Barratt, K. Howard, N. Houssami, and L. Irwig. 2007. Effects of study methods and biases on estimates of invasive breast cancer overdetection with mammography screening: A systematic review. *Lancet Oncology* 8:1129–1138.

Bird, R. E., T. W. Wallace, and B. C. Yankaskas. 1992. Analysis of cancers missed at screening mammography. *Radiology* 184:613–617.

Birdwell, R. L. The preponderance of evidence supports computer-aided detection for screening mammography. 2009. *Radiology* 253:9–161.

Birdwell, R. L., D. M. Ikeda, K. F. O'Shaughnessy, and E. A. Sickles. 2001. Mammographic characteristics of 115 missed cancers later detected with screening mammography and the potential utility of computer-aided detection. *Radiology* 219:192–202.

Blamey, R. W., A. R. Wilson, and J. Patnick. 2000. ABC of breast diseases: Screening for breast cancer. *British Medical Journal* 321:689–693.

Blanks, R. G., S. Moss, and J. Patnick. 2000. Results from the United Kingdom NHS breast screening programme 1994–1999. *Journal of Medical Screening* 7:195–198.

Blanks, R. G., M. G. Wallis, and R. M. Given-Wilson. 1999. Observer variability in cancer detection during routine repeat (incident) mammographic screening in a study of two versus one view mammography. *Journal of Medical Screening* 6:152–158.

Blanks, R. G., M. G. Wallis, and S. M. Moss. 1998. A comparison of cancer detection rates achieved by breast cancer screening programmes by number of readers, for one and two view mammography: Results from the UK National Health Service Breast Screening Programme. *Journal of Medical Screening* 5:195–201.

Brancato, B., N. Houssami, D. Francesca et al. 2007. Does computer-aided detection contribute to the performance of digital mammography in a self-referred population. *Breast Cancer Research and Treatment* 111:373–376.

Brem, R. F., J. W. Hoffmeister, G. Zisman, M. P. DeSimio, and S. K. Rogers. 2005. A computer-aided detection system for the evaluation of breast cancer by mammographic appearance and lesion size. *American Journal of Roentgenology* 184:893–896.

Brenner, R. J., M. J. Ulissey, and R. M. Wilt. 2006. Computer-aided detection as evidence in the courtroom: Potential implications of an appellate court's ruling. *American Journal of Roentgenology* 186:48–51.

Brewer, N. T., T. Salz, and S. E. Lillie. 2007. The long-term effects of false-positive mammograms. *Annals of Internal Medicine* 146:502–510.

Castells, X., E. Molins, and F. Macià. 2006. Cumulative false positive recall rate and association with participant related factors in a population based breast cancer screening programme. *Journal of Epidemiology and Community Health* 60:316–321.

Chersevani, R., S. Ciatto, and C. Faveroetal. 2010. "CADEAT": Considerations on the use of CADe (computer-aided diagnosis) in mammography. *La Radiologia Medica* 115:563–570.

Cho, N., S. J. Kim, H. Y. Choi et al. 2010. Features of prospectively overlooked computer-aided detection marks on prior screening digital mammograms in women with breast cancer. *American Journal of Roentgenology* 95:1276–1282.

Ciatto, S., D. Ambrogetti, G. Risso et al. 2005. The role of arbitration of discordant reports at double reading of screening mammograms. *Journal of Medical Screening* 12:125–127.

Cupples, T. E., J. E. Cunningham, and J. C. Reynolds. 2005. Impact of computer-aided detection in a regional screening mammography program. *American Journal of Roentgenology* 185:944–950.

Dean, J. C. and C. C. llvento. 2006. Improved cancer detection using computer-aided detection with diagnostic and screening mammography: Prospective study of 104 cancers. *Radiology* 187:20–28.

D'Orsi, C. J. 2001. Computer-aided detection: There is no free lunch. *Radiology* 221:585–586.

Dowling, E. C., C. Klabunde, J. Patnick, and R. Ballard-Barbash. 2010. Breast and cervical cancer screening programme implementation in 16 countries. *Journal of Medical Screening* 17:139–146.

Duffy, S. W., L. Tabar, A. H. Olsen et al. 2010. Absolute numbers of lives saved and overdiagnosis in breast cancer screening, from a randomized trial and from the Breast Screening Programme in England. *Journal of Medical Screening* 17:25–30.

Duncan, K. A., G. Needham, F. J. Gilbert, and H. E. Deans. 1998. Incident round cancers: What lessons can we learn? *Clinical Radiology* 53:29–32.

Elmore, J. G., C. Y. Nakano, T. D. Koepsell, L. M. Desnick, C. J. D'Orsi, and D. F. Ransohoff. 2003. International variation in screening mammography interpretations in community-based programs. *Journal of the National Cancer Institute* 95:1384–1393.

Elmore, J. G., K. Armstrong, C. D. Lehman, and S. W. Fletcher. 2005. Screening for breast cancer. *Journal of American Medical Association* 293:1245–1256.

Elmore, J. G., M. B. Barton, V. M. Moceri, S. Polk, P. J. Arena, and S. W. Fletcher. 1998. Ten-year risk of false positive screening mammograms and clinical breast examinations. *New England Journal of Medicine* 338:1089–1096.

Elmore, J. G., C. K. Wells, C. H. Lee, D. H. Howard, and A. R. Feinstein. 1994. Variability in radiologists' interpretations of mammograms. *New England Journal of Medicine* 331:1493–1499.

European Cancer Observatory accessed April 12, 2011, http://eu-cancer.iarc.fr/cancer-13-breast-screening.html,en#block-20–70.

Fenton, J. J., S. H. Taplin, P.A Carney et al. 2007. Influence of computer-aided detection on performance of screening mammography. *New England Journal of Medicine* 356:1399–1409.

Fletcher, S. W. and J. G. Elmore. 2003. Clinical practice. Mammographic screening for breast cancer. *New England Journal of Medicine* 348:1672–1680.

Freer, T. W. and M. J. Ulissey. 2001. Screening mammography with computer-aided detection: Prospective study of 12,860 patients in a community breast center. *Radiology* 220:781–786.

Gabe, R. and S. W. Duffy. 2005. Evaluation of service screening mammography in practice: The impact on breast cancer mortality. *Annals of Oncology* 16:153–162.

Gale, A. G. 2003. PERFORMS: A self assessment scheme for radiologists in breast screening. *Seminars in Breast Disease* 6:148–152.

Gilbert, F. J., S. M. Astley, M. G. C. Gillan et al. 2008a. Single reading with computer-aided detection for screening mammography. *New England Journal of Medicine* 359:1675–1684.

Gilbert, F. J., S. M. Astley, C. R. M. Boggis et al. 2008b. Variable size computer-aided detection prompts and mammography film reader decisions. *Breast Cancer Research* 10:R72.

Given-Wilson, R. M. and R. G. Blanks. 1999. Incident screening cancers detected with a second mammographic view: Pathological and radiological features. *Clinical Radiology* 54:724–735.

Gotzsche, P. C. and M. Nielsen. 2011. Screening for breast cancer with mammography. *Cochrane Database of Systematic Reviews* 6:CD001877.

Greenberg, J. S. 2006. An appellate court ruling and potential implications for CADe technology in the courtroom. *American Journal of Roentgenology* 186:52–53.

Guerriero, C., M. G. C. Gillan, J. Cairns, M. G. Wallis, and F. J. Gilbert. 2011. Is computer aided detection (CADe) cost effective in screening mammography? A model based on the CADET II study. *BMC Health Services Research* 11:11.

Gur, D., A. I. Bandos, C. S. Cohen et al. 2008. The "laboratory" effect: Comparing radiologists' performance and variability during prospective clinical and laboratory mammography interpretations. *Radiology* 249:47–53.

Hakama, M., M. P. Coleman, D. Alexe, and A. Auvinen. 2008. Cancer screening: Evidence and practice in Europe 2008. *European Journal of Cancer* 44:1404–1413.

Helvie, M. 2007. Improving mammographic interpretation: Double reading and computer-aided diagnosis. *Radiologic Clinics of North America* 45:801–811.

Hirsch, B. R. and G. H. Lyman. 2011. Breast cancer screening with mammography. *Current Oncology Reports* 13:63–70.

Hofvind, S., S. Thoresen, and S. Tretli. 2004. The cumulative risk of a false-positive recall in the Norwegian Breast Cancer Screening Program. *Cancer* 101:1501–1507.

Holland, R., H. Rijken, and J. Hendricks. 2007. The Dutch population-based mammography screening: 30-year experience. *Breast Care* 2:12–18.

Houssami, N. and R. Given-Wilson. 2007. Incorporating new technologies into clinical practice without evidence of effectiveness in prospective studies: Computer-aided detection (CADe) in breast screening reinforces the need for better initial evaluation. *Breast* 16:219–221.

Houssami, N., R. Given-Wilson, and S. Ciatto. 2009. Early detection of breast cancer: Overview of the evidence on computer-aided detection in mammography screening. *Journal of Medical Imaging & Radiation Oncology* 53:171–176.

Humphrey, L. L., M. Helfand, B. K. Chan, and S. H. Woolf. 2002. Breast cancer screening: A summary of the evidence for the U.S. Preventive Services Task Force. *Annals of Internal Medicine* 137:347–360.

Huynh, P. T., A. M. Jarolimek, and S. Daye. 1998. The false-negative mammogram. *Radiographics* 18:1137–1154.

Ikeda, D. M., R. L. Birdwell, K. F. O'Shaughnessy, E. A. Sickles, and R. J. Brenner. 2004. Computer-aided detection output on 172 subtle findings on normal mammograms previously obtained in women with breast cancer detected at follow-up screening mammography. *Radiology* 230:811–819.

International Agency for Research on Cancer. 2002. Use of breast cancer screening. In: Vainio H, Bianchini F (eds.), *Breast Cancer Screening*. IARC Handbooks of Cancer Prevention, Vol. 7. Lyon, France: International Agency for Research on Cancer.

Jons, K. 2006. Europe is showing the way. *Breast Care* 1:402–404.

Jorgensen, K. J. and P. C. Gotzsche. 2009. Overdiagnosis in publicly organised mammography screening programmes: Systematic review of incidence trends. *British Medical Journal* 339: b2587.

Kalager, M., M. Zelen, F. Langmark, and H.-O. Adami. 2010. Effect of screening mammography on breast-cancer mortality in Norway. *New England Journal of Medicine* 363:1203–1210.

Kim, S. J., Moon W. K., N. Cho, J. H. Cha, S. M. Kim, and J. G Im. 2006. Computer-aided detection in digital mammography: Comparison of craniocaudal, mediolateral oblique, and mediolateral views. *Radiology* 241:695–701.

Kim, S. J., Moon W. K., N. Cho, J. H. Cha, S. M. Kim, and J. G. Im. 2008. Computer-aided detection in full-field digital mammography: Sensitivity and reproducibility in serial examinations. *Radiology* 246:71–80.

Klabunde, C. N. and R. Ballard-Barbash. 2007. Evaluating population-based screening mammography programs internationally. *Seminars in Breast Disease* 10:102–107.

Ko, J. M., M. J. Nicholas, J. B. Mendel, and P. J. Slanetz. 2006. Prospective assessment of computer-aided detection in interpretation of screening mammography. *American Journal of Roentgenology* 187:483–1491.

Krupinski, E. A. 2004. Computer-aided detection in clinical environment: Benefits and challenges for radiologists. *Radiology* 231:7–9.

Krupinski, E. A. et al. 2005. Visual search of mammographic lesions. *Academic Radiology* 12:965–969.

Lampic, C., E. Thurfjell, J. Bergh, and P. O. Sjödén. 2001. Short- and long-term anxiety and depression in women recalled after breast cancer screening. *European Journal of Cancer* 37:463–469.

Larsson, L. G., I. Andersson, N. Bjurstam et al. 1997. Updated overview of the Swedish randomized trials on breast cancer screening with mammography: Age group 40–49 at randomization. *Journal of the National Cancer Institute Monographs* 22:57–61.

Lederman, R., I. Leichter, E. Ratner et al. 2010 Should CADe be used as a second reader? Exploring two alternative reading modes for CADe in screening mammography. In: Marti J et al. (eds.), *Digital Mammography IWDM 2010, Lecture Notes in Computer Science 6136*. Heidelberg, Germany: Springer, pp. 161-167.

Lee, C. H., D. Dershaw, D. Kopans et al. 2010. Breast cancer screening with imaging: Recommendations from the society of breast imaging and the ACR on the use of mammography, breast MRI, breast ultrasound, and other technologies for the detection of clinically occult breast cancer. *Journal of American College of Radiology* 7:18–27.

Leon, S., L. Brateman, J. Honeyman-Buck, and J. Marshall. 2009. Comparison of two commercial CADe systems for digital mammography. *Journal of Digital Imaging* 22:421–423.

Lindfors, K. K., M. C. McGahan, C. J. Rosenquist, and G. S. Hurlock. 2006. Computer-aided detection of breast cancer: A cost-effectiveness study. *Radiology* 239:710–717.

Malich, A., D.R. Fischer, and J. Bottcher. 2006. CADe for mammography; the technique, results, current role and further developments. *European Radiology* 16:1449–1460.

McCann, J., D. Stockton, and S. Godward. 2002. Impact of false-positive mammography on subsequent screening attendance and risk of cancer. *Breast Cancer Research* 4:R11.

Morton, M. M., D. H. Whaley, K. R. Brandt, and K. K. Amrami. 2006. Screening mammograms: Interpretation with computer-aided detection-prospective evaluation. *Radiology* 239: 425–437.

National Institute for Health and Clinical Excellence. CG41 Familial breast cancer: Full guideline (the new recommendations and the evidence they are based on), accessed March 30, 2010. http://guidance.nice.org.uk/cg41/guidance/pdf/English.

NHS Breast Screening Programme (NHSBSP). 2005. Quality assurance guidelines for breast cancer screening radiology. In: Liston J., Wilson R. (eds.), *Quality Assurance Guidelines for Breast Cancer Screening Radiology*, Vol. 59. Sheffield, England: NHSBSP Publication, pp. 1–26.

Noble, M., W. Bruening, S. Uhl, and K. Schoelles. 2009. Computer-aided detection mammography for breast cancer screening: Systematic review and meta analysis. *Archives of Gynecology and Obstetrics* 279:881–890.

Nodine, C. F., H. L. Kundel, S. C. Lauver, and L. C. Toto. 1996. Nature of expertise in searching mammograms for breast masses. *Academic Radiology* 6:575–585.

Nodine, C. F., C. Mello-Thoms, S. P. Weinstein et al. 2001. Blinded review of retrospectively visible unreported breast cancers: An eye-position analysis. *Radiology* 221:122–129.

Paquerault, S., N. Petrick, H. P. Chan, B. Sahiner, and M. A. Helvie. 2002. Improvement of computerized mass detection on mammograms: Fusion of two-view information. *Medical Physics* 29:238–247.

Patnick, J. 2004. NHS breast screening: The progression from one to two views. *Journal of Medical Screening* 11:55–56.

Pauli, R., S. Hammond, J. Cooke, and J. Ansell. 1996. Comparison of radiographer/radiologist double film reading with single reading in breast cancer screening. *Journal of Medical Screening* 3:18–22.

Perry, N., M. Broeder, C.de Wolf, S. Törnberg, R. Holland, L. von Karsa. 2006. *European Guidelines for Quality Assurance in Breast Cancer Screening and Diagnosis*, 4th edn. Luxembourg: Office for Official Publications of the European Communities.

Philpotts, L. E. 2009. Can computer-aided detection be detrimental to mammographic interpretation? *Radiology* 253:17–22.

Pisano, E. D., C. Gatsonis, E. Hendrick E. et al. 2008. Diagnostic accuracy of digital versus film mammography: Exploratory analysis of selected population subgroups in DMIST. *Radiology* 246:376–383.

Puliti, D. and E. Paci. 2009. The other side of technology: Risk of overdiagnosis of breast cancer with mammography screening. *Future Oncology* 5:481–491.

Rao, V. M., D. C. Levin, L. Parker, B. Cavanaugh, A. Frangos, and J. H. Sunshine. 2010. How widely is computer-aided detection used in screening and diagnostic mammography? *Journal of the American College of Radiology* 7:802–805.

Saarenmaa, I., T. Salminen, U. Geiger et al. 2001. The visibility of cancer on previous mammograms in retrospective review. *Clinical Radiology* 56:40–43.

Sadaf, A., P. Crystal, A. Scaranelo, and T. Helbich. 2011. Performance of computer-aided detection applied to full-field digital mammography in detection of breast cancers. *European Journal of Radiology* 77:457–461.

Sahiner, B., H. P. Chan, L. M. Hadjiiski et al. 2006. Joint two-view information for computerized detection of microcalcifications on mammograms. *Medical Physics* 33:2574–2585.

Sala, M., M. Comas, F. Macià, J. Martinez, M. Casamitjana, X. Castells. 2009. Implementation of digital mammography in a population-based breast cancer screening program: Effect of screening round on recall rate and cancer detection. *Radiology* 252:31–39.

Sala, M., D. Salas, F. Belvis et al. 2011. Reduction in false-positive results after introduction of digital mammography: Analysis from four population-based breast cancer screening programs in Spain. *Radiology* 258:388–395.

Samulski, M., R. Hupse, C. Boetes, R. D. M. Mus, G. J. den Heeten, and N. Karssemeijer. 2010. Using computer-aided detection in mammography as a decision support. *European Radiology* 20:2323–2330.

Sanders, M. E., P. A. Schuyler, W. D. Dupont, and D. L. Page. 2005. The natural history of low-grade ductal carcinoma in situ of the breast in women treated by biopsy only revealed over 30 years of long-term follow-up. *Cancer* 103:2481–2484.

Schell, M. J., B. C. Yankaskas, R. Ballard-Barbash et al. 2007. Evidence-based target recall rates for screening mammography. *Radiology* 243:681–689.

Scott, H. J. and A. G. Gale. 2006. Breast screening: PERFORMS identifies key mammographic training needs. *British Journal of Radiology* 79:S127–S133.

Scott, H. J., A. G. Gale, and C. E. Griffiths. 2004. Breast screening radiographers and radiologists: Performance and confidence levels on the PERFORMS film sets. *Breast Cancer Research* 6:P10.

Sinnatamby, R. and P. D. Britton. 2007. Breast screening in the UK—A national quality assured programme. *Breast Care* 2:6–10.

Skaane, P. 2009. Studies comparing screen-film mammography and full-field digital mammography in breast cancer screening: Updated review. *Acta Radiologica* 50:3–14.

Skaane, P., A. Kshirsagar, S. Stapleton, K. Young, and R. A. Castellino. 2007. Effect of computer-aided detection on independent double reading of paired screen-film and full-field digital screening mammograms. *American Journal Roentgenology* 188:377–384.

Smith-Bindman, R., R. Ballard-Barbash, D. L. Miglioretti, J. Patnick, and K. Kerlikowske. 2005. Comparing the performance of mammography screening in the USA and the UK. *Journal of Medical Screening* 12:50–54.

Taylor, P. 2002. Computer aids for detection and diagnosis in mammography. *Imaging* 14:472–477.

Taylor, P. 2010. Modelling the impact of changes in sensitivity on the outcomes of the UK breast screening programme. *Journal of Medical Screening* 17:31–36.

Taylor, P., J. Champness, R. Given-Wilson, K. Johnston, and H. Potts. 2005. Impact of computer-aided detection prompts on the sensitivity and specificity of screening mammography. *Health Technology Assessment* 9(6):1–58.

Taylor, P. M., J. Champness, R. M Given-Wilson, H. W. W. Potts, and K. Johnston. 2004a. An evaluation of the impact of computer-based prompts on screen readers' interpretation of mammograms. *British Journal of Radiology* 77:21–27.

Taylor, P., R. Given-Wilson, J. Champness, H. W. Potts, and K. Johnston. 2004b. Assessing the impact of CADe on the sensitivity and specificity of film readers. *Clinical Radiology* 59:1099–1105.

Taylor, P. and H. W. Potts. 2008. Computer aids and human second reading as interventions in screening mammography: Two systematic reviews to compare effects on cancer detection and recall rate. *European Journal of Cancer* 44:798–807.

Taylor, P., S. Wilson, H. Potts, L. Wilkinson, L. Khoo, and R. Given-Wilson. 2009. Evaluation of CADe with full field digital mammography in the NHS breast screening programme. NHSBSP Equipment Report 0910. NHS Cancer Screening Programmes, Sheffield, U.K.

Taylor, P. M., H. W. W. Potts, L. Wilkinson, and R. M. Given-Wilson. 2010. Impact of CADe with full field digital mammography on workflow and cost. In: Martí J, Oliver A, Freixenet J, and Marti R (eds.), *Proceedings 10th International Workshop on Digital Mammography*, IWDM 2010, Girona, Spain, Lecture Notes in Computer Science, Springer, 6136, pp. 1–8.

The, J. S., K. J. Schilling, J. W. Hoffmeister, E. Friedmann, R. McGinnis, and R. G. Holcomb. 2009. Detection of breast cancer with full-field digital mammography and computer-aided detection. *American Journal of Roentgenology* 192:337–340.

U.S. Preventive Services Task Force. 2009. Screening for breast cancer: U.S. preventive services task force recommendation statement. *Annals of Internal Medicine* 151:716–726.

Van Den Biggelaar, F., A. G. H. Kessels, J. M. A. van Engelshoven, C. Boetes, and K. Flobbe. 2010. Computer-aided detection in full-field digital mammography in a clinical population: Performance of radiologist and technologists. *Breast Cancer Research and Treatment*.120:499–506.

van Engeland, S. and N. Karssemeijer. 2007. Combining two mammographic projections in a computer aided mass detection method. *Medical Physics* 34:898–905.

Vinnicombe, S., S. M. Pinto Pereira, V. A. McCormack, S. Shiel, N. Perry, and I. M. dos Santos Silva. 2009. Full-field digital versus screen-film mammography: Comparison within the UK breast screening program and systematic review of published data. *Radiology* 251:347–358.

Wald, N. J., P. Murphy, P. Major, C. Parkes, J. Townsend, and C. Frost. 1995. UKCCCR multicentre randomised controlled trial of one and two view mammography in breast cancer screening. *British Medical Journal* 311:1189–1193.

Warren, R. and A. Eleti. 2006. Overdiagnosis and overtreatment of breast cancer: Is overdiagnosis an issue for radiologists? *Breast Cancer Research* 8:205.

Warren Burhenne, L. J., S. A. Wood, C. J. D'Orsi et al. 2000. Potential contribution of computer-aided detection to the sensitivity of screening mammography. *Radiology* 215:554–562.

Wei, J., H. P. Chan, C. Zhou et al. 2011. Computer-aided detection of breast masses: Four-view strategy for screening mammography. *Medical Physics* 38:1867–1876.

Wivell, G., E. R. Denton, C. B. Eve, J. C. Inglis, and J. Harvey. 2003. Can radiographers read screening mammograms? *Clinical Radiology* 58:63–67.

Yang, S., W. K. Moon, N. Cho et al. 2007. Screening mammography-detected cancers: Sensitivity of a computer-aided detection system applied to full-field digital mammograms. *Radiology* 244:104–111.

Yankaskas, B. C., C. N Klabunde, R. Ancelle-Park et al. 2004. International comparison of performance measures for screening mammography: Can it be done? *Journal of Medical Screening* 11:187–193.

Zheng, B., R. G. Swensson, S. Golla, C. M. Hakim, R. Shah, L. WallaceL, and D. Gur. 2004. Detection and classification performance levels of mammographic masses under different computer-aided detection cueing environments. *Academic Radiology* 11:398–406.

Chapter 24

Clinical Utility of CAD Systems for Lung Cancer

Matthew T. Freedman

CONTENTS

LIST OF ABBREVIATIONS

AUC	Area under the ROC curve
CADe	Computer-aided detection
CADx	Computer-aided diagnosis
CT	Computed tomography
CXR	Chest x-radiograph
FP/I	False positives per image
NCI	National Cancer Institute
NLST	National Lung Screening Trial
NSCLC	Non-small-cell lung cancer
PACS	Picture archiving and communication system
PCP	Primary care practitioners
PLCO	Prostate, Lung, Colorectal, and Ovarian Cancer Screening Trial
ROC	Receiver operating characteristic

24.1 INTRODUCTION

Medicine continues to evolve, and the important changes that are currently promoted are the result of what is called evidence-based medicine. Evidence-based medicine is based on a consensus decision based on the best available science to guide clinical care. For lung cancer computer-aided detection (CADe) and computer-aided diagnosis (CADx), there has been no such consensus decision. For CADe for lung cancer, there is evidence obtained from well-designed cohort or case control studies; these are all almost based on retrospectively assembled cases, but with reinterpretations by radiologists using the CADe programs. The studies are sufficient, but not optimal to indicate full acceptance for clinical use. The level of risk from routine clinical implementation is not yet established.

For the purposes of this chapter, a more appropriate name would be *outcome-based medicine*. Is what a physician does effective in helping the patient? In the past and continuing into the present, clinicians expected that the diagnosis of cancer and its staging was the most important contributions that lung imaging could provide. The clinical questions now evolving are who should be screened and whether finding an abnormality, and even cancer itself, benefits the patient by decreasing morbidity and mortality. This is a different task of simply identifying a cancer, but one that now should underlie the questions of the clinical utility of CADe and CADx systems for lung cancer. It questions if one should use CADe and CADx for all patients or only some; if only some, how should those be selected? It points toward approaches to the evaluation of a patient with a CADe-identified abnormality. It raises questions of the cost–benefit–injury trade-offs that exist within medicine.

There are commercial systems for CADe of lung cancer and lung nodules to aid in the interpretation of chest radiographs and lung CTs. These have been shown to have probable effectiveness in small-scale studies that used selected cases comparing the detection rates of lung cancers or lung nodules interpreted first, without and then with computer assistance. Unlike studies of mammography CADe, to date, no report of the effectiveness of these systems in more than minimal clinical use appears to have been published.

This chapter discusses the background clinical information of importance to physicians caring for people with possible lung cancer and the degree of benefit reported for several CADe systems. It discusses this from the vantage of outcome-based medicine, though recognizing that medical practice is only starting to evolve in that direction.

24.2 EPIDEMIOLOGY OF LUNG CANCER

Lung cancer is the most frequent cancer and the most frequent cause of cancer deaths in the United States and in the world. Worldwide, there are 1.1 million new cases per year in men with 0.95 million deaths and 0.51 million new cases per year in women with 0.43 million deaths (Jemal et al. 2011).

The frequency of lung cancer increases with age and with the degree of smoking history. Only a few cases are seen before age 40 (age 35–39: 3.2/100,000). The frequency increases with increasing age; for example, age 45–49: 25.3/100,000; age 60–64: 172.4/100,000; age 70–74: 371.4/100,000 (National Cancer Institute).

The frequency of lung cancer also increases with increasing smoking history. In the NCI Prostate, Lung, Colorectal and Ovarian (PLCO) Cancer Screening Trial (Hocking et al. 2010, 722–731), the incidence rates were 2.8/10,000 person years in never smokers, 12.2/10,000 person years in smokers who quit more than 15 years ago, 40.6/10,000 person years in smokers who quit less than 15 years ago, and 70.9/10,000 person years in current smokers (Hocking et al. 2010). Thus, in current smokers over age 55, one would expect there to be one individual with lung cancer for every 141 smokers studied, though not all of these are detectable.

Almost all primary lung cancer cases occur in current or former smokers. In the NCI PLCO study, 18.3% of cancers occurred in smokers who quit 15 or more years ago, 34.3% in former smokers who quit less than 15 years before, and 41.3% in current smokers. In never smokers, 6.1% occurred.

This indicates that the level of suspicion that an abnormality identified on a chest radiograph or lung CT is cancer should be much greater in current and former smokers than in never smokers. It gives an incomplete guide to who should be screened with CADe.

24.3 LUNG CANCER DETECTION

Lung cancers are not always detected. Austin (Austin et al. 1992) reported on 27 lung cancer cases that were missed by radiologists. All 27 were originally missed by a board-certified radiologist. In the study of these chest x-rays (CXRs), 18 radiologists failed to detect 27 potentially resectable bronchogenic carcinomas revealed retrospectively on serial chest radiographs. Six consultant radiologists, who were biased by knowledge that the cases were of missed bronchogenic carcinoma, were individually shown the radiographs in 22 of the cases. Each consultant missed a mean of 26% (5.8 ± 1.7) of the lesions. One of the six consultants missed the lesion in 16 (73%) of the cases. Even when the consultants knew they were reading missed lung cancer cases, many were missed.

Quekel (Quekel et al. 1999) reported the analysis of all consecutive patients with pathologically proven non-small-cell lung cancer (NSCLC) between 1992 and 1995 in a 700-bed community hospital. In a retrospective review of N = 495 patients, 396 had available x-rays and 259 had visible nodules. Forty-nine lung cancers were definitely missed. Before it was detected, the tumor changed from T1 stage to T2 in 21 of the 49 patients (43%). The authors estimated a 23% drop in 5-year survival for those patients.

Lung CT does detect neither all lung nodules nor all lung cancers. Peldschus (Peldschus et al. 2005) reported on 100 patients whose scans were initially interpreted as normal. Of that, 33 (33%) had focal lung lesions identified by a prototype CADe system. There were a total of 53 lesions of which 5 were greater than or equal to 10 mm in diameter, 21 were 5–9 mm, and 27 were 4 mm or less.

Armato (Armato et al. 2002) reports on the performance of a CADe system on lung nodules missed in a CT lung cancer screening program. The CADe program detected 32 of 38 lung cancers that had not been prospectively detected.

24.3.1 Approaches for Detecting Lung Cancer

Lung cancer can be detected using four different approaches: case finding, screening, incidental to some other medical evaluation, and surveillance of those with identified risk factors. In addition, unsuspected lung cancers can be found at autopsy.

24.3.1.1 Case Finding
Case finding occurs mainly in the evaluation of a higher-risk individual and/or in the evaluation of symptoms that could be caused by lung cancer. In these settings, the physician is concerned that lung cancer could explain the patient's symptoms or findings and orders a chest radiograph or CT to confirm or exclude that suspicion. This is likely the method by which most lung cancers are found today (Klabunde et al. 2010).

24.3.1.2 Screening
Screening is the process of looking to a disease in asymptomatic individuals who may or may not have specific risk factors for the disease of interest.

When screening is underway, cancers can be detected by the screening process or between screening exams. Those cases detected between screening exams are called interval cancers because they are detected in the interval between screenings. Interval cancers represent two groups: those that can be identified in retrospect on the screening examination and those that cannot. Since many of the interval cancers can be seen in retrospect, the use of CADe should decrease the frequency of interval cancers.

24.3.1.3 Incidental Detection
Incidental detection occurs when the patient is under evaluation for some other suspected disease process and evidence of lung cancer is identified. This is sometimes called serendipitous detection because one finds something not being searched for. An example would be the detection of a

lung cancer in someone undergoing CT angiography where the lung cancer is incidentally detected on the images (Moore et al. 2011).

24.3.1.4 Surveillance***

Surveillance is the oversight of certain groups of individuals with increased risk for lung cancer where they are regularly examined for the disease. Individuals identified with a lung nodule on a chest radiograph or CT are often then placed in surveillance, looking for growth in the nodule over time; if growth is detected, further investigation to exclude cancer is indicated. In the United States, surveillance is also used in those with occupational lung disease from, for example, exposure to asbestos, looking for progression of the underlying disease and the development of lung and pleural neoplasia. For breast cancer, those with prior chest wall radiation therapy used, for example, to treat Hodgkin disease may be placed under surveillance for the development of breast or lung cancer at a younger age.

When groups of individuals whose cancer was detected under these different approaches are compared, those detected with screening are more likely to have smaller cancers of lower stage (Hocking et al. 2010). The interval cases where the cancer cannot be identified on the screening examination are more likely to be undifferentiated and to be small-cell lung cancer, rather than NSCLC. Those detected with symptoms of lung cancer are more likely to have advanced disease, though some presenting with mild symptoms may still have stage 1 disease (Tammemagi et al. 2004).

24.3.2 Cancer Symptoms

The presence of lung cancer symptoms is considered by some to be a sign of advanced disease. This is not always the case (Tammemagi et al. 2004). Of those with symptoms of lung cancer, 24.2% were at stage 1. Certain symptoms including hoarseness, hemoptysis, dyspnea, noncardiac chest pain, extrathoracic pain, neurologic symptoms, weight loss, and weakness/fatigue were associated with more advanced disease and/or worse prognosis.

24.4 BENEFIT FROM FINDING LUNG CANCER

Screening for lung cancer with chest radiographs has not been shown to provide a benefit when compared to usual care (not otherwise defined). Low-dose lung CT screening, when compared to screening with a chest radiograph, has been shown to result in a 20% decrease in mortality over a 7-year period in men and women over age 55 with a history of at least moderate current or prior smoking. There

has been no comparison of either CT or chest radiographs to no chest radiographs. The data for the chest radiographs could still be distorted by a process called contamination, where individuals in the usual care group had chest radiographs as part of usual care. While PLCO states that this is only a small factor (estimated 11% of the usual care group), its published results do not indicate separate groups of nonsmokers, former smokers, and current smokers in relation to chest radiographs obtained in the usual care arm (Hocking et al. 2010). An estimated 44%, of the routine care group, were never smokers, so the actual contamination rate among current and former smokers could be higher.

Another reason to expect that the contamination rate could be higher is that primary care practitioners (PCPs) do order tests to look for lung cancer in current and former smokers over age 50 (Klabunde et al. 2010). Among the PCPs surveyed, 66.6% would test for lung cancer given appropriate age (50+) and smoking history; 17.2% would recommend imaging with LDCT and 45% with CXR. This means, of those who would test (the 66.6% of the total), 25% would test with LDCT and 67% would test with CXR. This suggests that the rate of contamination in the usual care arm of PLCO could be higher, perhaps 66%.

PLCO compared screening with CXRs to usual care. It showed no difference between the arms in long-term mortality, but substantial improvement in survival compared to historic controls (1975–2007) recorded in the NCI Surveillance, Epidemiology and End Results (SEER) Program (National Cancer Institute). There were two arms in the PLCO—screened and usual care. The 5-year survival using CXR screening was 45%, usual care 35%, and SEER data 16.4%; 10-year survival was 33% screened, and 30% unscreened, SEER 10%. At 13 years (final year of PLCO), it was 28% screened, 24% unscreened, and SEER 9%. Lung cancers detected by CXR have a substantially better survival than shown by the published data from SEER. In the screened group, this could represent lead-time bias (see Section 24.5.2.1), but that should not apply to the usual care group.

In the early years of the PLCO study (up to 10 years), one finds a reduction in the mortality rate (not statistically significant for this sample size) (Oken et al. 2011). At 5 years, the mortality rate reduction was 11%, decreasing to 5% at 10 years. At 11 years, the difference essentially disappears. Screening with chest radiographs does appear to offer some potential intermediate term benefit, though the results were not statistically significant.

In the National Lung Screening Trial (NLST; National Lung Screening Trial Research Team et al. 2011, 395–409), publicity has stressed the improvement with CT but has not emphasized the actual mortality rate over 6+ years since randomization. There were, cumulative to January 15, 2009, in the CT group, 427 lung cancer deaths among 1865 cancers (22.9%), so 77.1% survived or died of other causes. In the CXR group, there were 503 lung cancer deaths among 1991 cases of lung cancer (25.3%), so 74.7% survived or died of other causes. As of this publication, it is not possible to compare this to historic or other controls because the actual period of follow-up (while balanced between the CT and CXR arms of the study) varies for different enrollees based on the time the cancer was detected, from a maximum of 7 years to a minimum of 2 years. The SEER data report a 2-year survival of 28.6% and a 7-year survival of 13.6%. This suggests that screening with CT or chest radiograph results in a better survival rate than the SEER historic data.

The SEER data are drawn from different populations (likely more diverse) than the PLCO and NLST study populations, so these data cannot be accurately compared; however, the results indicate that cancers detected by chest radiographs are still associated with long-term survival.

24.5 LUNG CANCER RISK ASSESSMENT

The risk of developing lung cancer varies among individuals. CADe programs should not be used for all chest radiographs or lung CTs. In low-risk populations, the potential harms from false-positive interpretations may exceed the benefit from finding the rare lung cancer. In addition, the cost of screening and follow-up of abnormalities in low-risk individuals may distort the allocation of health-care funding away from other health-care tasks of greater relative value.

24.5.1 People Who Should Be Screened

The level of risk necessary before one is screened is currently not settled. While it is clear that the risk of lung cancer increases with age and with smoking history, there is no general consensus on the age and degree of smoking history that should prompt a decision to screen. It is expected that future analysis of the data from the NCI NLST will provide estimates of cost–risk–benefit trade-offs for different cancer risk strata; these risk strata will be limited within those used for the selection of subjects for the NLST (over age 55, current or former smoker).

To determine whether or not to screen, it is important to compare risks and benefits. There are two broad different categories of risk: the risk of an individual to develop cancer and the risks occurring from the correct or incorrect assignment of cancer to an individual. The risks for an individual of developing lung cancer have been detailed in Section 24.1. They include smoking history, age, family history, and certain industrial exposures.

The risks of detecting a potential lung cancer are several and depend, in part, on whether or not the abnormality identified by imaging (or other methods) is or is not a cancer.

If the imaging finding is not a lung cancer, the risks are of two types: psychological (related to being labeled as possibly having a lung cancer) and the physical effects of any diagnostic procedure that may be used to exclude the cancer. If the imaging abnormality is a cancer, the issues are more complex and are related to the concept of overdiagnosis. Overdiagnosis is one of the biases that can occur with cancer detection and screening and is discussed in Section 24.6.2.3.

At present, no specific recommendations can be made defining who should be screened.

Case finding is different from screening. Case finding in those with symptoms of lung cancer can be done whenever such symptoms are present. Most people with symptoms consistent with lung cancer do not have lung cancer. The main associated symptoms are dyspnea, noncardiac chest pain, extrathoracic pain, neurologic symptoms, weight loss, weakness, and fatigue (Tammemagi et al. 2004).

24.5.2 Estimated Cost of Screening

Detailed estimates of the cost of screening per cancer case found and per life saved are expected to come from the future analysis of the NLST. *Society* as represented by the government puts limits on the total amount of health-related expenditures that are acceptable. Within these limits, spending for one aspect of health care should decrease the spending for a different aspect of health care. For example, if lung cancer screening becomes policy, that could require an offset of spending for another disease, for example, pancreatitis. Cost–benefit analysis is a method of ranking the *value* to society of different approaches to health care. Once the detailed analysis is completed, it is this writer's opinion that screening for lung cancer will be found to be of higher value than some competing health-care expenditures.

24.6 MEASURING THE SUCCESS OF CANCER DETECTION

24.6.1 Measures of Success

At the elementary level, the identification of cancer is a sign of success. This provides only partial evidence of success. The purpose of cancer detection is twofold: first to identify the cancer and second to provide some benefit to the patient by lowering the potential morbidity or mortality outcome of the cancer.

There are several measures of outcome that are slightly different when describing the outcome of an individual compared to the outcomes of a group of individuals.

For an individual, the outcomes are cancer detection, improved duration of survival, decreased morbidity, and decreased mortality.

When applied to a group of people, the outcomes are test sensitivity and specificity, survival that can be measured at 1, 3, 5, and 10 years of duration (e.g., percent 5-year survival), measures of morbidity, and measures of mortality. These can be supplemented by measures of quality of life and cost effectiveness of the detection and treatment process.

24.6.2 Measurement Biases

Cancer detection measurements are subject to several biases, each of which can falsely elevate the apparent benefit of earlier detection. These biases are usually considered to be related to screening biases but apply somewhat more broadly.

24.6.2.1 Lead-Time Bias

If a person has a cancer that will kill him or her in 10 years (because of an absence of any curative treatment), then it does not matter whether the cancer is detected after 2, 5, or 10 years; death occurs at the same time no matter when the cancer is detected. The cancer may have been detected earlier, but this earlier detection has no benefit. There is more *lead-time* from detection to death, but no change in outcome.

24.6.2.2 Length-Time Bias

Cancers of different cell types and the same type in different people can grow at different speeds. If you look for cancers once a year, there will be fast-growing cancers that can appear after the initial search and that kill the patient before the next cancer search. At the same time, slower-growing cancers will remain and can be detected. Thus, screening at any interval will result in the detection of fewer of the fast-growing cancers. This means that survival will appear to be improved because the fast-growing cancers are not detected. This bias has its greatest effect the first time a person or group is studied because, in that setting, a greater percentage of the cancers will be slow growing. This is called length-time bias.

24.6.2.3 Overdiagnosis Bias

Overdiagnosis bias occurs when cancer is identified that would not have affected the patient during his or her lifetime. When a cancer is detected that will have no effect on the patient's symptoms or survival, that is considered to be overdiagnosis. For example, there are many older men with prostate cancer who will never have symptoms from their cancer and will die from some other cause. This indicates that finding cancer is not the end goal of patient management, but we need to find only those cancers that will affect the patient's health and life. Some people with lung cancer will die of diseases unrelated to the lung cancer. From the perspective of outcome-based medicine, these cancers are overdiagnosed. At present, in general, it is not possible to tell which lung cancers would affect the patient if they remained untreated and which would, eventually, kill the patient.

24.6.2.4 Confirmation Bias/Verification Bias

Confirmation bias is when one incorrectly assigns a cause of death because of something known about the patient. When a patient is known to have cancer, and the patient dies, that cancer may or may not be the cause of death. Once someone has cancer, the person can die from cancer, with cancer with a different cause of death, after having survived cancer with a different cause of death, or from a different disease. If the cause of death is assigned to the cancer without additional proof that the cancer caused the death, that is an example of confirmation bias. This will affect the statistical measures of the success of a cancer detection method.

Each of these biases affects measures of the outcome of cancer detection methods. In general, for the radiologists, improved cancer detection is what they are seeking. For the epidemiologist and those practicing evidence-based medicine, more can be required to assure them that these biases are not giving a false indication of the benefit of a cancer detection strategy.

24.6.3 CADe Measures of Success

There are different methods that can be used to measure the success of a lung nodule/cancer CADe program. To understand the reported results, it is important to understand the measure of success used to generate the results. At the simplest level, a CADe program should mark the location of lung nodules. Since some primary lung cancers can be more difficult for the human observer to detect than benign lung nodules, a study of the detection of primary lung cancers is likely a better measure of success when primary lung cancer is the target. In the same way, metastases can be easier to detect than some primary lung cancers (Way et al. 2010). If all a CADe system can do is detect more benign lung nodules (but not more cancers), it is not likely to be a clinically useful system.

The goal of CADe should be to aid the radiologist or other observer to identify nodules/cancers that would otherwise not be detected. If the radiologist can detect the lung nodules/cancers without the CADe system, then CADe provides limited benefit. Thus, a better method of measuring success is to show that radiologists improve their detection when using CADe.

Two CADe programs can have different cancer detection sensitivities; the better of the two programs is the one where radiologists using it detect more cancers, even if the detection rate of the program is less.

CADe and CADx articles mainly report measures of changes in cancer detection sensitivity (improved sensitivity) and specificity (usually decreased) and often some measurements of false positives. These measures are usually summarized using one of the forms of receiver operating characteristic (ROC) analysis; however, measures of sensitivity, specificity, false positives, and ROC findings give only part of the answer of whether or not CADe and CADx are or would be effective in clinical practice. Additional measures of effectiveness can be presented such as the size of the cancer, clinical stage, and location. Measures of survival, changes in morbidity and mortality, and cost–benefit analysis are usually considered beyond the scope of CAD studies but are helpful to the clinician in deciding their clinical benefit.

24.7   SCREENING METHODS

There are several screening methods that can be used for the detection of lung cancer. These include radiographic methods (the chest radiograph, enhanced chest radiograph with CADe and image processing, and lung CT) and nonradiographic methods (sputum cytology, bronchoscopy, light-assisted bronchoscopy, biochemical methods, and single-cell screening methods on sputum and blood). In considering these different methods, it is important to understand how success is measured.

24.7.1   Chest Radiograph

There have been a series of studies of the effectiveness of the chest radiograph in screening for lung cancer (Stitik and Tockman 1978, Muhm et al. 1983, Fontana et al. 1984, 1986, Stitik et al. 1985, Hocking et al. 2010, National Lung Screening Trial Research Team et al. 2011). In screening studies, the cases detected after screening with the chest radiograph are of lower stage than historic controls. There is no evidence of improvement in outcome, as measured by a decrease in mortality, when compared to usual care.

Prior to the wider use of CT screening for lung cancer, most of the cases of lung cancer that were cured would have been identified on chest radiographs, so it is clear that some cases found with the chest radiograph do have a good outcome, but identifying them in an organized screening program with annual chest radiographs does not present an advantage to the detection of cancer on chest radiographs obtained as part of the usual care of patients (case finding, incidental detection, and, for a much smaller group, surveillance).

24.7.2   Lung CT

Lung CT, used in a systematic screening program, in male or female current or former smokers, age 55 or greater, has been shown to result in a decrease in lung cancer mortality and in all-cause mortality (National Lung Screening Trial Research Team et al. 2011). The decrease in lung cancer mortality recorded was 20%. In the NLST, screening was performed for 3 years. This author considers it likely that the decrease in mortality would have been greater if screening had been continued throughout the multiyear period of follow-up.

24.7.3   Other Methods

Sputum cytology, bronchoscopy, and light-assisted bronchoscopy are important methods to be considered as an add-on to CT screening in high-risk individuals. While the results released by NLST are not yet sufficient to be certain, lung CT is most sensitive in the aerated parts of the lungs. Sputum cytology, bronchoscopy, and light-assisted bronchoscopy screen the trachea and main bronchi extending into the hila. Many of the tumors in these locations are squamous cell carcinomas, whereas most of the lung cancers detected with CT are adenocarcinomas (National Lung Screening Trial Research Team et al. 2011).

Biochemical methods based on measures of breath chemicals and plasma chemicals are newer methods under development. They appear to be able to detect the molecular signature of lung cancer in the breath or plasma. One can also identify single cancer cells in the blood. These methods identify cancer or potential for cancer but do this without the localization of the tumor. These may become important methods of screening in the future.

24.8   WHAT DOES A POSITIVE SCREEN MEAN FOR THE SUBJECT/PATIENT?

One of the critical questions facing the radiologist and other physicians following a positive screening test for lung cancer is whether the nodule is benign or malignant. Most identified lung nodules are indeterminate, but some predictions can be made based on the demographic features of the patient, some based on image analysis, and some based on contrast enhancement parameters on CT or MRI. In addition, certain predictive factors appear to exist to group patients as those more like to have early metastasizing lung cancer. These will be discussed in sequence.

24.8.1   Demographic Predictors

As indicated in Section 24.1, not everyone is at equal risk of developing lung cancer. Increasing age, smoking history, family history of lung cancer, and family history of other cancers are each indicators of increased risk. Dyspnea, noncardiac chest pain, extrathoracic pain, neurological symptoms, weight loss, and weakness or fatigue are all signs of lung cancer, and many are signs of cancer in general. None of these by themselves or in combination indicate that a patient has lung cancer but should raise the level of suspicion.

An interesting approach is offered by Tammemagi (Tammemagi et al. 2009), who reviewed the PLCO data and identified independent predictors of cancer in those with a finding suspicious for lung cancer. These predictors were older age, lower education, heavier and longer duration of smoking, body mass index less than 30, family history of lung cancer, lung nodule, lung mass, unilateral hilar or mediastinal adenopathy, lung infiltrate, and upper or middle chest lesion location.

The model using these variables had an ROC AUC of 86.4%. Excluding smoking variables, it had and ROC AUC of 77.1, and excluding all nonradiologic variables, it had an ROC AUC of 77.3%.

Swensen et al. (1997) reported a model for determining the likelihood of malignancy. Six hundred and twenty-nine patients with radiologically indeterminate solitary pulmonary nodules 4–30 mm in diameter, of which 23% were confirmed lung cancer, were entered into the study. The model included smoking history, history of extrathoracic cancer, diameter of the nodule, and spiculation of the edge and upper lobe location. The ROC AUC was 83.3% (Swensen et al. 1997).

Spitz (Spitz et al. 2007) reports on a model developed at M.D. Anderson Cancer Center. Based on factors associated with lung cancer including exposure to tobacco smoke (environmental and from smoking), dust exposure, family history of lung or other cancers, and prior respiratory disease, the 1-year individual risk of developing lung cancer can be estimated.

While these reports indicate those more likely to have lung cancer, they are not able to tell that someone does not have cancer.

When a patient is found with a lesion suspicious for lung cancer, we can determine whether the individual is at a greater or lesser risk that the lesion is cancer, but we cannot confirm that it is benign based on these approaches.

24.8.2 Is a Person in a High-Risk Category for Early Metastasizing Lung Cancer?

There are some individuals who, if they have lung cancer, appear to be at greater risk of having one that may metastasize early. Tammemagi (Tammemagi et al. 2007) reported on factors associated with human small aggressive NSCLC. Based on an analysis of the PLCO study data, based on a limited number of cases, and requiring confirmation with additional cases, this study found that these

small aggressive NSCLCs were inversely associated with the use of ibuprofen use and were associated with younger age (but above age 55, a PLCO entry criterion), female gender; the association with female gender was more pronounced in those with a family history of lung cancer; males did not show this association with family history. Adenocarcinoma was more frequent in this group, and there was a lighter smoking history.

These findings need confirmation from a larger study but suggest that those suspected of having a possible lung cancer should have a more aggressive follow-up or workup if they were younger, female, and had a family history of lung cancer. In addition, the degree of current or prior smoking may not be as great.

24.8.3 Image Analysis Parameters

Certain patterns seen on chest radiographs and CTs increase the likelihood that an identified finding is caused by lung cancer. The classic findings include nodule with an irregular border and lobar collapse with a mass visible in the hilum (e.g., Golden's reverse S sign).

Several groups have performed computer image analysis of nodules and have shown that partial differentiation of benign and malignant nodules was achievable. While these methods have not been incorporated into a CADx system, there is potential for such future development.

While a detailed discussion is not warranted here, the methods include spatial gray-level dependence methods (Cavouras et al. 1992, McNitt-Gray et al. 1999b); nodule CT density, size, shape, and texture features (McNitt-Gray et al. 1999a, Shiraishi et al. 2003, Li et al. 2004); as well as 2D and 3D features such as eccentricity, circularity, compactness, and histogram (Armato et al. 2003, Reeves et al. 2006). Wavelet analysis of nodules have also shown some promise (Osicka et al. 2006, 2007).

24.8.4 Use of Follow-Up to Determine Malignancy

One of the more common methods used to determine the likelihood of malignancy, whether detected with or without CADe, is to obtain follow-up studies after some period of time—ranging from 1 to 12 months. For example, the Fleischner Society (MacMahon et al. 2005) in 2005 recommended that the evaluation of people with an identified small lung nodule on CT be divided into those at low risk and high risk. High risk is based on smoking history, age, and other known risk factors. Nodules are then considered based on size. The intervals recommended for follow-up vary from none needed for nodules 4 mm or less in low-risk patients to follow-up at 3–6, 9–12, and 24 months for larger nodules and in higher-risk individuals. Greater detail and discussion is given in the article. As data from NLST are analyzed, these recommendations may change.

The American College of Chest Physicians (Gould et al. 2007) has published its recommendation for the evaluation of pulmonary nodules. They generated separate lists of recommendations for nodules measuring at least 8 mm in diameter, for those smaller than 8 mm, and multiple nodules when these are identified incidentally in evaluating solitary pulmonary nodules. The recommendations are based on considerations of the risk that the individual has cancer and the risk and benefits of various management strategies; the preferences of patients should also be considered. This approach includes measures of pretest probability of malignancy, evaluation of the nodule appearance on the single and, if available, prior and follow-up images (evaluating for changes in the nodule), contrast-enhanced CT for larger nodules, and FDG-PET for nodules 8 mm or larger. Then, needle biopsy should be considered. In those nodules that remain indeterminate, follow-up with repeat CT scans at 3, 6, 12, and 24 months is recommended. Readers are referred to the article for caveats and greater detail.

Based on the published research, there is no evidence that follow-up in less than 6 months affects stage or survival. There is some evidence that delays of 1 year will allow some cases to change to a more advanced stage. Several studies have looked at the possible effect of delays less than 6 months from lesion identification and others at delays longer than 1 year. Several studies (Bozcuk and Martin 2001, Aragoneses et al. 2002, Pita-Fernandez et al. 2003, Quarterman et al. 2003, Discussion 113–114, Myrdal et al. 2004) demonstrated no effect of delays less than 6 months. One paper (Christensen et al. 1997) provides data that the authors interpret as showing an effect on cancer stage of delays less than 6 months, but their data can be interpreted differently to show that no deleterious effect was demonstrated. Three papers, discussing cancer overlooked and then detected on a later radiograph (Quekel et al. 1999, Kashiwabara et al. 2002, 2003), show that some patients had progressed in stage between the two time points. In general, the interval of delay in these cases is 12 months or greater. Quekel (Quekel et al. 1999) reports that tumor size increased from T1 to T2 in 43% of their 49 patients. Kashiwabara (Kashiwabara et al. 2002, 2003) reports that those screened subjects whose missed tumors were 20 mm or larger at the time they were overlooked had a worse survival than a matched set of patients with tumors of similar size that were not overlooked.

24.8.5   Emotional Impact of an Indeterminate Screening Result

There are several downsides to CADe. Most lung nodules found by CADe will not be cancer. Cancer is, in clinical practice, far less common than lesions that can mimic the patterns of cancer. These true findings, but false positive for cancer, can create anxiety (Taylor et al. 2004, van den Bergh et al. 2010) and affect future willingness of people to undergo future screening (Taylor et al. 2004). Thus, the results of CADe and the subsequent evaluation must be presented in such a way that the individual does not decide to stop screening.

24.9   KEY FINDINGS ON CHEST RADIOGRAPHS OR LUNG CT THAT MAY BE ENHANCED BY CADe AND CADx

24.9.1   Patterns of Lung Cancer on Images

There are several patterns of lung cancer as seen on chest radiographs and CTs. On chest radiographs and CTs, the most frequent finding depends on how early it is detected. Patterns include nodules, masses, lung parenchymal opacities (consolidation and ground-glass opacities), areas of lung collapse (local segmental and lobar and lung), and rarer findings. Theros (Theros 1977) provides a detailed review of the patterns seen in 1267 peripheral lung neoplasms referred to the Armed Forces Institute of Pathology. The upper lobes were the most common locations. The average size of the lesions was approximately 5 cm. Forty-two percent were peripheral in location. Common patterns included lobulation (21%), sharp definition of edge (10%), shaggy margin (12%), poorly defined margin (10%), ball or coin lesion (5%), cavitation (6%), and calcification in lesion (1%). Most CADe programs for chest radiographs have been designed to identify lung nodules that are solid or semisolid; CADe for CT has been designed to identify lung nodules that may be solid, semisolid, or nonsolid.

With early lung cancer, the most frequent finding is that of a nodule or a mass. This nodule may be solid, nonsolid, or semisolid. According to the Fleischner Society definitions (Hansell et al. 2008), a lung nodule is a rounded opacity up to 3 cm in diameter. It can be well or poorly defined. On CT (and infrequently on chest radiographs), it can appear nonsolid, allowing one to see vessels and bronchial margins through it. Some nodules are partially solid and partially nonsolid. A mass has the same description as a nodule but is greater than 3 cm in diameter. Less often, lung cancer can appear with consolidation; this is an area of homogeneous increase in the opacity of the lung parenchyma.

24.9.2   Finding Multiple Nodules

Most CADe programs have been designed with the primary focus to identify solitary lung nodules. Such programs will also identify several lung nodules, though CADe programs may have been designed with a maximum cutoff of sites identified to decrease the number of false positives.

Single nodules and multiple nodules in the chest point to different diseases. Most solitary nodules are due to nonmalignant causes including certain types of infections and noninfectious inflammatory disease. Uncommonly, they are due to intra-lung lymph nodes, vascular abnormalities, and congenital malformations. While a lung nodule can be a cancer, this is less common. Most focal findings on chest radiographs suspicious for cancer, after evaluation, are found not to represent cancer. In the NLST, 39.1% of the CT group and 16% of the chest radiography group had at least one positive screening exam. Of these, 96.4% in the CT group and 94.5 in the chest radiography group were false positives (National Lung Screening Trial Research Team et al. 2011).

When there are multiple lung nodules, these can be due to infectious disease, noninfectious inflammatory disease, and metastases to the lung of various neoplasms.

Once multiple lung nodules are identified, there is likely little benefit in the identification of all of them. The search of the image, in that setting, should be to identify changes in the nodules and, importantly, any new nodule. The identification of change is important because it can indicate progression, stabilization, or regression of the disease. A new nodule indicates progression.

24.9.3   Measurements of the Size of Nodule

The measurement of the size of a nodule is of great importance clinically. The clinical imperative is to determine whether the nodule has increased (or decreased) in size. Either type of change indicates that the nodule is active and, therefore, more likely to require some type of action: A nodule increasing in size could indicate infection or cancer; a nodule decreasing in size indicates a resolving process but must be followed to make sure that the disease does not again become active. On occasion, cancers can decrease in size and then, later, start to increase in size.

The measurement of the size of a nodule, especially when small changes are important, is a nontrivial task (Shah et al. 2005, Gavrielides et al. 2009, McNitt-Gray et al. 2009). Nodules are 3D objects that are seen in a 2D projection on chest radiographs but can be seen either as multiple slices

or as 3D-generated objects on CT. The difficulties in measuring a nodule occur because of several factors: (1) The edges of nodules are not sharp; this is more frequent in malignant nodules. (2) There is partial pixel or partial voxel (volume) effect at their edges. (3) There are often structures touching or incorporated into the nodule that need to be *deleted* from the measurement to obtain a valid size. (4) Nodules can change their orientation (e.g., by rotation or slight differences in projection) so that their appearance is not always consistent. (5) There are machine settings and algorithm differences. The best measurement needs to be designed to at least partially overcome these problems. For the detection of minimal changes, 3D reconstruction and 3D volume measurement are greatly beneficial (Yankelevitz et al. 2000, Reeves et al. 2006).

24.10   KEY RECENT CLINICAL TRIALS OF LUNG CANCER SCREENING IN THE ABSENCE OF CADe

Over time, there have been a series of clinical trials testing the effectiveness of lung cancer screening on the outcome of the disease. Three prominent studies in the 1970s had results that were generally interpreted as showing that screening with chest radiographs and sputum CT resulted in a shift in the stage of the lung cancers toward a lower stage but did not affect lung cancer mortality (Stitik and Tockman 1978, Muhm et al. 1983, Stitik et al. 1985). In the study from the Mayo clinic (Fontana et al. 1984, 1986), lung cancer mortality was greater in the screened group. None of these large clinical trials incorporated CADe or CADx.

In 1993, the National Cancer Institute started a study of the effectiveness of screening for 4 cancers in those 55 through 74 years at age: the PLCO Screening Trial. As related to lung cancer, this enrolled 77,445 subjects assigned to have an annual screening chest radiograph for 3 years (4 years for current or former smokers) and 77,456 subjects assigned to have usual care (i.e., no specific screening examinations) (Oken et al. 2005, 1832–1839, 2011, 1865–1873, Hocking et al. 2010).

Starting in 1993, the Early Lung Cancer Action Project (ELCAP) started a nonrandomized study of the effectiveness of CT for lung cancer screening. The initial report on this (Henschke et al. 1999) detailed the results from the initial 1000 subjects. At its start, subjects were to be 60 years of age, or older, be asymptomatic, and have at least a 10-year smoking history. In this trial, each CT was interpreted independently by two radiologists with agreement reached by consensus. The study is ongoing and is international in scope. The International Early Lung Cancer

Action Project (I-ELCAP) had enrolled over 31,000 subjects as of a 2006 publication (International Early Lung Cancer Action Program Investigators et al. 2006). The initial and continuing studies showed that CT could detect many more lung cancers than could be seen on the concurrent chest radiographs; therefore, the chest radiographs were discontinued. It showed that the stage of the lung cancers detected was substantially more favorable than historic controls. Their data, while not obtained in a randomized study, showed a strong shift toward lower cancer stage and improved survival. In their design, they could neither test for change in mortality nor control for lead-time bias. I-ELCAP did use 3D reconstructions and 3D measurements in assessing change in nodule size that could lead to biopsy (Reeves et al. 2006).

Starting in 2002, the National Cancer Institute initiated the NLST, where subjects were randomized to have either a chest radiograph or a lung CT for 3 years. This study enrolled 53,454 subjects who were followed to the end of 2009. Results of this study showed a 20% relative decrease in lung cancer mortality with CT screening as compared to chest radiographic screening. The chest radiographs were obtained with either screen-film or digital methods. The CTs were performed with multidetector CTs. No CADe or 3D image processing was used (National Lung Screening Trial Research Team et al. 2011).

24.11 RESULTS FROM SMALL CLINICAL TRIALS OF EFFECTIVENESS OF CADe

24.11.1 CADe and the Chest Radiograph

CADe uses pattern recognition software that is developed to aid radiologists to detect solitary pulmonary nodules, which could represent early stage lung cancer. CADe software exists for both chest radiographs and lung CTs. For chest radiographs, most systems described here (OnGuard™) were developed by Riverain Medical Group (Miamisburg, OH) and its predecessor Deus Technologies (Rockville, MD). Two other commercial systems are also described. The Riverain systems were tested on primary lung cancers. These commercial systems place circles around the regions of interest to reduce oversight errors. There are a series of reports on the effectiveness of these systems, starting with the initial system (Freedman 2004, Freedman and Osicka 2005) and continuing to more advanced systems.

Li (Li et al. 2008) reported that OnGuard™ 1.0 detected (i.e., circled) 37% of actionable nodules that were missed by radiologists. Chen (Chen and White 2008) reported that 36% of x-rays with nodules that were visible in retrospect,

but missed clinically, were marked by OnGuard™ 1.0. Freedman (Freedman 2004, Freedman and Osicka 2005) reported the results of OnGuard™ 1.0 where 15 radiologists interpreted 180 cases of which 60 contained solitary primary lung cancer. The area under the ROC curve increased from 0.829 to 0.865 (4.3%). The radiologists' sensitivity for cancer detection increased from 71% to 78%, 7 percentage points (9.9% increase). White (White et al. 2008, 2009) reported that the OnGuard™ 3.0 CADe system detected 47% of 89 cancers that had been originally overlooked. Meziane (Meziane et al. 2010) compared four versions of OnGuard™ developed between 2001 and 2010. These four versions showed increasing machine sensitivity for the detection of lung cancer and a decreasing number of false positives per image (FP/I). The newest version they tested, OnGuard™ 5.0, on their cases had the machine sensitivity of 64.4% with 2.0 FP/I. More recently, OnGuard™ 5.1 was approved by the FDA. On the test data submitted to the FDA, there was a substantial difference in the machine sensitivity between OnGuard™ 1.0 and OnGuard™ 5.1. On the set of cancer cases used for these tests, OnGuard™ 1.0 provided a cancer detection sensitivity of 49.38% and OnGuard™ 5.1 provided a cancer detection sensitivity of 74.07%. Despite this difference in machine performance, the effect of this difference on the radiologists was small, but significant; radiologists using OnGuard™ 1.0 detected 66% when location-correct was required and when using OnGuard™ 5.1 detected 70%. When case-correct, correct location not required, was the criterion, radiologists using OnGuard™ 1.0 detected 76% of cancers and those using OnGuard™ 5.1 detected 79%. This indicates that machine performance is only one factor in the effectiveness of CADe devices.

In the 2001 study of OnGuard™ 1.0, the number of FP/I was 5.3. On the 2010 set of cases, it was 5.03. For OnGuard™ 5.1 in 2010, there were 1.26 FP/I. This difference in FP/I did not result in differences in specificity (90% for both OnGuard™ 1.0 and OnGuard™ 5.1).

These results show that the major trend over time is a decrease in the number of FP/I, associated with a long-term increase in sensitivity, but not for every version.

There are few tests of other commercial systems on cancer cases. In 2003, Shingo Kakeda (Kakeda et al. 2004, 505–510) reported the results of a reader trial of a chest radiograph CADe system developed by Mitsubishi Space Software (Tokyo, Japan). They tested this system on CR chest radiographs. There were 45 cases containing a single lung cancer and 45 normal cases. Eight readers interpreted the cases using a sequential reader design. The average area under the ROC curve increased from 0.924 without to 0.986 with the CADe. The difference was statistically significant. There were 3.15 FP/I on the CT-confirmed normal cases.

EDDA Technology (Princeton, NJ) has its system, IQQA-Chest™, for lung nodule enhancement. Moore (Moore et al. 2011) determined machine sensitivity and specificity with secondary interpretation by a radiologist that reviewed the findings of IQQA-Chest™. Baseline sensitivity for nodules 0.5–1.5 cm in diameter was 70% with specificity 50%. After a radiologist indicated which machine generated false-positive locations to remove, the specificity increased to 78%. van Beek et al. reported in 2008 (van Beek et al. 2008) that radiologists working without IQQA-Chest™ with dual reading (resident and staff radiologist) reviewed 324 DR chest radiographs (214 eligible for inclusion), interpreting them first without and then with the use of IQQA-Chest™. IQQA-Chest™ was not used for all patients' chest radiographs; criteria for inclusion and exclusion of specific cases are not included in the report. All radiographs were in patients with a known primary cancer (other than primary lung cancer). Without the use of IQQA-Chest™, 35 cases were identified with confirmed lung nodules. With the use of IQQA-Chest™, 51 cases were identified with confirmed lung nodules. Sensitivity increased from 63.8% to 92.7%. Specificity decreased from 98.1% to 96.2%. Five of the sixteen (31%) of the newly detected nodules were cancer. Overall, there were 55 nodules (detected and not detected), 17 (31%) of which were confirmed malignant. The number of false-positive interpretations increased from three to six cases with the use of IQQA-Chest™. This reports the actual online use of a computer aid system for lung nodule detection.

These reports indicate that radiologists using CADe systems can increase their detection of malignant lung nodules. It also shows that these systems are improving over time, both in machine performance and in the number of new cancers detected by radiologists using these systems.

24.11.2 CADe and Lung CT

CADe systems have been developed to aid in the detection of lung nodules on lung CTs.

Armato (Armato et al. 2002) reported on the rate of detection of lung cancers missed on CT in a lung cancer screening program using a University of Chicago–developed system. The system detected 32 of 38 (84%) of the missed cancers with a false-positive rate of 1 FP per CT section.

Armato in 2005 reported on a University of Chicago CADe system for lung CT. For malignant nodules, at 0.85 false positives per CT section, sensitivity was 80%. No reader study was used.

Li (Li et al. 2005) in 2005 reported a reader study using 14 radiologists reading 17 patients with a CT missed cancer and 10 control subjects. A University of Chicago–developed CADe system was used. Sensitivity increased from 52% to 68%. The area under the ROC curve increased from 0.763 to 0.854. Specificity was decreased, but the amount of decrease is not given.

Peldschus (Peldschus et al. 2005) showed the potential benefit of such a system. A prototype CADe system from R2 (R2 Technologies, Sunnyvale, CA) was tested on 100 patients whose CTs were originally interpreted as normal. In 33 patients, a total of 53 significant lesions were detected by the CADe system and confirmed by an expert panel. There were 125 false-positive lesions (1.25 per case, range 0–11 FP marks). There were also 107 lesions considered to be not significant lesions (calcified lesions and apical or pleural scars). No reader study was performed with the CADe system.

Marco Das (Das et al. 2006) reported a study where three radiologists were tested on 25 CTs with a total of 116 pulmonary nodules. Two CAD systems—ImageChecker™ CT (R2 Technologies, Sunnyvale, CA) and Nodule Enhanced Viewing (NEV) (Siemens Medical Solutions, Forchheim, Germany)—were compared. The radiologist observers interpreted the CTs initially without the CADe systems. They were then tested 6–12 weeks later when using the first of two CADe systems and then, after an additional 6–12 weeks, with the second CADe system. Ground truth was established by the consensus of a panel consisting of the three tested radiologists and a more senior radiologist as adjudicator, as needed. Sensitivity for radiologist 1 was 68%, which increased to 79%; for radiologist 2, sensitivity without CADe was 78% and increased to 90% with CADe; and for radiologist 3, sensitivity was 82% and increased to 86% with CADe. The number of machine false positives was 6 for one of the CADe systems and 8 for the others. After a short period of follow-up, one case of cancer had been diagnosed. The other nodules had shown no growth.

Hirose (Hirose et al. 2008), using ZIOCAD software (Ziosoft, Inc., Tokyo, Japan), performed a reader study using six radiologists. Included were 21 patients, 6 without and 15 with lung nodules. Nodules ranged from 1.5 to 15 mm in diameter, average 4.5 mm. Twenty-five of the forty-nine nodules were 4 mm or larger. The CADe software showed the sensitivity of 71.4% with 0.95 FP per case. Radiologists improved from an unaided 39.5% sensitivity to 81.0%, CADe aided, with an increase in FP per case from 0.14 to 0.89. JAFROC figure of merit increased from 0.390 without to 0.845 with the use of ZIOCAD.

24.11.3 Computer-Aided Diagnosis

The systems described earlier are CADe systems; CADx systems are also under development.

Shiraishi reported in 2003 and 2006 the results of two different reader studies of CADx programs for chest radiographs from the University of Chicago. The earlier study (Shiraishi et al. 2003) used 53 chest radiographs with nodules,

31 primary lung cancers, and 22 benign nodules. Sixteen radiologists served as readers. The mean area under the ROC curve increased from 0.743 to 0.817. The performance of the program itself exceeded that of the radiologists with AUC = 0.889. The second study (Shiraishi et al. 2006) used 150 chest radiographs, including 108 with solitary pulmonary nodules and 42 cases without nodules. In the reader study, there were 48 cases: 24 with primary lung cancer, 12 with benign nodules, and 12 without nodules. For the 24 malignant cases, the CADx program was beneficial, on average, for 3.9 cases; detrimental for 0.9 cases; 21.6 cases were correctly marked without CADx. For the 12 benign nodule and 12 nonnodule cases, the program was beneficial for an average of 4.3 cases and detrimental for 2.1.

Way (Way et al. 2010) reports on a lung CT CADx system developed at the University of Michigan. Six readers reviewed 256 CT-detected lung nodules (124 malignant and 132 benign). The readers first assessed their decision on the likelihood of malignancy. The CADx results were then presented graphically. The graph displayed the Gaussian frequency distribution of benign and malignant nodules for each score. The radiologist then records the likelihood of malignancy based on their inclusion of the CADx information. Higher results, both without and with CADx, were seen for metastatic than for primary lung cancer. Overall, AUC increased from 0.833 to 0.853. Changes in scoring occurred with more changes in the correct direction than the incorrect direction (95.0 vs. 31.0). Decision for or against further evaluation (CT follow-up, immediate action) of a nodule was made more often in the correct direction (6.8 vs. 4.0).

24.12 COMMENTS ON READER FALSE-POSITIVE AND READER FALSE-NEGATIVE DECISIONS

24.12.1 False-Positive Decisions

False-positive detections are those where the radiologist or the software marks a location as suspicious that is not caused by the disease suspected. So if the machine or radiologist mark a location as suspicious for cancer, but the location is not that of cancer, then it is a false positive.

Radiologists working without CADe identify many locations that are false positives. For example, in the PLCO study, among the 77,464 subjects in the intervention arm (chest radiographs), there were, over 3–4 years of screening, 17,643 (23%) subjects with suspicious findings; of these subjects, 20.3% had positive follow-up CT scans, 3.0% had biopsies, and 1.7% had biopsies positive for cancer (Hocking et al. 2010). All of those with positive screens, not found to have cancer, were false positives. This was in the absence of CADe.

When using CADe for lung cancer, radiologists increase their frequency of false-positive detections. Sometimes, this is reported as a decrease in specificity and other times as an increase in false-positive rate. In the study comparing OnGuard™ 1.0 to OnGuard™ 5.1, radiologists decreased their specificity from 94% (unaided) to 90%, when aided by either OnGuard™ 1.0 or OnGuard™ 5.1. Sensitivity without CADe was 62%, increasing to 66% with OnGuard™ 1.0 and 70% with OnGuard™ 5.1. With the SoftView™ bone suppression–soft issue enhancement software (Riverain Medical Group, Miamisburg, OH) (Freedman et al. 2011), the specificity decreased from 96.1% to 91.8%; this occurred as the readers' average sensitivity increased from 49.5% to 66.3%.

False positives marked by CADe software are considered to be undesirable. There are several proposed reasons for this. First, the CADe mark may mislead the radiologist to also mark the same location as suspicious; this would potentially increase the cost for the follow-up of the suspect abnormality and increase patient anxiety. Second, if there are too many false positives, the radiologist may lose confidence in the quality of the software and then ignore the marks, resulting in missed lesions that should be evaluated for, for example, cancer. Third, a false positive, agreed to by the radiologist, may result in biopsy or other physical harm to the patient (Silvestri 2011). Reviewing the literature, I have not found experimental proof that any of these undesirable effects have been identified with the use of CADe for chest radiographs or lung CTs.

24.12.2 Increase in False-Negative Decisions/Detections

In the SoftView™ study (Freedman et al. 2011), radiologists removed their marks from correct locations in 2% of cases when using SoftView™; for 1.4%, the correct mark was removed, and no other suspicious location was marked; for 0.6% of cases, the mark was moved from a correct location to an incorrect location. This should be compared to a 16.8% increase in cancer detection sensitivity.

24.12.3 Effect of Decreases in Software False-Positive Detections and Radiologist Detection Specificity and the Effect of Increased Software True-Positive Detections

There is an expectation that an increase in software CADe detections will result in an increase in the radiologist's cancer detections and that a decrease in software CADe detections will result in a decrease in radiologist false-positive detections. In a comparison of OnGuard™ 1.0 and

OnGuard™ 5.1, there was a substantial increase in software sensitivity from 49.4% (OnGuard™ 1.0) to 74.1%; but the radiologists' cancer detection sensitivity increased from 62% without CADe to 66% with OnGuard™ 1.0 and 70% with OnGuard™ 5.1. This is a much smaller increase than one would have expected given the large difference in the CADe software sensitivity. The CADe software FP/I were, for OnGuard™ 1.0, 5.3 for the cases used in 2001 and 5.03 for the cases used in 2010. For OnGuard™ 5.1, on the 2010 cases, the false-positive marks per image were 1.26. The specificity of the radiologists, on the 2010 cases, was 90% for both versions of the CADe software compared to 94% without CADe.

The lack of change in specificity in this single study suggests that the number of false positives produced by the CADe software, within this range, does not affect radiologists' false-positive detections; they were able to distinguish most of the machine marks into true positives and false positives.

Regarding the great difference in the CADe software cancer detections compared to a much smaller improvement in radiologists' detections with OnGuard™ CADe, it is apparent that the cases marked by the CADe software do not always result in the radiologists changing their decisions; if the cases are easy enough so that the radiologists can detect the cancer without CADe, then CADe does not help them improve. It is only with the cases that radiologists fail to detect and CADe does that CADe can help the radiologists.

24.13   INTEGRATION OF LUNG CANCER CADe AND CADx INTO CLINICAL WORK FLOW

CADe devices for lung cancer have been integrated into several different picture archiving and communication system (PACS) vendors' systems and into CT workstations. Although there have been many successful implementations, the integration requires the cooperation of the PACS vendor and the CADe manufacturer. For chest radiograph CADe, the device can create an overlay to the original image so that the CADe marks are displayed, either as a new image or as a toggle on–off. The CADe software can also send the coordinates of the marks so that the PACS system can display the marks within its own display framework. For CT, the systems have been designed to be integrated into various manufacturers' workstations.

As important are questions of when the systems should be used clinically. There may not be a need to run and review the CADe system on every image that the radiologist interprets. For systems designed to detect primary lung cancer, younger patients have such a low likelihood of having lung cancer that CADe is not likely to be of benefit. A method of filtering which images should be processed by CADe would be a useful clinical development.

24.14   CONCLUSION

Currently, there has been no report of a large-scale prospective clinical trial of CADe or CADx for lung cancer detection or diagnosis. For this reason, the clinical utility of CAD systems is still not established. Commercial systems tested in small studies show definite improvement in lung cancer detection, and, in the future, these or other systems will likely be shown to be important in routine clinical care.

CADe systems can, because of false-positive detections accepted by the radiologist, lead to unnecessary workups with exposures to additional radiation and, perhaps, a few biopsies. If a radiologist changes a true-positive detection without CADe to a false-negative decision because the CADe program did not detect an abnormality, this could harm the patient. For these reasons, a true prospective trial of these systems should be encouraged.

It is probably not useful to use the CADe software for all chest radiographs and lung CTs; their use should be more selective and based on patient risk factors. Formulas to estimate the individual risk for lung cancer have been developed but need further validation. Eventually, a combination of the submitted indication for the chest radiograph combined with individual risk information drawn from the electronic medical record could indicate when CADe should be used. Below some as yet unquantified level of risk, CADe, because of false-positive decisions, may represent more risk than benefit.

CADx programs are still in the development stage. Initial results show that these have great potential, and further development is strongly encouraged. Such systems could combine image analysis with the incorporation of nonimage information about the patients, such as smoking history, age, and family history of cancer. Combining CADe with CADx should enhance the benefit–risk trade-offs.

REFERENCES

Aragoneses, F. G., N. Moreno, P. Leon, E. G. Fontan, and E. Folque. 2002. Influence of delays on survival in the surgical treatment of bronchogenic carcinoma. *Lung Cancer* 36 (1): 59–63.

Armato, S. G. 3rd, M. B. Altman, J. Wilkie, S. Sone, F. Li, K. Doi, and A. S. Roy. 2003. Automated lung nodule classification following automated nodule detection on CT: A serial approach. *Medical Physics* 30 (6): 1188–1197.

Armato, S. G. 3rd, F. Li, M. L. Giger, H. MacMahon, S. Sone, and K. Doi. 2002. Lung cancer: Performance of automated lung nodule detection applied to cancers missed in a CT screening program. *Radiology* 225 (3): 685–692.

Austin, J. H., B. M. Romney, and L. S. Goldsmith. 1992. Missed bronchogenic carcinoma: Radiographic findings in 27 patients with a potentially resectable lesion evident in retrospect. *Radiology* 182 (1): 115–122.

Bozcuk, H. and C. Martin. 2001. Does treatment delay affect survival in non-small cell lung cancer? A retrospective analysis from a single UK centre. *Lung Cancer* 34 (2): 243–252.

Cavouras, D., P. Prassopoulos, and N. Pantelidis. 1992. Image analysis methods for solitary pulmonary nodule characterization by computed tomography. *European Journal of Radiology* 14 (3): 169–172.

Chen, J. J. and C. S. White. 2008. Use of CAD to evaluate lung cancer on chest radiography. *Journal of Thoracic Imaging* 23 (2): 93–96.

Christensen, E. D., T. Harvald, M. Jendresen, S. Aggestrup, and G. Petterson. 1997. The impact of delayed diagnosis of lung cancer on the stage at the time of operation. *European Journal of Cardiothoracic Surgery* 12 (6): 880–884.

Das, M., G. Muhlenbruch, A. H. Mahnken, T. G. Flohr, L. Gundel, S. Stanzel, T. Kraus, R. W. Gunther, and J. E. Wildberger. 2006. Small pulmonary nodules: Effect of two computer-aided detection systems on radiologist performance. *Radiology* 241 (2): 564–571.

Fontana, R. S., D. R. Sanderson, W. F. Taylor, L. B. Woolner, W. E. Miller, J. R. Muhm, and M. A. Uhlenhopp. 1984. Early lung cancer detection: Results of the initial (prevalence) radiologic and cytologic screening in the mayo clinic study. *The American Review of Respiratory Disease* 130 (4): 561–565.

Fontana, R. S., D. R. Sanderson, L. B. Woolner, W. F. Taylor, W. E. Miller, and J. R. Muhm. 1986. Lung cancer screening: The mayo program. *Journal of Occupational Medicine: Official Publication of the Industrial Medical Association* 28 (8): 746–750.

Freedman, M. 2004. State-of-the-art screening for lung cancer (part 1): The chest radiograph. *Thoracic Surgery Clinics* 14 (1): 43–52.

Freedman, M. T., S. C. Lo, J. C. Seibel, and C. M. Bromley. 2011. Lung nodules: Improved detection with software that suppresses the rib and clavicle on chest radiographs. *Radiology* 260 (1): 265–273.

Freedman, M. T. and T. Osicka. 2005. Computer aided diagnosis for decision support in thoracic imaging. In *Decision Support in the Digital Medical Environment*, E. Siegel, B. Reiner, and B. Erickson (eds.), Vol. Primer 6, pp. 53–68. Leesburg, VA: SCAR (Society for Computer Applications in Radiology).

Gavrielides, M. A., L. M. Kinnard, K. J. Myers, and N. Petrick. 2009. Noncalcified lung nodules: Volumetric assessment with thoracic CT. *Radiology* 251 (1): 26–37.

Gould, M. K., J. Fletcher, M. D. Iannettoni, W. R. Lynch, D. E. Midthun, D. P. Naidich, D. E. Ost, and American College of Chest Physicians. 2007. Evaluation of patients with pulmonary nodules: When is it lung cancer?: ACCP evidence-based clinical practice guidelines (2nd edition). *Chest* 132 (3 Suppl): 108S–130S.

Hansell, D. M., A. A. Bankier, H. MacMahon, T. C. McLoud, N. L. Muller, and J. Remy. 2008. Fleischner society: Glossary of terms for thoracic imaging. *Radiology* 246 (3): 697–722.

Henschke, C. I., D. I. McCauley, D. F. Yankelevitz, D. P. Naidich, G. McGuinness, O. S. Miettinen, D. M. Libby et al. 1999. Early lung cancer action project: Overall design and findings from baseline screening. *Lancet* 354 (9173): 99–105.

Hirose, T., N. Nitta, J. Shiraishi, Y. Nagatani, M. Takahashi, and K. Murata. 2008. Evaluation of computer-aided diagnosis (CAD) software for the detection of lung nodules on multidetector row computed tomography (MDCT): JAFROC study for the improvement in radiologists' diagnostic accuracy. *Academic Radiology* 15 (12): 1505–1512.

Hocking, W. G., P. Hu, M. M. Oken, S. D. Winslow, P. A. Kvale, P. C. Prorok, L. R. Ragard et al. 2010. Lung cancer screening in the randomized prostate, lung, colorectal, and ovarian (PLCO) cancer screening trial. *Journal of the National Cancer Institute* 102 (10): 722–731.

International Early Lung Cancer Action Program Investigators, C. I. Henschke, D. F. Yankelevitz, D. M. Libby, M. W. Pasmantier, J. P. Smith, and O. S. Miettinen. 2006. Survival of patients with stage I lung cancer detected on CT screening. *The New England Journal of Medicine* 355 (17): 1763–1771.

Jemal, A., F. Bray, M. M. Center, J. Ferlay, E. Ward, and D. Forman. 2011. Global cancer statistics. *CA: A Cancer Journal for Clinicians* 61 (2): 69–90.

Kakeda, S., J. Moriya, H. Sato, T. Aoki, H. Watanabe, H. Nakata, N. Oda, S. Katsuragawa, K. Yamamoto, and K. Doi. 2004. Improved detection of lung nodules on chest radiographs using a commercial computer-aided diagnosis system. *American Journal of Roentgenology* 182 (2): 505–510.

Kashiwabara, K., S. Koshi, K. Itonaga, O. Nakahara, M. Tanaka, and M. Toyonaga. 2003. Outcome in patients with lung cancer found on lung cancer mass screening roentgenograms, but who did not subsequently consult a doctor. *Lung Cancer* 40 (1): 67–72.

Kashiwabara, K., S. Koshi, K. Ota, M. Tanaka, and M. Toyonaga. 2002. Outcome in patients with lung cancer found retrospectively to have had evidence of disease on past lung cancer mass screening roentgenograms. *Lung Cancer* 35 (3): 237–241.

Klabunde, C. N., P. M. Marcus, G. A. Silvestri, P. K. Han, T. B. Richards, G. Yuan, S. E. Marcus, and S. W. Vernon. 2010. U.S. primary care physicians' lung cancer screening beliefs and recommendations. *American Journal of Preventive Medicine* 39 (5): 411–420.

Li, F., M. Aoyama, J. Shiraishi, H. Abe, Q. Li, K. Suzuki, R. Engelmann, S. Sone, H. Macmahon, and K. Doi. 2004. Radiologists' performance for differentiating benign from malignant lung nodules on high-resolution CT using computer-estimated likelihood of malignancy. *American Journal of Roentgenology* 183 (5): 1209–1215.

Li, F., H. Arimura, K. Suzuki, J. Shiraishi, Q. Li, H. Abe, R. Engelmann, S. Sone, H. MacMahon, and K. Doi. 2005. Computer-aided detection of peripheral lung cancers missed at CT: ROC analyses without and with localization. *Radiology* 237 (2): 684–690.

Li, F., R. Engelmann, C. E. Metz, K. Doi, and H. MacMahon. 2008. Lung cancers missed on chest radiographs: Results obtained with a commercial computer-aided detection program. *Radiology* 246 (1): 273–280.

MacMahon, H., J. H. Austin, G. Gamsu, C. J. Herold, J. R. Jett, D. P. Naidich, E. F. Patz Jr, S. J. Swensen, and Fleischner Society. 2005. Guidelines for management of small pulmonary nodules detected on CT scans: A statement from the Fleischner society. *Radiology* 237 (2): 395–400.

McNitt-Gray, M. F., L. M. Bidaut, S. G. Armato, C. R. Meyer, M. A. Gavrielides, C. Fenimore, G. McLennan et al. 2009. Computed tomography assessment of response to therapy: Tumor volume change measurement, truth data, and error. *Translational Oncology* 2 (4): 216–222.

McNitt-Gray, M. F., E. M. Hart, N. Wyckoff, J. W. Sayre, J. G. Goldin, and D. R. Aberle. 1999a. A pattern classification approach to characterizing solitary pulmonary nodules imaged on high resolution CT: Preliminary results. *Medical Physics* 26 (6): 880–888.

McNitt-Gray, M. F., N. Wyckoff, J. W. Sayre, J. G. Goldin, and D. R. Aberle. 1999b. The effects of co-occurrence matrix based texture parameters on the classification of solitary pulmonary nodules imaged on computed tomography. *Computerized Medical Imaging and Graphics* 23 (6): 339–348.

Meziane, M., P. Mazzone, E. Novak, M. L. Lieber, O. Lababede, M. Phillips, and N. A. Obuchowski. 2010. A comparison of four versions of a computer-aided detection system for pulmonary nodules on chest radiographs. *Journal of Thoracic Imaging* 27 (1):58–64.

Moore, W., J. Ripton-Snyder, G. Wu, and C. Hendler. 2011. Sensitivity and specificity of a CAD solution for lung nodule detection on chest radiograph with CTA correlation. *Journal of Digital Imaging: The Official Journal of the Society for Computer Applications in Radiology* 24 (3):405–410.

Muhm, J. R., W. E. Miller, R. S. Fontana, D. R. Sanderson, and M. A. Uhlenhopp. 1983. Lung cancer detected during a screening program using four-month chest radiographs. *Radiology* 148 (3): 609–615.

Myrdal, G., M. Lambe, G. Hillerdal, K. Lamberg, T. Agustsson, and E. Stahle. 2004. Effect of delays on prognosis in patients with non-small cell lung cancer. *Thorax* 59 (1): 45–49.

National Cancer Institute. SEER cancer statistics in review: 1975–2007. In National Cancer Institute [database online]. Bethesda, MD. Available from http://seer.cancer.gov/csr/1975_2007/results_merged/sect_15_lung_bronchus.pdf Accessed December 21, 2011.

National Lung Screening Trial Research Team, D. R. Aberle, A. M. Adams, C. D. Berg, W. C. Black, J. D. Clapp, R. M. Fagerstrom et al. 2011. Reduced lung-cancer mortality with low-dose computed tomographic screening. *The New England Journal of Medicine* 365 (5): 395–409.

Oken, M. M., W. G. Hocking, P. A. Kvale, G. L. Andriole, S. S. Buys, T. R. Church, E. D. Crawford et al. 2011. Screening by chest radiograph and lung cancer mortality: The prostate, lung, colorectal, and ovarian (PLCO) randomized trial. *JAMA: The Journal of the American Medical Association* 306 (17): 1865–1873.

Oken, M. M., P. M. Marcus, P. Hu, T. M. Beck, W. Hocking, P. A. Kvale, J. Cordes et al. 2005. Baseline chest radiograph for lung cancer detection in the randomized prostate, lung, colorectal and ovarian cancer screening trial. *Journal of National Cancer Institute* 97 (24): 1832–1839.

Osicka, T., M. T. Freedman, and F. Ahmed. 2006. Characterization of pulmonary nodules features on computer tomography (CT) scans using wavelet coefficients and heat maps. *Proceedings of SPIE: Image Processing* 6144: 1946–1956.

Osicka, T., M. T. Freedman, and F. Ahmed. 2007. Characterization of pulmonary nodules features on computed tomography (CT) scans: The effect of additive white noise on feature selection and classification performance. *Proceedings of SPIE: Image Processing* 6512: 6512–6545.

Peldschus, K., P. Herzog, S. A. Wood, J. I. Cheema, P. Costello, and U. J. Schoepf. 2005. Computer-aided diagnosis as a second reader: Spectrum of findings in CT studies of the chest interpreted as normal. *Chest* 128 (3): 1517–1523.

Pita-Fernandez, S., C. Montero-Martinez, S. Pertega-Diaz, and H. Verea-Hernando. 2003. Relationship between delayed diagnosis and the degree of invasion and survival in lung cancer. *Journal of Clinical Epidemiology* 56 (9): 820–825.

Quarterman, R. L., A. McMillan, M. B. Ratcliffe, and M. I. Block. 2003. Effect of preoperative delay on prognosis for patients with early stage non-small cell lung cancer. *Journal of Thoracic Cardiovascular Surgery* 125 (1): 108,13, Discussion 113–114.

Quekel, L. G., A. G. Kessels, R. Goei, and J. M. van Engelshoven. 1999. Miss rate of lung cancer on the chest radiograph in clinical practice. *Chest* 115 (3): 720–724.

Reeves, A. P., A. B. Chan, D. F. Yankelevitz, C. I. Henschke, B. Kressler, and W. J. Kostis. 2006. On measuring the change in size of pulmonary nodules. *IEEE Transactions on Medical Imaging* 25 (4): 435–450.

Shah, S. K., M. F. McNitt-Gray, S. R. Rogers, J. G. Goldin, R. D. Suh, J. W. Sayre, I. Petkovska, H. J. Kim, and D. R. Aberle. 2005. Computer aided characterization of the solitary pulmonary nodule using volumetric and contrast enhancement features. *Academic Radiology* 12 (10): 1310–1319.

Shiraishi, J., H. Abe, R. Engelmann, M. Aoyama, H. MacMahon, and K. Doi. 2003. Computer-aided diagnosis to distinguish benign from malignant solitary pulmonary nodules on radiographs: ROC analysis of radiologists' performance—Initial experience. *Radiology* 227 (2): 469–474.

Shiraishi, J., H. Abe, F. Li, R. Engelmann, H. MacMahon, and K. Doi. 2006. Computer-aided diagnosis for the detection and classification of lung cancers on chest radiographs ROC analysis of radiologists' performance. *Academic Radiology* 13 (8): 995–1003.

Silvestri, G. A. 2011. Screening for lung cancer: It works, but does it really work? *Annals of Internal Medicine* 155 (8): 537–539.

Spitz, M. R., W. K. Hong, C. I. Amos, X. Wu, M. B. Schabath, Q. Dong, S. Shete, and C. J. Etzel. 2007. A risk model for prediction of lung cancer. *Journal of the National Cancer Institute* 99 (9): 715–726.

Stitik, F. P. and M. S. Tockman. 1978. Radiographic screening in the early detection of lung cancer. *Radiologic Clinics of North America* 16 (3): 347–366.

Stitik, F., M. Tockman, and N. Khouri. 1985. Chest radiology. In *Screening for Cancer*, A. B. Miller (ed.), pp. 163–191. New York: Academic Press.

Swensen, S. J., M. D. Silverstein, D. M. Ilstrup, C. D. Schleck, and E. S. Edell. 1997. The probability of malignancy in solitary pulmonary nodules: Application to small radiologically indeterminate nodules. *Archives of Internal Medicine* 157 (8): 849–855.

Tammemagi, C. M., M. T. Freedman, T. R. Church, M. M. Oken, W. G. Hocking, P. A. Kvale, P. Hu et al. 2007. Factors associated with human small aggressive non small cell lung cancer. *Cancer Epidemiology, Biomarkers & Prevention: A Publication of the American Association for Cancer Research, Cosponsored by the American Society of Preventive Oncology* 16 (10): 2082–2089.

Tammemagi, M. C., M. T. Freedman, P. F. Pinsky, M. M. Oken, P. Hu, T. L. Riley, L. R. Ragard, C. D. Berg, and P. C. Prorok. 2009. Prediction of true positive lung cancers in individuals with abnormal suspicious chest radiographs: A prostate, lung, colorectal, and ovarian cancer screening trial study. *Journal of Thoracic Oncology: Official Publication of the International Association for the Study of Lung Cancer* 4 (6): 710–721.

Tammemagi, C. M., C. Neslund-Dudas, M. Simoff, and P. Kvale. 2004. Lung carcinoma symptoms—An independent predictor of survival and an important mediator of African-American disparity in survival. *Cancer* 101 (7): 1655–1663.

Taylor, K. L., R. Shelby, E. Gelmann, and C. McGuire. 2004. Quality of life and trial adherence among participants in the prostate, lung, colorectal, and ovarian cancer screening trial. *Journal of the National Cancer Institute* 96 (14): 1083–1094.

Theros, E. G. 1977. 1976 caldwell lecture: Varying manifestation of peripheral pulmonary neoplasms: A radiologic-pathologic correlative study. *American Journal of Roentgenology* 128 (6): 893–914.

van Beek, E. J., B. Mullan, and B. Thompson. 2008. Evaluation of a real-time interactive pulmonary nodule analysis system on chest digital radiographic images: A prospective study. *Academic Radiology* 15 (5): 571–575.

van den Bergh, K. A., M. L. Essink-Bot, G. J. Borsboom, E. Th Scholten, M. Prokop, H. J. de Koning, and R. J. van Klaveren. 2010. Short-term health-related quality of life consequences in a lung cancer CT screening trial (NELSON). *British Journal of Cancer* 102 (1): 27–34.

Way, T., H. P. Chan, L. Hadjiiski, B. Sahiner, A. Chughtai, T. K. Song, C. Poopat et al. 2010. Computer-aided diagnosis of lung nodules on CT scans: ROC study of its effect on radiologists' performance. *Academic Radiology* 17 (3): 323–332.

White, C. S., T. Flukinger, J. Jeudy, and J. J. Chen. 2009. Use of a computer-aided detection system to detect missed lung cancer at chest radiography. *Radiology* 252 (1): 273–281.

White, C. S., R. Pugatch, T. Koonce, S. W. Rust, and E. Dharaiya. 2008. Lung nodule CAD software as a second reader: A multicenter study. *Academic Radiology* 15 (3): 326–333.

Yankelevitz, D. F., A. P. Reeves, W. J. Kostis, B. Zhao, and C. I. Henschke. 2000. Small pulmonary nodules: Volumetrically determined growth rates based on CT evaluation. *Radiology* 217 (1): 251–256.

Chapter 25

Clinical Utility of CADe Systems for Colon Cancer

Farid Dahi and Abraham H. Dachman

CONTENTS

Computed tomographic colonography (CTC) is a rapidly developing method that is gaining acceptance for colorectal screening for polyps and masses. Because of variable sensitivities reported for CTC, computer-aided detection and diagnosis (CAD) has been developed to help readers, especially novice readers, and increase the test sensitivity. There are two abbreviations: CADe (computer-aided detection), which refers to the software that looks for only polyp candidates without any histological analysis, and CADx (computer-aided diagnosis), which differentiates benign from malignant lesions (Suzuki and Dachman, 2011). We discuss only CADe in this chapter.

In this chapter, we provide information about colorectal cancer (CRC) epidemiology, pathogenesis, screening methods, and guidelines followed by a brief description of CTC technique, preparation, and major CTC clinical trials, and then we discuss the CADe utility in CTC, CADe clinical trials, false negatives (FNs) and false positives (FPs), and integration of CADe systems into visualization.

25.1 EPIDEMIOLOGY OF COLORECTAL CANCER

CRC is the third most commonly diagnosed cancer in males and the second in females. Over 1.2 million new cancer cases and 608,700 deaths are estimated to have occurred in 2008 (Jemal et al., 2011). Most cases occur in average-risk individuals, those without family or predisposing medical history. Higher incidence has been seen with increased age, male gender, and black race. Among all racial and ethnic subgroups, black persons have the highest incidence and mortality rates from CRC, about double the mortality rate compared with other ethnic minorities (Whitlock et al., 2008). Modifiable risk factors for CRC include smoking, physical inactivity, overweight and obesity, red and processed meat consumption, and excessive alcohol consumption (Jemal et al., 2011). If CRC is diagnosed at an early stage (confined to the wall of the bowel), 5-year survival is 90%; the survival decreases to 68% for regional disease (lymph node involvement) and reaches to 10% if distant metastases are present (Levin et al., 2008).

In terms of geographic distribution, Australia and New Zealand, Europe, and North America have the highest incidence, whereas the lowest rates are reported in Africa and South–Central Asia (Jemal et al., 2011). However, the incidence of CRC is rapidly increasing in some areas previously found to be at low risk, including Spain and several countries within Eastern Asia and Eastern Europe. This may be due to a combination of factors including changes in dietary patterns, obesity, and an increased prevalence of smoking. The United States is the only country with a significant decrease in CRC incidence both in males and in females. In comparison, the CRC incidence in the United States decreased 1.8% per year during the time period between 1985 and 1995 and then stabilized through 2000. Similarly, the CRC death rates have decreased since 1980 because of both reduction in CRC incidence and 5-year survival rate improvement up to 60%. Conversely, the trend in CRC incidence in all European countries showed a steady increase from 1960 to 2006. Therefore, the increase in CRC incidence in Europe together with low 5-year survival rate (<50%) resulted in an increased death rate (Hassan et al., 2011; Jemal et al., 2011). The declining trend in CRC incidence and mortality in the United States likely reflects the effect of reduced exposure to risk factors, screening and early detection and prevention through polypectomy, and treatment improvement. Despite the favorable recent trends reported in the United States, studies have demonstrated that although mortality reduction is dependent on early detection of invasive disease and early removal of adenomatous polyps, a majority of U.S. adults still are not receiving regular age- and risk-appropriate and many have not been screened at all (Levin et al., 2008).

The burden of CRC on society worldwide is related not only to the incidence and mortality rate but also to the huge cost of therapy. Annual CRC-associated expenditure in the United States was estimated to be $8.4 billion in 2005 (with an assumption of $45,000 per CRC treatment), while the treatment costs are increasing as chemotherapy regimens improve (Hassan et al., 2011). Studies published around mid-1920s showed that the achievement of 7 more months of survival (up from 14 to 21 months) through developing new chemotherapy regimens has been resulted in 340-fold increase in the cost of drugs for CRC treatment. Moreover, the total cost of treatment, which was estimated to be $7.49 billion in 2000, is expected to reach $14.03 billion by 2020 (Lansdorp-Vogelaar et al., 2009). This huge expenditure of financial resources could potentially be diverted to implementation of a widespread CRC screening, which result in savings of both life and expense.

25.2 UNDERSTANDING POLYP HISTOLOGY AND SIZE

Colonic polyps are common with a variable nature from benign with no malignancy potential to frank advanced cancers. About 50% of people over age 60 are estimated to have one adenomatous polyp ≥1 cm in size. In a study performed on 100 patients who underwent screening colonoscopy (CSPY), the average age of patients with polyps was 61 years, and 35% were under 60. Among 181 excised polyps, 40% were tubulovillous, 35% tubular, 14% metaplastic, and 1% villous. Low-grade dysplasia was seen in 85%, and 8% showed high-grade dysplasia (HGD; Hunter et al., 2011).

The natural history observed in CRC development in average-risk individuals is the *adenoma–carcinoma sequence*. Adenomas are nonmalignant precursor lesions seen in polypoid (often) pedunculated or flat shapes. Small percentages of these adenomas undergo histological alteration with increased villous component and marked cellular dysplasia, which may eventually progress to adenocarcinoma. A small portion of CRC cases, estimated as 20%–30%, arise directly from the mucosa without adenomatous precursor (Hassan et al., 2011). According to the Paris classification, colorectal neoplasms are classified as polypoid and nonpolypoid (elevated <2.5 mm above the level of mucosa). Nonpolypoid tumors account for <5% of all CRCs. They are hard to detect and may be found during postpolypectomy follow-up (Lorenzo Zúñiga et al., 2011).

A national polyp study performed on 1400 patients with adenomatous polyps showed a decrease of 76%–90% of CRC incidence, 6 years after the removal of all polyps. Several other studies also confirmed the protective effect of polypectomy that suggests the slow progression of polyps to CRC. However, considering the high prevalence of polyps (50%–60% of people over age 50) and low prevalence of CRC (0.1%–1%), only a small fraction of adenomas progress to cancer (Hassan et al., 2011).

Histology and size of polyps are two main determinants of their clinical importance. Concerning the histology, adenomatous polyps that comprise one-half to two-thirds of colorectal polyps are associated with a higher risk for CRC (Levin et al., 2008). A fivefold increased risk of rectal polyps has been reported in patients with HGD compared with the general population (Atkin et al., 1992). Also, a mathematical simulation calculated a conversion rate to CRC of 17% for polyps with HGD vs. 0.25% risk in those with more favorable histology (Gschwantler et al., 2002).

There is a positive relationship between polyp size and presence of unfavorable histology. It has been reported that polyps >10 mm are more prone to accumulate oncogenic mutations compared with smaller lesions, and HGD or malignancy is more prevalent among lesions ≥10 mm (Hassan et al., 2011). Ahlawat et al. demonstrated a 1.72 times greater likelihood for invasive carcinoma in polyps >40 mm compared with polyps between 20 and 40 mm in size (31% vs. 9%, p = 0.02) (Ahlawat et al., 2011). In a systemic review of data from screening cohort studies performed on a total number of 20,562 asymptomatic subjects, the prevalence of advanced adenoma (defined as adenomas with HGD or a prominent villous component) was 5.6%. The frequency of advanced adenoma in patients whose largest polyps were diminutive (≤5 mm), small (6–9 mm), subcentimeter (<10 mm), and large (≥10 mm) was reported as 0.9%, 4.9%, 1.7%, and 73.5% respectively. Furthermore, 95% of subjects with advanced adenomas had polyps ≥6 mm, whereas 88% were seen in patients with polyps >10 mm. Assuming a 5.6% prevalence of advanced adenomas and a 3.3% per year progression of advanced adenomas into cancer (Brenner et al., 2007), the 5-year CRC risk in patients with ≤5, 6–9, and ≥6 mm polyps was calculated as 0.04%, 0.07%, and 0.88%, respectively (Hassan et al., 2010).

25.3 COLORECTAL CANCER SCREENING METHODS

The main purposes of CRC screening, as a secondary prevention, are detection and removal of premalignant lesions and early diagnosis of CRC in its initial stages that result in better survival. Considering the cost for CRC prevention, it compares favorably with other screening plans such as those of breast and cervical cancers (Pignone et al., 2002). There are several screening tests including (1) stool blood tests (g-FOBT and fecal immunochemical test [FIT]), (2) sDNA, (3) flexible sigmoidoscopy (FS), (4) CSPY, (5) double-contrast barium enema (DCBE), and (6) CTC. None of these tests are perfect for either cancer or adenoma detection, and each has shown to have unique advantages, but each also has associated limitations and risks.

25.3.1 Stool Blood Tests: g-FOBT and FIT

Guaiac-based fecal occult blood test (g-FOBT) is the most common CRC screening test, which detects blood in the stool through the pseudoperoxidase activity of hem or hemoglobin. Blood in stool is nonspecific and may originate from large polyps (>1–2 cm) or CRC. The usual protocol consists of a collection of two samples from each of three consecutive bowel movements at home. It is a safe and simple test, but the limitation is low sensitivity under best

circumstances, which may be further reduced by incomplete specimen collection or improper processing and interpretation (Levin et al., 2008). Sensitivity and specificity of g-FOBT for CRC have been reported to be 40% and 97%, respectively, with 7.4% positive predictive value and <20% accuracy for advanced adenoma (Mandel et al., 1993). This limitation could be related to small adenomas, which do not tend to bleed, and due to the intermittent nature of bleeding from CRC or large polyps (Levin et al., 2008). Patients with a positive test are recommended to undergo CSPY, which has reported a 96.5% sensitivity for lesions detected by g-FOBT (Hassan et al., 2011).

FIT, or immunochemical-based i-FOBT, has been suggested for screening more recently, and with more technological advantages, it is specific for human hemoglobin and has more accuracy. The spectrum of benefits, limitations, and harms is similar to g-FOBT, but a higher sensitivity has been reported for i-FOBT for detection of advanced adenoma and cancer compared with g-FOBT (Levin et al., 2008; Hassan et al., 2011). Other advantages include the fact that no restricted diet is required for testing, and because globin is degraded by digestive enzymes in the upper gastrointestinal (GI) tract, FIT is more specific for lower GI bleeding, which improves the specificity. Moreover, for some variants of FIT, stool sampling requires fewer samples or less direct handling of stool (Levin et al., 2008). Despite the limitations of stool blood tests, a review of four randomized controlled trials demonstrated a 16% reduction in the relative risk of CRC mortality through FOBT screening, either g-FOBT or i-FOBT (Hewitson et al., 2011).

25.3.2 sDNA

In sDNA tests, the stool is evaluated for the presence of known DNA alterations during adenoma–carcinoma sequence in the adenoma and carcinoma cells, which are continuously shed into the large bowel. The current available sDNA test requires the entire stool specimen (30 g minimum) to ensure adequate sample of stool for evaluation. Several studies on sDNA test for CRC screening showed that sensitivity ranged from 52% to 91% with specificity ranging from 93% to 97%. Currently, sDNA testing is considered an acceptable option and has been included in CRC screening (Levin et al., 2008).

25.3.3 Flexible Sigmoidoscopy

FS is a safe and relatively painless endoscopy of the distal colon, which has a very low complication rate and is performed with no sedation. The advantage of FS is that it can be performed with a more limited bowel preparation than standard CSPY. The complication of FS, even without performing biopsy or polypectomy, includes colonic perforation, which occurs in <20,000 examinations. The chief limitation of FS is that only the rectum, sigmoid, and descending colon can be evaluated. Also, since no sedation is used, patients experience more discomfort, which results in a greater reluctance to undergo further screening exams (Levin et al., 2008; Hassan et al., 2011). Evidence showed that there is a risk of twofold or higher for proximal colon neoplasia if a patient has an adenoma of any size in the distal colon (Imperiale et al., 2000; Lieberman and Weiss, 2001). Moreover, in recent studies, FS was able to detect over 70% of advanced neoplasia throughout the colon in male patients who underwent CSPY after FS found any adenoma in the distal colon (Lieberman et al., 2000). Despite several studies that showed reduction in CRC mortality by screening with FS, there is still a concern for missing right-sided lesions that are not seen with FS (Hassan et al., 2011).

25.3.4 Colonoscopy

CSPY is widely performed in the United States. The entire colon can be directly inspected, and any suspected lesion can be biopsied or removed (polypectomy) during the same procedure. In a comparison study between CSPY and FS, CRC incidence reduction reported is 60% for CSPY compared with 40% for FS (Winawer et al., 1993). One of the CSPY limitations is the need for full bowel preparation, which requires one or more days of dietary preparation and bowel cleansing. Also, due to sedation, patients need a chaperone for transportation after the procedure. After all, it is an invasive procedure, and according to surveys, most adults prefer other noninvasive options for CRC screening. Complications may be perforation, postpolypectomy hemorrhage, and subsequent hospitalization. The risk of perforation increases with age and the presence of diverticular disease (Levin et al., 2008). Despite all limitations, CSPY allows a full structural evaluation of the colon and rectum. Patients at average risk for CRC who are screened with CSPY have a 0.05%–1% chance of colon cancer, and 5%–10% have advanced neoplasia, which can be detected and removed during the procedure (Hassan et al., 2011).

25.3.5 Double-Contrast Barium Enema

DCBE, which has been adopted as a CRC screening option, evaluates the entire colon after coating the mucosal surface with high-density barium and distending the colon with air through a flexible catheter inserted into the rectum. The procedure requires bowel preparation through a 24 h dietary and laxative regimen. There is no sedation, and the whole procedure takes 20–40 min on average. The advantage of DCBE is its potential to evaluate the entire colon especially when CSPY has failed or is contraindicated. Studies reported a sensitivity of 85%–97% for CRC detection. Some limitations include need for extensive colonic preparation, discomfort in some patients during and after the procedure, no opportunity for biopsy or polypectomy, and being operator dependent. Overall, it is relatively safe, and the risk of perforation is 1 of 25,000 compared with 1 of 1,000–2,000 for CSPY. If any polyp >6 mm is found on DCBE, the patient should undergo CSPY (Levin et al., 2008). In the United States, the number of DCBEs performed has dropped making it increasingly difficult to train new residents.

25.3.6 CT Colonography

CTC, also referred to as virtual CSPY, has been rapidly developing since its introduction in the mid-1990s. It is a minimally invasive imaging modality for the evaluation of the entire colon and rectum. Helical CT images are used to create standard axial and reformatted two-dimensional (2D) and three-dimensional (3D) images of the colon. It provides the visualization of 3D endoscopic flight paths through the inside of the colon accompanied with simultaneous interactive 2D images, which allows polyp detection and characterization of lesion density and location. A limited evaluation of extracolonic structures is also possible through 2D images. The residual stool and fluid are tagged with barium and/or iodine oral contrast agents. Also, bowel preparation and gaseous distention of the colon through a CO_2 insufflator are required for a successful examination (Levin et al., 2008).

The advantages of CTC are time efficient, minimally invasive, and no sedation is utilized, so the patient can return to work on the same day. In terms of radiation exposure, the standard CTC results in a radiation dose of 4–10 mSV, which is much lower than the threshold defined for the health effects of low-dose radiation (50–100 mSV). However, there is controversy over the potential harm of long-term radiation dose effect (Nadel et al., 2005; Levin et al., 2008). Recently, dose reductions in CTC have dropped the exam dose to 2–4 mSV. There are some limitations for CTC. It requires full bowel preparation, although reduced (or non-) cathartic preparations have been successfully employed (Johnson et al., 2011). Therapeutic intervention is not possible, so the patient should be referred to CSPY if a suspected lesion is detected. In such cases, same-day polypectomy can be offered to avoid the need for additional bowel preparation. Moreover, reimbursement for CTC screening is limited and is mostly offered for diagnostic CTC where the clinical indication is limited to incomplete CSPY (Levin et al., 2008). Knudsen et al. used microsimulation models to evaluate the cost-effectiveness of CTC screening for CRC. They showed that if CTC screening was reimbursed at $488 per scan (slightly less than the reimbursement for a CSPY without polypectomy), it would be the most costly strategy (Knudsen et al., 2010). Cost-effectiveness studies are highly subject to the input variables that often do not take into account the cost of FP biopsies and their complications and sometimes use outdated data for the exam performance features of CTC. For example, when diminutive polyps are not reported, CTC was found to be the most cost-effective and safest screening option (Pickhardt et al., 2007). Patient acceptance of CTC has been excellent.

Despite reimbursement limitations, a growth of adoption of CTC by U.S. hospitals has been reported as 17% in 2008 compared with 13% in 2005. Motivating factors included elderly patients and patients with failed CSPY, long waiting list for CSPY, desire to provide an alternative screening option for frail patients, and promising evidence on CTC in literature (McHugh et al., 2011). Currently, there is a consensus that all patients with one or more polyps ≥10 mm or three or more polyps ≥6 mm should be referred for CSPY. There is still controversy for referring patients with <3 polyps in which the largest polyp is 6–9 mm (Levin et al., 2008).

25.4 COLORECTAL CANCER SCREENING GUIDELINES

There are two independent and updated guidelines for CRC screening, first proposed by a joint commission formed by the American Cancer Society (ACS), the US Multisociety Task Force on Colorectal Cancer, and the American College of Radiology (Levin et al., 2008). The second was prepared by US Preventive Services Task Force (USPSTF) (Whitlock et al., 2008). The main difference between the two screening guidelines is that USPSTF does not recommend stool test and CTC because of their varying degrees of uncertainty. Regarding CTC, the authors of USPTF guidelines decided not to include CTC largely based on low positive predictive value reported by the American College of Radiology Imaging Network (ACRIN) study, limitation in detection polyps <10 mm, the risk of radiation, and extracolonic findings. However, the authors of first guideline found ACRIN study data adequate for the acceptance of CTC for large polyps. Indeed, the ACS has focused on CRC incidence reduction as a high priority by emphasizing the role of sensitivity over all other variables. In contrast, USPTF guidelines tend to emphasize the specificity of the tests (Hassan et al., 2011).

The ACS guidelines have two phases. The first phase focuses on the stool tests (g-FOBT, FIT, and sDNA), and the second phase focuses on the structural exams (CSPY, FS, DCBE, and CTC). The target population is average-risk individuals over the age 50. The important factors for selecting screening tests are availability of resources and patient preferences. Some patients are not willing to undergo invasive tests, are not comfortable with bowel preparation, or may prefer to do screening in the privacy of their home. Also, there may be limited access to invasive tests. Therefore, all options and their risks and benefits should be discussed with patients. The recommended repetition intervals for average-risk individuals between 50

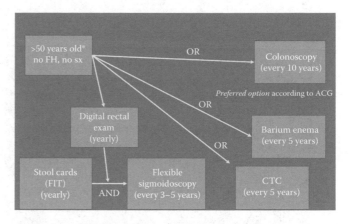

Figure 25.1 Recommendations for screening for CRC for average-risk individuals based on the multiple society guidelines (American Gastroenterological Association and American Cancer Society). *African Americans start at 45 per ACG. (From Levin, B. et al., *Gastroenterology*, 134(5), 1570, 2008; Rex, D.K. et al., *Am. J. Gastroenterol.*, 104(3), 739, 2009, doi: 10.1038/ajg.2009.104.)

and 80 years old are 10 years for CSPY; 5 years for sigmoidoscopy, CTC, and DCBE; and 1 year for both g-FOBT and i-FOBT (Figure 25.1). There are also different guidelines for screening and surveillance for adenomas and CRC in people at increased or high risk. Individuals at increased risk are those that have a history of adenomatous polyps, a personal history of curative-intent resection of CRC, or colorectal adenomas diagnosed in a first-degree relative before 60 years. High-risk group includes individuals with a history of inflammatory bowel disease of significant duration or patients having either/both of familial adenomatous polyposis and hereditary nonpolyposis colon cancer (Levin et al., 2008).

25.5 PATIENT PREPARATION AND EXAM TECHNIQUE

To have persistent high-quality CTC examinations several factors before the exam are required to be considered, such as proper patient preparation and tagging. Currently, there is no single best suggested method for preparation and tagging, and controversies are mostly about diet, timing, and duration of bowel preparation. A combination of cathartic and purgation cleansing and some form of fecal tagging has shown high performance in large clinical trials (Pickhardt and Choi, 2003; Johnson et al., 2008b).

Some centers recommend fiber-restricted diet for 1–2 days before exam to reduce the amount of stool in colon. Also for further cleaning, liquid diet (water, juice, broth, popsicles, and Jell-O) has been suggested, for at most 1 day before the exam. Cathartic preparation has been described by patients as one of the most unpleasant portions of bowel

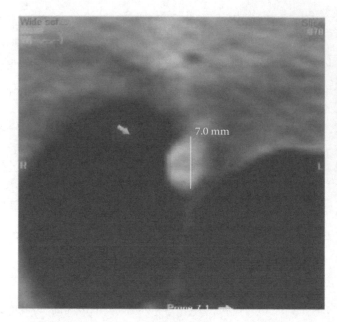
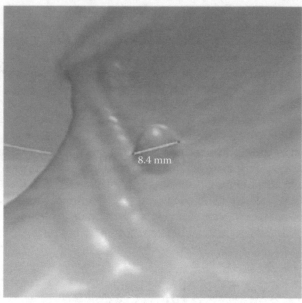

Figure 25.2   Density of polyp can be confused for tagging, particularly with an intermediate soft tissue window/level setting. Although the polyp's density is similar to muscle, by narrowing the windows, it will look denser. Weak tagging of stool and fluid can cause densities that overlap between stool and true polyps.

preparation (Ristvedt et al., 2003; van Gelder et al., 2004). Several cathartic formulations are available, including (1) polyethylene glycol (PEG)–based electrolyte solution, which is an iso-osmolar nonabsorbable solution, and is required to ingest a large amount of 2 or 4 L orally, which may reduce patient compliance. Therefore, many centers prefer to use other cathartics or at least a reduced form of PEG solution (HalfLytely), which does not contain sulfate and requires only 2 L of ingestion. (2) Bisacodyl sodium, a stimulatory cathartic, often used combined with other cathartics (PEG, sodium phosphate, and magnesium phosphate). (3) Sodium phosphate, which is a hyperosmolar agent and draws fluid from circulation into the bowel. A small dose of 45 or 90 mL is used. Due to the risk of acute phosphate nephropathy, it is no longer available as an over-the-counter drug and is accessible only by prescription in a tablet form. (4) Magnesium citrate is hyperosmolar and contains 18 g of magnesium citrate and very low sodium, so it is preferred for patients susceptible to electrolyte imbalances from fluid shifts (Lenhart et al., 2011).

In regards to fecal and fluid tagging, retained stool and fluid are tagged by consuming a small amount of either barium- or iodine-based contrast material (1–2 days prior to CTC) in order to be distinguished from polyps. Since the radiopaque contrast does not incorporate into polyps, they show soft tissue attenuation in cross-sectional view, while fluid and feces demonstrate a high attenuation. A key factor to have a better visualization and fewer artifacts

is the dilution of contrast material. Both very dilute and concentrate contrasts yield to inappropriate digital subtraction and presence of artifacts or missing true polyps (Figure 25.2). Barium sulfate agents are in forms of 2% or 2.1% concentrations. Since they have lower water solubility, they have limited ability to tag fluid, but they tag stool very well. Therefore, they are usually used with ionic iodine-based agents for a better tagging. Ionic iodine-based agents consist of diatrizoate meglumine and diatrizoate sodium. Due to hyperosmolarity, they may cause diarrhea and cramps. To overcome this issue, nonionic iodine-based agents with lower osmolarity were introduced, such as iopromide, iohexol, and iodixanol (Lenhart et al., 2011).

In general, appropriate bowel preparation is essential for a meticulous CTC examination. Several studies have been working on different techniques for preparation and tagging concerning the contrast dose, timing, etc., in order to get closer to patient acceptance and compliance (Faccioli et al., 2011; Liedenbaum et al., 2011a).

25.6   KEY CLINICAL TRIALS

Since the introduction of CTC in the early 1990s, there have been several studies mostly focused on the capability of CTC compared with CSPY. The main concern was whether CTC could demonstrate a polyp that had been identified through CSPY, and if so, was there any size threshold? And could it be used as a new screening tool? (Geertruyden et al., 2011). The earliest clinical trials for screening appeared in peer-reviewed literature in 1997 and 1998 (Royster et al., 1997; Dachman et al., 1998). Subsequent early clinical trials yielded mixed results. Some reported high sensitivity of >90% for the detection of polyps >1 cm, but they were countered by other less appealing results. The discrepancy among the results of various studies was due to the type of patient cohort, training and experience of readers, and 2D vs. 3D image analysis techniques (McFarland et al., 2011). In 1999, Felon et al. demonstrated a sensitivity of 90% for polyps ≥6 mm and 67% for those ≤5 mm for CTC screening of 100 cases who were at high risk for CRC. Residual stool, diverticular disease, poor colonic distention, and thickened haustral folds were the most common causes of FPs (Fenlon et al., 1999).

In a meta-analysis performed in 2003, the results of 14 studies were evaluated and showed per-patient sensitivity of 65% and per-polyp sensitivity of 43% for polyps ≤5 mm. The numbers were higher as the polyps' sizes increased. Per-patient sensitivities for polyps sized 6–9 and ≥10 mm were 84% and 88%, and per-polyp sensitivities were 62% and 81%, respectively. The overall specificity was reported as 95% (Sosna et al., 2003). At the same year, the US Department of Defense's (DOD) large multicenter study not only demonstrated an impressive result but also introduced two novel CTC techniques, which were fecal tagging and primary use of 3D *fly-through* polyp detection. Previously, 3D views were reserved only for problem solving. They performed CRC screening of 1233 asymptomatic adults with CTC followed by same-day CSPY. For polyps ≥10 mm, per-patient sensitivity and specificity were 93.8% and 96%, respectively, while the calculated sensitivity of CSPY for the same patients was 87.5%. Per-patient sensitivity and specificity for polyps 8–10 mm were 93.9% and 92.2%, respectively, compared with 91.5% sensitivity of CSPY for similar-sized polyps. For polyps sized 6–8 mm, per patient sensitivity and specificity were 88.7% and 79.6%, respectively. Sensitivity of CSPY for the same group was 92.3% (Geertruyden et al., 2011).

The results of DOD were reinforced by a larger trial performed by ACRIN. Two thousand and six hundred asymptomatic patients 50 years or older were involved in this trial. Similar to DOD study, they employed stool and fluid tagging and mechanical insufflation. They used multidetector-row CT scanners (≥ 16 rows). Fifteen expert radiologists reviewed the cases. The main goal was to detect histologically confirmed large (≥10 mm) adenomas and adenocarcinomas that had been detected by CSPY. Also, detection rate for polyps between 6 and 9 mm was evaluated. Per-patient sensitivity and specificity of CTC for polyps ≥10 mm were 90% and 86%, respectively. For smaller polyps, the size-stratified per-patient sensitivities were reported as 90%, 87%, 84%, and

78% for lesions ≥9, ≥8, ≥7, and ≥6 mm, respectively. For the same size series, per-patient specificities were 86%, 87%, 87%, and 88%, respectively (Johnson et al., 2008a). In a comparison study, Graser et al. compared the sensitivity of CTC with CSPY for the detection of advanced colonic neoplasia in 307 average-risk adults. They showed a sensitivity of 96.7% for CTC compared with 100% for CSPY (Graser et al., 2008).

Most recent studies also provided favorable results for CTC screening. de Haan et al. performed a meta-analysis on prospective CTC clinical trials and cohort studies in individuals who were predominantly (≥95%) average risk and over 50 years old. The estimated per-patient sensitivity and specificity of CTC for adenomas ≥6 mm were 82.95% and 91.4% in asymptomatic adults. The estimated per-patient sensitivity and specificity for adenomas ≥10 mm were 87.9% and 97.6%, respectively. For colorectal polyps, the estimated sensitivity and specificity were slightly lower. Also, all CRC cases were detected by CTC. In comparing with CSPY, they concluded that CTC provides a good sensitivity for advanced adenomas ≥10 mm and somewhat lower sensitivity for adenomas ≥6 mm (de Haan et al., 2011). Moreover, Regge et al. evaluated the performance of CTC in a population of 937 individuals who were at increased risk of CRC (with family history of advanced neoplasia in first-degree relatives, personal history of colorectal adenomas, or FOBT positive test). They found a sensitivity of 85.3% for CTC in the detection of advanced neoplasia 6 mm or larger in size. Also, they reported an overall negative predictive value of 96.3% (Regge et al., 2009).

Although there are many reports favoring CTC potentials for CRC screening, it should be taken into account that *training* plays a great role in CTC sensitivity. Several studies highlighted the importance of training on readers performance (Dachman et al., 2008; Fletcher et al., 2010; Haycock et al., 2010; Liedenbaum et al., 2011b). Fletcher et al. demonstrated significantly improved performance in inexperienced radiologists (defined interpretations for fewer than 500 CTC examinations correlated with CSPY) after a 1-day educational course (Fletcher et al., 2010). Dachman et al. also performed a formative evaluation of the effect of a 1-day comprehensive training program on seven novice readers. After training, 60 cases were interpreted by participants, which resulted in an overall high sensitivity and good specificity. For polyps ≥10 mm, mean sensitivity and specificity were 98% and 92%, respectively (Dachman et al., 2008).

High sensitivity for CRC is crucial for both asymptomatic screening and symptomatic patients. Although, a 10-fold difference in cancer prevalence has been reported between asymptomatic screening and symptomatic study population (<0.5% vs. 6%), the sensitivity of CTC has shown to remain high regardless of disease prevalence (Pickhardt et al., 2011). Despite the evidence of high sensitivities for CTC screening, there are still variations in numbers across different studies. CADe systems have evolved to help reduce the inconsistency (Yoshida and Näppi, 2007). A standard comprehensive training may also reduce inter-reader variability in interpretation accuracy.

25.7 PRIMARY, SECONDARY, AND CONCURRENT CADe USE

CADe has been developed for CTC as a potential tool to increase diagnostic accuracy in the detection of polyps, decrease reader variability, and reduce interpretation time by focusing only on regions highlighted by CADe (i.e., a first reader) or mainly on the small number of regions suggested by CADe. The most common problems in CTC interpretation include failure to detect a polyp that is visible in retrospect, and also mischaracterizing a polyp candidate as stool or fold. CADe automatically detects polyps in CTC and marks the suspected areas in CTC for the reader's review. It is particularly helpful in finding polyp candidates ≥6 mm (Suzuki and Dachman, 2011). CADe has been expected to overcome the problem of variable detection sensitivity and high interobserver variance in CTC. Several CADe systems have been reported to detect retrospectively visible colorectal lesions in CTC with high sensitivity and shown a high potential to increase the detection sensitivity and reduce interobserver variance of human readers, especially in inexperienced readers (Näppi and Nagata, 2011).

There are three different reading paradigms with using CADe. In the *secondary-reader* paradigm, which is the classic CADe implementation, CADe is applied after the case is thoroughly read. By reviewing CADe hits, missed abnormalities during unassisted reading may be revealed. The interpretation time increases in this mode. The other paradigm is *concurrent reader*, in which the CADe hits are revealed initially and the reader performs a full read with the CADe marks shown on the screen. The last paradigm, *primary reader*, means the reader first goes through CADe hits to evaluate if they are true positives (TPs) or FPs and then he/she reads the remaining areas for any additional findings.

As a comparison, the primary-reader paradigm introduces the most bias since the areas suggested by CADe allows reader to have less vigilance for a comprehensive evaluation, which results in a lower sensitivity. This may also happen in the secondary-reader paradigm since the reader expects the CADe hits to be revealed later (Suzuki and Dachman, 2011). Using CADe as a concurrent reader is more time efficient than secondary reader, and it showed similar sensitivity for polyps 6 mm or larger. However, secondary-reader mode maximizes sensitivity, particularly for smaller lesions (Taylor et al., 2008). Most researchers recommend using CADe in second-reader mode, which provides a less biased interpretation. In our opinion, a comprehensive read should be done, regardless of the CADe output.

Recommended steps for CTC reading are (1) reading the case using CADe as a second-reader mode. A primary 3D fly-through is fast and can be done in each direction on both supine and prone to maximize polyp detection; (2) searching for flat lesions, large masses, and in segments not well seen on 3D by using 2D images; and (3) turning CADe off and evaluating each CADe polyp candidate, as necessary using lesion texture, interactive window/level adjustment, multi-planar 2D image comparison (MPR), 2D–3D image comparison, or supine–prone comparison.

25.8 CTC CADe OBSERVER TRIALS

Several studies have shown that CADe improves the readers performance not only in the detection of easy and difficult polyps but in the detection of polyps missed by readers as well (Suzuki and Dachman, 2011). In one of these studies, four observers with different levels of reading skills (two experienced radiologists, a gastroenterologist, and a radiology resident) read 20 CTC scans (including 11 polyps 5–12 mm in size) without and with CADe. The detection rate increased for all readers after using CADe, regardless of their reading skill. The areas under receiver operating characteristic (ROC) curve (AUCs) before and after using CADe were 0.70 and 0.85, respectively. This value was the largest for the gastroenterologist. The study results indicated that CADe can improve human reader performance (Okamura et al., 2004).

In a similar study, Mang et al. evaluated the efficacy of CADe on the performance of readers with different levels of expertise. Four radiologists (two were expert and two were inexperienced in CTC) independently evaluated a total of 52 CTC patient datasets (37 patients with 55 endoscopically confirmed polyps ≥0.5 cm and 7 cancers; 15 patients with no abnormalities) in second-reader mode. Their performance was analyzed with and without the supplemented use of CADe through the calculation of sensitivity and reading time. The overall sensitivity of two expert readers increased from 91% each to 96% (p = 0.25) and 93% (p = 1), when CADe was integrated as a second reader. Overall detection rates for two nonexpert readers increased significantly from 76% to 91% (P = 0.008) and from 75% to 95% (P = 0.001). However, CADe findings had no influence on the performance of all four readers in the detection of carcinomas. CADe increased reading time by an average of 2.1 min. The study highlighted the potential role of CADe as a second reader to increase polyp detection rates especially for nonexpert readers. The low detection rate was seen in stenotic carcinomas, which indicated the need for improvement in CADe algorithm before wide clinical application (Mang et al., 2007).

Petrick et al. designed a screening cohort on 60 patients to evaluate the benefit of using CADe in a second-reader mode to investigate only neoplastic polyps (size ranges: 6 mm or larger, 6–9 and 10 mm or larger). Four radiologists initially read CTCs without CADe, then CADe hits were revealed and they were allowed to reconsider and modify their initial diagnosis. All four radiologists achieved higher performance using CADe with the increased sensitivity by 0.15, 0.16, and 0.14 for respective groups, with a corresponding decrease in the specificity of 0.14. They concluded that by using CADe as a second reader, there would be an increased sensitivity and decreased specificity for detecting polyps ≥6 and 6–9 mm in size (Petrick et al., 2008).

The largest multicase, multireader trial was performed on 100 CSPY cases in which 19 readers were included to assess the effect of CADe (as a second reader) on readers' accuracy (Dachman et al., 2010). The 100 cases were from screening CTC examinations but chosen to enrich the number of patients with polyps such that the ratio of small-to-large polyps was 3:2. The final sample of 52 positive patients included 35 patients with polyps ≥6 mm and no polyps ≥10 mm and 17 patients with polyps ≥10 mm (four with one and one with two synchronous 6–9 mm polyps) and 48 negative patients. The polyps ranged in size from 6 to 20 mm. Among the 52 patients with polyps, there were a total of 74 polyps in 65 colon segments. Fifty-three polyps were sessile, thirteen pedunculated, and eight flat. There were 36 patients with adenomatous polyps with 47 adenomatous polyps in 44 colon segments. Thirty-two of the adenomatous polyps were small (6–9 mm) and 15 large (≥10 mm). There were 48 negative cases. Nineteen blinded readers interpreted each case with and without using a commercial CADe system (VeraLook, iCAD, Inc.) (a total of 200 readings for each reader). ROC curve analysis was performed in segment level and patient level. The readers' average segment-level AUC with CADe was significantly higher than the average AUC in unassisted group. Higher reading accuracy was seen in 68% of readers. Readers' per-segment, per-patient, and per-polyp sensitivities were higher for all polyps ≥6 mm (P < 0.011, 0.007, and 0.005, respectively) in CADe-assisted group compared with unassisted (0.517 vs. 0.465, 0.521 vs. 0.466, and 0.477 vs. 0.422, respectively). Also, a higher sensitivity was seen in patients with at least one large polyp ≥10 mm with CADe than without (0.777 vs. 0.743). The average reader sensitivity improved by >0.08 for small adenomas. Although there was a small reduction of 0.025 in specificity (p = 0.050) and increase in reading time, the CADe system resulted in a significant improvement in overall reader performance. The software used had been first *trained* on a separate cohort of 437 cases and then tested on 355 cases (184 with positive findings and 171 with negative findings). In a stand-alone testing, the CADe was 94.4% sensitive for patients with at least one polyp >10 mm and 90.2% sensitive for patient with small polyps between 6 and 10 mm. The average number of false marks for all cases with positive findings was 5.07 and 4.08 for negative cases.

In another large-scale study, 10 readers trained in CT (without special expertise in CTC) interpreted 107 CTC cases first with and then without CADe after temporal separation of 2 months. There were 142 polyps overall (62 polyps ≥6 mm) in 60 patients, 14 patients with a polyp ≥10 mm, 40 patients with a polyp ≥6 mm, and 26 patients with polyps 6–9 mm. Per-patient sensitivity increased significantly for 70% of CADe-assisted readers. Per-polyp sensitivity also increased significantly. Small (≤5 mm) and medium-sized (6–9 mm) polyps were significantly more likely to be detected when prompted correctly by CADe. However, overall performance was relatively poor; even with CADe, and on average, readers detected only 10 polyps (51.0%) ≥10 mm and 24 (38.2%) ≥6 mm. The results showed that despite the higher detection rate by using CADe as a supporting tool, CADe cannot substitute for adequate CTC training since the inexperienced readers did not achieve a satisfactory outcome even with CADe (Halligan et al., 2006).

25.9   CADe OBSERVER FALSE-NEGATIVE AND FALSE-POSITIVE INTERPRETATION

CADe has shown a high sensitivity in stand-alone trials (Yoshida et al., 2002; Bogoni et al., 2005; Summers et al., 2005; Park et al., 2009; Lawrence et al., 2010). When employed by human readers, the reader may accept or reject a CADe hit; thus, the ultimate benefit of CADe depends on whether it helps or hinders the radiologist interpreting the exam (Petrick et al., 2008; Taylor et al., 2009). The knowledge of the most common causes of CADe FNs and FPs may help readers to have a more accurate interpretation of CADe hits.

25.9.1   CADe False Negatives

CADe FNs are typically similar to radiologists. CADe techniques mostly depend on shape analysis. Cap-like shapes or lesions protruding substantially into the lumen are considered polypoid lesions. Therefore, CADe systems can be confused when they encounter diminutive (<5 mm), small (5–9 mm), and flat polyps, since they lose their margin due to partial volume effect. Also, large lesions with a significant deviated shape from polypoid can result in FNs. Other possibilities include polyps located in collapsed region on the colon or submerged in fluid (untagged) (Yoshida and Näppi, 2007).

CADe techniques for lesion detection play an important role in reducing FNs, which results in a higher sensitivity. Suzuki and colleagues at the University of Chicago evaluated their CADe scheme, massive-training artificial neural network (MTANN) scheme, in the detection of polyps that were missed by human reader due to the perceptual errors. Twenty-four FN cases (who had at least one missed polyp) with twenty-three polyps were included. Polyp sizes ranged from 6 to 15 mm, with an average of 8.3 mm. An experienced radiologist reviewed the CTC cases and determined the locations of polyps with reference to a CSPY report and also determined the difficulty in detection for each polyps/mass as difficult, moderate, and easy. Both conventional CADe scheme with linear discriminant analysis (LDA) and MTANN scheme were applied. MTANN CADe scheme achieved a sensitivity of 58% (14/24) with 8.6 FPs per patient for 24 missed lesions, while conventional LDA scheme showed a sensitivity of 25% at the same FP rate. Analyzing the polyps detected by MTANN CADe scheme, in terms of difficulty category, showed that it would be helpful in the detection of *difficult* polyps (Suuzuk et al., 2010).

25.9.2 CADe False Positives

Despite the great advantages of current CADe schemes for improving polyp detection, still one of the major limitations is a relatively large number of FPs that tend to be much more than FPs reported by human readers (Roehrig, 2005). This could confound the reader interpretation and may lead to unnecessary further workup. Knowledge about the patterns of CADe FPs helps readers to ignore them during image interpretation. Most of the FPs detected by CADe systems are easy to differentiate from true lesions, and only 10%–20% are challenging to dismiss (Yoshida and Näppi, 2007). In a recent analysis of 50 cases, the incidence of various causes of CADe FPs is shown in Table 25.1 (Dachman et al., 2010, Appendix).

The most common causes of CADe FPs are thickened haustral folds and retained stool (Yoshida and Näppi, 2007). Thickened haustral folds can be caused by suboptimal colon distention or sigmoid muscular hypertrophy. Looking at nearby folds helps to dismiss as FP if they have similar appearance to the detected fold. Other challenging folds include nodular folds, which may be caused by movement or reconstruction artifacts and convergence of two or more normal folds (Figure 25.3). Reconciliation between 2D and 3D views helps for a confident differentiation (Näppi and Nagata, 2011).

Untagged or poorly tagged stool is also a significant source of CADe FPs. In such cases, internal mottled texture pattern or irregular angulated contour can allow recognition as a FP. Also, internal diffuse gas or internal positive contrast tagging may be seen in 2D view with an optimal soft tissue window-level setting or 3D view with a translucency or color map tool. It is important not to confuse enhancement of internal density that favors for tagged stool with a lesion covered by a layer of tagging (O'Connor et al., 2006;

TABLE 25.1   ANALYSIS OF SOURCES OF CADe FPS IN 50 CASES

	Prone View	Supine View
No. of FPs	224	210
Colonic fold	94 (42.0%)	69 (32.9%)
Small bump <6 mm	36 (16.1%)	24 (11.4%)
Ileocecal valve	29 (13.0%)	36 (17.1%)
Poor distension	14 (6.3%)	19 (9.1%)
Stool	11 (4.9%)	6 (2.9%)
Rectal tube	2 (0.9%)	1 (0.5%)
Flexural pseudotumor	1 (0.5%)	3 (1.4%)
Extrinsic compression	1 (0.5%)	0
Fluid artifact	1 (0.5%)	8 (3.8%)
Motion artifact	1 (0.5%)	0
Other	34 (15.2%)	44 (21.0%)
Easy to dismiss FP	156 (69.6%)	160 (76.2%)
Average difficulty to dismiss	62 (27.7%)	47 (22.4%)
Hard to dismiss	6 (2.7%)	3 (1.4%)

Source: Dachman, A.H., et al., *Radiology*, 256, 827, 2010.

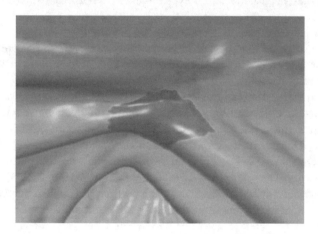

Figure 25.3   CADe FP caused by convergence of folds.

Näppi and Nagata, 2011). Moreover, visual correspondence analysis between prone and supine views helps to distinguish polyps from stool, if the stool is mobile (Figure 25.4) (Yoshida and Näppi, 2007).

Other sources of CADe FPs include (1) ileocecal valve (ICV), which is a frequent source of CADe FPs, but it is relatively easy to dismiss because of its characteristic image pattern and location near cecum. However, there might be challenging cases due to variation of the ICV shape and density, polyps growing on ICVs, or lesions imitating the shape of ICV. Therefore, readers should confirm the location and extent of the true ICV when reviewing CADe detection similar to the ICV (Figure 25.5c and d)

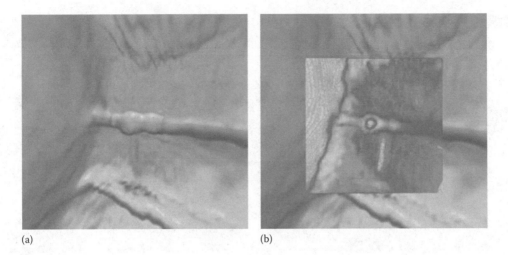

Figure 25.4   (See color insert.) CADe reader FP caused by a small focus of tagged stool. (a) CADe detected a small raised area caused by stool on a fold. In the translucency view (b), a color map of the HU distribution shows central white consistent with tagged stool. This should have been recognized by the reader. Stool may be correctly identified by internal gas, tagging, or movement when comparing supine and prone views.

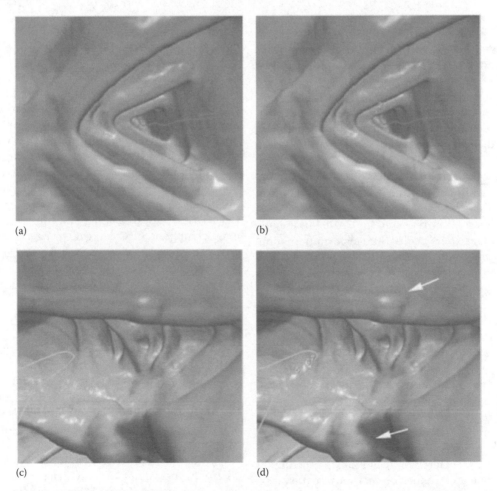

Figure 25.5   (See color insert.) Top panel (a) (CADe off) and (b) (CADe on) show two FP marks on a shallow or <5 mm diminutive foci. The bottom panel ((c) with CADe off and (d) with CADe on) show a true-positive polyp on the apex of a fold (upper arrow) and fatty ileocecal valve (lower arrow).

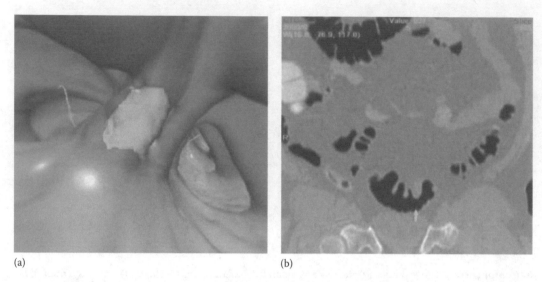

(a)   (b)

Figure 25.6   (See color insert.) CADe FP caused by *flexural pseudotumor*. (a) Endoluminal view and (b) coronal 2D view show (arrow) a prominent fold mimicking a polyp at the inside of a sharp turn in the sigmoid colon. Note how all the adjacent folds appear thinner and normal.

(Näppi and Nagata, 2011). (2) Electrical cleansing (EC), which is subtracting tagged materials (as a potential source of FPs) before the application of the CADe, can also result in a large number of small residual subtraction artifacts (Cai et al., 2008) and more FPs. Therefore, the application of EC with CADe may be limited to the detection of larger lesion and/or to cathartic bowel preparations with clearly tagged fluid (Näppi and Nagata, 2011). (3) Rectal tubes are other sources for CADe FPs that are easy to dismiss, but readers should still be cautious and confirm that detected area is not caused by a true adjacent lesion. (4) Other potential sources reported for CADe FPs include small bumps (Figure 25.5a and b), extrinsic compression, extracolonic regions, anal papillae, flexural pseudotumors (Figure 25.6), high-density objects within abdomen such as hip prosthesis, diverticular fecaliths, movement artifacts such as peristalsis, coarse mucosa, sharp turns or bending of the colon, and inverted diverticula. In many of them, reconciliation between 2D and 3D views and between different scan views helps to dismiss CADe FPs (Näppi and Nagata, 2011).

To reduce CADe FPs, several methods have been developed based on 3D pattern processing (Göktürk et al., 2001), volumetric features (Näppi and Yoshida, 2002), supine–prone correspondence (Näppi et al., 2005), quadratic discriminant analysis (Acar et al., 2002), standard neural network (ANN) (Jerebko et al., 2003), etc. Suzuki et al. also developed a FP reduction technique called mixture of 3D MTANNs to reduce various types of FPs such as rectal tubes, stool, haustral folds, and ICV (Suzuki et al., 2006, 2008).

25.10   INTEGRATION OF CADe INTO VISUALIZATION

For practical use, CADe output must be integrated into clinical workflow in a user-friendly fashion (Figures 25.7a and 25.8). The first step is the integration of CTC and postprocessed images into picture archive and communication system (PACS). Current workstations provide 2D multiplanar reconstruction views with a real-time 3D view with endoluminal fly-through capability. For CADe implementation, recently developed computer networks allow the original digital imaging and communications in medicine, compliant CTC images, to be transmitted to PACS gateway, where they are routed to a CADe server for lesion detection. The CADe processing software is most commonly integrated into the visualization computer. Sometimes, it can be a separate computer connected to the visualization computer to permit rapid simultaneous processing, and reading of cases is a busy CTC practice. CADe processing can also be done in web-based applications as can visualization software.

The reader can see CADe-detected areas, *CADe marks*, in the form of color-highlighted areas or arrows pointing to polyp candidates on 2D and 3D views (Figure 25.7b and c). Different options are available on different software programs. Some provide a list of polyp candidates, which the user can toggle through sequentially by mouse click or keyboard hot key and then problem-solve and mark as a TP or reject as an FP. Some software also shows the polyp diameter and volume. The CADe evaluation can then be integrated into the visualization reporting software.

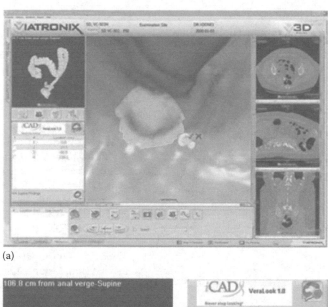

(a)

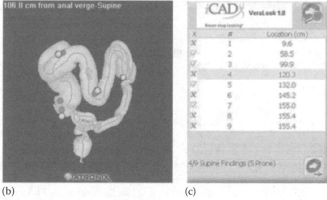

(b)   (c)

Figure 25.7   (See color insert.) (a) CADe integrated into visualization software. CADe marks displayed as *Blue Caps* on the virtual colon wall in the 3D view. The green checkmark and red "X" marks displayed near each CADe mark in the 3D view enable users to accept or reject CADe marks as polyps. CADe marks are displayed as yellow circles on image slices in the 2D views. (b) CADe marks are displayed as yellow circles on the *full colon* view. (c) CADe findings are numbered and displayed in a list that indicates the distance from the anal verge and whether or not each CADe mark has been accepted or rejected as a polyp. The icon to the right of the logo enables users to toggle CADe marks on/off (defaulted off), as does the "C" key on the keyboard.

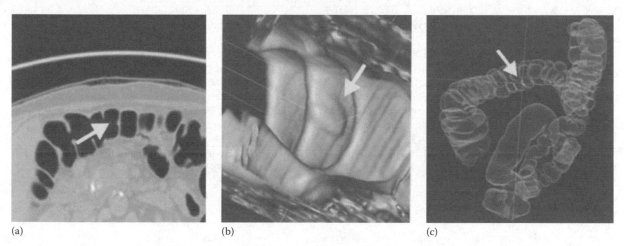

(a)   (b)   (c)

Figure 25.8   Screen shots of 2D axial view (a) with 3D endoluminal (b) and colon (c) views of a CADe-detected flat adenoma in transverse colon.

For example, when viewing a polyp candidate, the user can click to accept or reject the polyp candidate by clicking on a *check* or "x" mark that appears near the candidate on the 3D view or on the list of polyp candidates.

25.10.1   Summary

In summary, CADe adds only a few minutes to the reading time and improves reader performance based on peer-reviewed data. However, we believe that with practice, the added time to use CADe reduces and the impact on *confidence of interpretation* may be an additional benefit that is hard to objectively quantify. We hope CADe will help encourage radiologists to incorporate CTC into their daily practice.

REFERENCES

Acar, B, Beaulieu, CF, Göktürk, SB et al. (2002). Edge displacement field-based classification for improved detection of polyps in CT colonography. *IEEE Transactions on Medical Imaging* 21 (12), 1461–1467.

Ahlawat, SK, Gupta, N, Benjamin, SB et al. (2011). Large colorectal polyps: Endoscopic management and rate of malignancy: Does size matter? *Journal of Clinical Gastroenterology* 45 (4), 347–354.

Atkin, WS, Morson, BC, Cuzick, J (1992). Long-term risk of colorectal cancer after excision of rectosigmoid adenomas. *The New England Journal of Medicine* 326 (10), 658–662.

Bogoni, L, Cathier, P, Dundar, M et al. (2005). Computer-aided detection (CAD) for CT colonography: A tool to address a growing need. *The British Journal of Radiology* 78 (Spec. No. 1), S57–S62.

Brenner, H, Hoffmeister, M, Stegmaier, C et al. (2007). Risk of progression of advanced adenomas to colorectal cancer by age and sex: Estimates based on 840,149 screening colonoscopies. *Gut* 56 (11), 1585–1589.

Cai, W, Zalis, ME, Näppi, J et al. (2008). Structure-analysis method for electronic cleansing in cathartic and noncathartic CT colonography. *Medical Physics* 35 (7), 3259–3277.

Dachman, AH, Kelly, KB, Zintsmaster, MP et al. (2008). Formative evaluation of standardized training for CT colonographic image interpretation by novice readers. *Radiology* 249 (1), 167–177.

Dachman, AH, Kuniyoshi, JK, Boyle, CM et al. (1998). CT colonography with three-dimensional problem solving for detection of colonic polyps. *American Journal of Roentgenology* 171 (4), 989–995.

Dachman AH, Obuchowski NA, Hoffmeister JW, Hinshaw LJ, Frew MI, Van Uitert, RL Summers RM, Hillman BJ. (2010). Impact of computer aided detection for CT colonography in a multireader, multicase trial. *Radiology* 256, 827–835.

de Haan, MC, van Gelder, RE, Graser, A et al. (2011). Diagnostic value of CT-colonography as compared to colonoscopy in an asymptomatic screening population: A meta-analysis. *European Radiology* 21 (8), 1747–1763.

Faccioli, N, Foti, G, Barillari, M et al. (2011). A simplified approach to virtual colonoscopy using different intestinal preparations: Preliminary experience with regard to quality, accuracy and patient acceptability. *La Radiologia Medica* 116 (5), 749–758.

Fenlon, HM, Nunes, DP, Schroy, PC et al. (1999). A comparison of virtual and conventional colonoscopy for the detection of colorectal polyps. *The New England Journal of Medicine* 341, 1496–1503.

Fletcher, JG, Chen, M-H, Herman, BA et al. (2010). Can radiologist training and testing ensure high performance in CT colonography? Lessons from the national CT colonography trial. *American Journal of Roentgenology* 195 (1), 117–125.

Göktürk, SB, Tomasi, C, Acar, B et al. (2001). A statistical 3-D pattern processing method for computer-aided detection of polyps in CT colonography. *IEEE Transactions on Medical Imaging* 20 (12), 1251–1260.

Graser, A, Stieber, P, Nagel, D et al. (2008). Comparison of CT colonography, colonoscopy, sigmoidoscopy and faecal occult blood tests for the detection of advanced adenoma in an average risk population. *Gut.* 58 (2), 241–248.

Gschwantler, M, Kriwanek, S, Langner, E et al. (2002). High-grade dysplasia and invasive carcinoma in colorectal adenomas: A multivariate analysis of the impact of adenoma and patient characteristics. *European Journal of Gastroenterology & Hepatology* 14 (2), 183–188.

Halligan, S, Altman, DG, Mallett, S et al. (2006). Computed tomographic colonography: Assessment of radiologist performance with and without computer-aided detection. *Gastroenterology* 131 (6), 1690–1699.

Hassan, C, Lang, GD, Rubin, DT (2011). Epidemiology and screening of colorectal cancer. In: Dachman AH, Laghi A (eds). *Atlas of Virtual Colonoscopy*, 2nd edn., Springer-Verlag, Inc., New York, NY, pp. 55–63.

Hassan, C, Pickhardt, PJ, Kim, DH et al. (2010). Systematic review: Distribution of advanced neoplasia according to polyp size at screening colonoscopy. *Alimentary Pharmacology & Therapeutics* 31, 210–217.

Haycock, A, Burling, D, Wylie, P et al. (2010). CT colonography training for radiographers—A formal evaluation. *Clinical Radiology* 65 (12), 997–1004.

Hewitson, P, Glasziou, P, Irwig, L et al. (2011). Screening for colorectal cancer using the faecal occult blood test, hemoccult. *Cochrane Database of Systematic Reviews.* Jan 24 (1), CD001216.

Hunter, J, Harmston, C, Hughes, P et al. (2011). What is the nature of polyps detected by the NHS bowel cancer screening pilots? *Colorectal Disease: The Official Journal of the Association of Coloproctology of Great Britain and Ireland* 13 (5), 538–541.

Imperiale, TF, Wagner, DR, Lin, CY et al. (2000). Risk of advanced proximal neoplasms in asymptomatic adults according to the distal colorectal findings. *The New England Journal of Medicine* 343 (3), 169–174.

Jemal, A, Bray, F, Center, MM et al. (2011). Global cancer statistics. *CA: A Cancer Journal for Clinicians* 61 (2), 69–90.

Jerebko, AK, Summers, RM, Malley, JD et al. (2003). Computer-assisted detection of colonic polyps with CT colonography using neural networks and binary classification trees. *Medical Physics* 30 (1), 52–60.

Johnson, CD, Chen, MH, Toledano, AY et al. (2008a). Accuracy of CT colonography for detection of large adenomas and cancers. *The New England Journal of Medicine* 359 (12), 1207–1217.

Johnson, CD, Manduca, A, Fletcher, JG et al. (2008b). Noncathartic CT colonography with stool tagging: Performance with and without electronic stool subtraction. *American Journal of Roentgenology* 190 (2), 361–366.

Johnson, CD, Scott Kriegshauser, J, Lund, JT et al. (2011). Partial preparation computed tomographic colonography: A feasibility study. *Abdominal Imaging* 36 (6), 707–712.

Knudsen, AB, Lansdorp-Vogelaar, I, Rutter, CM et al. (2010). Cost-effectiveness of computed tomographic colonography screening for colorectal cancer in the medicare population. *Journal of the National Cancer Institute* 102 (16), 1238–1252.

Lansdorp-Vogelaar, I, van Ballegooijen, M, Zauber, AG et al. (2009). Effect of rising chemotherapy costs on the cost savings of colorectal cancer screening. *Journal of the National Cancer Institute* 101 (20), 1412–1422.

Lawrence, EM, Pickhardt, PJ, Kim, DH et al. (2010). Colorectal polyps: Stand-alone performance of computer-aided detection in a large asymptomatic screening population. *Radiology* 256 (3), 791–798.

Lenhart, DK, Johnston, RP, Zalis, ME (2011). Patient preparation and tagging. In: Dachman, AH, Laghi, A (eds.), *Atlas of Virtual Colonoscopy*. New York: Springer, pp. 79–86.

Levin, B, Lieberman, DA, McFarland, B et al. (2008). Screening and surveillance for the early detection of colorectal cancer and adenomatous polyps, 2008: A joint guideline from the American Cancer Society, the US Multi-Society Task Force on Colorectal Cancer, and the American College of Radiology. *Gastroenterology* 134 (5), 1570–1595.

Lieberman, DA, Weiss, DG (2001). One-time screening for colorectal cancer with combined fecal occult-blood testing and examination of the distal colon. *The New England Journal of Medicine* 345 (8), 555–560.

Lieberman, DA, Weiss, DG, Bond, JH et al. (2000). Use of colonoscopy to screen asymptomatic adults for colorectal cancer. Veterans Affairs Cooperative Study Group 380. *The New England Journal of Medicine* 343 (3), 162–168.

Liedenbaum, MH, Bipat, S, Bossuyt, PMM et al. (2011b). Evaluation of a standardized CT colonography training program for novice readers. *Radiology* 258 (2), 477–487.

Liedenbaum, MH, Denters, MJ, Zijta, FM et al. (2011a). Reducing the oral contrast dose in CT colonography: Evaluation of faecal tagging quality and patient acceptance. *Clinical Radiology* 66 (1), 30–37.

Lorenzo-Zúñiga, V, Moreno de Vega, V, Boix, J (2011). Changing trends in polypoid colorectal cancer diagnosed by colonoscopy. *Colorectal Disease* 13 (3), e37–e41.

Mandel, JS, Bond, JH, Church, TR et al. (1993). Reducing mortality from colorectal cancer by screening for fecal occult blood. Minnesota Colon Cancer Control Study. *The New England Journal of Medicine* 328 (19), 1365–1371.

Mang, T, Peloschek, P, Plank, C et al. (2007). Effect of computer-aided detection as a second reader in multidetector-row CT colonography. *European Radiology* 17 (10), 2598–2607.

McFarland, EG, Keysor, KJ, Vining, DJ (2011). Virtual colonoscopy: From concept to implementation. In: Dachman, AH, Laghi, A (eds.), *Atlas of Virtual Colonoscopy*. New York: Springer, pp. 3–7.

McHugh, M, Osei-Anto, A, Klabunde, CN et al. (2011). Adoption of CT colonography by US hospitals. *Journal of the American College of Radiology* 8 (3), 169–174.

Nadel, MR, Shapiro, JA, Klabunde, CN et al. (2005). A national survey of primary care physicians' methods for screening for fecal occult blood. *Annals of Internal Medicine* 142 (2), 86–94.

Näppi, JJ, Nagata, K (2011). Sources of false positives in computer-assisted CT colonography. *Abdominal Imaging* 36 (2), 153–164.

Näppi, J, Okamura, A, Frimmel, H et al. (2005). Region-based supine-prone correspondence for the reduction of false-positive CAD polyp candidates in CT colonography. *Academic Radiology* 12 (6), 695–707.

Näppi, J, Yoshida, H (2002). Automated detection of polyps with CT colonography: Evaluation of volumetric features for reduction of false-positive findings. *Academic Radiology* 9 (4), 386–397.

O'Connor, SD, Summers, RM, Choi, JR et al. (2006). Oral contrast adherence to polyps on CT colonography. *Journal of Computer Assisted Tomography* 30 (1), 51–57.

Okamura, A, Dachman, AH, Parsad, N et al. (2004). Evaluation of the effect of CAD on observers' performance in detection of polyps in CT colonography. *International Congress Series* 1268, 989–992.

Park, SH, Kim, SY, Lee, SS et al. (2009). Sensitivity of CT colonography for nonpolypoid colorectal lesions interpreted by human readers and with computer-aided detection. *American Journal of Roentgenology* 193 (1), 70–78.

Peter Geertruyden, MAJ, Richard Choi, J, Alex Galifianakis, LCDR (2011). Implementation and clinical trials in the United States. In: Dachman, AH, Laghi, A (eds.), *Atlas of Virtual Colonoscopy*. New York: Springer, pp. 65–73.

Petrick, N, Haider, M, Summers, RM et al. (2008). CT colonography with computer-aided detection as a second reader: Observer performance study. *Radiology* 246 (1), 148–156.

Pickhardt, PJ, Choi, J-HR (2003). Electronic cleansing and stool tagging in CT colonography: Advantages and pitfalls with primary three-dimensional evaluation. *American Journal of Roentgenology* 181 (3), 799–805.

Pickhardt, PJ, Hassan, C, Halligan, S et al. (2011). Colorectal cancer: CT colonography and colonoscopy for detection—Systematic review and meta-analysis. *Radiology* 259, 939–405.

Pickhardt, PJ, Hassan, C, Laghi, A, Zullo A, Kim DH, Morini S (2007). Cost-effectiveness of colorectal cancer screening with computed tomography colonography: The impact of not reporting diminutive lesions. *Cancer* 109, 2213–2221.

Pignone, M, Saha, S, Hoerger, T et al. (2002). Cost-effectiveness analyses of colorectal cancer screening: A systematic review for the U.S. Preventive Services Task Force. *Annals of Internal Medicine* 137 (2), 96–104.

Regge, D, Laudi, C, Galatola, G et al. (2009). Diagnostic accuracy of computed tomographic colonography for the detection of advanced neoplasia in individuals at increased risk of colorectal cancer. *JAMA* 301 (23), 2453–2461.

Rex, DK, Johnson, DA, Anderson, JC et al. (2009). American College of Gastroenterology guidelines for colorectal cancer screening 2009 [corrected]. *The American Journal of Gastroenterology* 104 (3), 739–750, doi: 10.1038/ajg.2009.104.

Ristvedt, SL, McFarland, EG, Weinstock, LB et al. (2003). Patient preferences for CT colonography, conventional colonoscopy, and bowel preparation. *The American Journal of Gastroenterology* 98 (3), 578–585.

Roehrig, J (2005). The manufacturer's perspective. *The British Journal of Radiology* 78 (Spec. No. 1), S41–S45.

Royster, AP, Fenlon, HM, Clarke, PD et al. (1997). CT colonoscopy of colorectal neoplasms: Two-dimensional and three-dimensional virtual-reality techniques with colonoscopic correlation. *American Journal of Roentgenology* 169 (5), 1237–1242.

Sosna, J, Morrin, MM, Kruskal, JB et al. (2003). CT colonography of colorectal polyps: A metaanalysis. *American Journal of Roentgenology* 181 (6), 1593–1598.

Summers, RM, Yao, J, Pickhardt, PJ et al. (2005). Computed tomographic virtual colonoscopy computer-aided polyp detection in a screening population. *Gastroenterology* 129 (6), 1832–1844.

Suuzuk, K, Rockey, DC, Dachman, AH (2010). CT colonography: Advanced computer-aided detection scheme utilizing MTANNs for detection of "missed" polyps in a multicenter clinical trial. *Medical Physics* 37 (1), 12–21.

Suzuki, K, Dachman, AH (2011). Computer-aided diagnosis in computed tomographic colonography. In: Dachman, AH, Laghi, A (eds.), *Atlas of Virtual Colonoscopy*. New York: Springer, pp. 163–182.

Suzuki, K, Yoshida, H, Näppi, J et al. (2006). Massive-training artificial neural network (MTANN) for reduction of false positives in computer-aided detection of polyps: Suppression of rectal tubes. *Medical Physics* 33 (10), 3814–3824.

Suzuki, K, Yoshida, H, Näppi, J et al. (2008). Mixture of expert 3D massive-training ANNs for reduction of multiple types of false positives in CAD for detection of polyps in CT colonography. *Medical Physics* 35 (2), 694–703.

Taylor, SA, Charman, SC, Lefere, P et al. (February 2008). CT colonography: Investigation of the optimum reader paradigm by using computer-aided detection software. *Radiology* 246 (2), 463–471.

Taylor, SA, Robinson, C, Boone, D et al. (2009). Polyp characteristics correctly annotated by computer-aided detection software but ignored by reporting radiologists during CT colonography. *Radiology* 253 (3), 715–723.

van Gelder, RE, Birnie, E, Florie, J et al. (2004). CT colonography and colonoscopy: Assessment of patient preference in a 5-week follow-up study. *Radiology* 233 (2), 328–337.

Whitlock, EP, Lin, JS, Liles, E et al. (2008). Screening for colorectal cancer: A targeted, updated systematic review for the U.S. Preventive Services Task Force. *Annals of Internal Medicine* 149 (9), 638–658.

Winawer, SJ, Zauber, AG, Ho, MN et al. (1993). Prevention of colorectal cancer by colonoscopic polypectomy. The National Polyp Study Workgroup. *The New England Journal of Medicine* 329 (27), 1977–1981.

Yoshida, H, Näppi, J (2007). CAD in CT colonography without and with oral contrast agents: Progress and challenges. *Computerized Medical Imaging and Graphics* 31 (4–5), 267–284.

Yoshida, H, Näppi, J, MacEneaney, P et al. (2002). Computer-aided diagnosis scheme for detection of polyps at CT colonography. *Radiographics* (A Review Publication of the Radiological Society of North America, Inc.) 22 (4), 963–979.

Chapter 26

Future Perspectives

CAD to Quantitative Image Biomarkers, Phenotypes, and Imaging Genomics

Maryellen L. Giger

CONTENTS

Medical imaging in disease detection, diagnosis, and treatment continues to expand with advances in image quality regulations (e.g., the ACR mammography accreditation program), image acquisition systems (e.g., digital radiography, tomosynthesis, and automated 3D ultrasound), and computerized image analysis (e.g., computer-aided detection [CADe]). The benefit of a medical imaging exam depends on both image quality and interpretation quality. Interpreting medical images is the main undertaking of radiologists. However, image interpretation by humans can be limited by incomplete visual search patterns, the potential for fatigue and distractions, the presence of structure noise (camouflaging normal anatomical background) in the image, the presentation of subtle and/or complex cancers that require integration of both image data and clinical information, the vast amount of image data in a screening program with low cancer prevalence, and the physical quality of the image itself.

The chapters in this book have carefully detailed the development and clinical implementation of CAD in various diseases, with the most translated ones being in breast cancer, lung diseases, and colon cancer. A daily check of the literature reveals more and more algorithms, newer fields, and expanded disease states for CAD developers and clinical users. Research in CAD is still, however, in its infancy with most radiological interpretation remaining within the realm of human interpretation and decision making [1–8].

Impediments to clinical translation still exist. However, gone are the days when a new CAD algorithm results in yet another CAD workstation, adding to the display device overload in the reading room. Researchers are more aware now of the need to address efficiency in addition to just the effectiveness of their algorithms—user friendliness and integration into the clinical workflow. Successful CAD output will need to show both efficacy and efficiency.

26.1 QUANTITATIVE IMAGE ANALYSIS: BEYOND CAD

The role of quantitative medical image analysis in the detection and diagnosis of disease continues to increase, with methods being developed and evaluated for use in CADe and computer-aided diagnosis (CADx), as well as

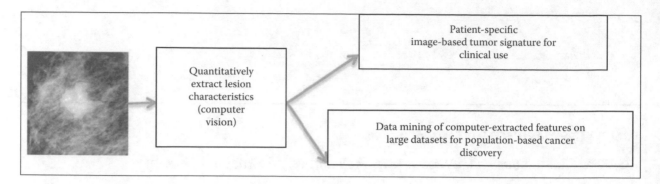

Figure 26.1 Schematic demonstrating the expansion of CAD into personalized quantitative medicine and into population-based disease discovery with multidisciplinary contributions from clinical, histopathological, and genomic aspects, i.e., radiomics and radiogenomics.

for prognostic markers, for predictive markers, and in the assessment of risk and/or response to therapy.

The extraction of features from digital medical images without the association with disease characteristics is basically only extracted information. Through investigations into the applications of these computer vision techniques, within CAD and beyond, knowledge is gained in (1) the management of the (cancer) patient (as in CAD) and in (2) the understanding of the disease (i.e., discovery). See Figure 26.1.

26.2 ROLE IN PATIENT MANAGEMENT

As more and more information is extracted from imaging data, computer output will potentially move from being a radiologist's aid to an expert reader and from a second reader to a concurrent reader to a primary reader. Various observer studies of breast CADx have yielded performance results, showing that the performance of the computer alone is similar to or exceeds the performance level of the radiologists in the task of distinguishing between cancerous and noncancerous lesions [9–11]. This implies that CADx might be better used as a concurrent reader than as a second reader. An analogy may be made to the incorporation of blood tests and ECG analyses, giving quantitative values along with ranges of normal, into a physician's assessment of a patient's condition.

As promoted by the Quantitative Imaging Biomarkers Alliance (QIBA), quantitative imaging biomarkers are becoming effective tools for clinical decision making in patient management—building *measuring devices* rather than *imaging devices* [12]. Research efforts from scientists working in CAD are being combined with efforts from those working on quantitative imaging systems to yield information on morphology, function, molecular structure, and more. The potential goal here is twofold: (1) output from the quantitative analysis of an image might be used as an image-based biomarker, and (2) such output might be used as a means with which to validate biomarkers in pharmaceutical discovery studies.

Quantitative biomarkers may be used to characterize tumors as well as surrounding tissue. Depending on the task, image-based biomarkers may include volumetric, morphological, textural, kinetics (physiologic), and/or metabolic characteristics of the disease as presented on single or multimodality medical images [3,7]. While many quantitative image analysis methods are developed for specific imaging modalities, methods have been presented for merging lesion characteristics from multimodality images [13–18].

Computer analyses may also be performed on normal tissue such as the parenchyma on breast images. In addition to mammographic breast density, the relationship between mammographic parenchymal patterns and the risk of developing breast cancer is being studied by various investigators [19–25]. Parenchymal pattern (texture) and enhancement (kinetics) can be assessed on FFDM and MRIs, respectively. It has been shown that women at high risk have dense breasts with parenchymal patterns that are coarse and of low contrast [21,23]. In addition, women with dense breasts had more parenchymal enhancement at their peak time point than those women with fatty breasts, and thus, breast parenchymal enhancement may be associated with breast density and may be potentially another characteristic for assessing breast cancer risk [26,27].

26.3 COMPUTER-AIDED PROGNOSIS AND ASSESSMENT OF THE RESPONSE TO THERAPY

The CAD approach and its algorithms are being extended from the diagnostic discrimination task for malignant and benign lesions to prognostic tasks, for example, in distinguishing between cancer subtypes, and noninvasive and invasive lesions, thereby yielding, for example, MRI-based prognostic markers [28,29]. In other studies, the computer analyses of imaged lesions are being related to the molecular

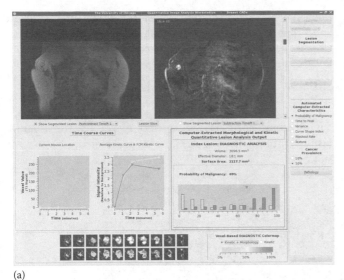

(a)

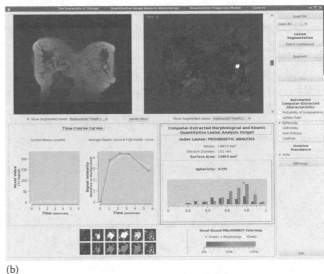

(b)

Figure 26.2   University of Chicago (a) diagnostic and (b) prognostic workstations for breast MRI. (From Giger, M.L. et al., Intelligent search workstation for computer-aided diagnosis, *Proc. of Computer Assisted Radiology and Surgery (CARS'2000)*, pp. 822–827, 2000; Bhooshan, N. et al., *Radiology*, 254, 680, 2010; Bhooshan, N. et al., *PMB*, 45, 5995, 2011; Shimauchi A. et al., *Radiology*, 258, 696, 2011.)

classifications, for example, ER status or existence of triple negative case. In this role, the computer-extracted features of the tumor can potentially be used to assess the aggressiveness of the tumor. For example, in the assessment of the prostate on MRI, the computer output could potentially be used along with clinical indicators to yield noninvasive methods, that is, *virtual biopsies*, that will help to determine the next steps in patient management [30–32].

Dynamic contrast-enhanced breast MRI is an example of an imaging biomarker with quantitative analysis that has been studied through lab investigations, cooperative group (e.g., American College of Radiology Imaging Network [ACRIN]) evaluation as with the I-SPY trials, and clinical usage [33–35]. An example of a workstation for the quantitative imaging of breast MRI is shown in Figure 26.2.

Quantitative image analysis for advancing future patient management also resides in the use of imaging biomarkers in the preclinical imaging of animal models, especially in the evaluation of preventive and therapeutic pharmaceuticals, for example, in the assessment of chemotherapy for prostate cancer [36]. In order to improve effectiveness and efficiency for high-throughput evaluations, advanced computer vision techniques can be even translated from the medical clinical domain to the preclinical domain.

If the imaging and subsequent image analyses are successful in indicating the underlying biology of cancer (or other diseases), then computerized image analyses of the types used in CAD may play a role in triaging patients for appropriate therapy regimens (such as neoadjuvant therapy in the treatment of breast cancer) or in terminating or modifying a regimen if image-based analyses indicate a lack of response.

26.4   CAD AND PATHOLOGY

Digital pathology lends itself well to CAD as did digital radiography decades ago. The use of computers to analyze histopathological data occurs at both the specimen level and the individual cellular level [37–40] as well as on DNA array autoradiographs [41]. Many of the techniques of tumor analysis, such as morphological characterization, are applicable at different scales as with digital pathology.

26.5   ROLE IN DISCOVERY: IMAGING GENOMICS AND *IMAGE-OMICS*

26.5.1   Machine Learning and Data Mining of Imaging Data

Just as radiologists are trained from the viewing of many cases as residents, so can a computer. In fact, a computer may "see" more cases than does a resident in training. Throughout the various chapters, many investigators have noted the training of classifiers for specific tasks, for example, in distinguishing between malignant and benign lung nodules. With machine learning, computers can learn to distinguish categories of images based on either supervised or nonsupervised methods. In addition, data mining enables the content-based retrieval of images [42,43].

Data reduction methods is a part of machine learning in which a large number of mathematical descriptors that characterize lesions across modalities (i.e., features) undergo data reduction techniques to yield information on the data structure of the feature space, as well as potentially serve as a complementary approach to feature selection.

Investigators have applied principal component analysis as well as recently developed nonlinear dimension reduction techniques to computer-extracted lesion features across databases from mammography, ultrasound, and MRI [44].

The development of successful CADx methods depends on the collection of large databases. While establishing a well-documented database requires careful collection, review, annotation, and time, unlabeled image data may be readily obtained. Thus, machine learning with unlabeled data may augment the understanding of feature space and subsequently improve the overall performance of quantitative image analysis techniques [45].

26.5.2 Computers Learning from Images Directly

An alternative to having the computer extract specific lesion features (e.g., margin sharpness) from the lesion

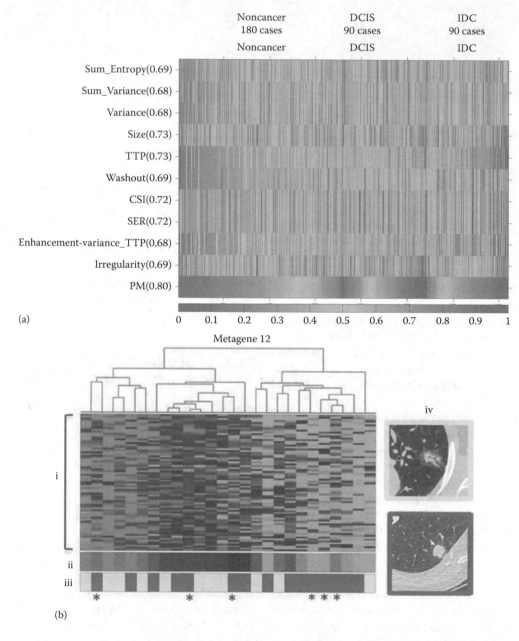

Figure 26.3 (a) Rapid high-throughput image-based phenotyping yielding an MRI prognostic array for breast tumors. (From Giger, M.L. et al., Visualization of image-based breast cancer tumor signatures, in: *Radiological Society of North America Annual Meeting*, 2012.) (b) Radiogenomics correlation map of NSCLC—association between metagene 12 and the image feature for the internal air bronchogram. (From Gevaert, O. et al., *Radiology*, 264(2), 387, 2012.)

image is to input the image data to the computer and have the computer learn directly from the image data. Learning directly from the image data has led to methods for content-based retrieval, CAD, and data mining [46].

26.5.3 Image-Based Phenotyping and Imaging Genomics

Beyond using CAD techniques for aiding in the management of the patient, computer output from quantitative image analysis is expected to aid in understanding disease, by yielding high-throughput image-based phenotyping [47], or *radiomics* [48]. Such procedures may effectively and efficiently analyze large populations and enable personalized medicine. Investigators have developed various methods for presenting such outputs [47–50]; some are shown in Figure 26.3a and b.

Association studies between breast cancer phenotypes from image-based biomarkers and genomic studies may yield new noninvasive means to localize and/or characterize the cancer. Initial associations had been investigated between image-based phenotypes (density and parenchymal texture) and SNPs for the UGT2B gene clusters in order to examine the genetic contribution of UGT2B genes for interindividual variation in breast density and mammographic parenchymal patterns [51], while more are being investigated in conjunction with NCI's the Cancer Genome Atlas (TCGA) and the Cancer Imaging Archive (TCIA) [52,53,55].

26.6 EXPEDITING DEVELOPMENTS, VALIDATIONS, AND TRANSLATION

As with any medical test, rigorous evaluation is necessary prior to broad-based clinical usage, and many such methods have been presented throughout the various chapters. Given that this aspect is crucial along all components in the research and translation chain, it is worth noting again. Various organizations are addressing this issue and only a few are mentioned here.

As more imaging biomarkers are studied through cooperative groups, such as the ACRIN [54] and Cancer and Leukemia Group B groups, datasets should be made available for expediting the evaluation of additional CAD and quantitative image analysis methods, perhaps via a sequestered system for the technology assessment that would maintain the integrity of the datasets. The American Association of Physicists in Medicine has been promoting the establishment of an institute for technology assessment. The TCGA [52] and Cancer Imaging Archive [55] groups of the NCI have developed open access methods for investigators to efficiently collaborate and share data, including both user-friendly policies and downloading mechanisms.

Such complementary efforts are expected to help expedite the advancement of imaging genomics.

Appropriate methods of metrology should also be utilized, and efforts from the RSNA QIBA Metrology group have been focused on the comparison of computer algorithms for quantitative biomarkers [56,57]. In their review, they provide a framework and statistical methods for algorithm comparisons.

26.7 SUMMARY

In summary, the current goals of CAD are to reduce search errors, reduce interpretation errors, reduce variation between and within observers, and/or improve the efficiency of the breast imaging interpretation process. These goals can be achieved if the computer's output is presented in an effective and efficient manner and if the computer output is used appropriately by the radiologist. However, the potential of various developments in CAD goes beyond the radiologist's interpretation process to future roles as image-based biomarkers (phenotypes) for assessing progrnosis and estimating response to therapy as well as in imaging genomics and cancer (disease) discovery.

ACKNOWLEDGMENTS

Research in the Giger Lab at the University of Chicago has been supported in the past by various funding sources, including NIH R33 113800, P50 CA125183, and P30 CA14599, DOE grant DE-FG02-08ER6478, NIH S10 RR021039, and DOD grant W81XWH-10-1-0216.

M.L.G. is a stockholder in R2 Technology/Hologic, is a cofounder of and has equity in Quantitative Insights, Inc., and receives royalties from Hologic, GE Medical Systems, MEDIAN Technologies, Riverain Medical, Mitsubishi, and Toshiba. It is the University of Chicago Conflict of Interest Policy that investigators disclose publicly actual or potential significant financial interest that would reasonably appear to be directly and significantly affected by the research activities.

REFERENCES

1. Giger ML. Computer-aided detection/computer-aided diagnosis. In: *Advances in Medical Physics 2008*. Wolbarst AB, Mossman KL, Hendee WR (eds.), Medical Physics Publishing, Madison, WI, 2008 (Chapter 10), pp. 143–168.
2. Giger ML, Chen W. CAD: An image perception perspective. In: *The Handbook of Medical Image Perception and Techniques*. Samei E, Krupinski E (eds.), Cambridge University Press, New York, NY, 2010.
3. Giger ML, Chan H-P, Boone J. Anniversary paper: History and status of CAD and quantitative image analysis: The role of Medical Physics and AAPM. *Medical Physics* 35: 5799–5820, 2008.

4. Giger ML, Drukker K. The computer vision and artificial intelligence of CAD. In: *Advances in Medical Physics 2010*. Wolbarst AB (ed.), Medical Physics Publishing, Madison, WI, 2010.

5. Giger ML, Karssemeijer N, Schnabel J. Breast image analysis for risk assessment, detection, diagnosis, and treatment of cancer. *Annual Review of Biomedical Engineering* 15: 327–357, 2013.

6. Giger ML. Update on the potential of computer-aided diagnosis for breast cancer. *Future Oncology* 6: 1–4, 2010.

7. Chan H-P, Hadjiiski L, Zhou C, Sahiner B. Computer-aided diagnosis of lung cancer and pulmonary embolism in computed tomography—A review. *Academic Radiology* 15: 535–555, 2008.

8. van Ginneken B, Hogeweg L, Prokop M. Computer-aided diagnosis in chest radiography: Beyond nodules. *European Journal of Radiology* 72: 226–230, 2009.

9. Jiang Y, Nishikawa RM, Schmidt RA, Metz CE, Giger ML, Doi K. Improving breast cancer diagnosis with computer-aided diagnosis. *Academic Radiology* 6: 22–33, 1999.

10. Shimauchi A, Giger ML, Bhooshan N, Lan L, Chen W, Lee J, Abe H, Newstead G. Evaluation of clinical breast MR imaging performed with prototype computer-aided diagnosis breast MR imaging workstation: Reader study. *Radiology* 258: 696–704, 2011.

11. Chan H-P, Sahiner B, Helvie MA, Petric N, Roubidoux MA, Wilson TE, Adler DD, Paramagual C, Newman JS, Sanjay-Gopal S. Improvement of radiologists' characterization of mammographic masses by using computer-aided diagnosis: An ROC study. *Radiology* 212: 817–827, 1999.

12. Buckler AJ, Bresolin L, Dunnick NR et al. A collaborative enterprise for multi-stakeholder participation in the advancement of quantitative imaging. *Radiology* 258: 906–914, 2011.

13. Drukker K, Horsch K, Giger ML. Multimodality computerized diagnosis of breast lesions using mammography and sonography. *Academic Radiology* 12: 970–979, 2005.

14. Horsch K, Giger ML, Vyborny CJ, Lan L, Mendelson EB, Hendrick RE. Classification of breast lesions with multimodality computer-aided diagnosis: Observer study results on an independent clinical data set. *Radiology* 240: 357–368, 2006.

15. Horsch K, Giger ML, Metz CE. Potential effect of different radiologists reporting methods on studies showing benefit of CAD. *Academic Radiology* 15: 139–152, 2008.

16. Yuan Y, Giger ML, Li H, Bhooshan N, Sennett CA. Multimodality computer-aided breast cancer diagnosis with FFDM and DCE-MRI. *Academic Radiology* 17: 1158–1167, 2010.

17. Giger ML, Huo Z, Lan L, Vyborny CJ. Intelligent search workstation for computer-aided diagnosis. In: *Proceedings of Computer Assisted Radiology and Surgery (CARS'2000)*, San Francisco, CA, pp. 822–827, 2000.

18. Sahiner B, Chan H-P, Hadjiiski LM et al. Multi-modality CADx: ROC study of the effect of radiologists' accuracy in characterizing breast mass on mammograms and 3D ultrasound images. *Academic Radiology* 16: 810–818, 2009.

19. Byng JW, Yaffe MJ, Lockwood GA et al. Automated analysis of mammographic densities and breast carcinoma risk. *Cancer* 80: 66–74, 1997.

20. Huo Z, Giger ML, Wolverton DE, Zhong W, Cumming S, Olopade OI. Computerized analysis of mammographic parenchymal patterns for breast cancer risk assessment: Feature selection. *Medical Physics* 27: 4–12, 2000.

21. Huo Z, Giger ML, Olopade OI, Wolverton DE, Weber BL, Metz CE, Zhong W, Cummings S. Computerized analysis of digitized mammograms of BRCA1/BRCA2 gene mutation carriers. *Radiology* 225: 519–526, 2002.

22. Li H, Giger ML, Olopade OI, Chinander MR. Power spectral analysis of mammographic parenchymal patterns of digitized mammograms. *Journal of Digital Imaging* 21: 145–152, 2008.

23. Li H, Giger ML, Lan L, Bancroft Brown J, MacMahon A, Mussman M, Olopade OI, Sennett CA. Computerized analysis of mammographic parenchymal patterns on a large clinical dataset of full-field digital mammograms: Robustness study with two high risk datasets. *Journal of Digital Imaging* 25: 591–598, 2012.

24. Manduca A, Carston MJ, Heine JJ et al. Texture features from mammographic images and risk of breast cancer. *Cancer Epidemiology, Biomarkers & Prevention* 18: 837–845, 2009.

25. Wei J, Chan HP, Wu YT et al. Association of computerized mammographic parenchymal pattern measure with breast cancer risk: A pilot case-control study. *Radiology* 260: 42–49, 2011.

26. Jansen SA, Lin VC, Giger ML, Li H, Karczmar GS, Newstead GM. Normal parenchymal enhancement patterns in women undergoing MR screening of the breast. *European Radiology* 21: 1374–1382, 2011.

27. Li H, Giger ML, Yuan Y, Jansen SA, Lan L, Bhooshan N, Newstead GM. Computerized breast parenchymal analysis on DCE-MRI. In: *Proceedings of SPIE Medical Imaging Conference*, 2009, Vol. 7260, 72600N1-6.

28. Bhooshan N, Giger ML, Jansen S, Li H, Lan L, Newstead G. Image-based prognostic markers from computerized characterization of a clinical breast MRI database. *Radiology* 254: 680–690, 2010.

29. Bhooshan N, Giger ML, Edwards E, Yuan Y, Jansen S, Li H, Lan L, Sattar H, Newstead G. Computerized three-class classification of MRI-based prognostic markers for breast cancer. *PMB* 45: 5995–6008, 2011.

30. Hylton N. Dynamic contrast-enhanced magnetic resonance imaging as an imaging biomarker. *Journal of Clinical Oncology* 24(20): 3293–3298, 2006.

31. Galban CJ, Chenevert TL, Meyer CR et al. The parametric response map is an imaging biomarker for early cancer treatment outcome. *Nature Medicine* 15(5): 572–576, 2009.

32. Peng Y, Jiang Y, Yang C, Bancroft Brown J, Antic T, Sethi I, Schmid-Tannwald C, Giger ML, Eggener SE, Oto A. Quantitative analysis of multiparametric prostate MR images: Differentiation between prostate cancer and normal tissue and correlation with Gleason Score—A computer-aided diagnosis development study. *Radiology* 267: 787–796, 2013.

33. Esserman LJ, Berry DA, Cheang MCU et al. Chemotherapy response and recurrence-free survival in neoadjuvant breast cancer depends on biomarker profiles: Results from the I-SPY 1 TRIAL (CALGB 150007/150012; ACRIN 6657). *Breast Cancer Research and Treatment* 132: 1049–1062, 2012.

34. Hylton N, Blume JD, Bernreuter WK et al. Locally advanced breast cancer: MR imaging for prediction of response to neoadjuvant chemotherapy—Results from ACRIN 6657/I-SPY TRIAL. *Radiology* 263(3): 663–672, 2012.

35. McLennan G, Clarke L, Hohl RJ. Imaging as a biomarker for therapy response: Cancer as a prototype for the creation of research resources. *Clinical Pharmacology & Therapeutics* 84(4): 433–436, 2008.

36. Lee KC, Sud D, Meyer CR, Moffat BA, Chenevert TL, Rehemtulla A, Pienta KJ, Ross BD. An imaging biomarker of early treatment response in prostate cancer that has metastasized to the bone. *Cancer Research* 67: 3524–3528, 2007.

37. Alexe G, Monaco J, Doyle S, Basavanhally A, Reddy A, Seiler M, Ganesan S, Bhanot G, Madabhushi A. Towards improved cancer diagnosis and prognosis using analysis of gene expression data and computer aided imaging. *Experimental Biology and Medicine* 234: 860–879, 2009.

38. Peng Y, Jiang Y, Chuang S-T, Yang XJ. Computer-aided detection of prostate cancer on tissue sections. *Applied Immunohistochemistry & Molecular Morphology* 17: 442–450, 2009.

39. Peng Y, Jiang Y, Liarski VM, Kaverina N, Clark MR, Giger ML. Computerized image analysis of cell-cell interactions in human renal tissue by using multi-channel immunoflourescent confocal microscopy. *Proceedings of SPIE* 83153F, 2012.

40. Petushi S, Garcia FU, Haber MM, Karsinis C, Tozeren A. Large-scale computations on histology images review grade-differentiation parameters for breast cancer. *BMC Medical Imaging* 6: 14, 2006.

41. Pelizzari CA, Khodarev NN, Gupta N, Calvin DP, Weichelbaum RR. Quantitative analysis of DNA array autoradiographs. *Nucleic Acids Research* 28: 4577–4581, 2000.

42. Müller H, Michoux N, Bandon D, Geissbuhler A. A review of content-based image retrieval systems in medical applications—clinical benefits and future directions. *International Journal of Medical Informatics* 73:1–23, 2004.

43. Tourassi GD, Harrawood B, Singh S, Lo JY, Floyd CE. Evaluation of Information-theoretic similarity measures for content-based retrieval and detection of masses in mammograms. *Medical Physics* 34:140–150, 2007.

44. Jamieson A, Giger ML, Drukker K, Li H, Yuan Y, Bhooshan N. Exploring non-linear feature space dimension reduction and data representation in breast CADx with Laplacian eigenmaps and t-SNE. *Medical Physics* 37: 339–351, 2010.

45. Jamieson AR, Giger ML, Drukker K, Pesce L. Enhancement of breast CADx with unlabeled data. *Medical Physics* 37: 4155–4172, 2010.

46. Jamieson AR, Drukker K, Giger ML. Breast image feature learning with adaptive deconvolutional networks. In: *Proceedings of SPIE Medical Imaging Conference*, 2012, Vol. 8315, 831506-1.

47. Giger ML, Li H, Lan L. Visualization of image-based breast cancer tumor signatures. In: *Radiological Society of North America Annual Meeting*, 2012.

48. Kuo MD, Rutman AM. Radiogenomics: Creating a link between molecular diagnostics and diagnostic imaging. *European Journal of Radiology* 70: 232–241, 2009.

49. Gevaert O, Xu J, Hoang CD, Leung AN, Xu Y, Quon A, Rubin DL, Napel S, Plevritis SK. Non-small cell lung cancer: Identifying prognostic imaging biomarkers by leveraging public gene expression microarray data—Methods and preliminary results. *Radiology* 264(2): 387–396, 2012.

50. Segal E, Sirlin CB, Ooi C et al. Decoding global gene expression programs in liver cancer by noninvasive imaging. *Nature Biotechnology* 25(6): 675–680, 2007.

51. Li H, Giger ML, Sun C, Ponsukcharoen U, Huo D, Lan L, Olopade OI, Jamieson AR, Bancroft Brown J, Di Rienzo A. Pilot study demonstrating association between breast cancer image-based risk phenotypes and genomics biomarkers. *Medical Physics* 41, 031917, 2014.

52. http://cancergenome.nih.gov.

53. The Cancer Genome Atlas Network. Comprehensive molecular portraits of human breast tumours. *Nature* 490: 61–70, 2012.

54. http://www.acrin.org.

55. http://imaging.cancer.gov/informatics/thecancerimaging archive.

56. http://www.rsna.org/QIBA.aspx.

57. Obuchowski NA, Reeves AP, Huang EP, Wang XF, Buckler AJ, Kim HJ, Barnhart HX, Jackson EF, Giger ML, Pennello G, Toledano AY, Kalpathy-Cramer J, Apanasovich TV, Kinahan PE, Myers KJ, Goldgof DB, Barboriak DP, Gillies RJ, Schwartz LH, Sullivan AD. Quantitative imaging biomarkers: A review of statistical methods for computer algorithm comparisons. *Statistical Methods in Medical Research*, June 11, 0962280214537390, 2014.

Index